Meramour's™ Guide to

The Body-Feedback Acupuncture System

Volume I

A New Approach to Holistic Medicine

Meramour™
Body-Feedback for Health, LLC

Meramour's Guide to The Body-Feedback Acupuncture System

First edition December 2020

Body-Feedback for Health, LLC
2014 Yahara Place, Madison, WI 53704
www.body-feedback.com

For information about special discounts available for bulk purchases, sales promotions, fund-raising, and educational needs, contact Body-Feedback for Health, LLC at info@body-feedback.com or **608-535-9144**.

Interior design, cover design, and illustrations by Miroslava Sobot

ISBN 978-0-9992069-4-2

Library of Congress Control Number 2020919733
A catalog record for this book is available from the Library of Congress

Acknowledgments

The pioneers of Traditional Chinese Medicine (TCM) in the West have created the opportunity for the current generation of acupuncturists to become mainstream and recognized as a valid form of holistic medicine. I acknowledge those teachers who influenced my early education and guided me down my path as a healer.

From Kiiko Matsumoto and David Euler, I learned the art of palpation-style acupuncture and a deeper understanding of classical Chinese medical theory. Nicholas J. Lacarrubba, Jr. introduced me to the Korean four-point treatment approach combined with Dr. George Goodheart's Applied Kinesiology approach. To them, I am grateful.

I want to thank my team of editors and designers who brought structure and form to my treatment style: Peggy Joque Williams for editing and coaching, Patricia Whalen and Tim Walsh for content editing, Miroslava Sobot for creating the illustrations and a beautiful textbook, and Kit Timmerman for proofreading and designing the anatomical diagrams.

Table of Contents

SECTION 2

FOREWORD

For over 20 years, I have been searching the narrow landscape where what has yet to be known emerges into being. In this quest, I look for tools and techniques that can help me achieve optimal health. I have searched throughout both conventional and esoteric sciences. My search has included a bachelor's degree in biology, a master's degree in Oriental medicine, certifications in bioenergetic medicine and functional biochemistry as well as advanced training in Qi Gong and meditation. I have worked as part of an integrative medicine team alongside three medical doctors, a nutritionist, a homeopath, and multiple yoga, massage, and energetic practitioners striving to provide very high quality medical and wellness care. However, the pinnacle of my search did not occur in California–the mecca of integrative medical thought where I have spent most of the past two decades–it took place in the Wisconsin Dells at a functional medicine conference where a mutual friend introduced me to Michelle Meramour. Michelle offered to treat my wife and I using her Body-Feedback system, and there I recognized the profound difference between knowledge and wisdom.

Since meeting Michelle, I have been fortunate to witness firsthand her drive to manifest powerful healing that reaches beyond the walls of her clinic to the larger community of medical practitioners and the countless clients who stand to benefit. Michelle is precise in her information, generous in her desire to help others, and appropriately urgent in her mission to advance her valuable methods. *Meramour's Guide to The Body-Feedback Acupuncture System* is everything I wish I had learned in acupuncture school and more. The theory upon which her system is built is profound and elegant. Her Body-Feedback method for confirming the best points, oils, or remedies generates undeniably positive results. The point prescriptions are precise and well supported by theory. The ability to round out treatments to include essential oils, herbs, and supplements is dynamic in its capacity to promote a full orchestra of biogenic forces. Reading *Meramour's Guide to The Body-Feedback Acupuncture System* is akin to discovering a manuscript that somehow contains the totality of the ancient past, the present, and a glimpse into the future. Whether you were led to this text by a friend or through happenstance, prepare to give thanks for your good fortune. You are about to gain confidence and see the possibilities for success that come from peering into the *sanctum sanctorum* where knowledge and wisdom unite.

Body-Feedback is part of a new paradigm of medical care, and those on the front line of this progress will reap the rewards decades before mainstream medicine adopts these principles. Conventional medicine is oriented to the masses. Extensive double-blind studies are the gold standard for determining the treatment outcomes of drugs or other medical interventions. However, a positive outcome across an entire group cannot predict success for you as one single individual. You are unique, and your very complex biological system may not respond obediently to the "standard of care." I used to work with a medical doctor who would say, "Her body didn't read the textbook," as if the burden is on the patient to respond predictably to treatment, rather than on the medical practitioner to seek an approach capable of addressing the exception as well as the rule. Most of my patients are seeking alternative treatments because they did not fit neatly within the well-defined treatment protocols of conventional medical care: an unwanted side effect, a lack of symptom resolution, or a presentation of symptoms that didn't fit neatly within the "textbook."

I applaud the successes of modern medicine, but medical assessments and laboratory tests do not have the ability to anticipate the body's response to the selected remedy, be it a drug, herb, or supplement. The exponentially increasing knowledge of medicine is a somewhat futile effort to comprehend the unfathomable wisdom of the human body logically. Left out of all the findings and test results is you, your own body, and its infinite wisdom. *Meramour's Guide to The Body-Feedback Acupuncture System* is an invitation to step beyond the limitations of what is known and into the realm of discovery.

Body-Feedback is a dialogue in which you ask the body why it is suffering from disease and what remedies it needs. Like any new language, you will need to learn the rules and practice to become proficient. Through this conversation you will begin to clearly "hear" what will promote healing. How monumental would it be to know what will improve your health or what will do harm? In your hands, you hold the key to access the wisdom of the body. This is the promise of the Body-Feedback system.

May your life and health expand with possibility.

Tim Walsh, BS, MS, LAc
Licensed Acupuncturist

PREFACE

Discovering Body-Feedback

In 1999, just before I started acupuncture school, a friend strongly suggested I take a weekend workshop on acupressure for massage therapists and receive an acupuncture treatment from Nicholas J. Lacarrubba, Jr. in Tampa, Florida. After my acupuncture session with Dr. Lacarrubba, he explained to me that he found the most effective acupuncture treatments were rooted in the four-point approach attributed to the Korean monk Sa-am. The weekend workshop used these Korean four-point combinations with palpation techniques to release tight muscle groups associated with the acupuncture meridians based on the Applied Kinesiology teachings of the chiropractor Dr. George Goodheart. I filed this information in the back of my brain and focused on my classes at acupuncture school.

When I started acupuncture school, I gravitated to an acupuncture system taught by Kiiko Matsumoto that used hands-on palpation techniques to check the accuracy of the chosen acupuncture points and treatment results. My first career had been as an accountant, where I always learned to check my work, and Kiiko's style of double-checking the points before needling felt natural to me. Kiiko's system is complex and requires participation from the person receiving the acupuncture to report changes in tenderness. At times this system was difficult to follow, and my clients experienced confusion and stress when deciding if an area felt more or less tender.

After a few years in practice and struggling with difficult cases, I remembered Dr. Lacarrubba's comment on the Korean four-point treatments. I began analyzing the Korean four-point and Chinese six-point approaches looking for an efficient way to integrate this system with Kiiko's palpation style of diagnosing and double-checking the correct point selection.

Over the course of my next 16 years in practice, I developed the Body-Feedback style of acupuncture. This style combines palpation techniques that assess specific muscle groups, connective tissues, and master points with needling acupoint prescriptions based on the five-element controlling cycle and supporting abdominal, scalp, and facial acupoint combinations. These palpation techniques are used to frequency-test essential oils, herbs, and nutritional supplements. Kiiko Matsumoto and the Applied Kinesiology theory strongly influenced my early education, and you will see aspects of these pioneers in the Body-Feedback System.

The Body-Feedback techniques provide both a diagnosing system and a treatment approach. The Body-Feedback testing techniques, special point prescriptions, and essential oil blends can identify root dysfunctions compromising health. The ability to diagnose a root dysfunction with objective palpation techniques provides valuable information and confirmation when choosing herbs and supplements, making lifestyle recommendations, and monitoring diet choices.

Each Body-Feedback treatment can continue to improve health for three to four weeks with a supportive lifestyle. If treating the root is not achieving the desired outcomes or the corrections are not holding, further investigation of personal care products, diet, and at times functional medicine laboratory testing is recommended.

In this system, clients actively feel changes in their muscle tightness and tension as part of the treatment process. People today are looking for confirmation that their healthcare choices are correct. Clients find the release of tension in specific muscle groups and the reduction of discomfort in the master points that correlate with their symptoms both reassuring and somewhat magical. When a new client feels the immediate release of pain and discomfort and deep relaxation occurs, they often say their treatment experience enabled them to understand this elevated level of healing. It is exciting to witness the transformation that happens with the alignment of the body, mind, and spirit.

After the initial course of treatment has taken care of their immediate needs, the majority of clients request to continue maintenance acupuncture treatments, supplements, or herbs to keep their constitution strong and slow the aging process. Other clients become accustomed to feeling healthy and balanced, and at the first sign of discomfort, emotional distress, or digestive difficulties, they schedule a follow-up treatment.

Carrie's Search for Answers

Carrie came for a consultation after seeing a different acupuncturist for infertility, a chiropractor for chronic neck and shoulder pain, and her physician for an annual physical. The physician recommended seeing me for infertility as I had helped several of her other patients. Carrie had been trying to conceive for eight years, and after undergoing a series of tests from the fertility clinic, she had received a diagnosis of unexplained infertility. Carrie had tried medicated cycles a few years ago and detested how the hormones had made her feel. A year prior, she had conceived naturally, but that pregnancy had ended in a miscarriage.

Carrie proceeded to tell me how she had seen another acupuncturist about a year ago who gave her several different nutritional supplements and Chinese herbs that didn't make her feel better, and she disliked taking multiple pills. She said she felt anxious and frustrated at the end of her acupuncture sessions, and she couldn't tell if they were doing any good. Carrie was concerned that she would be wasting her money and time by seeing me.

Meramour's Endocrine Funnel

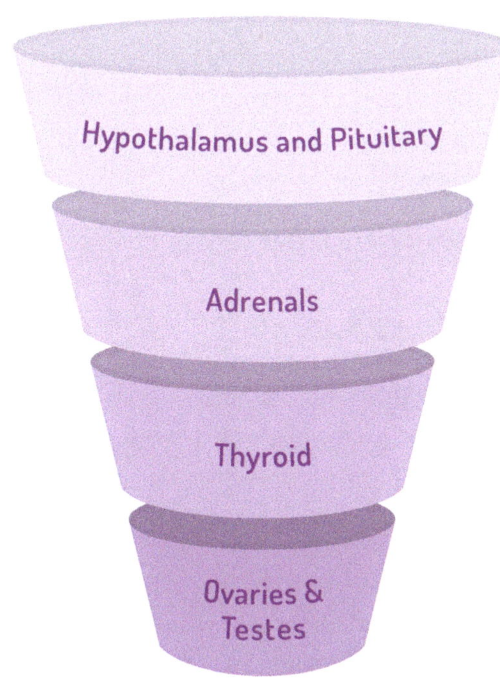

I noticed that Carrie's complexion was blotchy, which is consistent with imbalanced hormones. I explained to Carrie that I would use her body as a feedback system to tell me what the root of her hormone imbalance was. Once we knew the source of her problem, we could look at critical supplements and lifestyle changes to support her fertility. I next explained my version of the endocrine funnel, which categorizes the endocrine gland functions into four distinct layers.

The top layer of the funnel consists of the hypothalamus and pituitary. The hypothalamus-pituitary axis, or HP axis, describes the synchronized communication between these glands that controls all of the hormonal activity in the body. If the hypothalamus and pituitary are miscommunicating, it will disrupt the entire endocrine system and hormonal balance.

The second layer of the funnel contains the adrenals. The adrenals depend on proper communication from the hypothalamus and pituitary to function. The hypothalamus-pituitary-adrenal axis, or HPA axis, is a delicate balance of hormonal activity that impacts every cell in the body. Stress, allergies, infections, and environmental toxins easily disturb the synchronized HPA axis and disrupt the thyroid and reproductive functions that depend on the adrenals working correctly.

The third layer of the funnel consists of the thyroid. The thyroid depends on a healthy HPA axis to function optimally. Thyroid activity can fluctuate between hypo and hyper, compromising thyroid hormones when the HPA axis is dysfunctional. Thyroid hormones directly impact the reproductive system, which comprises the lowest level of the funnel.

The lowest layer of the funnel contains the ovaries, testes, and reproductive hormones. The reproductive system depends upon the thyroid, adrenals, and HP axis to function normally. With infertility or sub-fertility, any one of the endocrine funnel layers could be disrupting the reproductive system. I explained to Carrie that I would check her Body-Feedback testing locations for each segment of the funnel to see if we could identify the root imbalance affecting her ability to conceive.

Following the Body-Feedback testing methods, it was apparent that Carrie's chronic neck and shoulder pain were the muscle associations for the hypothalamus and pituitary. She had been receiving chiropractic care for this pain. However, Carrie was unsure if she should continue seeing the chiropractor because the adjustment results did not hold. I explained that acupuncture and chiropractic care support each other and could help shift her health rapidly. I recommended that she alternate acupuncture and chiropractic care weekly. The Body-Feedback approach identified Carrie's hypothalamus and pituitary dysfunction as the root cause of the neck and shoulder pain and her infertility.

Next, I checked her adrenal testing locations. They were very painful and tight, so I inquired about her amount of stress, exercise, and relaxation. Carrie explained that she had a low-stress lifestyle and practiced yoga regularly, which indicated her adrenals were unable to work correctly because of the hypothalamus and pituitary dysfunction. I then checked her thyroid and ovary testing locations, which were both overly tight and uncomfortable. Carrie understood that these testing locations were reflecting the dysfunction affecting her endocrine system.

We started testing the Meramour's essential oil blends associated with the hypothalamus and pituitary, as they were the uppermost dysregulated level of her endocrine funnel. The Heart Meridian Balancing Blend tested remarkably well, so I applied it to her forehead because the hypothalamus and pituitary glands are located behind there. Applying this blend to this area is most effective when addressing the HP axis. The tightness in Carrie's shoulder and neck diminished by 70-80% instantly.

Using Body-Feedback techniques, I determined that the heart meridian was the root dysfunction. I then rechecked the testing locations with discomfort relating to the endocrine funnel, and they showed an average of 70% improvement just by having the proper essential oils applied to the appropriate area. Carrie's testing locations responded best to the heart balancing and sedation prescriptions (HT3, HT4, HT7, LU8, KD10, SP3) with added facial points to calm the stress response and a uterus supporting point (LV5).

After the treatment, Carrie's testing locations associated with the endocrine funnel were 100% improved and free of all pain and discomfort. New clients are often astonished by pain, tension, or discomfort that suddenly disappears, but after years of treating thousands of clients with the Body-Feedback system, I expect to see rapid improvements.

Based on this information I knew that Carrie needed to correct the hypothalamus-pituitary connection before we could determine if there were any other disruptions in the endocrine funnel affecting her fertility. Because Carrie didn't like taking pills, I recommended she apply the Meramour's Heart Meridian Balancing Blend to her face and forehead twice daily. The effects of essential oils generally last six to eight hours, so using the blend twice a day was needed to balance the hypothalamus and pituitary.

From Carrie's initial appointment she found answers to the questions she had been asking for more than five years. She understood how the chronic neck and shoulder pain was related to her endocrine system. She learned to monitor treatments she was receiving for fertility by assessing improvements in the chronic neck and shoulder pain. I explained how the heart meridian controlled the implantation sites in the uterus and the first trimester of pregnancy, and that it was critical to support this meridian to achieve pregnancy.

Carrie left her first Body-Feedback treatment feeling confident that the acupuncture was strengthening her fertility, and the plan of care made sense to her. For the first time, Carrie understood and could feel in her body the challenges of the endocrine system. With this knowledge, she could find treatment options to improve her chances of conceiving a healthy child.

Carrie experienced a miracle between her first and second Body-Feedback acupuncture sessions. Her cycle was a day late and she had several pregnancy tests that registered positive. At her second appointment her facial appearance looked healthier from the essential oil blend, which she told me she loved. Her hypothalamus and pituitary held the treatment well and the testing locations showed a 75% improvement from continuing the essential oils and chiropractic care. I recommended increasing the application of the Heart Meridian Balancing Blend to three times daily. The point prescription that improved Carrie's testing locations continued to be the heart balancing and sedation prescriptions (HT3, HT4, HT7, LU8, KD10, SP3) with added facial points to calm the stress response and a uterus supporting point (LV5).

Carrie's healthy lifestyle of eating organic foods, practicing yoga, and exercising regularly, along with the chiropractic care, prepared her body to conceive naturally when the endocrine system was balanced and supported. She merely needed the accurate diagnosis and treatment of the acupuncture meridian system to correct the hypothalamus-pituitary axis. After the first treatment, the implantation sites in the uterus reset, and her body then believed it was safe to carry a pregnancy. Continuing the acupuncture, essential oils, and maintaining a low-stress lifestyle during the pregnancy allowed her to deliver a healthy baby boy, full-term, naturally.

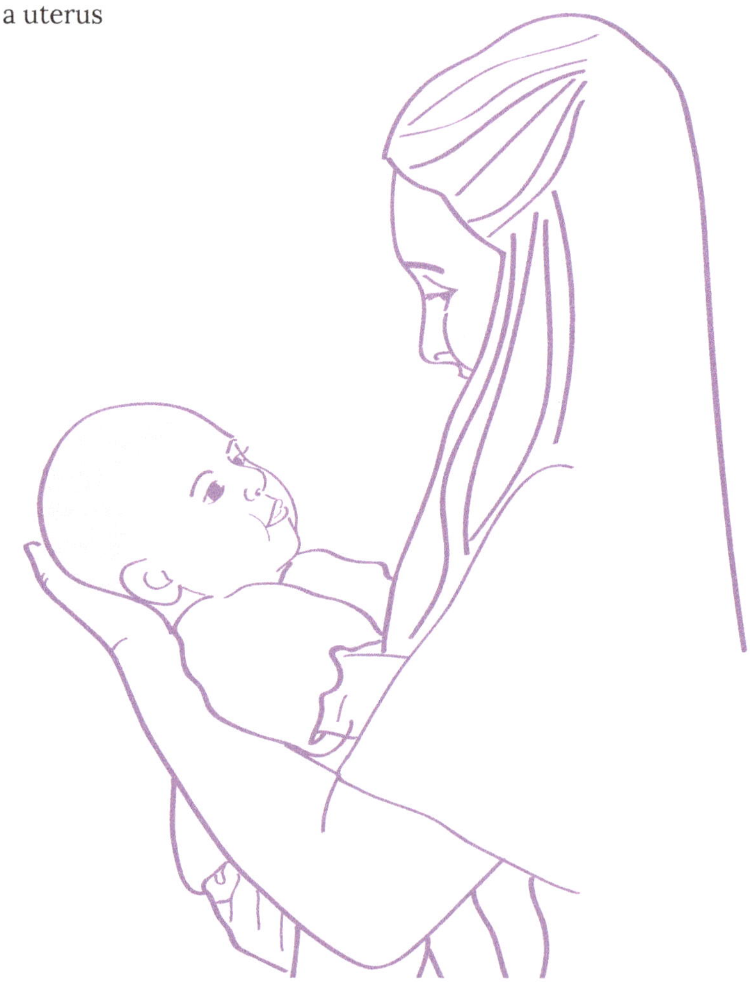

INTRODUCTION

Introduction to The Body-Feedback System

Meramour's Body-Feedback style of acupuncture is a complete system for diagnosing and treating meridian imbalances and organ dysfunction. This system relies on involuntary responses in a client's body that initiate on a cellular level. The cells carry a person's life-force, which is instinctively aware of health issues and what can hinder or encourage healing. Whether the root cause of a health condition is physical, emotional, or spiritual, the Body-Feedback system can identify its impact and the solutions for healing.

According to the *Yellow Emperor's Classic of Medicine*, "In diagnosis, there are five areas that deserve close examination. They are the pulses, the channels that correspond to the organs, the muscles, the tendons, and the acupoints. In general, close scrutiny of these five areas will provide sufficient information to make a proper diagnosis; however, there are cases that display inconsistent pulse patterns, making accurate diagnosis difficult." [1]

The Body-Feedback system incorporates Chinese pulse diagnosis, palpation techniques of the muscles, tendons, and key acupuncture points (the Body-Feedback testing locations), and frequency assessment of the meridians and organs. Everything in this world expresses a particular frequency based on how rapid the energy associated with it is moving. Frequency is how energy, or qi, travels throughout the universe. Every organ and meridian in the body, along with essential oils, Chinese herbs, and nutritional supplements, vibrates to a specific frequency. The Body-Feedback system makes use of the interaction of these frequencies to determine the most efficient ways to support self-healing.

Energy, or qi, travels through the acupuncture meridians and organs, and each expresses a specific frequency when it is healthy and able to self-heal. Checking the different frequencies of key acupoints, essential oils, Chinese herbs, and supplements to the testing locations provides insight for promoting health and longevity. By knowing what supports self-healing and what hinders it, you can help your clients create a lifestyle that supports their individual needs. You can even use Body-Feedback techniques to test different foods, music, colors, clothing, and personal care products. Color is how the body sees frequency. Sound is how the body hears frequency. Both of these significantly impact how energy flows through the meridian system.

Cellular communication occurs rapidly in the nervous system. A positive or negative response to any stimulus first registers as a change in emotions, tension, or tightness in the body. A negative emotional shift causes disrupted or shallow breathing patterns. Negative stimulus instantly causes pain or tightness in the Body-Feedback testing locations. Improved emotions and breathing patterns occur when the meridian system regains balance and indicates a positive physical response.

When clients are aware of the subtle changes in emotional and physical health and breathing patterns, they will better understand their path to improved health and well-being. The acupuncture meridian system addresses physical, emotional, and mental health on an energetic level within the cells. Learning how to communicate with the life-force inside the cells is the key to the exceptional tool called the Body-Feedback System.

Self-Care Using Body-Feedback

The Body-Feedback system easily adapts for self-care, for both the practitioner and the client. Lifestyle choices and home therapies that support the meridian system will significantly improve any holistic care received, including acupuncture, chiropractic, and massage therapy. Clients enjoy self-care at home using the Body-Feedback system because they feel shifts in their body and see results. Most clients choose to do self-care with herbs, nutritional supplements, and therapeutic-grade essential oils because they can quickly check them to testing locations or the pulse and determine if they will be beneficial. They can also check these testing locations after eating to help identify food intolerances and create a supportive diet.

Self-care for the practitioner is critical. I believe that healers must continually work on themselves if they are to be a conduit of healing for others. Holistic healthcare providers are at their best when they regularly work on their own physical, emotional, and spiritual health while incorporating Body-Feedback self-care techniques for themselves.

People often ask why I use the term clients instead of patients. According to Merriam-Webster, "A patient is a person awaiting or receiving medical care. A client is a person who engages in the professional advice or service of another." My approach to healthcare is to address any symptoms of dysfunction as they arise. Then I work with my clients on a regular basis to keep their body, mind, and spirit as healthy as it can be. This approach strengthens their constitution so people can quickly overcome health crises as they arise. A person whose meridian system is balanced and strong will overcome trauma, pathogens, and emotional upsets more quickly than someone with a weakened and stagnant meridian system.

It can be challenging to objectively choose the best points to needle on yourself when depending on subjective symptoms alone. The Body-Feedback system objectively reads and assesses the meridian system independent of subjective symptoms and complaints. I have found it easy to accurately diagnose organ dysfunctions in myself and needle or use magnets to stimulate the point prescriptions. I routinely check testing locations that are my weaknesses and determine my simple point prescription before inserting my first needle. Needling myself in a recliner is most comfortable, and I use magnetic pellets as needed. My self-care routine includes daily Body-Feedback testing of nutritional supplements, foods, and essential oils incorporated with meditation, acupuncture, chiropractic care, and massage to support physical, emotional, and spiritual health.

Learning the Body-Feedback system takes a commitment to excellence. You will gain a new level of understanding of some of the basics you learned in acupuncture school. Memorizing the point prescriptions and practicing the palpation techniques, along with learning to check the pulse for accurate point location will ensure success. Body-Feedback is the language the body speaks and, as you learn this new language, it is essential to study, have patience, and practice to master it.

Lessons from Case Studies

Treatment with the Body-Feedback system is a conversation between the practitioner and the client in which the primary objective is to listen to the wisdom of the body. This dialogue is achieved with palpation of specific muscle groups and acupuncture points, along with monitoring the pulse. The theory underlying the Body-Feedback system provides you with logical steps to evaluate your clients' symptoms and assess their organs and meridians before, during, and after each session. In addition, I use my intuition and instincts to guide each client's session and unify their body, mind, and spirit to maximize their healing potential. This unspoken connection between practitioner and client is challenging to fully convey through written case studies and theory. Integrating the palpation techniques and treatment steps with your insights and hunches are the skills you will master by taking the time to study and practice this system.

At times, I have a clear understanding of why a client's body needs certain point combinations, and at other times it becomes clear in the future. In rare cases, it may never make sense why someone tests positive for certain point combinations and why they have the healing response that they do. However, when I double-check my work using the Body-Feedback techniques, I know with confidence that the treatment will make a positive impact on their overall health.

When reading through the case studies in this book, remember that with experience your intuition and instincts flourish as a practitioner. The Body-Feedback system will confirm for you when you are on the right path and when you need to adjust your treatment approach. This system requires you to memorize the map of the body and the Body-Feedback point combinations to work efficiently. Then, with experience, your insights will guide you, your clients will become your teachers, and you will witness everyday miracles in your practice just as I have.

Taking a few minutes at the beginning of each session to plan the treatment will allow you to move through the needling process quickly. The Body-Feedback treatment style relies less on subjective symptoms and more on palpatory findings at each session. I spend several minutes talking with my clients and then, as quickly as possible, encourage them to lie on the table. I always ask how they felt after their last treatment, how much improvement they had in their main symptoms, and if they have any new symptoms. I will ask questions during the pre-treatment planning stage that relate to the Body-Feedback testing locations I am treating.

The case studies are outlined in three stages: pre-treatment planning, treatment steps, and post-treatment assessment.

1. **Pre-Treatment Planning**
    - a) Identify asymmetry
    - b) Determine treatment position (supine or prone) to balance the autonomic nervous system
    - c) Test and choose Body-Feedback Balancing Acupoints
    - d) Test and choose Body-Feedback Sedation or Tonification Acupoints
    - e) Palpate and assess the corresponding Body-Feedback testing locations for the root treatment
    - f) Test and apply essential oils
2. **Treatment Steps for the four types of treatment approaches**
    - a) Symmetrical Supine Treatment Session
    - b) Asymmetrical Supine Treatment Session
    - c) Symmetrical Prone Treatment Session
    - d) Asymmetrical Prone Treatment Session
3. **Post-Treatment Assessment**
    - a) Apply magnets, pellets, ear-seeds, or press-tacks as needed
    - b) Test nutritional supplements and Chinese herbs
    - c) Check foods and personal care products as needed

Following these steps will ensure your acupuncture practice rises above client expectations. Allowing a client's body to communicate with you changes the focus of your practice from alleviating individual symptoms to whole-body wellness. Your clients will experience long-lasting improvements, which build a foundation of communication and trust. This book, with its step-by-step instructions and specific case studies, enables you to confidently interact with your clients on a deeper level to direct the healing process. Approaching clients as guides will bestow you with lifelong teachers!

With a sea of love,
Michelle Meramour

SECTION

1

Body-Feedback Theory

CHAPTER 1

The Body-Feedback Trisections

> *The five elemental phases and the six atmospheric influences [fire, dampness, summer-heat, dryness, cold, and wind] have a definite pattern and rhythm. This knowledge is very profound. If one grasps it, one can know the changes that will transpire in the natural world. One who masters this science can enjoy eternal health... Please learn, understand, and apply this knowledge carefully.*[2]

A master acupuncturist can treat many patients, but form and structure are necessary to teach many masters. In the Body-Feedback system, the trisections are the framework. The Body-Feedback trisections group together related organs by integrating yin-yang theory, the five elemental phases, and the six levels of the body. Treating organ dysfunction by harmonizing the trisections provides immediate results and a deeper understanding of how pathogens affect health. The organs within a trisection work together to create the larger systems of the body, such as respiratory, digestive, nervous, endocrine, skeletal, and so on. The trisections guide a practitioner in choosing the most appropriate acupoints, essential oils, herbs, and supplements for every client. The ability to optimize health occurs when the body's systems and organs are functioning properly, and the meridian system is balanced. Harmonizing the trisections provides constitutional support and long-term benefits.

The Body-Feedback system uses acupuncture points in different ways. Acupuncture points treated with needles, press tacks, or magnetic pellets are identified as *acupoints*. Acupuncture points that are palpated for pain, tightness, or discomfort during Body-Feedback testing are identified as *points*. Point categories, such as he-sea or fire-element, which can be used for both testing and treatment, are referred to as *point designations*. Throughout this text, the acupuncture points will be classified as acupoints, points, or point designations to indicate their use. The *Body-Feedback balancing, sedation, and tonification prescriptions* are unique acupoint combinations based on the five-element theory used to both diagnose and treat traditional Chinese medical pathology and trisection discord.

1.1 Separation of Yin and Yang into Six Levels and Twelve Pairs

According to Chinese philosophy, everything in the universe arises from the original separation of pure energy, known as chaos, which systematically arranged itself into yin and yang. After this first separation, unlimited possibilities of creation can occur as long as it follows the laws that govern yin and yang. For instance, the rotation of the planet earth around the sun provides for day (yang) and night (yin) and the four seasons; spring (yang), summer (yang), fall (yin), and winter (yin). The seasons in combination with the rotation of the planet generate the five elements (wood, fire, earth, metal, and water) and six atmospheric influences (wind, cold, summer heat, dampness, dryness, and fire). As long as the earth's rotation and the four seasons follow the laws of yin and yang, genesis can exist on earth.

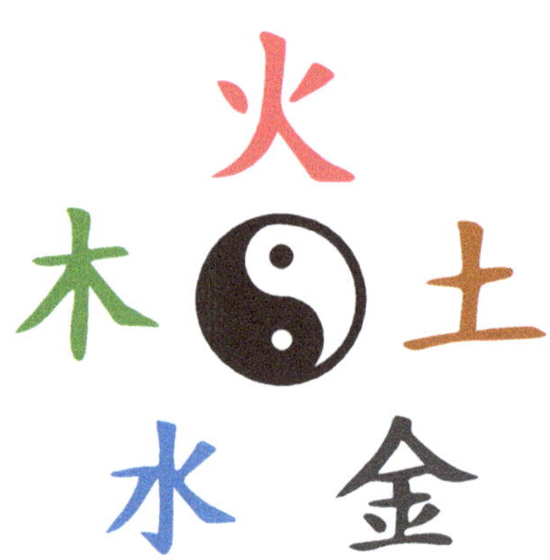

ID 107164152 © Miceking | Dreamstime.com

Grouping the twelve major organs of the body into three sections (trisections) is based on *The Yellow Emperor's Classic of Medicine*. According to Qi Bo, "Yin provides form. Yang provides growth."[3] Qi Bo explains that in the body, the initial separation of yin and yang simultaneously creates the three yang and yin levels. The three yang levels are *yang-ming*, *tai-yang*, and *shao-yang*. The three yin levels are *tai-yin*, *shao-yin*, and *jue-yin*. These six levels couple together in a specific order, and the three resulting pairs (trisections) contain "yang within yin."[4]

The Separation of Yin and Yang into Six Levels

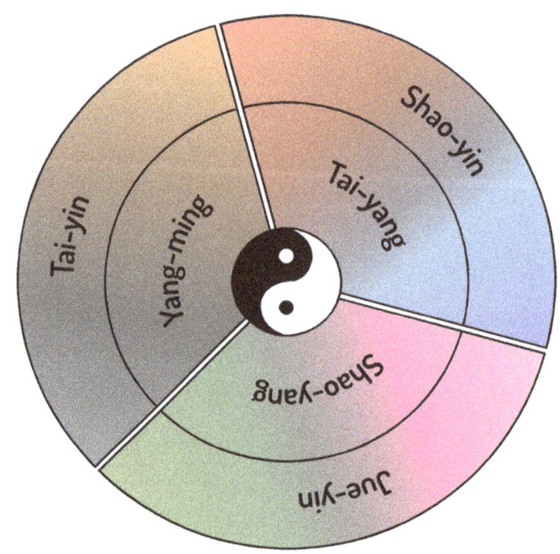

Yang-ming couples inside of and with **tai-yin** (the first trisection).

Tai-yang couples inside of and with **shao-yin** (the second trisection).

Shao-yang couples inside of and with **jue-yin** (the third trisection).

The next separation of the original three yin and yang levels further divides the body into the twelve main organs and corresponding meridians. This creates six sets of upper (hand) organs/meridians paired with lower (foot) organs/meridians of the same yin or yang level:

THE FIRST TRISECTION

Hand tai-yin (lung) pairs with foot tai-yin (spleen).

Hand yang-ming (large intestine) pairs with foot yang-ming (stomach).

THE SECOND TRISECTION

Hand shao-yin (heart) pairs with foot shao-yin (kidney).

Hand tai-yang (small intestine) pairs with foot tai-yang (urinary bladder).

THE THIRD TRISECTION

Hand jue-yin (pericardium) pairs with foot jue-yin (liver).

Hand shao-yang (triple burner) pairs with foot shao-yang (gallbladder).

This second separation establishes the order in which the twelve primary meridians connect to create a complete circuit. The twenty-four-hour organ clock divides the day into two-hour segments identifying when organs and their corresponding meridians are most active. The order of peak organ activity flows around the body throughout the day following the succession of the meridian system circuit. The flow of peak organ activity is different from the order in which *qi*, the body's circulating energy and life force, flows through the six-levels of the body from exterior to interior and back to exterior. The six-level theory is detailed later in this chapter.

Each trisection starts with the yin six-level hand organ/meridian, and then transitions to the yang six-level hand organ/meridian of the same element. For example, the first trisection begins with hand tai-yin (lung organ/meridian) and transitions to hand yang-ming (large intestine organ/meridian). Next in order is the yang six-level foot organ/meridian, which transitions to the yin six-level foot organ/meridian of the same element to complete the trisection. In this example, foot yang-ming (stomach organ/meridian) transitions to foot tai-yin (spleen organ/meridian) to end the first trisection. The hand and foot yang level pairs inside, or between, the hand and foot yin level.

Twenty-Four-Hour Clock of Peak Organ Times by Trisection

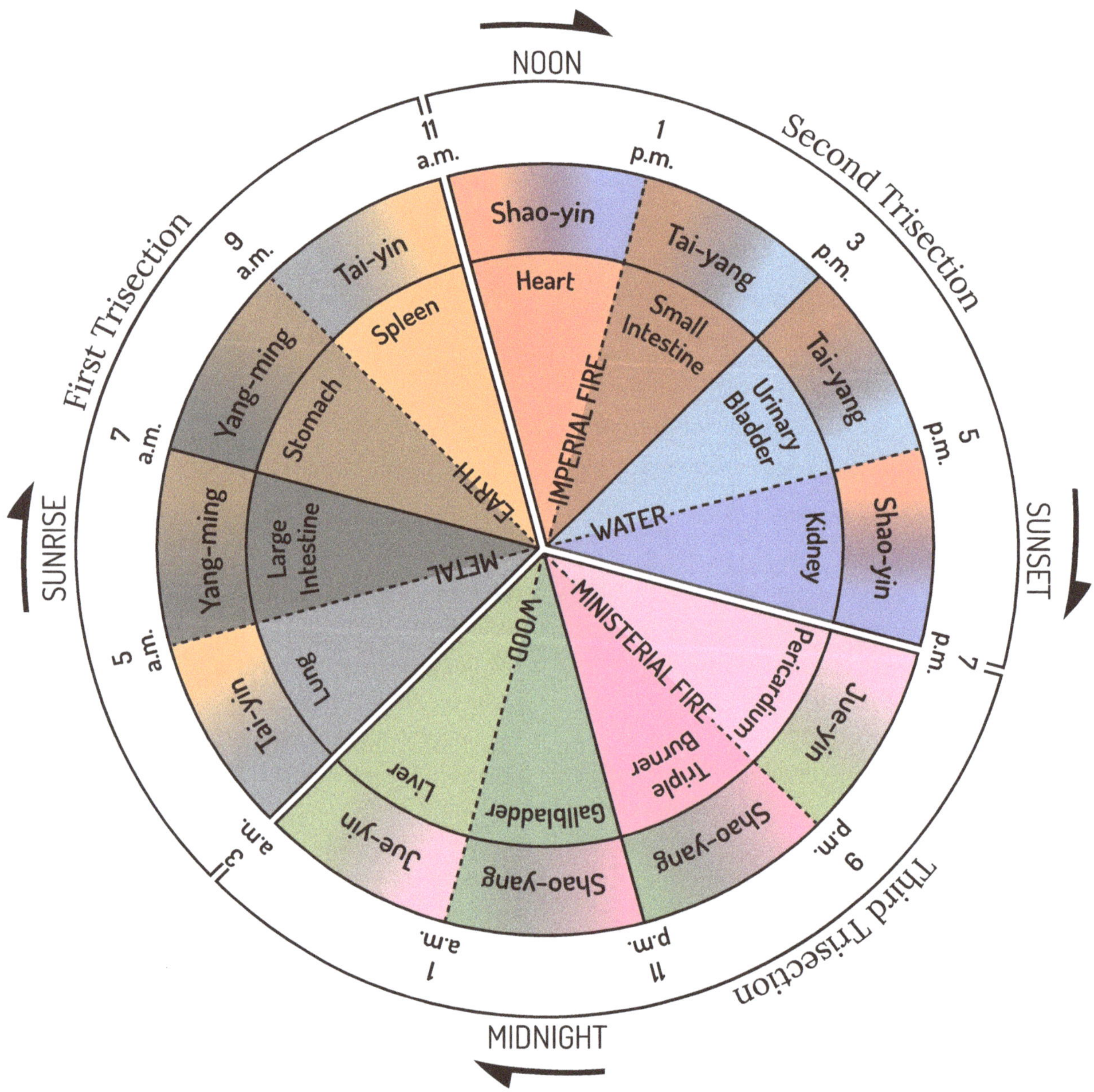

The trisection model organizes the twelve organs and corresponding meridians from the first and second separations of yin and yang. The first separation creates three groupings of yang coupling within yin that result in six levels. The second separation organizes these six levels into hand and foot pairs, which results in twelve organs and their associated meridians coupling in order based on the six-level and five-element theory.

The trisections separate the twenty-four-hour day into three eight-hour groupings: from 3 a.m. to 11 a.m., from 11 a.m. to 7 p.m., and from 7 p.m. to 3 a.m. The four organs and meridians within a trisection operate together to carry out their corresponding six-level and five-elemental functions. These combined functions within a trisection influence specific activity as described below.

The first trisection, occurring from 3 a.m. to 11 a.m., includes the lung, large intestine, stomach, and spleen organs and meridians. This trisection influences the respiratory system, energy production through respiration and digestion, the beginning and end stages of digestion, the majority of the immune and circulatory systems, and the elimination of waste via the colon.

The second trisection, occurring from 11 a.m. to 7 p.m., includes the heart, small intestine, urinary bladder, and kidney organs and meridians. This trisection influences the brain and nervous system, emotional well-being, the endocrine glands, aspects of the circulatory system, the reproductive, skeletal, and excretory systems, the aging process, and the elimination of waste via the kidneys and bladder.

The third trisection, occurring from 7 p.m. to 3 a.m., includes the pericardium, triple burner, gallbladder, and liver organs and meridians. This trisection influences the middle stages of digestion in which the body creates cholesterol, collagen, and hormones from fats. It also influences the lymph, muscular, and fascia systems and the detoxification of blood. Together the third trisection meridians connect the exterior (yang) and interior (yin) functions of the body.

Grouping body systems within the trisections exhibits why and how a root organ/meridian dysfunction manifests in multiple areas of health. Treating the root dysfunction within a trisection restores harmony between the four related organ/meridians and their corresponding body systems. Balancing the organ/meridians within a trisection, along with harmonizing the three trisections, accelerates healing, strengthens constitutional weaknesses, diminishes cellular aging, and encourages longevity.

With the Body-Feedback approach, a standard TCM diagnosis and evaluation includes the trisection discord and harmonizing the trisection within the treatment plan. The trisection framework associates individual endocrine glands with their functions to specific meridians through their related body systems. Analyzing health and the endocrine glands using the trisections is a new paradigm in TCM and a vital component of the Body-Feedback system.

1.2 Interaction of Yin and Yang within the Trisections

> *The law of yin and yang is the natural order of the universe, the foundation of all things, mother of all changes, the root of life and death. In healing, one must grasp the root of the disharmony, which is always subject to the law of yin and yang.*[5]

The Body-Feedback system uses the principles of yin and yang to treat organ dysfunction and meridian imbalance. This straightforward approach categorizes organ and meridian pathology as either an *excess* requiring *sedation*, or a *deficiency* requiring *tonification*. The meridians provide immediate access to the organs, and the ability to direct self-healing. By following the rules of five-element and six-level theory, the Body-Feedback system arranges traditional Chinese medical theory into trisections that guide diagnosis and provide treatment strategies.

The fundamental laws that govern the yin and yang state are:[6]

Yin and yang are rooted in each other and are interdependent.

Yin and yang counterbalance each other.

Yin and yang are divisible but inseparable.

Yin and yang are not fixed categories but relative ones.

In medicine, the interpretation of these fundamental laws of yin and yang include:[7]

Yin and yang attributes are used to categorize anatomical areas and physiological functions of the body.

In disease, a detriment to yang affects yin, and a detriment to yin affects yang.

Within the body, the natural ebb and flow of yin and yang is in constant fluctuation; as one expands the other contracts.

As pathology lingers, the excess of yin will change to an excess of yang, an excess of yang will change to an excess of yin, excess conditions will turn to deficiency, deficiency conditions will turn to excess, pathological heat will convert to pathological cold, and pathological cold will convert to pathological heat.

Each organ and its corresponding meridian within the trisection unite with three others for balance. When one organ/meridian becomes dysfunctional, the other three related organs/meridians adjust to balance the trisection based on the rules of yin-yang theory. For example, in the first trisection, when the large intestine is dysfunctional, the lung, stomach, and spleen compensate to keep the pathology contained within the trisection. The following chapter, "Trisection Imbalances," explains in detail the interaction of dysfunctional organs/meridians within a trisection.

1.3 Flow of Qi within the Six Levels

The Six Levels of Yin and Yang

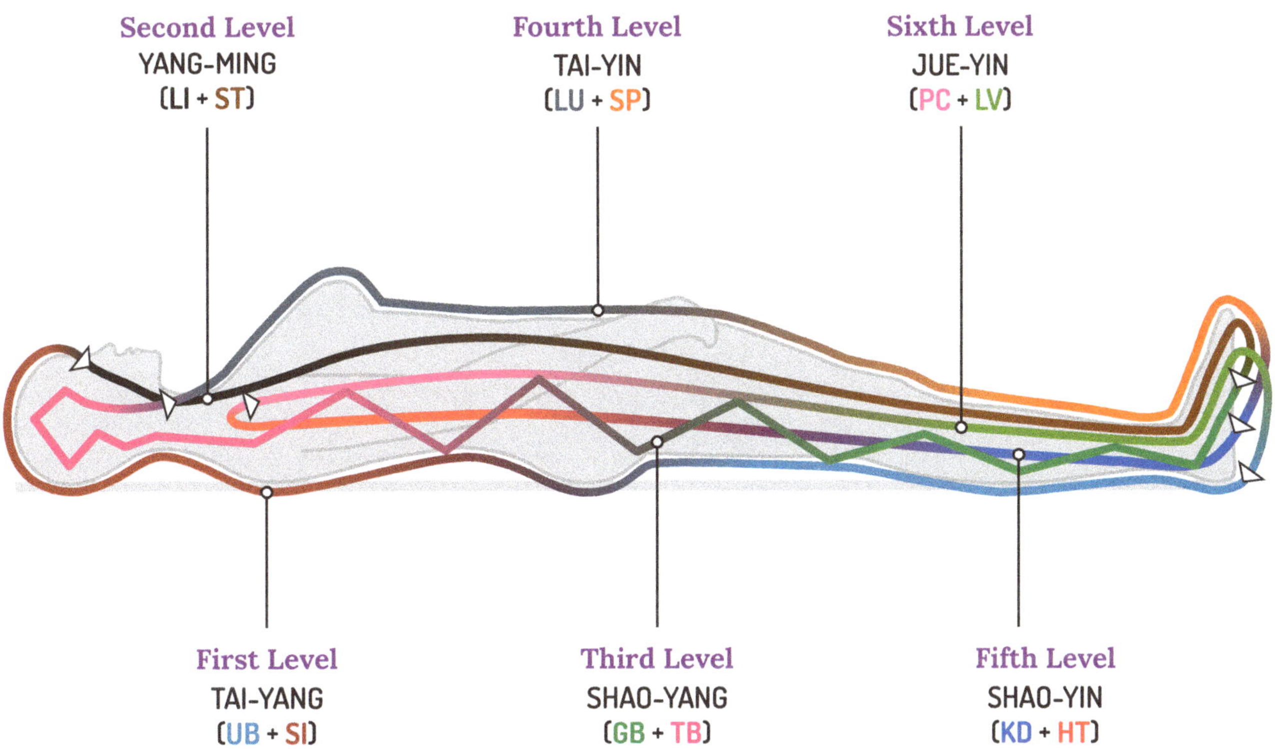

The daily cycle of qi flows through the levels as follows; tai-yang, yang-ming, shao-yang, tai-yin, shao-yin, and jue-yin.

"The qi of the five *zang* organs [the five-element yin organs include the lung, spleen, heart, kidney, and liver] circulates throughout the body in a continuous fashion, like the universe with its myriad galaxies." According to *The Yellow Emperor's Classic of Medicine*, daily qi flow begins on the back in tai-yang (urinary bladder and small intestine meridians). Then the qi flows onward to the front of the body through yang-ming (large intestine and stomach meridians), and then to the body's sides via shao-yang (gallbladder and triple burner meridians). The gallbladder and triple burner meridians transition qi flow into the yin levels. The first and outermost yin level qi passes through is tai-yin (lung and spleen meridians). Then the qi gathers in the deeper reservoirs of shao-yin (kidney and heart meridians) before it flows through jue-yin (pericardium and liver meridians), known as terminal (reverting) yin. Then the qi transitions back to the yang channels via the liver and pericardium meridians in a repeating cycle."[8]

- Tai-yang (second trisection) circulates qi and can spread pathology to yang-ming (first trisection).
- Yang-ming (first trisection) circulates qi and can spread pathology to shao-yang (third trisection).
- Shao-yang (third trisection) circulates qi and can spread pathology to tai-yin (first trisection).
- Tai-yin (first trisection) circulates qi and can spread pathology to shao-yin (second trisection).
- Shao-yin (second trisection) circulates qi and can spread pathology to jue-yin (third trisection).
- Jue-yin (third trisection) circulates qi and can spread pathology to tai-yang (second trisection), and the cycle repeats itself.

The circulation of qi through the six-levels is the method by which qi interacts directly between two trisections. Pathological qi, such as exterior-wind, qi stagnation, or unbalanced emotions, can disrupt a meridian's circulation within its level and into the following one. Within its level, if the meridian is unable to resolve the pathological qi, dysfunction can occur in the associated organ and imbalance the paired meridian. For example, qi stagnation with depressive heat affecting the liver meridian can spread to the liver organ and provoke liver blood deficiency, blood heat, or liver wind. The moment the liver meridian becomes excess or deficient, the pericardium meridian becomes imbalanced and can lead to organ pathology.

The six-level theory reflects how and where pathology challenges health utilizing the natural progression of energy flow from the superficial to the deepest levels of the body. The six-level approach applies to the whole body and the individual cells. For the body, skin creates a barrier from the outside world; for the cell, its wall creates a barrier for the inside microcosm. When qi pathology affects one of the six-levels, it can circulate and invade the following level. In this instance, the qi stagnation affecting jue-yin can invade tai-yang. Qi stagnation affecting tai-yang can cause qi deficiency that leads to exterior-wind pathogens entering the body or cells freely.

Pathogens disrupt the tai-yang and yang-ming levels, triggering an immune system response in the respiratory and digestive systems. As pathogens penetrate, they disturb the tai-yin and shao-yang levels and, in some cases, trigger autoimmune conditions. The deepest level, shao-yin, includes the nervous system, brain, and DNA sequencing, which together influence aging and the healthy replication of cells. If pathogens or autoimmune conditions afflict the shao-yin level, the brain and nervous system deteriorate, and abnormal cells can result. The jue-yin level releases toxins, including used hormone metabolites, cellular byproducts, and waste from pathogens, to be excreted from the body and cells.

As outlined above, the movement of qi through the body occurs from external to internal and then back to external in a continuous loop, while peak organ times flow around the daily clock. Therefore, the trisections concentrate on supporting organ function and harmonizing related organs via the meridians, and the six levels focus on pathogenesis and qi disruption that leads to diseases. The Body-Feedback balancing, sedation, and tonification acupoint prescriptions (see Chapters 9 and 10) treat pathology within a trisection while correcting qi flow. See Chapter 3, "Pathogenic Heat," for the Body-Feedback approach to the treatment of externally contracted diseases according to *Shang Han Lun*'s six-level theory.

1.4 Elemental Interactions within the Trisections

The five-element theory integrates with the Body-Feedback system in three fundamental ways. First, by establishing organ and meridian pairings within a trisection that operate different body systems. Second, by determining the Body-Feedback balancing, sedation, and tonification acupoint prescriptions. Third, by directing which supporting acupoints can be added to treatments. The five elements that guide the cycles in nature and life are fire, earth, metal, water, and wood.

Each trisection contains two sets of elemental pairs, which correspond with organs, glands, and meridians that work together within the related body systems. The fire element is subdivided into imperial-fire (heart and small intestine) and ministerial-fire (pericardium and triple burner). These six elemental pairs couple with the six levels to form the three trisections:

The first trisection contains the metal and earth pairs.

The second trisection contains the imperial-fire and water pairs.

The third trisection contains the ministerial-fire and wood pairs.

The pathological influences that negatively impact the elements and their corresponding organs are external pathogens, weather patterns, and unhealthy emotions. The five-element theory outlines the natural laws of the universe, identifying the critical *engendering* and *restraining* sequence for each element to regulate another. The engendering and restraining theories are the foundation for the Korean four-point and Chinese six-point acupoint combinations, lending to the creation of the Body-Feedback prescriptions.

The Body-Feedback style of acupuncture incorporates specific five-element principles to analyze and create a complete treatment approach. The Body-Feedback balancing, sedation, and tonification prescriptions use the Korean four-point and Chinese six-point combinations as a diagnostic tool and change their order to create a new treatment approach. Additional supporting acupoints enhance the foundational root Body-Feedback prescriptions following the rules of five-element theory. Scalp, facial, abdominal, and back acupoints optimize the autonomic nervous system to accelerate healing, and local needling addresses specific musculoskeletal symptoms.

The following charts organize the Body-Feedback trisections with the basic five-element correspondences.[9]

First Trisection

	METAL	EARTH
SEASON	AUTUMN	LATE SUMMER
YIN ORGAN	LUNG	SPLEEN
YANG ORGAN	LARGE INTESTINE	STOMACH
UNHEALTHY EMOTION	GRIEF/SADNESS	DISTRESS/WORRY
BODY REGION	SHOULDER/UPPER BACK	MID BACK
ORIFICE	NOSE	MOUTH
WEATHER PATTERN	DRYNESS	DAMPNESS
PATHOLOGICAL ACTION	COUGH	SPITTING

Second Trisection

	IMPERIAL-FIRE	WATER
SEASON	SUMMER	WINTER
YIN ORGAN	HEART	KIDNEY
YANG ORGAN	SMALL INTESTINE	URINARY BLADDER
UNHEALTHY EMOTION	(EXCESS) JOY (MANIA)	FEAR
BODY REGION	CHEST/RIBS	LOWER BACK/HIPS
ORIFICE	EAR	ANUS/URETHRA
WEATHER PATTERN	HEAT	COLD
PATHOLOGICAL ACTION	ANXIOUS LOOK	SHIVERING

Third Trisection

	MINISTERIAL-FIRE	WOOD
SEASON	SUMMER	SPRING
YIN ORGAN	PERICARDIUM	LIVER
YANG ORGAN	TRIPLE BURNER	GALLBLADDER
UNHEALTHY EMOTION	(EXCESS) JOY (MANIA)	ANGER
BODY REGION	CHEST/RIBS	NECK/HEAD
ORIFICE	EAR	EYES
WEATHER PATTERN	HEAT	WIND
PATHOLOGICAL ACTION	ANXIOUS LOOK	CLENCHED FIST/SPASMS

1.5 Daily Cycle of Peak Organ Times

The daily cycle of peak organ activity divides the day into two-hour segments for each of the twelve main organs. At 3 a.m., the liver organ ends the previous daily cycle and transitions to the lungs to start the new day. The two-hour segment in which each organ is most active will exacerbate any underlying organ pathology. The organ with the most severe pathology is called the root dysfunction and corresponds with the Body-Feedback balancing acupoint prescription that tests favorably. The root organ dysfunction will often fluctuate between excess and deficiency, requiring either sedation or tonification acupoints. The root organ dysfunction can change from session to session as health improves or deteriorates. The peak organ times and common symptoms include:

3 a.m. to 5 a.m. with lung issues such as sleep apnea, snoring, or waking early

5 a.m. to 7 a.m. with large intestine or colon issues such as diarrhea, constipation, or irritable bowel symptoms

7 a.m. to 9 a.m. with stomach issues such as indigestion after breakfast, ravenous upon waking, or bleeding gums

9 a.m. to 11 a.m. with spleen or pancreas issues such as low energy, no desire for food, fatigue after breakfast, or sugar cravings

11 a.m. to 1 p.m. with heart organ or emotional issues such as arrhythmia, rapid pulse, or feeling anxious

1 p.m. to 3 p.m. with small intestine issues such as digestive bloating after lunch, constipation, or difficulty absorbing nutrients

3 p.m. to 5 p.m. with urinary bladder symptoms including frequent or incomplete urination or neurological issues affecting bladder control

5 p.m. to 7 p.m. with kidney or adrenal issues causing water retention, fatigue, or difficulty with end stages of detoxification

7 p.m. to 9 p.m. with pericardium symptoms such as indigestion, excessive nervous energy, or difficulty relaxing

9 p.m. to 11 p.m. with triple burner or lymph system issues such as excessive urination, swollen lymph nodes, or edema

11 p.m. to 1 a.m. with gallbladder symptoms such as indigestion, muscle cramps, or difficulty falling asleep

1 a.m. to 3 a.m. with liver issues such as headaches, dizziness, sleep disturbance, or nausea

The trisections provide structure to organize the interaction of qi flow, organ function, the five elements, the six levels, and the multitude of pathologies. The twenty-four-hour clock of peak organ activity creates the treatment structure for the body systems. The meridians provide access to alter organ physiology and improve health. The six levels establish protective layers for the body and individual cells, circulate qi, and initiate function within the cells. The five elements govern the laws of nature for healing and well-being in this world. The trisections offer an understanding of disease pathogenesis, the pathway for healing, and clues to identify the most critical lifestyle factors in supporting health. The trisection model creates a comprehensive framework for these universal forces and the foundation of the Body-Feedback system.

CHAPTER 2

Trisection Imbalances

A combination of internal and external factors can impede the health of an organ or meridian and cause dysfunction. A dysfunctional organ or meridian can become excess and therefore require sedation, or it can become deficient requiring tonification. The intimate relationship between an organ and its meridian causes them to operate as one unit. When one becomes excess or deficient, the other simultaneously follows suit. The reference to an *organ/meridian* implies that they are functioning as one unit. The organ/meridian that is most excess or deficient is the root dysfunction requiring treatment.

Within a trisection, when one organ/meridian becomes excess or deficient, it instantly impacts the other three organs/meridians. Each organ/meridian directly affects its elemental and six-level pair and indirectly affects its non-paired organ/meridian. The non-paired organ/meridian has an indirect relationship with the root pathology through its relationship with the root's elemental and six-level pairs. For example, in the first trisection, the lung pairs directly with the large intestine and the spleen, and indirectly interacts with the stomach. With a root lung deficiency, the stomach becomes deficient to accommodate the root pathology and maintain balance within the trisection.

The five-element theory describes how extreme weather patterns during any season challenge health by burdening the organs/meridians with external pathogens (wind in spring, heat in summer, dampness in late summer, dryness in autumn, and cold in winter). For example, during autumn, ruled by the metal element, the body is more susceptible to dryness and symptoms related to the lungs and large intestine such as dry skin, dry sinuses, dry stools, respiratory infections, allergies, and dehydration.

Internal causes that can negatively impact organ and meridian function include poor food choices, improper exercise, exposure to toxins, genetics, unbalanced emotions, and other lifestyle factors. Uncontrolled emotions negatively impact the qi of an organ and will contribute to the dysfunction and disharmony of the trisection. "Overindulgence in the five emotions--happiness, anger, sadness, worry or fear, and fright--can create imbalances."[10]

2.1 Pathogenesis of Trisection Discord

The laws of yin and yang govern how the organs within a trisection interact. Two different progressions can cause trisection discord. The first progression occurs when an organ/meridian becomes deficient; its elemental and six-level pairs simultaneously become excess. Then, the fourth non-paired organ/meridian in the trisection will become deficient. The second progression occurs when an organ/meridian becomes excess; its elemental pair and six-level pair become deficient. Then, the fourth non-paired organ/meridian in the trisection becomes excess.

The body attempts to confine pathology within a trisection to minimize possible negative health ramifications. When a discordant trisection lingers for too long or is too extreme, it can impact the other trisections. Often, the root organ/meridian dysfunction of the original imbalanced trisection will either disrupt the organ/meridian opposite it on the twenty-four-hour organ clock or affect the first organ/meridian in the next trisection.

When multi-trisection pathology continues, it will create the need for an asymmetrical treatment approach (see Chapter 7). The asymmetrical treatment approach effectively harmonizes complex patterns by treating the right and left sides of the body with different Body-Feedback acupoint prescriptions. Asymmetrical treatments can incorporate two different root organ/meridians from the same or different trisections. A common asymmetrical treatment within the first trisection is a lung sedation treatment on one side and a large intestine tonification treatment on the opposite side. A common asymmetrical treatment for root dysfunctions in two trisections is a spleen (first trisection) sedation treatment on one side of the body and a liver (third trisection) sedation treatment on the opposite side. In asymmetrical treatments, both root organs/meridians require treatment to restore health.

Body-Feedback testing illuminates the most pronounced root organ/meridian dysfunction causing trisection discord at any particular appointment. Depending on lifestyle choices, herbs, and supplements, the root dysfunction and Body-Feedback acupoint prescriptions will likely change from appointment to appointment. For example, a root lung dysfunction can transition to the large intestine elemental pair or the spleen six-level pair, or it can shift from lung excess to lung deficiency. When the same Body-Feedback balancing prescription tests best at multiple sessions, a client's root dysfunction is representing their constitutional or genetic weakness. See Chapter 6 for information on the Body-Feedback testing locations and Chapter 9 for the unique balancing prescriptions. In the example above, with a constitutional weakness affecting the colon, the client will most often test favorably for the large intestine balancing and sedation or tonification acupoints.

Balance and Discord within the First Trisection

FIRST TRISECTION IN A STATE OF BALANCE

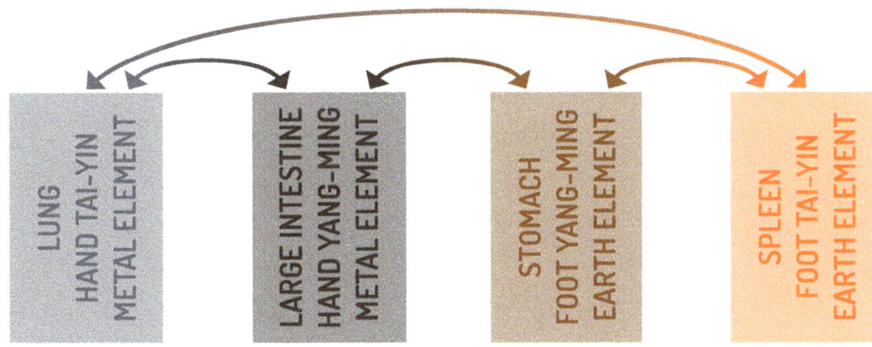

ROOT LUNG DEFICIENCY CAUSING DISCORD

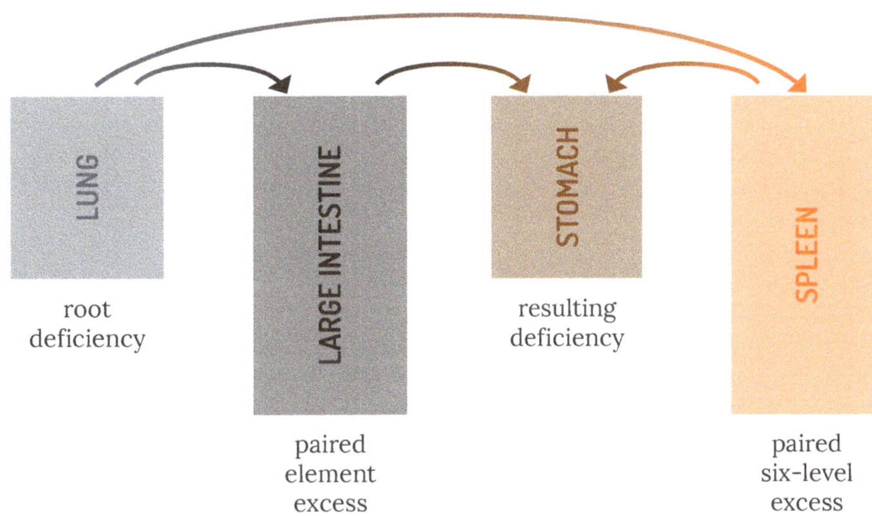

ROOT LUNG EXCESS CAUSING DISCORD

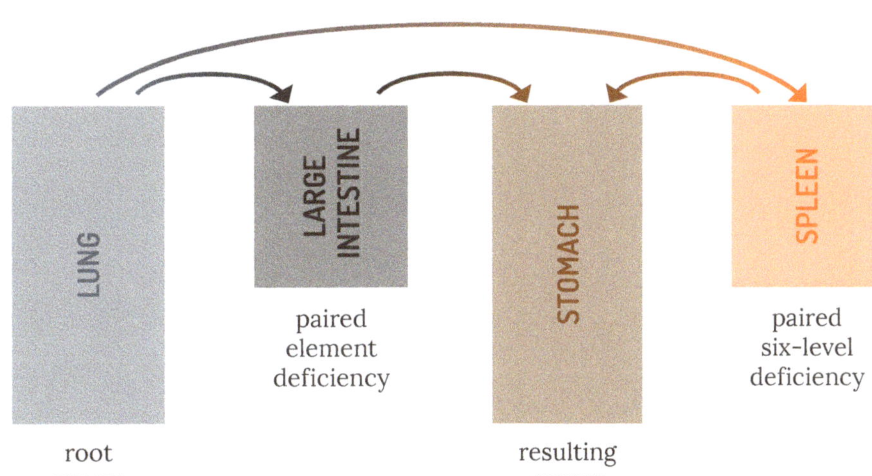

Balance and Discord within the Second Trisection

SECOND TRISECTION IN A STATE OF BALANCE

ROOT URINARY BLADDER DEFICIENCY CAUSING DISCORD

ROOT URINARY BLADDER EXCESS CAUSING DISCORD

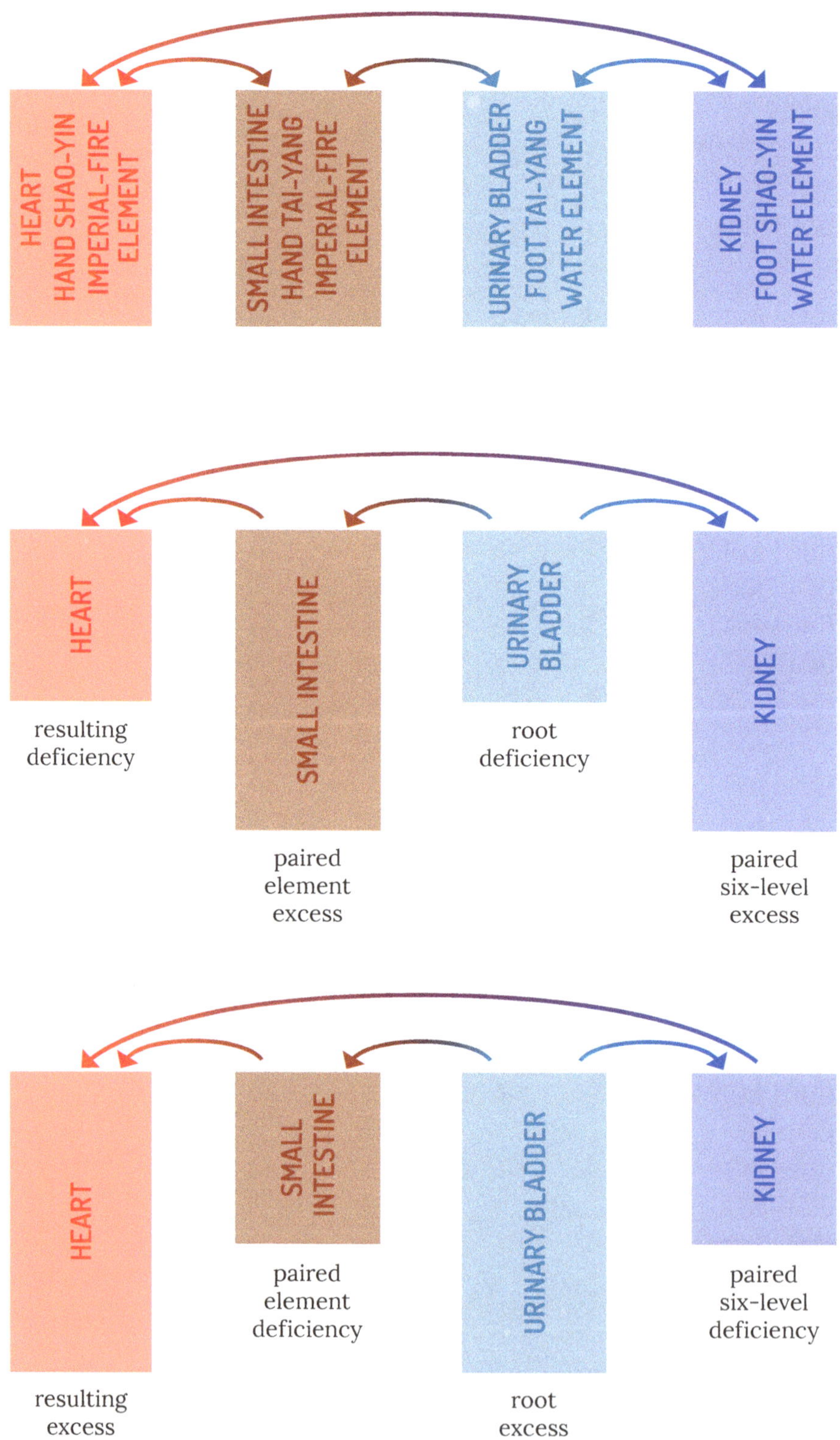

Balance and Discord within the Third Trisection

THIRD TRISECTION IN A STATE OF BALANCE

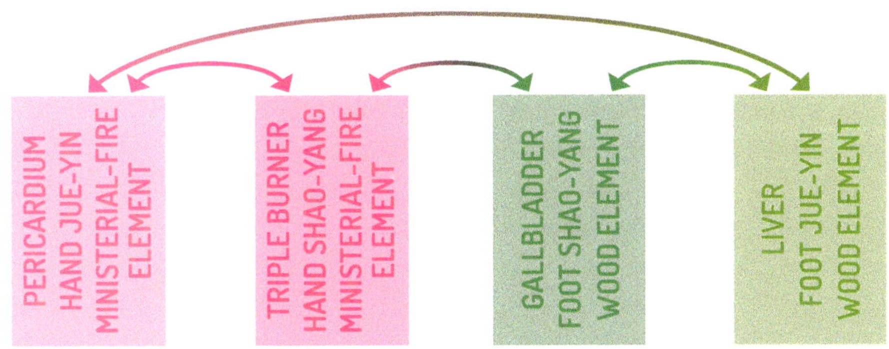

ROOT LIVER DEFICIENCY CAUSING DISCORD

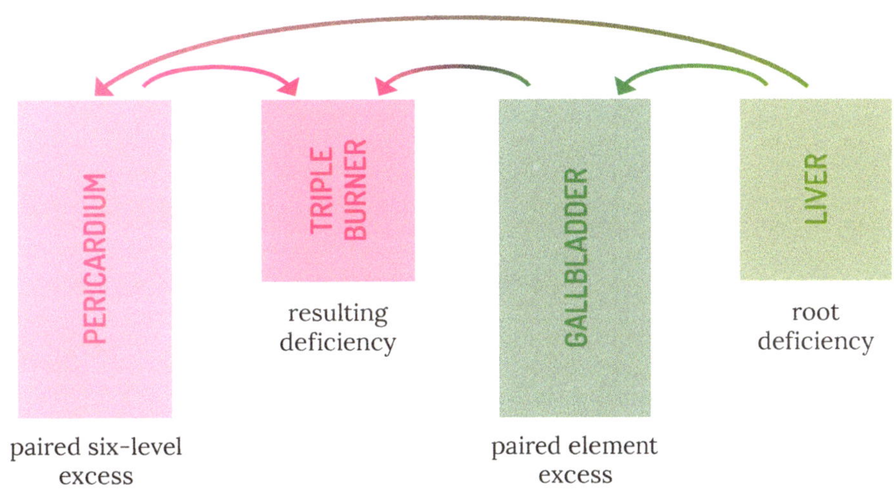

ROOT LIVER EXCESS CAUSING DISCORD

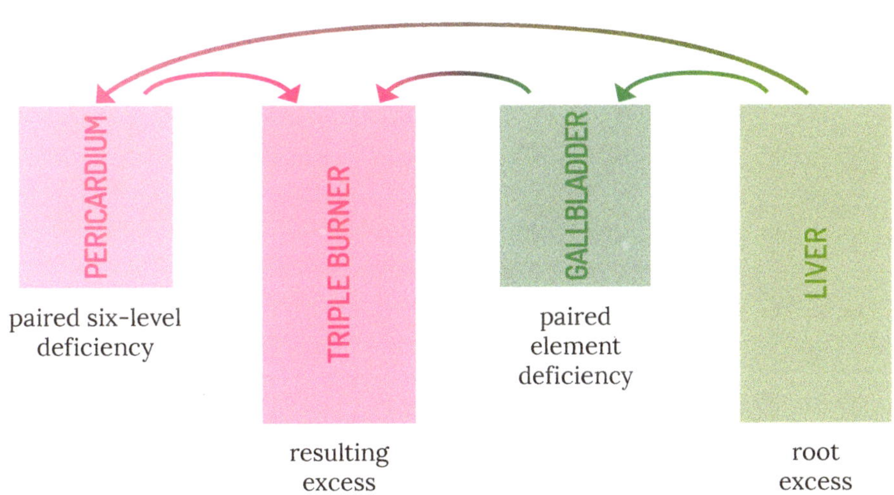

2.2 Imbalances Affecting the First Trisection

The first trisection organs/meridians include the tai-yin pair (lung and spleen), the yang-ming pair (large intestine and stomach), the metal element pair (lung and large intestine), and the earth element pair (stomach and spleen).

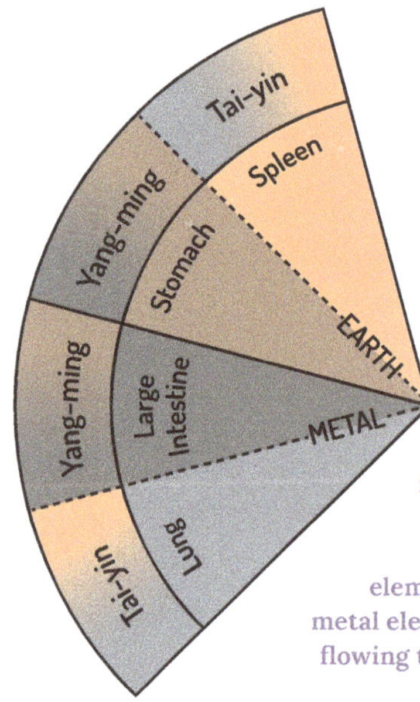

THE BALANCED FIRST TRISECTION

The lung, large intestine, stomach, and spleen are functioning efficiently. The earth element is engendering the metal element, and the qi is free flowing through the tai-yin and yang-ming levels.

FIRST TRISECTION IMBALANCE PATTERN ONE

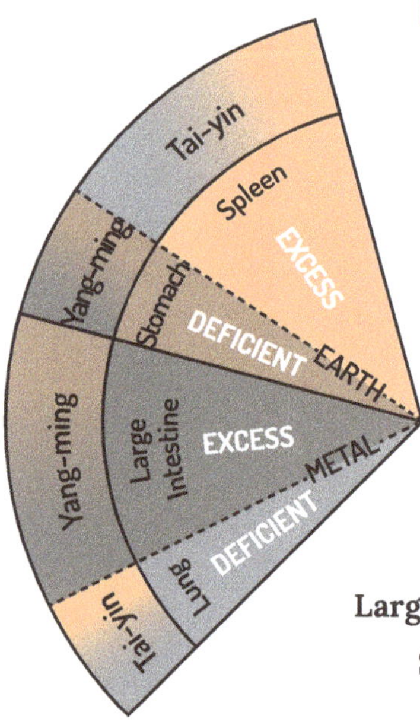

Lung: deficient

Large intestine: excess

Stomach: deficient

Spleen: excess

The lung and stomach are receiving insufficient qi, blood, yin, or yang. The large intestine and spleen are collecting qi stagnation, blood stasis, external pathogens, or negative emotions.

FIRST TRISECTION IMBALANCE PATTERN TWO

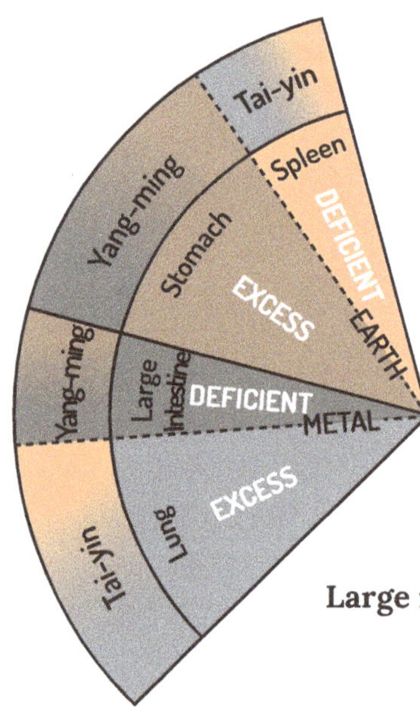

Lung: excess

Large intestine: deficient

Stomach: excess

Spleen: deficient

The large intestine and spleen are receiving insufficient qi, blood, yin, or yang. The lung and stomach are collecting qi stagnation, blood stasis, external pathogens, or negative emotions.

2.3 Imbalances Affecting the Second Trisection

The second trisection organs/meridians include the shao-yin pair (heart and kidney), the tai-yang pair (small intestine and urinary bladder), the imperial-fire element pair (heart and small intestine), and the water element pair (kidney and urinary bladder).

THE BALANCED SECOND TRISECTION

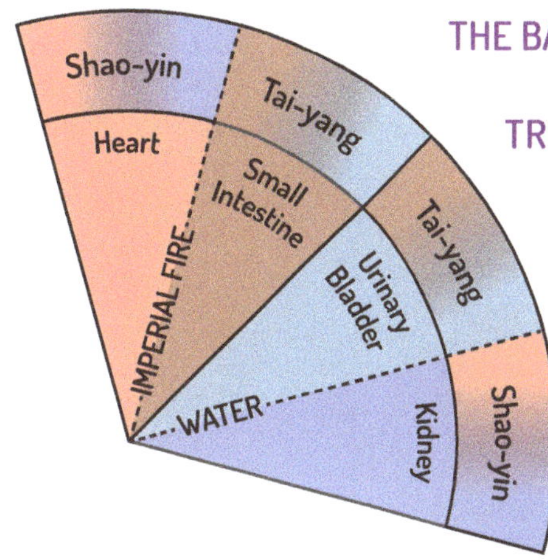

The heart, small intestine, urinary bladder, and kidney meridians are functioning efficiently. The water element is properly restraining the fire element, and the qi is free flowing through the shao-yin and tai-yang levels.

SECOND TRISECTION IMBALANCE PATTERN ONE

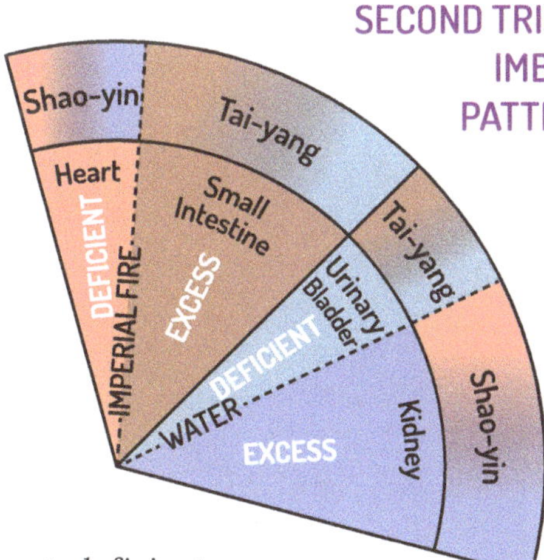

Heart: deficient

Small intestine: excess

Urinary bladder: deficient

Kidney: excess

The heart and urinary bladder are receiving insufficient qi, blood, yin, or yang. The small intestine and kidney are collecting qi stagnation, blood stasis, external pathogens, or negative emotions.

SECOND TRISECTION IMBALANCE PATTERN TWO

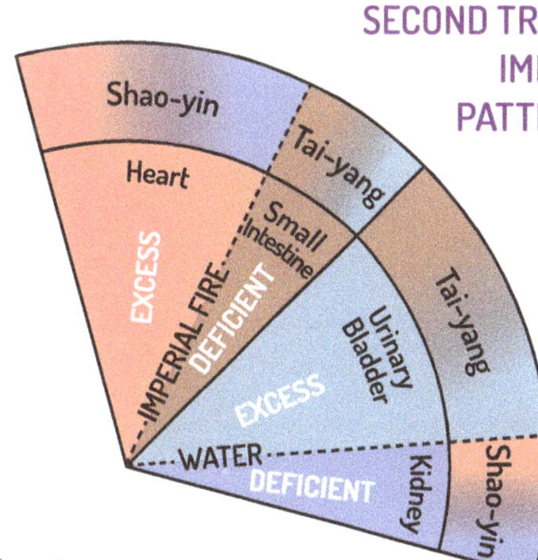

Heart: excess

Small intestine: deficient

Urinary bladder: excess

Kidney: deficient

The small intestine and kidney are receiving insufficient qi, blood, yin, or yang. The heart and urinary bladder are collecting qi stagnation, blood stasis, external pathogens, or negative emotions.

2.4 Imbalances Affecting the Third Trisection

The third trisection organs/meridians include the jue-yin pair (pericardium and liver), the shao-yang pair (triple burner and gallbladder), the ministerial-fire element pair (pericardium and triple burner), and the wood element pair (gallbladder and liver).

THE BALANCED THIRD TRISECTION

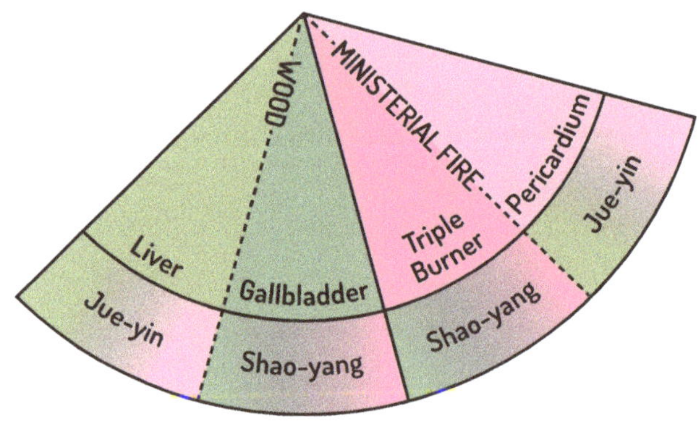

The pericardium, triple burner, gallbladder, and liver are functioning efficiently. The wood element is engendering the fire element, and the qi is free flowing through the jue-yin and shao-yang levels.

THIRD TRISECTION IMBALANCE PATTERN ONE

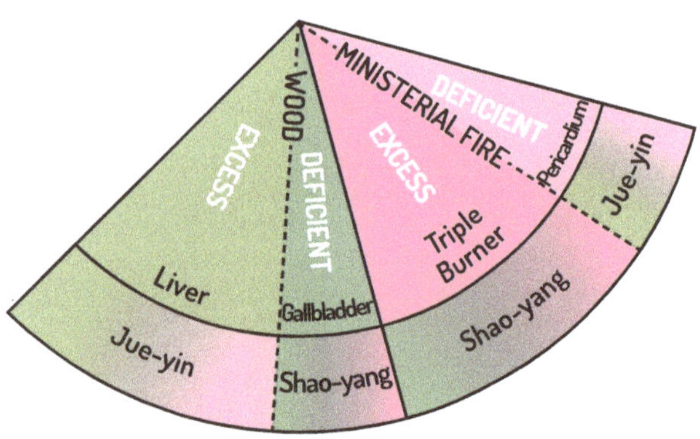

Pericardium: deficient

Triple burner: excess

Gallbladder: deficient

Liver: excess

The pericardium and gallbladder are receiving insufficient qi, blood, yin, or yang. The triple burner and liver are collecting qi stagnation, blood stasis, external pathogens, or negative emotions.

THIRD TRISECTION IMBALANCE PATTERN TWO

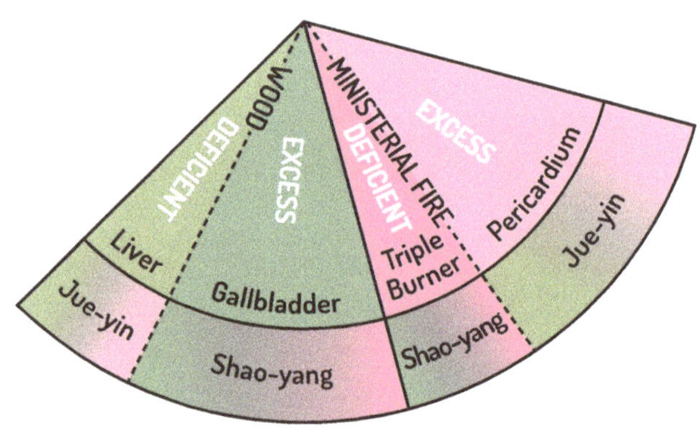

Pericardium: excess

Triple Burner: deficient

Gallbladder: excess

Liver: deficient

The triple burner and liver are receiving insufficient qi, blood, yin, or yang. The pericardium and gallbladder are collecting qi stagnation, blood stasis, external pathogens, or negative emotions.

2.5 Organ Relationships among Trisections

A severely compromised organ within a trisection can affect another trisection through one of three methods. First, by disrupting the organ opposite on the twenty-four-hour clock. Second, from interrupting the next element in the engendering cycle (wood engenders fire, fire engenders earth, earth engenders metal, metal engenders water, and water engenders wood). Third, by compromising qi flow through the six levels or carrying pathogens into subsequent levels. For example, a heart dysfunction (11 a.m. to 1 p.m.) in the second trisection and a gallbladder dysfunction (11 p.m. to 1 a.m.) in the third trisection create the heart-gallbladder disharmony pattern associated with insomnia. The pathogenesis of a heart-gallbladder disharmony pattern can occur through any one of the three forms above.

The gallbladder in a state of excess can provoke heart deficiency, or the heart in a state of excess can cause gallbladder deficiency. According to the five-element theory, wood engenders fire. A dysfunctional wood element (liver or gallbladder) can disrupt the fire element while negatively impacting any of the four fire element organs/meridians (heart, small intestine, pericardium, or triple burner). According to the six-level theory, shao-yin (the heart and second trisection) circulates qi and can spread pathology to jue-yin (the gallbladder and third trisection). Depending on the time of day, season, diet, and stress level, the root treatment for the gallbladder-heart disharmony will alternate between heart excess or heart deficiency and gallbladder excess or gallbladder deficiency.

Heart and Gallbladder Disharmony

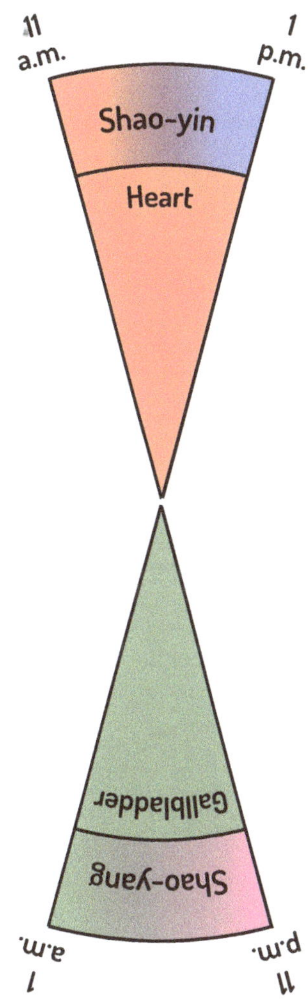

Heart and gallbladder organ dysfunction causing disharmony between the second and third trisections.

Another example of a two-trisection disharmony encompasses the metal element (lung and large intestine) in the first trisection and the water element (kidney and urinary bladder) in the second trisection. The metal and water elements are opposite each other on the twenty-four-hour peak organ activity clock. Metal engenders water; a lung and large intestine imbalance can disrupt the kidney and urinary bladder balance. Tai-yang circulates qi to yang-ming; a urinary bladder qi pathology can compromise the large intestine. Tai-yin circulates qi to shao-yin; a lung qi pathology can compromise the kidneys.

This two-trisection disharmony can manifest as immune and adrenal dysfunctions. Allergies can cause a maladapted stress response of excessive cortisol output, which eventually leads to adrenal fatigue. Stress can disrupt the immune system and cause low immunity or exacerbate autoimmune conditions. Again, depending on the time of day, time of year, diet, and stress level, the root treatment for this presentation will alternate between the lung, large intestine, kidney, or urinary bladder. Trisection analysis streamlines the Body-Feedback testing process to help identify the root dysfunctions.

Metal and Water Element Disharmony

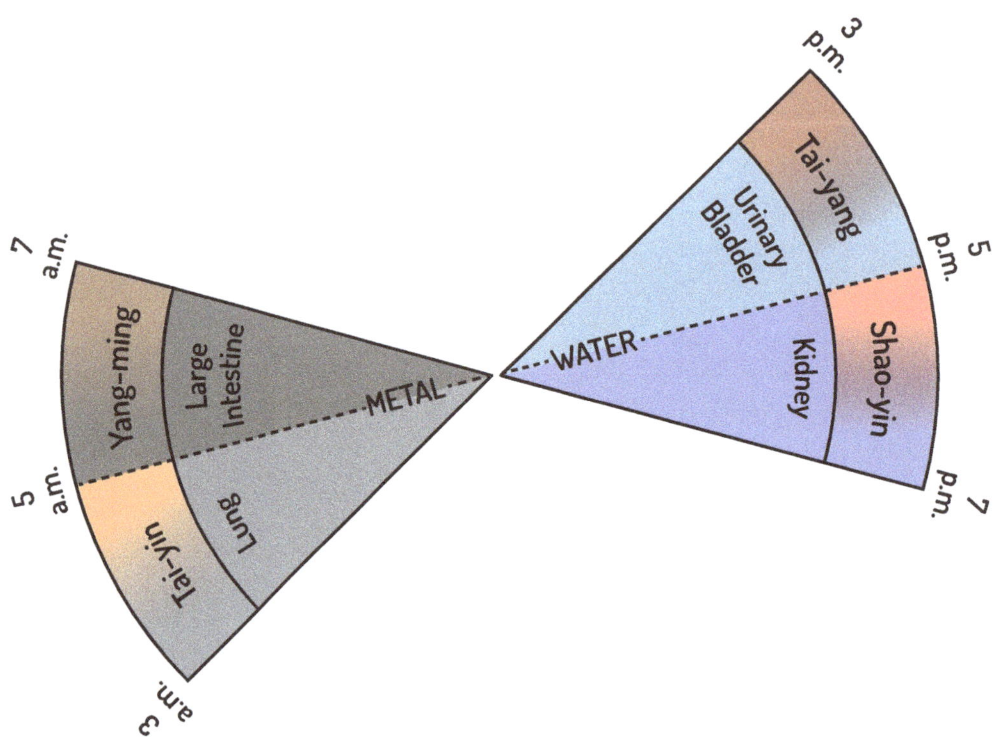

Organ dysfunction within the metal element (lung and large intestine) and the water element (kidney and urinary bladder) causing disharmony between the first and second trisections.

2.6 Practical Application Using Trisection Imbalances

The key to effective medicine is to determine the cause and rectify the imbalance of the yuan/original qi of the body. Study the ancient medical classics well. Follow the correct treatment principles and perform your healing with the utmost care and attention. Conduct yourself with the highest virtue and always have compassion towards your patients. In this way you will be outstanding in your cures and never cause malpractice. This is the way of the sage physicians.[11]

The trisection framework focuses treatments on the organs/meridians that need the most attention at any given time. By supporting the related organs/meridians within a trisection, the treatment approach will address both the root of compromised health and the branch symptoms. The trisections provide clarity in evaluating new clients and complex cases, along with creating concise treatment plans.

Analyzing health by way of the trisections identifies the following:

- the root organ/meridian dysfunction to support at the initial appointment
- the organs/meridians to check at future appointments based on the elemental and six-level pairs
- the organ/meridian to support a client's natural progression of healing (see Chapter 21)
- the root constitutional or genetic element or six-level pair weakness after clearing layers of dysfunction

Body-Feedback testing within the affected trisection can be utilized for checking acupoints, essential oils, herbs, and nutritional supplements. In most cases, a supplement that improves a testing location or pulse position for one organ/meridian within a trisection will benefit the other three related organs/meridians. If the Body-Feedback testing location for a root dysfunction has too much inflammation or is injured, use one of the other three related organ/meridian testing locations. If the testing results are unclear, use the other paired element's pulse positions within the same trisection. For example, with a first trisection root imbalance, check supplements and herbs for digestive or immune support to one of the testing locations for the lung, large intestine, stomach, or spleen, along with the first or second pulse positions on the right wrist.

Acupoints, essential oils, herbs, and supplements can test and affect the body differently depending on the time of day (morning, afternoon, and evening). For example, yang-boosting treatments to increase energy, motivation, metabolism, and circulation are most effective in the mornings or early afternoons. Yin-nourishing treatments to improve sleep, reduce stress, and cool deficient heat are most effective in the late afternoons to early evenings. It can be helpful to test yang and qi-boosting supplements in the morning, and test calming and yin-nourishing supplements in the evening.

In practice, a new client typically has liver dysfunction (excess or deficient) affecting the third trisection. By focusing on detoxing and clearing any liver congestion, the follow-up treatment may shift to a gallbladder presentation (excess or deficient). The gallbladder can cause abdominal bloating and indigestion as the liver releases toxins which pass through the gallbladder as they leave the body. Clients with autoimmune conditions may have compromised detoxification disrupting the metal element in the first trisection. With the number of toxins in our modern environment, new clients often have a liver or gallbladder dysfunction interrupting the first or second trisections.

The root treatment for menstruating women frequently shifts during different phases of their cycle. During the menstrual period, a root liver or gallbladder treatment can help detoxify and release the used hormones from the last cycle. During the follicular phase when the body is maturing the egg to release at ovulation, a root treatment in the second trisection is common because it includes the ovaries. During the luteal phase (post-ovulation), a wood or metal element root treatment is common. The liver and gallbladder organs (wood element) manage the higher hormone levels at this time of the cycle. The lung and large intestine organs (metal element) support the immune system to harmonize with the higher hormone levels and support implantation for a possible pregnancy.

The trisections provide a new paradigm for understanding symptoms that affect the meridians, organs, and endocrine glands. This new paradigm bridges TCM and allopathic medicine for a deeper understanding of today's health concerns. The combination of Body-Feedback testing, which allows for direct communication through the client's body, and trisection analysis of the root dysfunction is used to guide each treatment.

CHAPTER 3

Pathogenic Heat

Pathogenic heat generates quickly with exterior pathogens, such as bacteria, viruses, mold, fungi, and parasites, along with internal pathogens including qi stagnation, blood stasis, dampness, and yin deficiency. Pathogenic heat is an excess condition that can transform and progress to different organs, meridians, and regions of the body. To effectively supplement qi, blood, yin, and yang, a strategic release of heat pathogens is necessary. Heat is expansive by nature and can become destructive, like an out-of-control forest fire moving from one trisection to another, quickly causing dysfunction. Pathogenic heat accompanies chronic and autoimmune conditions, fueling ongoing tissue destruction.

Pathogenic heat in the body requires special attention as it can quickly intensify, spread, and compromise health. Frustration, irritability, anger, anxiety, and mania are early mental and emotional signs of excessive heat becoming pathogenic. With time, qi stagnation and blood stasis will transform excessive heat into a destructive fire, disrupting the self-healing process. Pathogenic heat can cause symptoms in various layers of the body, including:

- Skin becomes red, inflamed, itchy, cracked, and furfuraceous (flaky), and can even bleed or ooze white blood cells.
- Muscles tighten, retain fluid, easily cramp, and become painful.
- Tendons and ligaments lose their elasticity, limiting the range of motion of joints and injuring easily.
- Nerves at first feel hot, swell, become hyper-sensitive, and tingle. Over time, the myelin sheath can degenerate and desensitize the nerve causing numbness and atrophy in the surrounding tissue.
- Bones can become hot and sensitive to touch and eventually turn arthritic and change shape.
- Organs enlarge and reduce their function. Eventually, laboratory values become abnormal and reflect compromised organ functions.

The recurrence of pathogenic heat depends on several factors, including climate, food choices, activity, genetics, emotions, and the origin of the heat. Immediate relief of symptoms occurs with acupuncture and essential oils. Herbs and supplements can treat pathogenic heat between appointments. Clients with chronic conditions and autoimmune diseases respond best to regularly scheduled maintenance acupuncture and long-term support with herbs, supplements, and lifestyle changes to keep pathogenic heat to a minimum.

The Body-Feedback system corresponds the five elements with five forms of pathogenic heat. Body-Feedback testing and pulse diagnosis can identify the organs/meridians affected by pathogenic heat. The Body-Feedback prescriptions (balancing, sedation, and tonification) and metal + water combinations can release all forms of pathogenic heat. Body-Feedback testing can determine beneficial herbs and supplements to use between appointments for continued release of pathogenic heat.

3.1 Forms of Pathogenic Heat

The five forms of heat pathogens are exterior-wind heat, depressive heat, blood heat, damp heat, and yin-deficiency heat. Pathogenic heat can move between the six levels and the five elements changing in type and location. In complex and acute cases, several forms of pathogenic heat can occur in multiple levels, locations, and elements simultaneously. Each type of pathogenic heat has an affinity for a particular element. Organ/meridian dysfunction provides the mechanism for pathogenic heat to enter the body or generate internally. Once pathogenic heat occurs, it can transform and spread. For example, exterior-wind heat viruses inhaled through the lungs (metal element) can cause a sore throat, cough with phlegm, and yellow nasal discharge. If the exterior-wind heat lingers, it can damage the water element (next in the engendering cycle) causing lung yin-deficiency heat with symptoms of dry cough at night, dry throat at night, and a hoarse voice.

Pathogenic heat affecting one element can spread into the next element through the engendering cycle, or it can revert into the controlling element by disrupting the restraining cycle. For example, feelings of frustration or anger due to liver qi stagnation can follow the engendering cycle and provoke blood heat in the heart causing symptoms of anxiety, restless sleep, or insomnia. Feelings of frustration and anger disrupt the wood element's control of the earth element. Damp heat or excessive worry in the earth element can revert into the wood element through the controlling cycle, leading to loose stools or diarrhea after eating caused by a liver and spleen disharmony.

Five Types of Pathogenic Heat with Associated Elements

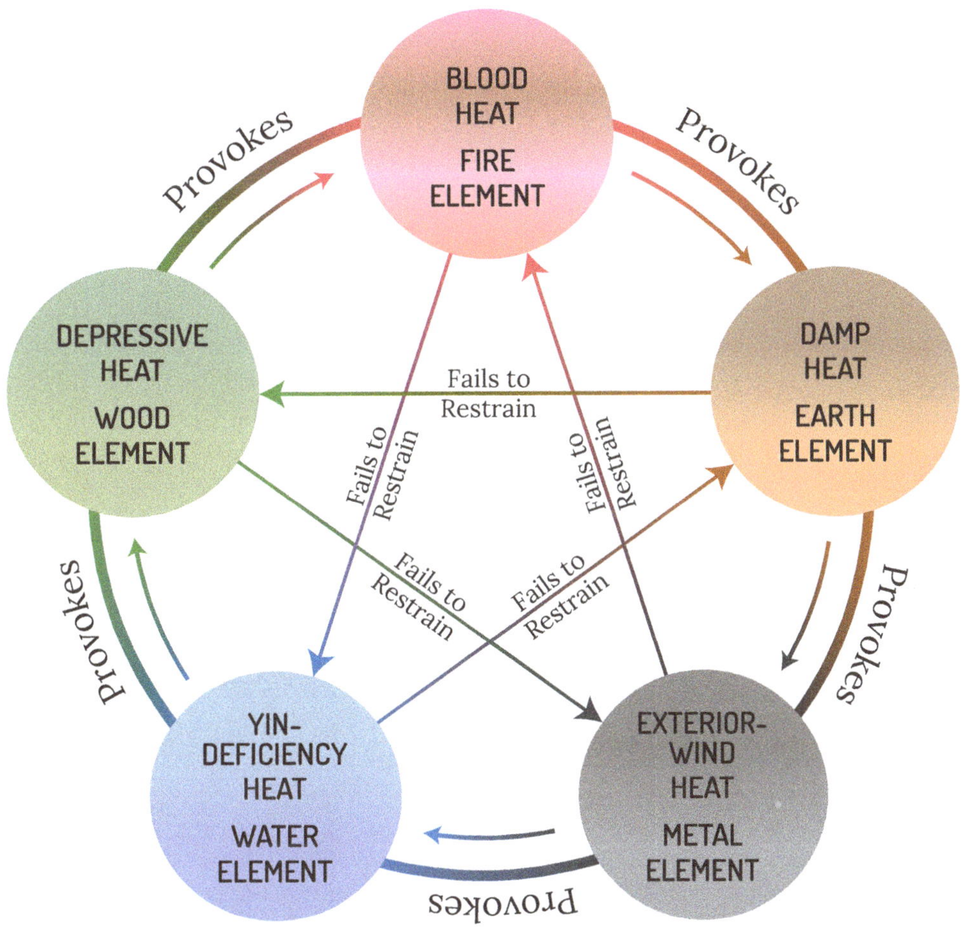

3.1.1 Exterior-Wind Heat

Exterior-wind heat includes the common cold, influenza, the initial stages of viral and bacterial infections, hives, vomiting, asthma, and wheezing due to outside factors. The tai-yang (small intestine and urinary bladder) and yang-ming (large intestine and stomach) levels protect the exterior borders of the body and are the first meridians affected by exterior-wind heat. If the surface layers fail to protect the body adequately, the expected progression of the pathogen follows the six-level stages by entering the shao-yang (gallbladder and triple burner) level and then the tai-yin (spleen and lung) level before settling in the deepest yin levels.

Exterior-wind heat can progress quickly to a deeper level depending on an individual's root or constitutional weakness. For example, when someone with a constitutionally weak yang-ming level catches a flu virus, it enters through the tai-yang level. The virus then quickly settles in the yang-ming level causing sore throat, thick yellow sinus congestion, sinus pressure, and constipation.

The Natural Progression of Exterior-Wind Pathogens

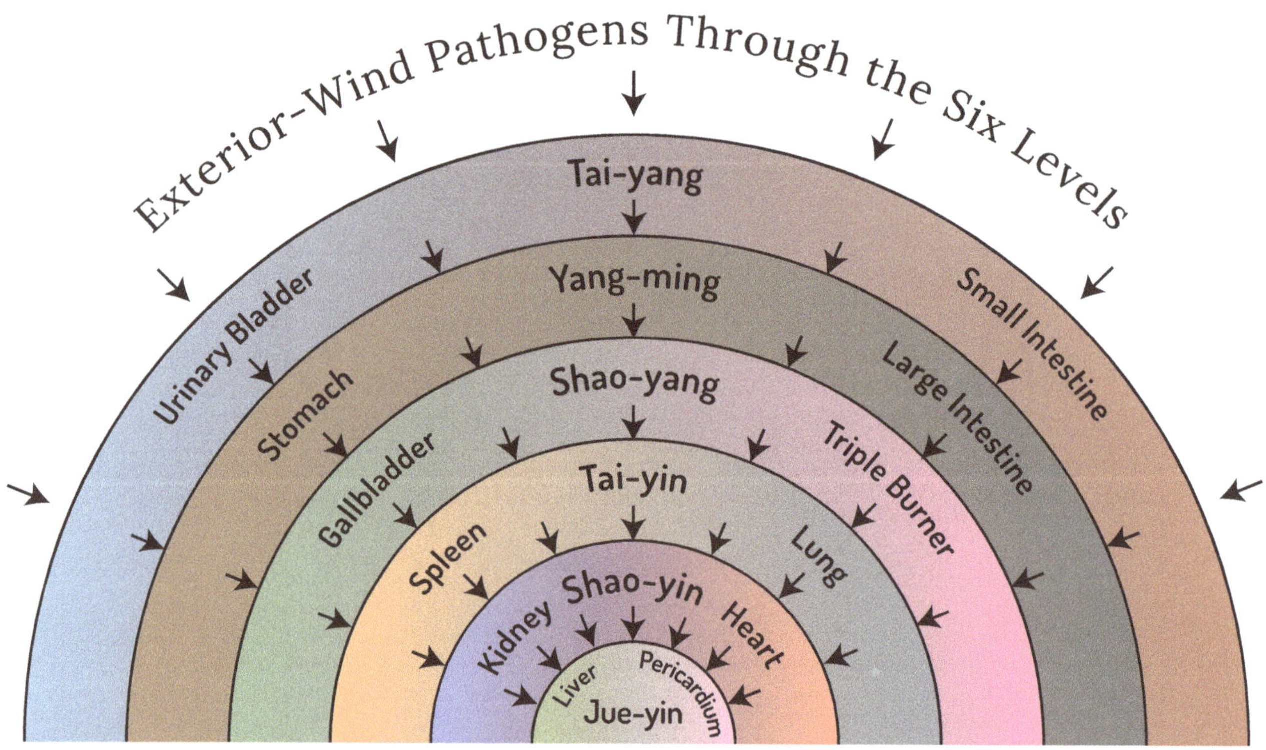

Diagnosing and treating the appropriate level allows the immune system to resolve the pathogen before it spreads or transforms. The Body-Feedback system follows the *Shang Han Lun* six-level theory[12] for treatment of externally contracted diseases. General symptoms for each level, along with the common pathogens and Body-Feedback pulse presentations are provided on the following page.

- Tai-yang experiences wind cold that transforms into wind heat with initial symptoms of stiff neck and back, headache, and a floating pulse (forceful in the left first or left third positions).
- Yang-ming channel (meridian) experiences the four great symptoms of heat–great sweating, great vexation, great thirst, and a large surging pulse (forceful in the right first and second positions).
- Yang-ming bowel (colon organ) experiences heat binding with food accumulation causing symptoms of tidal fever, constipation with abdominal fullness, distention, and pressure, and a forceful, deep, excess pulse (on the entire right side).
- Shao-yang experiences alternating fever and chills, vexation, retching, vomiting, bitter taste in mouth, lack of thirst and appetite, dizziness, and a string-like pulse (wiry and forceful in the middle left or third right positions).
- Tai-yin experiences wind cold or wind heat disturbing the digestive system (creating phlegm and dampness) with symptoms of vomiting, diarrhea, lack of thirst and appetite, and a weak pulse (difficult to detect in the right first and second positions).
- Shao-yin experiences severe cold weakening the heart and kidneys with symptoms of diarrhea with undigested food, cold limbs, insomnia, and dry mouth, and occasionally damages the yin causing yin-deficiency heat patterns (rapid, fine, and floating pulse in the first position on the left and deep in the third position on the left).
- Jue-yin experiences the most severe pathogens (such as parasites) causing heat in the upper-body and cold in the lower-body (a floating, wiry, and forceful pulse in the left middle and right third positions).

3.1.2 Depressive Heat

Depressive heat affects the body's superficial qi level. Like a compost pile, qi stagnation and blood stasis generate depressive heat. People who have fast metabolisms or run warm develop depressive heat easily in warmer climates. This form of heat can occur alone or combine with other pathogens:

- Exterior-wind cold with depressive heat can transform into exterior-wind heat.
- Dampness with depressive heat can turn into damp heat.
- Blood stasis with depressive heat can cause blood heat.
- Yin-deficiency with depressive heat can cause deficiency heat.

Common causes of qi stagnation leading to depressive heat include indigestion, trauma, and emotional constraints. Complex organ/meridian pathology always has a qi stagnation and depressive heat component. Because heat rises and expands, depressive heat will cause the pulse to become forceful and wiry in the positions associated with the affected organs or meridians. Blood stasis leading to depressive heat will cause the pulse to become choppy and forceful.

3.1.3 Blood heat

Blood heat can originate both inside and outside the body. The first trisection organs often generate blood heat from exposure to environmental toxins, food additives, preservatives, or infections. Lingering blood stasis with depressive heat, excessive inflammatory and histamine responses, or genetics can generate blood heat internally.

Blood heat can impact any of the three trisections. In the first trisection, the lungs oxygenate the blood, and the spleen generates and manages the blood. Airborne environmental toxins or pathogens can enter the blood through the lungs or skin. Food or waterborne toxins or pathogens can enter the blood through the spleen and stomach. In the second trisection, lingering blood heat carrying toxins can damage the nervous system (urinary bladder meridian) and delicate second trisection organs (heart, kidneys, and small intestine). In the third trisection, the liver, gallbladder, and triple burner (lymph system) cleanse the environmental toxins and pathogens from the blood. The pericardium protects the heart organ from pathogens in the blood.

The first trisection organs (lung, large intestine, stomach, and spleen) together have the most impact on the immune system and blood cells. White blood cells can generate pathogenic heat as a consequence of high levels of histamine or inflammation. Eosinophils and histamine occur in response to seasonal, environmental, and food allergens. Monocytes and basophils generate inflammation to initiate a healing response for a variety of reasons. The body's ability to moderate histamine and inflammation can become dysfunctional due to genetics or excessive consumption of high histamine and inflammatory foods. These cellular functions create excess blood heat when combined with other heat pathogens.

The third trisection organs (pericardium, triple burner, gallbladder, and liver) together cleanse and filter blood to release toxins, used hormone metabolites, and cellular by-products. Environmental toxins, toxins from pathogens, hormone-mimicking substances such as bisphenol A (BPA) found in plastics, and other endocrine-disrupting chemicals burden this trisection. The high level of toxins currently found in food, water, and clothing is challenging health daily. Heightened chemical sensitivities are increasing with each generation exposed to harmful toxins during the gestation period through umbilical cord blood. A 2016 study found higher levels of polychlorinated biphenyls (PCBs) and organochlorine pesticides (OCPs) in umbilical cord blood than maternal serum indicating fetuses may experience higher exposures of toxins than their mothers.[13]

When the first and third trisections fail to resolve blood heat, the second trisection organs (heart, small intestine, urinary bladder, and kidneys) suffer from the deep penetration of toxic influences affecting the endocrine and nervous systems. The increase in toxins over the decades corresponds with the increase in autoimmune conditions, infertility, autism spectrum disorders, and other severe health conditions affecting younger populations.

Blood heat combines with nutrients and oxygen, traveling through the cardiovascular system and into capillaries to affect the skin and connective tissues. Symptoms of blood heat include skin rashes such as hives, dermatitis, psoriasis, eczema, and darker patches from hormonal imbalances. Fungi, bacteria, viruses, and parasites can generate blood heat that leads to skin irritations.

Long-standing blood heat can cause blood deficiency, blood stasis, and eventually yin deficiency. The muscles and connective tissue rely on nourishment and fluids from blood. Overly taut, inflamed, or hot to the touch muscles, tendons, and ligaments indicate blood heat.

The pulse becomes rapid with blood heat. The more intense the heat, the faster the pulse becomes. In general, a resting pulse rate of 60 to 70 beats per minute (BPM) is healthy, and above 70 BPM indicates the presence of blood heat. Certain medications that treat high blood pressure and tachycardia, including beta blockers and calcium channel blockers, mask the presence of blood heat and cause the pulse to feel very thin with a reasonable rate. When blood stasis accompanies blood heat, the pulse will become choppy, thready, and rapid.

Menstruating women with blood heat will experience heavy bleeding or clotting during their menstrual periods. Signs of pathogenic heat affecting menstrual blood include a heavy bright red or crimson flow, thick or viscous-like menstrual blood, and passing clots. Many women today suffering from endometriosis and polycystic ovarian syndrome are struggling with blood heat caused by environmental toxins and endocrine disruptors.

3.1.4 Damp Heat

Damp heat occurs when dampness combines with the other forms of pathogenic heat, such as exterior-wind, depressive, blood, or yin-deficiency heat. Diets of high fat, sugar, and starch can cause damp heat and make it difficult to treat. Damp heat often reoccurs for people with sensitive digestion or who are overweight.

Damp heat affecting the first trisection organs (lung, large intestine, spleen, and stomach) causes thicker sinus congestion, loss of or excessive appetite, indigestion, diarrhea after eating, constipation, incomplete evacuation of bowels, and foul-smelling gas or stools. Sensations of heat, with or without perspiration on the face, can occur during or immediately after eating.

Damp heat affecting the second trisection organs (heart, small intestine, urinary bladder, and kidneys) causes back pain, urinary difficulty, vaginal discharge, difficulty absorbing nutrients, and brain fog. Damp heat may lead to neuralgia or neuropathy if the body is unable to repair nerves due to compromised fat absorption. The ingestion of unhealthy fats, such as trans fats or genetically modified fats, and an excess of omega-six in ratio to omega-three fats in the diet will cause damp heat. Prostate issues, blocked tubes, chronic yeast or bacterial infections, and certain types of infertility may indicate damp heat in the reproductive organs. Severe conditions such as high cholesterol, stroke, and heart attack reveal damp heat affecting the cardiovascular system.

Damp heat affecting the third trisection organs (pericardium, gallbladder, and liver) causes nausea, jaundice, abdominal bloating, discomfort in the rib cage area, bitter taste in the mouth, lack of appetite, and difficulty digesting high-fat foods. Damp heat affecting the triple burner (lymph system) causes swollen lymph nodes, water retention, fatigue, and short voiding of concentrated urine. Humid weather can exacerbate damp heat in the lymph system and transfer it to the other third trisection organs. Chronic bacterial, viral, mold, and fungal infections generate damp heat in the lymph system.

Damp heat causes intracellular fluid retention, which can confine the pulse and cause it to become less detectable in the individual radial positions. If the dampness is more pronounced than the heat, the pulse will be hard to detect, and more pressure will be needed to assess it. If the heat is more pronounced than the dampness, the pulse will be closer to the surface and overly slippery. The most forceful individual pulse position indicates the organ most affected by damp heat pathogens.

3.1.5 Yin-Deficiency Heat

In the body, lower levels of cooling fluids in proportion to its heat-generating functions create yin-deficiency heat. The excess of yang and insufficiency of yin produces deficiency heat symptoms, including hot flashes, uncontrollable sweating, and burning sensations. Common causes of yin-deficiency heat include chronic illness, autoimmune flare-ups, prolonged exposure to environmental and food toxins, a long-term diet of excessively spicy foods, and the peri-menopause transition time for women. The symptoms of yin-deficiency heat will eventually subside with the restoration of healthy levels of yin or the depletion of yang such that the levels match the reduced yin.

Hot flashes, also known as tidal fever, are surges of heat (with no signs of an elevated temperature) that feel like they originate deep within the body and expand to the surface. In ancient times, this type of heat was called steaming bone syndrome or tidal fever because it comes in waves and is generally worse in the afternoon and evening. Severe yin deficiency will cause episodes of uncontrollable sweating (often referred to as night-sweats, but which can also be present during the day) and sensations of heat in the hands, feet, and head. The time of day with increased symptoms can indicate the organ or multiple organs with yin deficiency. The organs directly affected by yin-deficiency heat include the lungs, stomach, heart, kidneys, and liver.

In the first trisection, excessive heat due to yin deficiency can damage the cooling functions of the lung and stomach. Common reasons for lung yin-deficiency heat include long-standing heat pathogens (viral, bacterial, mold, or fungal), exposure to smoke, air pollution, or uncontrolled asthma. The symptoms of lung yin-deficiency heat include tidal fever between 3 a.m. and 5 a.m., upon waking, or after a hot shower (because the lungs control the pores of the skin). Chronic dry mouth, burning sensations in the mouth or throat, hoarse voice, or dry phlegm that is challenging to cough up are also signs of lung yin-deficiency heat.

Insufficient stomach yin results in excessive heat damaging the throat, esophagus, and stomach. Bacterial infections, such as Helicobacter-pylori (H-pylori), Babesia, Bartonella, Ehrlichia, and Mycoplasma, injure the digestive tract causing inadequate cooling fluids needed to protect it from stomach acid. Yin-deficiency heat negatively impacts the down-bearing function of the stomach causing acid reflux, heartburn, burning sensations in the throat, slow stool transit time, and constipation. Stomach yin-deficiency heat compromises the early stages of digestion and nutrient absorption. Autoimmune conditions, such as Type-1 Diabetes, Celiac, and Crohn's damage the stomach yin and cause deficiency-heat symptoms in the first trisection organs.

In the second trisection, the heart and kidneys are often affected by yin-deficiency heat. The heart can suffer from yin deficiency due to long-standing heart blood deficiency, hyperthyroidism, Hashimoto's autoimmune thyroiditis, severe trauma, or post-traumatic stress syndrome. The symptoms of yin-deficiency heat affecting the heart include insomnia, palpitations, dizziness, anxiety, hot flashes and tidal fever during the day and night, and sensations of heat in the hands and feet.

The natural aging process and several autoimmune diseases deplete the cooling fluids, known as kidney yin, stored in the reservoir of the bones. Tidal fever originates in the bones as a sign of depleted kidney yin and is more pronounced during the evening when the yin is dominant. Acute flare-ups of rheumatoid arthritis, Sjögren's syndrome, lupus, and other autoimmune diseases cause yin-deficiency heat symptoms that damage bone and connective tissue for people of all ages.

In the third trisection, the liver is the only organ directly affected by yin-deficiency heat. Liver yin balances liver yang and is responsible for moistening the connective tissue, muscles, eyes, and reproductive organs. Yin-deficiency heat affecting the liver can cause muscle cramps, dry throat, unproductive cough, dry eyes, and vaginal dryness. Signs of excess liver yang due to deficient yin include headaches, red eyes, irritability, dizziness, insomnia, and excessive menstrual bleeding. Waking with hot flashes or night sweats between 1 a.m. and 3 a.m. indicates the presence of yin-deficiency heat affecting the liver.

Yin-deficiency heat spreads easily from organ to organ along the engendering and restraining cycles. Because of the combined deficiency and excess pathology, as yin becomes depleted, heat generates quickly and further consumes the cooling yin fluids causing more heat. With yin deficiency, the overall pulse will be thin, and a forceful, floating, or unrooted individual pulse position indicates the organ affected by yin-deficiency heat.

3.2 Techniques for Releasing Pathogenic Heat

The Body-Feedback acupoint prescriptions include unique heat-clearing combinations that address all forms of pathogenic heat. The Meramour Meridian Balancing and Organ Supporting essential oil blends provide immediate short-term relief of heat symptoms while enhancing acupuncture treatments. Body-Feedback testing ensures proper diagnosis and choice of herbs and supplements for ongoing support. Releasing pathogenic heat is addressed in every treatment stage throughout this book.

3.2.1 Acupuncture to Release Pathogenic Heat

In general, the jing-well, ying-spring, fire, water, and metal point designations release all forms of pathogenic heat. All of the balancing, sedation, and tonification prescriptions include some of these point designations to address pathogenic heat. The heat-clearing points are bolded in the chart below:

Heat-Clearing Acupoints

YIN MERIDIANS

	Jing-well	**Ying-spring**	Shu-stream	**Jing-river**	**He-sea**
	WOOD	**FIRE**	EARTH	**METAL**	**WATER**
LUNG	**LU11**	**LU10**	LU9	**LU8**	**LU5**
SPLEEN	**SP1**	**SP2**	SP3	**SP5**	**SP9**
HEART	**HT9**	**HT8**	HT7	**HT4**	**HT3**
KIDNEY	**KD1**	**KD2**	KD3	**KD7**	**KD10**
PERICARDIUM	**PC9**	**PC8**	PC7	**PC5**	**PC3**
LIVER	**LV1**	**LV2**	LV3	**LV4**	**LV8**

YANG MERIDIANS

	Jing-well	**Ying-spring**	Shu-stream	**Jing-river**	He-sea
	METAL	**WATER**	WOOD	**FIRE**	EARTH
LARGE INTESTINE	**LI1**	**LI2**	LI3	**LI5**	LI11
STOMACH	**ST45**	**ST44**	ST43	**ST41**	ST36
SMALL INTESTINE	**SI1**	**SI2**	SI3	**SI5**	SI8
URINARY BLADDER	**UB67**	**UB66**	UB65	**UB60**	UB40
TRIPLE BURNER	**TB1**	**TB2**	TB3	**TB6**	TB10
GALLBLADDER	**GB44**	**GB43**	GB41	**GB38**	GB34

The jing-well, ying-spring, and fire point designations effectively drain pathogenic heat. The metal + water point combinations provide nourishment while releasing heat. When yin-deficiency heat is present, the metal + water combination is the best option for nourishing the deficiency while clearing the heat. In the yang meridian Body-Feedback prescriptions, the jing-well and ying-spring acupoints are the metal + water combination. In the yin meridian Body-Feedback prescriptions, the he-sea and jing-river acupoints are the metal + water combination.

The heart requires special attention as the sacred yin organ that holds a person's spirit (shen). The heart often tests better for the metal + water combination as a substitution for the horary fire acupoint (HT8) in the Body-Feedback prescriptions. The HT4 metal + HT3 water combination tests well for the elderly, long-term pathogenic heat, or chronic stress affecting the heart. The fire acupoint (HT8) is more likely to test well with younger clients, high cortisol stress hormones, or acute pathogenic heat affecting the heart. Always check and compare the response to the pulse, master alarm points, or Body-Feedback testing locations of the HT4 metal + HT3 water combination to the fire acupoint (HT8) for possible substitution.

Clients who frequently require the same metal + water combinations to release pathogenic heat can use magnetic pellets on the acupoints between appointments. How long the magnetic pellets stay on depends on the location, exposure to water, and dryness of the skin. On the hands, apply the magnetic pellets to the metal and water acupoints at bedtime and remove them in the morning. On the feet, apply the magnetic pellets to the metal and water acupoints, and leave them on for up to five days if they stay on. At the end of a treatment, add magnetic pellets to the metal and water acupoints and take a picture with the client's phone so that they can reference it later to reapply at home.

Chart of Heat-Clearing Metal + Water Combinations

Meridian	Fire Shu-Point	Metal Shu-Point	Water Shu-Point
LUNG	LU10 FIRE	LU8 METAL	LU5 WATER
LARGE INTESTINE	LI5 FIRE	LI1 METAL	LI2 WATER
STOMACH	ST41 FIRE	ST45 METAL	ST44 WATER
SPLEEN	SP2 FIRE	SP5 METAL	SP9 WATER
HEART	HT8 FIRE	HT4 METAL	HT3 WATER
SMALL INTESTINE	SI5 FIRE	SI1 METAL	SI2 WATER
URINARY BLADDER	UB60 FIRE	UB67 METAL	UB66 WATER
KIDNEY	KD2 FIRE	KD7 METAL	KD10 WATER
PERICARDIUM	PC8 FIRE	PC5 METAL	PC3 WATER
TRIPLE BURNER	TB6 FIRE	TB1 METAL	TB2 WATER
GALLBLADDER	GB38 FIRE	GB44 METAL	GB43 WATER
LIVER	LV2 FIRE	LV4 METAL	LV8 WATER

In practice, substituting or adding the metal + water combination frequently occurs because long-standing pathogenic heat or deficiency affects most clients. The practical application sections throughout this book provide the step-by-step details for using this special metal + water acupoint combination.

3.2.2 Acupoint Designations that Increase Pathogenic Heat

When pathogenic heat is present, needling any acupoint that is not a jing-well, ying-spring, fire, water, or metal point has the potential to generate additional heat. When an acupoint tests well at first but then creates extra heat that becomes pathogenic, the Body-Feedback testing locations will become tight and painful during a treatment. The most precise way to test for low-level heat before inserting a needle is to apply pressure to the non-heat clearing acupoint for 10-30 seconds while checking the pulse for an increasingly wiry or forceful response. The radial pulse will shift from slippery or slightly slippery to wiry or wiry and forceful if an acupoint will cause excessive heat.

Another way to check non-heat clearing acupoints is testing them to GB21 (the master fire alarm point) or the individual Body-Feedback testing locations identified in the pre-treatment planning stage (see Chapter 12). It is vital to give the body adequate time to respond by holding the point for 10-30 seconds before rechecking. The pulse reacts faster than the muscles when testing for pathogenic heat. In practice, when a client has difficulty relaxing or feels an increase in pain or muscle tightness, it is because a non-heat clearing acupoint increased pathogenic heat during treatment. These clients usually respond best to needling only heat-clearing points.

There are three shu-transporting acupoints (ST36, SP3, and GB41) in the Body-Feedback balancing, sedation, and tonification prescriptions that require special attention because they will increase existing pathogenic heat. These are horary acupoints (an earth point on an earth meridian and a wood point on a wood meridian), which strongly tonify their associated element, meridian, and organ. ST36 (he-sea), along with SP3 and GB41 (shu-stream) are acupoints without any heat-clearing properties. Stimulating these acupoints with existing heat will cause the corresponding Body-Feedback testing locations to tighten up or experience discomfort, indicating a negative response.

The horary acupoints ST36, SP3, and GB41 often require substitutions when they are part of the Body-Feedback prescriptions. The five-element relationship between wood, earth, and fire naturally increases heat. In the engendering cycle, the wood element precedes and fuels the fire element. The earth element follows the fire element, allowing heat to build if not properly dispersed and regulated. In the restraining cycle, the interaction among the water, metal, and fire elements releases pathogenic heat. The metal element strengthens the water element to control heat.

Wood and Earth Horary Points that Increase Pathogenic Heat

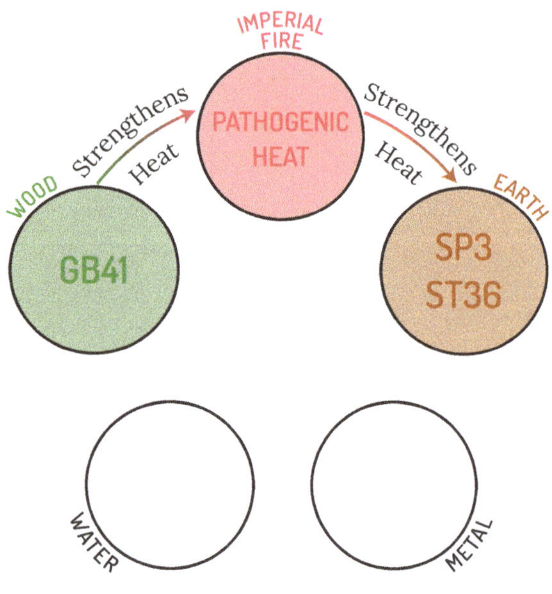

In the engendering cycle, the wood and earth horary shu-points strengthen pathogenic heat.

Metal and Water Shu-Points that Decrease Pathogenic Heat

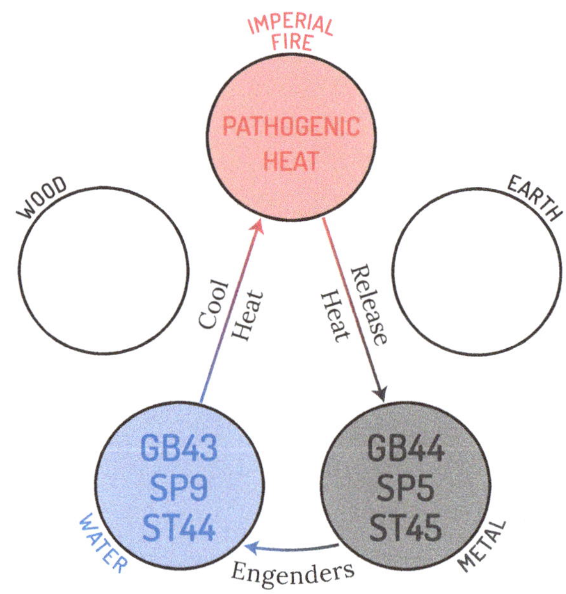

In the restraining cycle, the metal and water shu-points for the wood and earth elements release and cool pathogenic heat.

In detail, when the fire element (mother) is excess, the earth element (child) requires draining. Both ST36 (he-sea and earth point on earth meridian) and SP3 (shu-stream and earth point on earth meridian) will tonify earth and generate additional heat. To dissipate heat on the earth yang meridian, substitute the ST45 metal + ST44 water combination. To dissipate heat on the earth yin meridian, substitute the SP5 metal + SP9 water combination.

In addition, when the fire element (mother) is excess, the wood element requires heat clearing acupoints in order to cool the fire element. GB41 (shu-stream and wood point on wood meridian) will increase heat by tonifying the wood element (mother) to strengthen the fire element (child). To dissipate heat on the yang wood meridian, substitute the GB44 metal + GB43 water combination. LV1 (wood point on wood meridian) is a jing-well acupoint that naturally releases heat and therefore does not require substitution.

Conditions such as musculoskeletal diseases, acute traumas, and repetitive-use injuries can generate excessive amounts of pathogenic heat, causing inflammation, swelling, and redness that is warm or hot to the touch. Ashi acupoints, trigger points commonly used to treat musculoskeletal conditions, are painful upon palpation and differ from named and numbered traditional acupoints. Needling local ashi acupoints in regions with excessive pathogenic heat can further compromise healing and exacerbate the heat pathogens. Test local ashi acupoints to GB21 (master fire and inflammation point), TB15 (brain point), or the pulse to determine if needling them will be beneficial or should be avoided. If the local acupoints increase tightness in the master points or cause the pulse to become wiry or wiry and forceful, check the metal + water combinations for the meridians that travel in the region of the local ashi acupoints. With low-level pathogenic heat, such as depressive heat, needling the metal + water combination first can clear the heat for local ashi acupoints to test beneficial. With excessive blood heat, damp heat, or yin-deficiency heat, local ashi needling may need to wait until a future session when the heat pathogens have resolved.

During an acupuncture session, irritability or increased muscle tightness and discomfort in a Body-Feedback testing location can occur when energy builds in a meridian that is affected by pathogenic heat. Increased tightness in master points GB21 or TB15 will become apparent, along with a wiry and forceful pulse presentation, when pathogenic heat expands. When GB21 and TB15 become tighter, or the pulse becomes wiry and forceful, check any meridian with non-heat clearing acupoints by pressing the metal and water acupoints. For example, when pathogenic heat builds during treatment and SP3 is in the acupoint prescription, press on SP5 metal and SP9 water acupoints while checking GB21, TB15, or the pulse looking for improvement. If this does not help, check the metal + water combinations on the other meridians relating to the client's symptoms.

The client may have a difficult time relaxing during the session when pathogenic heat is not released. If this happens, check to see if the pulse became wiry and forceful during the treatment indicating an increase in heat. Check the metal + water combination on the spleen, stomach, and gallbladder meridians after removing the needles. If there are still signs of pathogenic heat in the pulse or Body-Feedback testing locations, check the metal + water combinations on the other meridians. Send the client home with magnet pellets on the metal and water acupoints and confirm improvement in the Body-Feedback testing locations and pulse before they leave. Explain to the client that a slight adjustment is needed due to heat building during treatment, and they can leave the magnetic pellets on overnight and should feel better in the morning.

3.2.3 Essential Oils to Release Pathogenic Heat

Essential oils contain fats, enzymes, and oxygen, which penetrate the body quickly and remove qi stagnation and blood stasis due to their active nature. Essential oils are cooling, neutral, or warming and have an affinity to target specific tissues of the body, such as muscles, bones, ligaments, blood vessels, and so on. Meramour's Meridian Balancing and Organ Supporting Blends (see Chapter 11) include carefully chosen essential oils to address heat pathogens that commonly affect a particular meridian or organ.

3.2.4 Herbs and Supplements to Release Pathogenic Heat

The five forms of pathogenic heat require an accurate differential diagnosis to select the appropriate herbs and supplements for self-care. Body-Feedback testing for herbs and supplements (see Chapter 18) before and after an acupuncture session will often provide different results. Testing after the application of oils and acupuncture will indicate the constitutional support acceptable for long-term use. Testing before an acupuncture session or application of essential oils will suggest short-term solutions for acute stages of pathogenic heat. When treating pathogenic heat, retest the recommended herbs and supplements weekly at first, and then retest before refilling or when there is a change in symptoms.

In some cases, herbs and supplements may need a month to take effect. Depending on the severity of the symptoms caused by pathogenic heat, weekly acupuncture for up to eight weeks may be required to relieve symptoms and promote self-healing. With complex cases or recurring pathogenic heat, determining the underlying causes may require further investigation.

3.2.5 Releasing Exterior-Wind Heat

The Body-Feedback acupoint prescriptions and essential oils can treat the first five levels of exterior-wind heat patterns (tai-yang, yang-ming channel, yang-ming bowel, shao-yang, and tai-yin). Chapter 17 instructs how to apply magnetic pellets, press tacks, or seeds after an acupuncture session to strengthen the heat-clearing treatment benefits. Children and the elderly with a weaker constitution should be closely monitored for dehydration and referred to the emergency room if needed. Refer the final two exterior-wind heat patterns (shao-yin and jue-yin) to urgent care physicians because they can become life-threatening.

In practice, most clients seek acupuncture and holistic treatments after the initial exterior-wind heat resolves and other lingering heat pathogens remain. In this scenario, the heat pathogen has transitioned to another form or multiple forms and has spread to other organs or systems of the body. Many autoimmune conditions start after the body is unable to resolve exterior-wind heat pathogens that transform to blood heat or damp heat in the deeper layers of the body.

3.2.6 Resolving Depressive Heat

Depressive heat is a common reason to substitute the metal + water combination in the balancing, sedating, and tonifying prescriptions. Additional metal + water supporting acupoints can resolve depressive heat in other meridians. After needling the Body-Feedback root prescriptions, check for any remaining wiry and forceful qualities in the individual pulse positions, pain at GB21, or tight muscles. Test additional metal + water combinations and needle the ones that normalize the pulse, release pain at GB21, or relax the tight muscles.

Depressive heat by itself is superficial and resolves more easily than other forms of pathogenic heat. Daily incorporation of cooling foods and beverages such as salads, smoothies, green vegetables, green tea, and healthy oils (fish, coconut, olive, and avocado) can help reduce depressive heat. Mindful practices such as yoga, meditation, creative visualization, affirmations, and journaling can help reduce emotional triggers and stress that frequently lead to depressive heat.

Depressive heat can move around the body or resolve itself, depending on lifestyle and constitutional health. The superficial nature of depressive heat affects individual meridians and often accompanies a person's genetic weaknesses. Depressive heat by itself will not cause organ dysfunction unless another form of pathogenic heat accompanies it. Many clients over consume sugar or carbohydrates, which causes depressive heat and dampness to combine into damp heat. The SP5 metal + SP9 water substitution for SP3 in the Body-Feedback prescriptions releases all forms of pathogenic heat affecting the spleen.

3.2.7 Cooling Blood Heat

When pathogenic heat settles in the blood level, additional supplementation, including cooling herbs and detoxification binders, is often necessary for a full recovery. Pathogenic blood-heat caused by bacterial, fungal, and other microbes responds best to a combination of acupuncture with a rotation of anti-pathogenic and anti-microbial supplements and herbs. In some cases, pathogens can manipulate the immune system to not recognize them, allowing microbes to multiply quickly. With some chronic infections, the immune system will discontinue fighting after years of unsuccessful eradication. Acupuncture helps restore a normal immune system response for complicated and chronic infections. Body-Feedback techniques help choose the best-tolerated supplements and herbs and identify when rotation is needed.

Environmental toxins and heavy metals can cause blood heat and burden the liver and kidneys. Supplements such as chlorella, activated charcoal, diatomaceous earth, fiber, and topical magnesium can bind with toxins to help safely remove them from the body. These binding supplements are best taken with a meal and away from other supplements and herbs. Chinese herbal formulas that resolve heat and support digestion are best taken on an empty stomach between meals for increased blood level concentration.

Functional medical tests can help identify the sources of chronic blood heat and monitor progress. Helpful tests include stool tests that use DNA pathogen identification, organic acid urine tests that look for byproducts of infections and toxin exposures, and heavy metal testing with hair and urine analysis. An acute episode of blood heat can resolve within two months, while chronic blood heat can take four to six months. Clients who repeatedly generate blood heat may require long-term cooling and blood cleansing supplements.

3.2.8 Transforming Damp Heat

Food choices and the health of the digestive system influence a body's tendency to generate damp heat internally. Acupuncture, essential oils, digestive enzymes, probiotics, and a diet of easy to digest high-quality fats and fiber, along with low-carbohydrate and low-sugar foods can all help resolve damp heat pathogens.

Humid climates cause the body to retain fluids that can generate damp heat if depressive or yin-deficiency heat are present. Traveling between hot and dry regions and humid ones can exacerbate pre-existing damp heat symptoms. Adjusting food choices to accommodate weather patterns can assist the body in adapting to the current environment.

Damp heat can affect the lungs, large intestine, and spleen organs in the first trisection, the small intestine, urinary bladder, and kidneys in the second trisection, and the triple burner, gallbladder, and liver in the third trisection. The heart, pericardium, and stomach organs are too dry to suffer from damp heat.

Damp heat becomes challenging to treat with herbs when it combines with yin-deficiency heat. Damp heat responds to drying herbs, and yin-deficiency heat requires moistening herbs. Menopausal women who are overweight may struggle with this combination of pathogenic heat that creates hot flashes and sweating after meals and during the night. These clients respond best to digestive support and damp-heat-clearing herbs during the day with yin-nourishing herbs at night before bed. Resolving this combined form of pathogenic heat may require a change in diet and weight reduction.

3.2.9 Nourishing Yin to Cool Deficiency Heat

Treatments for yin-deficiency heat require the proper balance of heat-clearing to alleviate symptoms and yin-nourishing to restore the body's natural cooling mechanism. Deficiency heat can be cooled quickly with acupuncture, essential oils, and herbs. Nourishing the yin also requires a supportive diet and lifestyle, time to relax in the evenings, and adequate sleep. Other forms of pathogenic heat can coincide with yin-deficiency heat and complicate the diagnosis. After a Body-Feedback acupuncture treatment, testing different herbal formulas can confirm the root of the pathogenic heat and affected organs when multiple forms of heat combine with yin-deficiency.

Long-term or severe blood deficiency causes yin deficiency. Therefore, carefully evaluate clients with yin-deficiency for accompanying signs of blood heat. The presence of blood heat can cause an increase in heat symptoms when using yin-nourishing herbs or acupuncture treatments. With complex cases, resolve blood heat before incorporating yin-nourishing therapies.

For menopausal women, multimineral supplements can cool blood to reduce hot flashes. Mineral deficiencies combined with low hormone levels cause yin-deficiency symptoms during the day and night for menopausal women. Using reverse osmosis to purify water removes all minerals, and occasionally low-grade calcium and magnesium are added back in. Always confirm the water source for menopausal women with yin-deficiency symptoms and recommend drinking high-quality spring water to nourish their blood and yin. Oral and topical pregnenolone and DHEA supplements provide the raw materials to produce estrogen, progesterone, and testosterone. Combining essential oils with these hormonal supplements can activate and cleanse hormone receptor sites to encourage one hormone's production over another.

3.3 True-Heat with False-Cold Pathogens

Testing acupoints can help identify the difficult-to-diagnose "true-heat with false-cold" pattern associated with long-standing pathogenic heat. For example, when pathogenic heat first affects the nerves, it causes inflammation; sensations of heat can be felt on the skin and nerve pathways. If the nerve inflammation persists, it can eventually damage the nerve and transform to false-cold, causing the skin to feel cold and numb. If left unresolved, the pathogenic heat (true-heat) will continue to damage the body, resulting in more false-cold symptoms. In this case, the metal + water combination releases tension and discomfort in the testing locations, while the horary shu-points SP3, ST36, and GB41 increase it.

True-heat with false-cold pathogens can occur with neurological diseases, peripheral neuropathy, reduced circulation to the capillaries (including diabetic neuropathy), intracellular infections, and chronic inflammation. Environmental toxins and chronic infections can cause autoimmune activity that permanently damages the body and results in true-heat with false-cold symptoms. In some cases, laboratory testing may identify contributing factors influencing these severe health challenges. A comprehensive approach of acupuncture, herbs, and supplements can encourage a healthy inflammatory cycle, optimize hormones, and promote regeneration. Resolving true-heat can slow the disease progression for some clients, and others may have substantial recovery of the false-cold symptoms.

3.4 Phlegm Nodules

The body stores environmental toxins, chronic low-grade infections, genetically modified foods, and fats that it cannot digest in phlegm nodules, which are sometimes called lipomas or fatty tumors. Artificial trans fats have been in use for decades and were banned by the FDA in 2018, but these harmful substances can still be distributed in some prepared foods through 2021.[14] Phlegm nodules are the body's way of removing toxins and pathogens from circulation by encapsulating them for storage when it cannot excrete them through sweat, urine, or stool.

When these benign phlegm nodules mix with pathogenic heat, the immune system dispatches cells to destroy the stored toxins and pathogens. The destructive immune cells can damage the healthy tissue surrounding a nodule and cause deterioration. Pain around the border of the nodule indicates there is immune system involvement with pathogenic heat. The Body-Feedback approach recommends using vigorous holistic treatments, including diluted topical essential oils (see Chapter 11), Chinese herbs (see Chapter 18), and surrounding the borders of the nodule(s) with needles (see Chapter 13), to resolve the phlegm nodules and pathogenic heat.

The body often stores phlegm nodules in different regions, for example:

- in the lower back on the spine and posterior iliac spine crest
- along muscles and connective tissue
- in the organ/meridian referral areas and muscle associations (see Chapter 6)
- inside lymph nodes
- at the site of previous injuries

Before attempting to dissolve phlegm nodules, work with the client to improve detoxification pathways and identify changes in the sourcing or quality of food and water. Multimineral supplements are beneficial for detoxifying heavy metals, and topical magnesium is useful for dissolving the phlegm coating. Reverse osmosis water depletes minerals in the body and over time will compromise detoxification. Quality spring water is naturally high in minerals that enhance detoxification pathways. Infrared saunas and infrared mattress pads safely accelerate detoxification and are beneficial for dissolving phlegm nodules. Essential oils contain enzymes and oxygen that, when applied topically, can consume the phlegm coating and neutralize the toxins.

The body will store phlegm nodules in the lower back because of the proximity to the colon. The nodules collect along the posterior superior border of the iliac spine crest (PSIS) and on the side of the lower lumbar vertebrae. This region is more likely to collect nodules when there has been a history of lower back pain with compromised detoxification.

Phlegm nodules along muscles and connective tissue respond well to a combination of *gua sha* (a Chinese medical massage) and essential oils. Because of the reduced blood flow to connective tissue, phlegm nodules in these locations can take longer to resolve.

Chronically swollen lymph nodes store pathogens or environmental toxins that the body cannot neutralize and release. Anything applied topically on the skin is absorbed into the lymph system. Adding a few drops of essential oils to an organic lotion and using as a moisturizer is an effective way to direct the essential oils into the lymph system. Lymph massage, along with infrared sauna therapy, can accelerate the detoxification process within the lymph system.

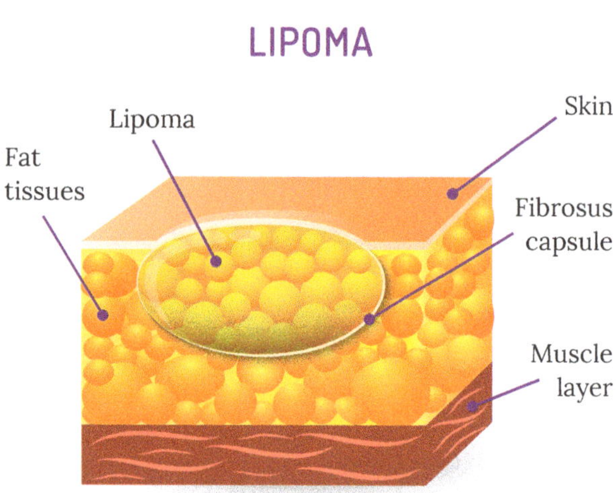

A lipoma is one example of a phlegm nodule.

ID 47829840 © Designua | Dreamstime.com

Phlegm nodule on a tendon at the site of a previous injury

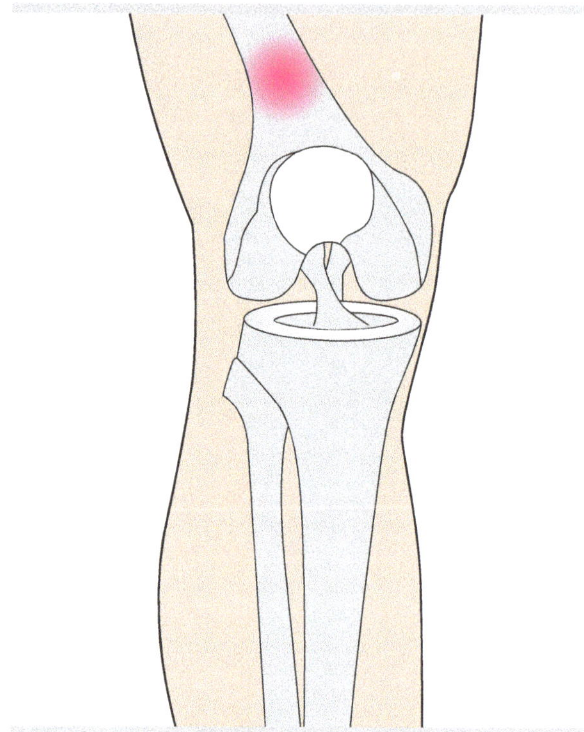

ID 56900888 © Pawel Graczyk | Dreamstime.com

Previous injuries leave the body with a weakened area and an immune system memory for that region. Pathogens are attracted to areas with reduced blood flow and scar tissue because the immune system has difficulty identifying and eradicating them. The immune system will encapsulate pathogens and environmental toxins in areas of reduced blood supply. Look for phlegm nodules when palpating previously injured areas and surround the outer border with needles to increase blood flow and initiate a new immune system response.

In general, phlegm nodules require patience and multiple treatment approaches. Palpate a nodule to feel if it is movable and if the surrounding tissue lacks muscle tone and integrity. For individual phlegm nodules, surround the outer edge with five or more needles depending on the size to improve the integrity of the surrounding tissue while reducing the size of the nodule. Swollen lymph nodes and phlegm nodules stored around the body or on tendons respond well to herbs that resolve phlegm. For clients with multiple phlegm nodules, apply diluted essential oils that test favorably over the nodules between appointments (see Chapter 11) and recommend extended herbal support to reduce the size of existing nodules and prevent new ones from forming.

Body-Feedback testing and acupoint prescriptions naturally prioritize complex symptoms caused by pathogenic heat. The Body-Feedback approach offers several treatment options aimed at providing immediate and long-term relief of symptoms. If treatments are only managing symptoms, investigate other reasons such as low-grade infections, food allergies, heavy metals, or dysbiosis that may be causing the chronic pathogenic heat. Changing the client's diet, water sources, and personal hygiene products may be needed to promote recovery.

CHAPTER 4

Body-Feedback Testing Techniques

For thousands of years, acupuncturists have been using palpation techniques to both assess and treat TCM pathology. Today, some of these practices are known as Chinese medical massage (*Tui Na* and *Gua Sha*), acupressure, Japanese Hara-diagnosis, and channel palpation. In ancient times, channel palpation played a significant role in diagnosing pathology and is discussed in both *The Inner Classic* (*The Nei Jing*) and *The Classic of Difficulties* (*The Nan Jing*). "Diagnostic palpation is particularly useful in the areas below the elbows and knees, where channel qi develops from the roots at the jing-well points on the fingers and toes, to its inward branching at the he-sea points."[15]

The integration of the acupuncture meridian system with Applied Kinesiology (AK) muscle testing is credited to both Dr. George Goodheart, a Chiropractor, and the German organization, Touch for Health. Both groups found that testing for muscle weakness and tension could be used to diagnose compromised organs and glands. Beneficial treatments reduced muscle weakness and tightness and therefore improved health. Both Dr. Goodheart and Touch for Health found that in practice the muscle-organ-gland and meridian-organ-gland correspondences agreed and produced similar results. The integration of eastern and allopathic holistic medicine began to flourish under these two healing modalities.

Many of the Body-Feedback testing locations overlap with regions defined by Dr. Goodheart and Touch for Health. However, Body-Feedback testing techniques differ significantly. Body-Feedback testing merges TCM palpation techniques, pulse analysis, and AK to communicate directly with the cells of the body. The Body-Feedback testing locations are comprised of specific acupuncture points, muscle groups, and areas surrounding the organs. The unique style of Body-Feedback testing is used to check acupoints, essential oils, herbs, supplements, foods, and personal care products.

Body-Feedback testing techniques use involuntary changes in muscle tension and pain to evaluate the potential effectiveness of treatment options. During the pre-treatment planning stage, testing acupoint prescriptions determines the root organ dysfunction and beneficial essential oils. In the treatment stage, testing confirms the exact location of the acupoints in the balancing, sedation, and tonification prescriptions, along with supporting acupoints. Immediately after acupuncture, checking herbs and supplements reveals the most effective options between appointments.

4.1 Origins of Body-Feedback Testing Techniques

In school, I gravitated towards Japanese styles of acupuncture that relied on abdominal and channel palpation techniques to choose acupoints. The non-verbal dialog with a client's body provided insights in choosing acupoints that resulted in immediate improvements for each client. Since beginning my practice, I have always relied on each client's body to guide the treatment process.

I am always looking for ways to improve my practice, and I began contemplating a method that would muscle test essential oils, herbs, and supplements directly to the meridian system using the Body-Feedback testing locations. My existing process of diagnosing root organ/meridian dysfunction and choosing acupoints needed to expand in order to incorporate testing of essential oils, herbs, and supplements.

Over the course of a few weeks, while I was contemplating how to broaden my testing techniques, several of my existing clients asked me the same question: "What makes an acupuncture point special?" I found this surprising because these clients had been seeing me for many years. After being asked a couple of times, I began responding with: "An acupuncture point is an area of low electrical resistance on the body; it's a place where the body can take in energy, or qi, to support physical, spiritual, or emotional health."

I also explained other important aspects about acupuncture, including:

- Acupuncture has been proven to create a healing response by regulating the nervous and endocrine systems, encouraging tissue regeneration, promoting healthy organ function, and enhancing brain function.
- Seven meridians travel vertically along the upper abdomen with closely grouped acupuncture points. The highest concentration of acupuncture points occurs on the upper abdomen creating the largest area of low electrical resistance on the body.
- All of the meridians either pass through or internally connect in the upper abdomen allowing for communication between the meridians, organs, and Body-Feedback testing locations.

I recognized that the responses I gave provided me with the direction I had been contemplating for expanding my testing techniques. After years of using palpation methods to check acupoints, I figured out how the unique hub-like qualities of the upper abdomen could communicate directly with the meridian system and Body-Feedback testing locations.

Quantum physics describes frequency as the measurement of energy (qi). Everything in this world vibrates to a specific frequency, including food, herbs, supplements, essential oils, and medications. We see frequency as color, we hear frequency as sound, and we feel frequency as emotions. Each meridian, muscle, gland, organ, and cellular function vibrates to a specific frequency. I pondered what would happen if I placed an essential oil blend, supplement, or herb on the upper abdomen in this area of low electrical resistance and how it would affect the meridian system. I knew I could monitor any changes this made to the meridian system by using my palpation and pulse assessment techniques.

The next client who asked me, "What makes an acupuncture point special?" received the full explanation above along with, "May I try muscle testing essential oils to your meridian system by placing the capped bottles on your upper abdomen?"

I discovered that particular essential oil blends released tension and pain in specific Body-Feedback locations while others increased the discomfort. Both my client and I felt the same release or increase of muscle tightness in the Body-Feedback testing locations when checking different blends. Then I compared the same essential oil blends one at a time while monitoring the pulse. The beneficial oils caused the pulse to be slightly slippery and balanced in all positions, and the disagreeable oils caused the pulse to be wiry and forceful, confirming the previous results in the Body-Feedback testing locations.

Before discovering this new way of checking essential oils, I would have clients smell the essential oils and then check the Body-Feedback testing locations for changes to determine which oils to use. I found that resting the capped bottles on the upper abdomen efficiently allowed for comparison of various oils or blends and didn't leave any lingering aroma in the sinuses. I immediately started testing essential oils on all my clients in this way.

Next, I decided to check supplements by placing the full bottles on the upper abdomen while evaluating changes in the Body-Feedback testing locations. I found that clients would respond differently to various forms, or quality, of raw materials used by manufacturers. For example, one client might test well for methylated B vitamins, and another might respond favorably for non-methylated, even when testing supplements made by the same manufacturer. I also found that about half of my clients needed a multi-mineral complex containing iodine and the other half a multi-mineral complex without iodine. This approach to choosing supplements using Body-Feedback testing created opportunities to fine-tune each client's supplement routine, and they noticed significant improvements in their health after changing to the recommended supplements.

Further testing in this manner brought to my attention that checking herbs and supplements at the end of a client's acupuncture session identifies those for long term use and constitutional support. Checking herbs, supplements, and essential oils before acupuncture indicates what the body needs most at that moment to address current symptoms. The time of day can also have an impact on testing. For example, testing supplements or herbs to support sleep in the late afternoon to evening is more effective than in the morning when a body's functions are gearing up for the day and cortisol is higher.

4.2 Body-Feedback Testing throughout the Treatment Stages

All stages of the Body-Feedback treatment approach include testing to communicate with the client's body at a cellular level via the meridian system. The practical application sections within the chapters listed below, along with the chapters that summarize the pre-treatment, treatment, and post-treatment stages, provide step-by-step details for the Body-Feedback testing techniques.

In the pre-treatment planning stage, Body-Feedback testing will be used to:

- Check for asymmetry (see Chapter 7).
- Determine the optimal treatment position (see Chapter 8).
- Identify the root dysfunction by checking the Body-Feedback prescriptions (see Chapters 9 and 10).
- Test essential oil blends (see Chapter 11).

In the treatment stage, Body-Feedback testing will be used to:

- Confirm the exact location of the acupoints (see Chapters 13 and 14).
- Choose supporting acupoints (see Chapter 15).

In the post-treatment stage, Body-Feedback testing will be used to:

- Test herbs and supplements (see Chapter 18).
- Check foods and personal care products (see Chapter 19).
- Monitor the progression of healing (see Chapter 21).

Body-Feedback testing is a skill that takes practice to master. With time, you will be able to discern the changes in muscle tone and tightness quickly. While learning this technique, I recommend spending extra time with a few regular clients that you can practice with and follow their progression of healing. Then start new clients with these techniques. I have found it easy to implement these techniques with new clients because they have fewer expectations and are usually open to trying something different. Finally, convert over clients who are open to trying a new system.

4.3 Communicating Body-Feedback Testing with Clients

Before beginning the palpation process, explain to the client how muscle testing the acupuncture meridian system works. This is the general information I provide to each client:

What makes an acupuncture point unique is that it is an area of low electrical resistance on the body where energy, or qi, can be added or adjusted to support health. Many studies have proven that acupuncture creates a healing response by regulating the immune, nervous, and endocrine systems, encouraging tissue regeneration, promoting healthy organ function, and enhancing brain function.

[Then I point to my upper abdomen and explain] *Seven meridians travel vertically along the upper abdomen, and their acupuncture points are closely grouped. The highest concentration of acupuncture points occurs here, and all of the meridians pass through this region creating a communication hub for the system. The upper abdomen contains the largest area of low electrical resistance on the body, and by placing essential oils, supplements, herbs, and foods in this area, the meridian system will respond after* 10-30 *seconds.*

If the items tested are beneficial, the muscle tension and areas of discomfort we identified earlier will release and feel more comfortable. When they are not helpful, the muscles will become tighter and more painful. Your body knows what will help it to self-heal, and through this testing process, together we can determine which essential oils, supplements, herbs, and foods will be the most beneficial for you.

Special acupuncture points called master points, located in the neck, shoulders, and upper back, monitor inflammation, hormones, and brain activity. These master points can help in determining which other acupoints to treat for the most beneficial approach. Other diagnostic points are found around the body and will be used throughout the session to help identify the root of your health challenges.

Do you have any questions before we get started? Do you feel comfortable, and are you able to relax in this position?

After confirming the client is in a relaxed and comfortable position, explain to them that you are going to check specific acupuncture points looking for pain or tenderness and muscle groups looking for tension.

I am going to press on specific areas of your body. Let me know if you experience any pain or discomfort during this process, and if the right and left sides of the body feel the same. Once I determine what needs attention, I will explain the meridians and organs that correspond with the areas of pain and tenderness. Just let me know if you find anything painful or uncomfortable.

Clients feel empowered along their healing journey when they are encouraged to participate in the Body-Feedback testing process. They will know that their treatments are useful, and that self-healing is occurring. The testing will identify the individual supplements and herbs that can provide a significant benefit and ensure that the client is spending their health care dollars wisely.

CHAPTER 5

Body-Feedback Pulse Assessment

The pulse provides direct access to monitor subtle changes within a client's meridian system while testing different acupoints, essential oils, herbs, and supplements. Each treatment option has the potential to enhance, diminish, or maintain the pulse quality. Body-Feedback pulse-testing monitors changes in the radial pulse while checking acupoints, essential oils, herbs, and supplements before use. Identifying how different treatment options affect individual pulse positions provides for a better understanding of how they will impact each element. Choosing treatment options that harmonize the five-element system and restore balance to the pulse maximizes healing potential.

Body-Feedback pulse assessment designates a pulse position for each of the six organ/meridian elemental pairs (wood, imperial-fire, ministerial-fire, earth, metal, and water). The first position is closest to the wrist crease and the third position is the most proximal to the wrist crease.

The length of each position is relative to the size of the client. The first position matches the width of the client's fingertip of the second metatarsal (index finger). The second position matches the width of the client's fingertip of the third metatarsal (middle finger). The third position matches the width of the client's fingertip of the fourth metatarsal (ring finger). Adjustments to accommodate clients with significantly smaller or larger hand and wrist sizes are needed to properly assess the individual positions. For smaller clients, shift the placement of your fingertips to assess each position individually, which accounts for the smaller surface size. For larger clients, slightly spread your fingertips to account for the larger surface length of each position.

When an organ/meridian is excess or deficient, its elemental pair instantly becomes the opposite, and the radial pulse will indicate the imbalance. The imbalanced pulse position can reflect the root dysfunction, the resulting excess or deficiency, or correspond with a region of the body affected by pathological heat, such as inflammation. Carefully choosing acupoints and essential oils with Body-Feedback testing techniques restores balance to all of the pulse positions, indicating accelerated self-healing.

Many styles of TCM include extensive pulse diagnosis. Practitioners who are well-versed in pulse diagnosis can expand their skills by incorporating the Body-Feedback pulse assessment and testing techniques into their practice. For practitioners new to pulse diagnosis, practicing the Body-Feedback testing techniques will build confidence and refine this valuable skill.

5.1 Radial Pulse and the Five Elements

Superimposing the five-element engendering cycle on the radial pulse positions creates the infinity symbol (a sideways figure eight). The engendering cycle repeats itself indefinitely in both nature and within the body to sustain life, foster growth, and promote healing. This infinity symbol signifies the vital role that the five elements have in the continuous cycle of life. By balancing all of the pulse positions, each element nourishes or generates the next.

The Engendering Cycle Superimposed on the Pulse Positions

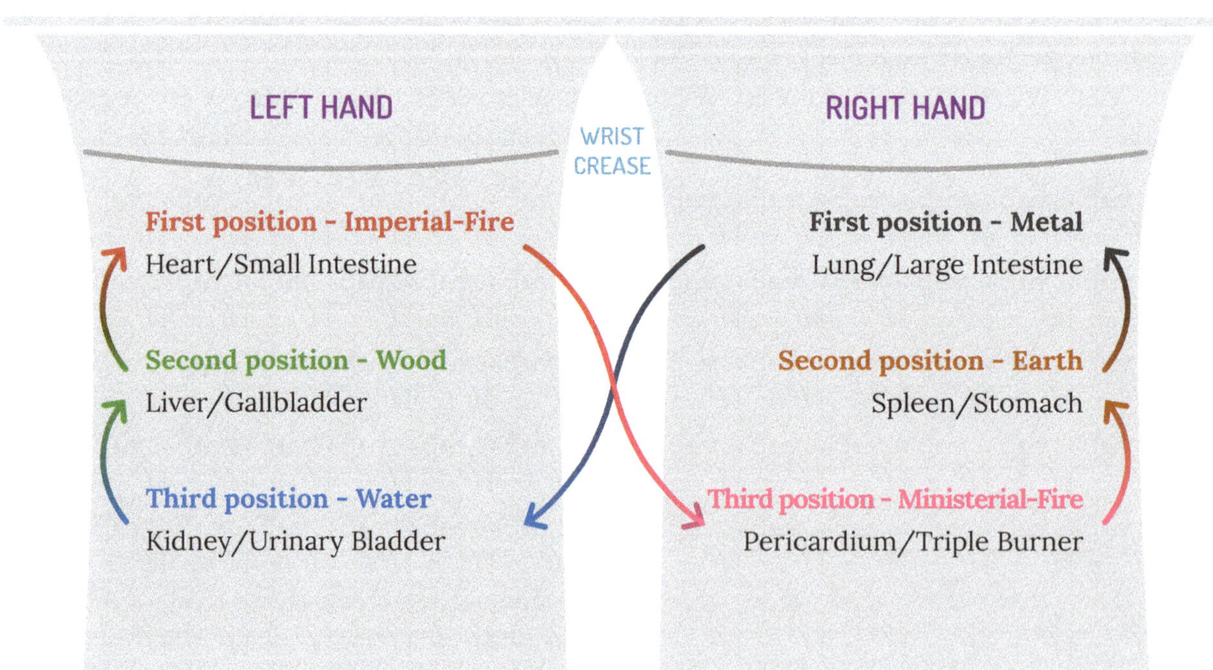

Checking Your Own Pulse

- The fire element's ashes fertilize the earth.
- The earth element's natural resources transform into metal.
- The metal element's condensation generates moisture.
- The water element's nourishment allows plants to grow.
- The wood element's timber feeds fire.

Monitoring the engendering cycle through the radial pulse while choosing acupoints and essential oils to correct the root five-element dysfunction ensures the most effective treatment approach at each session. Each beneficial acupoint, essential oil, herb, or supplement will gradually improve the pulse quality, optimizing the ability for one element to nourish the next.

5.2 Stomach of the Pulse

The proper depth to assess the pulse is the mid layer, which contains the *stomach of the pulse*. To find the stomach of the pulse, first locate the *bone* and *surface* layers of the pulse. Find the bone layer by slowly increasing the pressure to the depth at which the pulse becomes occluded. Then gradually release the pressure to find the surface layer where the pulse can no longer be detected. The location midway between the bone and surface layers is the stomach of the pulse, also referred to as the stomach level, which allows for the most accurate assessment.

The Three Layers of the Pulse

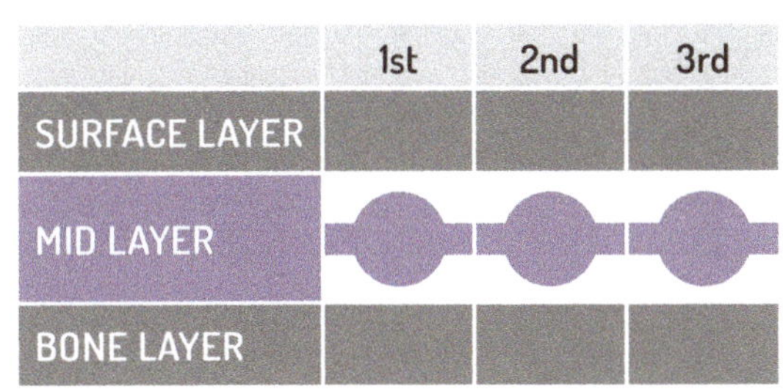

The mid layer contains the stomach of the pulse.

The radial pulse adapts to seasonal temperature changes to conserve or release heat from the body. In the summer, the radial artery rests just below the skin's surface to keep the blood cooler. In the fall, the radial artery descends and rests midway between the skin's surface and the radius bone. In the winter, the radial artery rests closest to the bone to keep the blood warmer. In the spring, the radial artery ascends and rests midway between the radius bone and the skin's surface. It is normal to adjust the amount of pressure needed to find the stomach of the pulse according to seasonal and temperature changes, with the lightest touch in the summer and the deepest force in the winter.

5.3 The Healthy Radial Pulse

The ideal pulse indicating the ability to self-heal and rejuvenate is slightly slippery and relatively balanced between the three positions. A balanced and slightly slippery pulse in the mid layer feels like a strand of round pearls or beads gliding under your fingertips. The artery's elasticity is apparent, and the roundness of each beat is distinguishable. A slightly slippery pulse is soft at the beginning and end of each beat and full in the middle. Locate a strand of round pearls or beads and allow your fingertips to glide lightly over the top to feel the individual roundness of each bead.

The Balanced Pulse

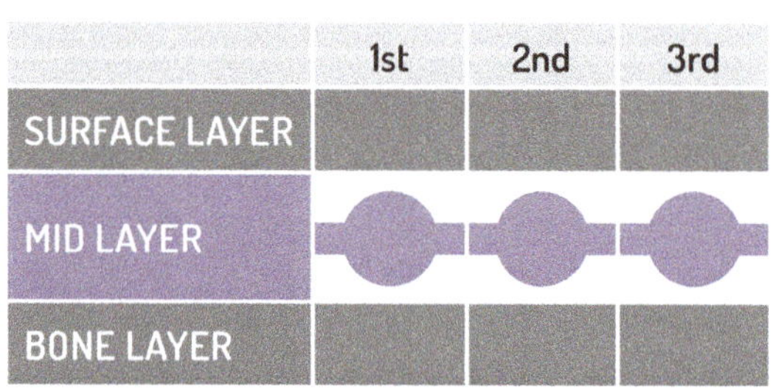

Pulse assessment utilizes multidimensional analysis to monitor the organ/meridian elemental pairs. The three layers of the pulse combine with the three positions starting at the wrist crease on each side (one position for each of the elemental pairs) to make an assessment. The first *(cun)* position will naturally be slightly closer to the surface layer when compared to the middle *(guan)* position, and the third *(chi)* position will be slightly deeper and closer to the bone layer. The vigor of a healthy radial pulse perfectly rolls under the practitioner's fingertips in the mid layer for easy assessment. A healthy pulse will feel more intense closer to the bone layer and softer closer to the surface layer.

5.4 Imbalanced Pulse Variations

Body-Feedback pulse assessment uses the basic TCM terms of *forceful, wiry, choppy, thin,* and *confined* to describe the imbalanced pulse variations that indicate compromised heath. A forceful quality in the pulse occurs when the radial artery is bounding aggressively from the bone layer into the surface layer. The forceful pulse aggressively pushes back against the practitioner's fingertips in the mid layer. This excessively strong quality indicates immune system involvement or pathogenic heat and can accompany a wiry, choppy, thin, or confined pulse.

The overall strength and elasticity of all three pulse positions can indicate the presence of systemic health challenges. Lifestyle choices, including types or sources of food, water, body washes, lotions, shampoo, laundry soaps, and dryer sheets, can have a significant impact on general health and pulse quality. Products applied directly to the skin, along with residue from clothes (laundry products and synthetic materials), absorb into the lymph and circulatory systems. If the client's pulse is not improving from session to session, look into the above lifestyle choices for hidden factors compromising health.

5.4.1 The Wiry Pulse

A wiry pulse reveals qi stagnation and is the first indication of an elemental imbalance. The pulse can feel wiry in each individual position or overall in all three positions on each wrist. A wiry presentation results from the artery's elasticity tightening, causing it to lose roundness and become taut like a guitar string. The individual beats lack differentiation and flow between the positions. The pulse slaps instead of rolling under the practitioner's fingertips. The wiry pulse can easily become too forceful and push outward, and is also the first sign of an acupoint, essential oil, herb, or supplement testing unfavorably.

The Wiry Pulse

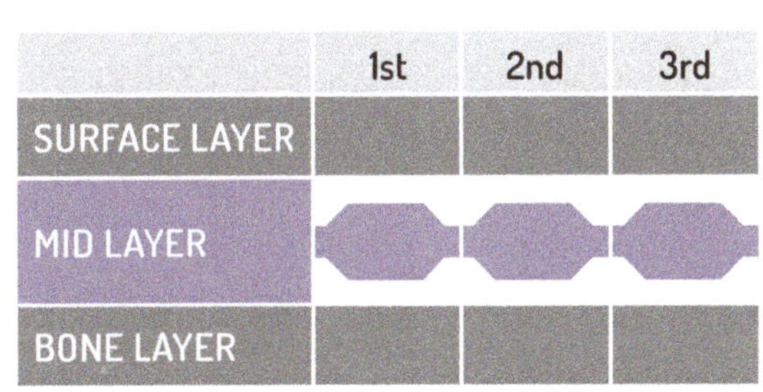

An overall wiry pulse implies compromised detoxification or immune system dysregulation. When all positions are tight and wiry, toxins or an excessive immune response can disrupt the endocrine, digestive, or hepatic-renal systems. A wiry, forceful, and floating pulse in the surface layer of all positions signifies an immune response pushing out external pathogens, causing excessive inflammation, or triggering an autoimmune flare-up.

The Wiry and Forceful Pulse

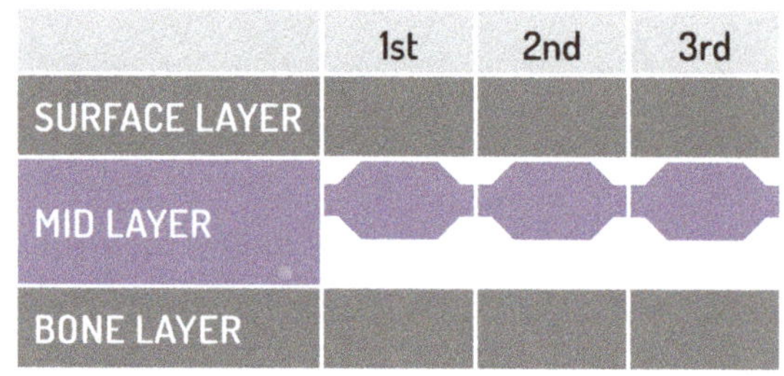

Several forms of pathogenic heat, including exterior-wind, depressive, blood, and yin-deficiency, can cause a single pulse position to feel wiry and forceful. When an autoimmune condition is impacting an organ, its pulse position can become wiry and forceful. Always check the metal + water combination to release heat as supporting acupoints for the organs/meridians with a wiry or wiry and forceful pulse presentation.

5.4.2 The Choppy Pulse

When pathology affects the internal organs, the body's ability to generate and maintain nourishing blood diminishes, resulting in a choppy pulse. The blood thickens, causing hardness in the individual beats with rough edges. The beat is abrupt with no lead-in and collides into the practitioner's fingertips. A choppy pulse is similar to a speedboat hitting rough waves head on. This pulse often accompanies long-standing pain, improperly digested proteins or fats, hardening of the arteries, varicose veins, or a build-up of toxins.

The Choppy Pulse

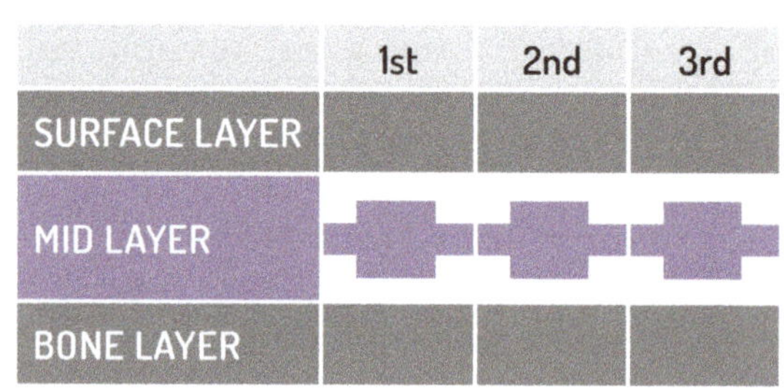

When all pulse positions feel choppy, the client's blood is too thick and congested. Examples of substances that can congest the blood include environmental toxins, undigested proteins from the diet, elevated cholesterol, and pathogenic infections. Menstruating women who have an excessively choppy pulse may experience viscous-type clots or a shiny, mucous film within their menstrual blood.

A choppy pulse in an individual pulse position indicates blood stasis (congestion of blood) is affecting one or both of the paired organs/meridians. Blood stasis causing the pulse to feel choppy signifies long-term pathology and can take several weeks to months to rectify. After an injury, a choppy pulse can occur in the individual positions that correspond with the affected meridians as the body heals. A choppy and forceful pulse can indicate blood stasis accompanying immune dysfunction, including autoimmune conditions that affect a specific organ/meridian.

5.4.3 The Thin Pulse

A thin pulse in all positions can occur with low blood volume, dehydration, or anemia. As people age, their blood volume naturally reduces, and intracellular fluid levels decline. An overall thin pulse is commonly seen in the elderly due to low blood volume or not drinking enough water. A thin pulse can accompany a smaller (narrow, less thick, or short) tongue that also appears thin.

A thin pulse in an individual position reveals the client's genetic or constitutional weakness. It can take several months of herbs and nutritional support, targeting the corresponding organ to improve a thin pulse. During maintenance treatments, the individual thin pulse position usually corresponds with the balancing acupoint prescription that tests the best to support the root organ dysfunction.

The Thin Pulse

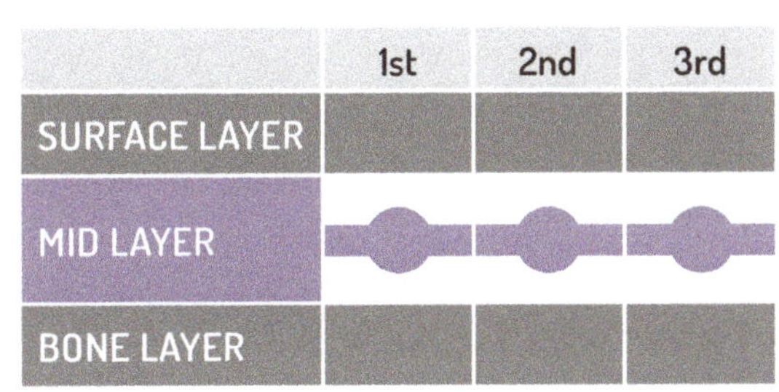

Reverse-osmosis and purified water have little to no naturally occurring minerals and will cause symptoms of chronic dehydration and decreased blood volume. Without adequate supplementation of a mineral complex and trace minerals, the body will leach minerals from the bones and teeth to offset the low mineral content of the water. Also, contemporary farming practices are resulting in foods with low mineral content. Clients who drink reverse-osmosis or purified water may unknowingly be creating additional health problems due to the lack of minerals. Using Body-Feedback testing methods, check samples of the client's water to determine if the quality is acceptable.

5.4.4 The Confined Pulse

A confined pulse feels similar to a thin pulse; however, the causes are very different. A confined pulse results from excessive intracellular fluids making the pulse hard to detect. Dampness, damp heat, and phlegm cause fluid retention that compresses the radial pulse. A confined pulse will accompany an enlarged or swollen tongue with scallops or teeth marks on the sides, indicating fluid retention. A thick white or yellow coating on the tongue signifies dampness or damp heat is confining the pulse. Obesity (excessive phlegm) can also hide the pulse, making it difficult to detect.

The Confined Pulse

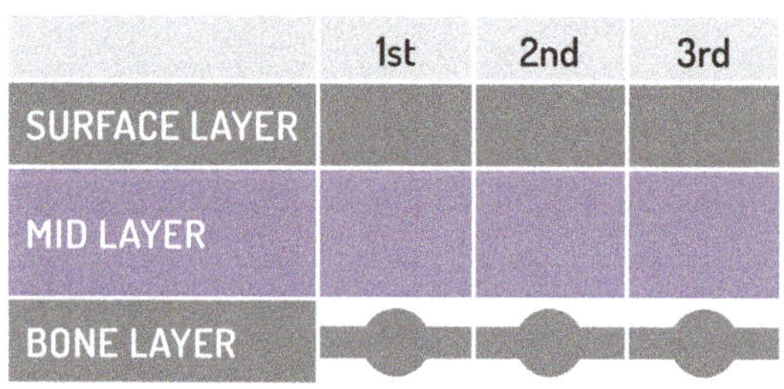

Improvements in the overall pulse quality and the individual positions at each session indicate that the client's lifestyle supports their health. When the pulse quality is not improving between sessions, further investigation into lifestyle factors, hidden infections, and genetics may be needed to improve health. The acupuncture sessions will have lasting results for clients who consistently progress towards a healthier pulse.

5.5 Imbalanced Pulse Positions

A root excess or deficiency condition will cause the radial pulse to become a combination of wiry, choppy, forceful, thin, or confined in the corresponding individual position. The position with the most imbalance reflects the root dysfunction at the time of the assessment. When other meridians, organs, or glands are affected by the root dysfunction, their corresponding pulse positions will also become imbalanced. The most imbalanced individual positions indicate which balancing acupoint prescriptions to test during each session.

Any of the pulse abnormalities can indicate either an excess or deficient condition. Health is dynamic, and the client's root dysfunction will often change as health improves or declines and with phases of the menstrual cycle. This variation is evident with changes in the pulse presentation at each session, indicating the need for different balancing, sedating, or tonifying prescriptions.

During maintenance acupuncture sessions, it is common to have the same pulse presentation with the acupoint prescriptions alternating between sedation and tonification. For example, a person with an overall choppy pulse and a thin second position on the left (liver/gallbladder pair) may test best for a liver tonification prescription at some sessions and a liver sedation prescription at others, depending on diet, hydration, activity, food choices, and stress.

On occasion, the pulse will not match the root dysfunction for clients with complex symptoms. For example, a client with autoimmune thyroid symptoms due to excessive exposure to environmental toxins may require liver detoxification support first even though the initial pulse assessment indicates a root dysfunction in the first trisection (lung/large intestine/stomach/spleen). After this client focuses on detoxification and reducing exposure to environmental toxins, the root dysfunction will match the pulse assessment of wiry and forceful in the first and second positions on the right hand. After a few months of detoxing, this client will transition from liver balancing acupoint prescriptions to spleen or stomach root balancing acupoint prescriptions.

When a pulse is forceful, wiry, choppy, thin, or confined in two specific positions, it often corresponds with a trisection imbalance or body system dysfunction.

FIRST TRISECTION IMBALANCE

	1st (*cun*)	2nd (*guan*)	3rd (*chi*)
RIGHT WRIST	LU/LI	SP/ST	
LEFT WRIST			

SECOND TRISECTION IMBALANCE

	1st (*cun*)	2nd (*guan*)	3rd (*chi*)
RIGHT WRIST			
LEFT WRIST	HT/SI		KD/UB

THIRD TRISECTION IMBALANCE

	1st (*cun*)	2nd (*guan*)	3rd (*chi*)
RIGHT WRIST			PC/TB
LEFT WRIST		LV/GB	

IMMUNE SYSTEM DYSFUNCTION AFFECTING THE SMALL AND LARGE INTESTINES

	1st (*cun*)	2nd (*guan*)	3rd (*chi*)
RIGHT WRIST	LU/LI		
LEFT WRIST	HT/SI		

DIGESTIVE SYSTEM DYSFUNCTION DUE TO EXCESSIVE FATS, SUGAR, OR CARBOHYDRATES

	1st (*cun*)	2nd (*guan*)	3rd (*chi*)
RIGHT WRIST		SP/ST	
LEFT WRIST		LV/GB	

ENDOCRINE SYSTEM IMBALANCE DUE TO COMPROMISED DETOXIFICATION

	1st (*cun*)	2nd (*guan*)	3rd (*chi*)
RIGHT WRIST			
LEFT WRIST		LV/GB	KD/UB

ADRENAL DYSFUNCTION

	1st (*cun*)	2nd (*guan*)	3rd (*chi*)
RIGHT WRIST			PC/TB
LEFT WRIST			KD/UB

ENDOCRINE SYSTEM DYSFUNCTION DUE TO COMPROMISED DIGESTION

	1st (*cun*)	2nd (*guan*)	3rd (*chi*)
RIGHT WRIST		SP/ST	PC/TB
LEFT WRIST			

IMMUNE SYSTEM DYSFUNCTION AFFECTING THE UPPER DIGESTIVE TRACT

	1st (*cun*)	2nd (*guan*)	3rd (*chi*)
RIGHT WRIST			
LEFT WRIST	HT/SI	LV/GB	

HYPOTHALAMUS-PITUITARY DYSFUNCTION AFFECTING THE ENDOCRINE SYSTEM

	1st (*cun*)	2nd (*guan*)	3rd (*chi*)
RIGHT WRIST			PC/TB
LEFT WRIST	HT/SI		

LONG-TERM IMMUNE DYSFUNCTION OR INFECTIONS

	1st (*cun*)	2nd (*guan*)	3rd (*chi*)
RIGHT WRIST	LU/LI		PC/TB
LEFT WRIST			

IMMUNE SYSTEM DYSFUNCTION AFFECTING THE ADRENALS, REPRODUCTIVE ORGANS, OR KIDNEYS

	1st (*cun*)	2nd (*guan*)	3rd (*chi*)
RIGHT WRIST	LU/LI		
LEFT WRIST			KD/UB

5.6 Practical Application of Pulse Assessment

The pulse responds to energy flow changes in the meridian system within 10-60 seconds. These immediate changes provide valuable information from the client's body to guide the treatment process. Throughout the session, a combination of pulse assessment and other Body-Feedback palpation testing methods guide the diagnosis and choice of acupoints, essential oils, herbs, and supplements. In certain situations, such as paralysis, hyper-sensitivity, or autism, formulating a treatment using only pulse assessment techniques is best. With taller clients, it is easier to check the acupoints on the lower body to the pulse for convenience. Several stages of the treatment process utilize pulse assessment to:

- Identify meridian, organ, or endocrine gland dysfunction.
- Determine the root dysfunction and corresponding balancing, sedating, and tonifying acupoint prescriptions.
- Find organs/meridians affected by pathogenic heat.
- Check supporting acupoints.
- Confirm the accuracy of acupoint locations.
- Determine if magnetic pellets or ear seeds are beneficial for use at home.
- Test essential oils, herbs, supplements, foods, and other personal care products.

The fingertips, as the most sensitive part of fingers, are the easiest to use to feel pulse subtleties for assessment. When assessing the pulse, feel the difference when you use your fingertips versus the pads of your fingers. If you have calluses or neuropathy in the fingertips, using the pads of your fingers may increase your sensitivity.

Finger Positions for Assessing the Pulse

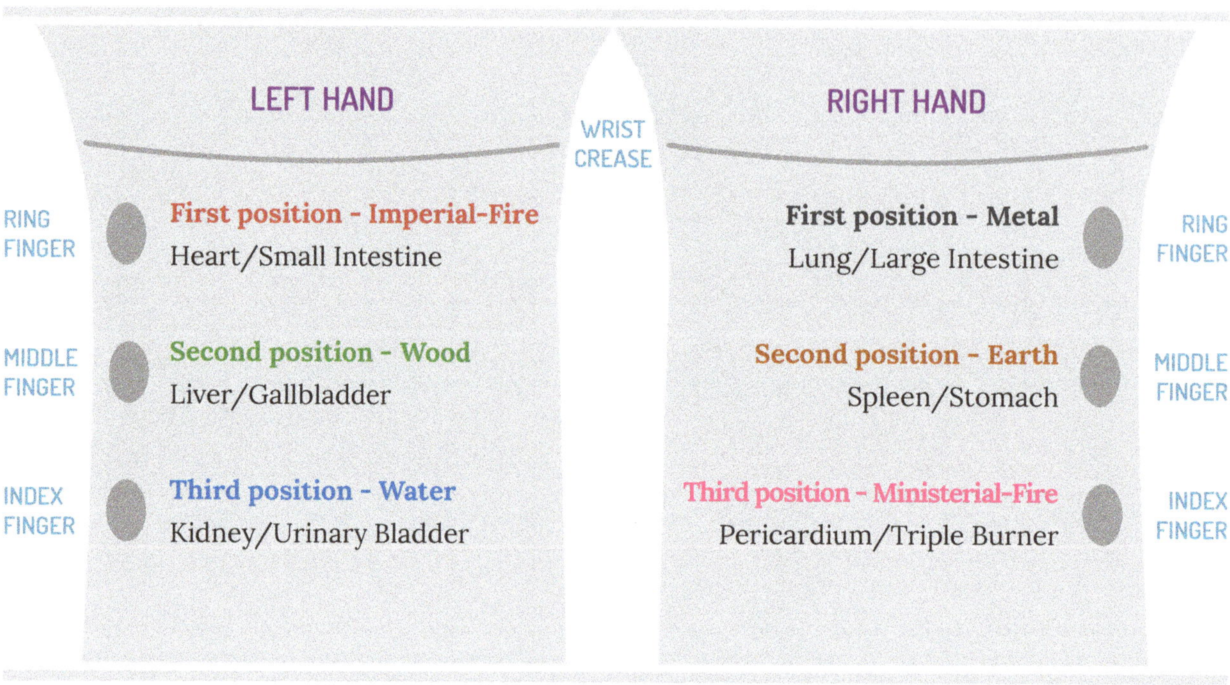

Checking Your Own Pulse

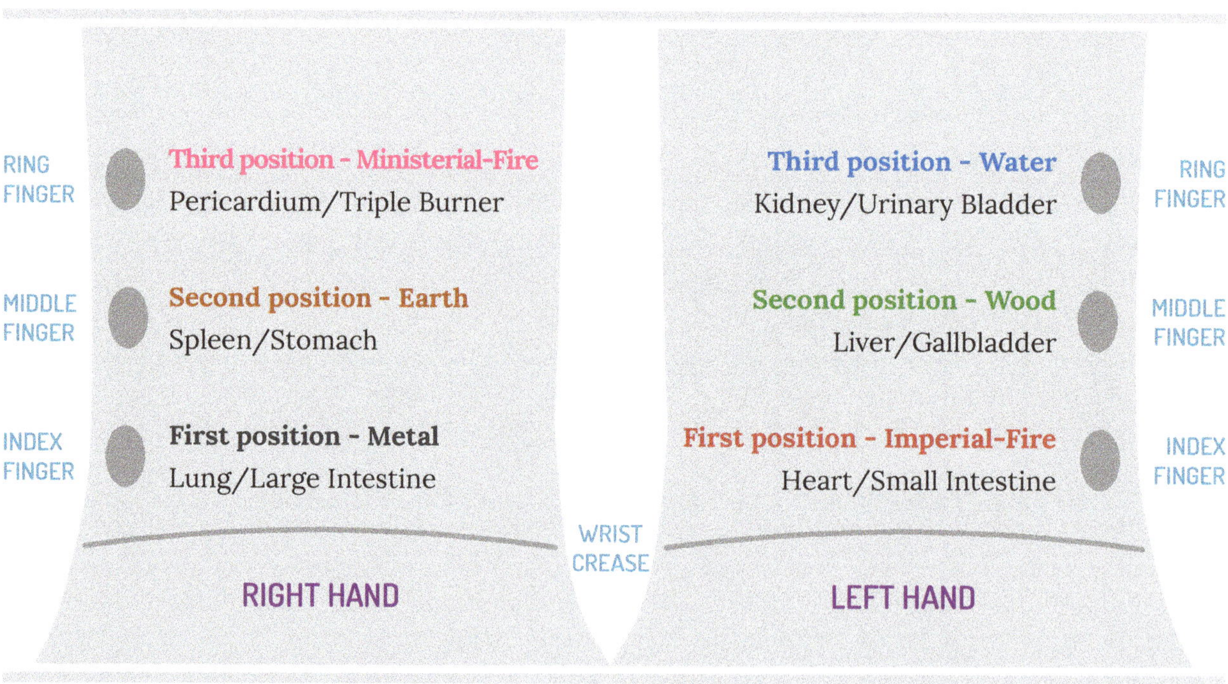

Checking Someone Else's Pulse

The first step to assess the radial pulse is to find the three pulse positions on each wrist and the proper depth. The first pulse position is at the crease of the wrist, the second position is at the level of the styloid process, and the third position is slightly further up the forearm. Start with finding the second pulse position by locating the styloid process, and let your middle finger glide from the middle of the styloid process to the inside of the wrist until you feel the pulse.

Proper Assessment of the Pulse

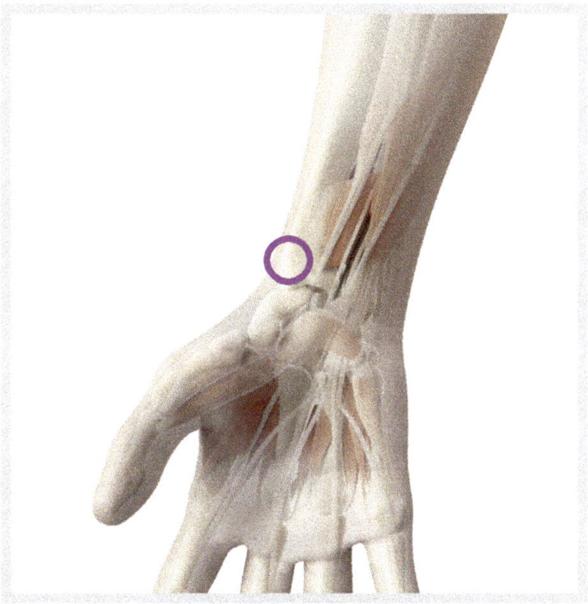

First locate the styloid process of the wrist to line up with the second pulse positions.

When testing yourself and someone similar in size, you can let your fingers naturally place themselves next to one another to find the first and third positions. If you are assessing a pulse of someone taller than you, you will need to slightly spread your fingers to find the first and third positions. If you are evaluating someone shorter than you, adjust your fingers to be tight and close. The length of the radial pulse that you can feel is relative to the height of the person you are checking.

Now find the stomach of the pulse by locating the surface and bone layers at the second position. Start with lightly pressing on the skin's surface until you feel the pulse meet your fingertip. Then press down until you no longer feel each beat. The stomach of the pulse occurs in the mid layer, between the surface and bone layers. For some people, the mid layer will be closer to the surface, while for others it is lower. Again, this is the proper depth to assess the pulse.

Start by assessing overall pulse quality (stomach of the pulse) at the mid layer to observe general health. When all the pulse positions are excessively wiry, choppy, forceful, thin, or hidden at multiple sessions, additional factors are compromising a client's ability to heal. Ongoing improvements in health occur when the global pulse quality improves from session to session.

Next, feel each position individually at the mid layer. Start by releasing the pressure but holding the placement by letting the fingers rest on the skin's surface. Compare the middle position on each wrist. Then compare the first and third positions. Note the positions that feel relaxed and slightly slippery versus wiry, choppy, forceful, thin, and confined.

Check the pulse while sitting across from a client during the intake process, and again with them lying on the treatment table. The feel of the radial pulse will change slightly from sitting to lying down. Checking the pulse with a client sitting provides information about health in an active, sitting, or walking position. Checking the pulse with the client lying on the treatment table gives insights about health while resting. Because the acupuncture session occurs in a resting state, it is best to check the acupoints with the client relaxing on the treatment table.

On occasion, a client may feel a positive or negative shift in their energy that agrees with the changes in their pulse. Choosing a treatment approach based on pulse assessment alone is optional; however, testing acupoints and essential oils to the pulse alone may leave the average client unaware of the immediate treatment results. Testing the master points, muscles, and organ/meridian associations engages a client to experience the reduced discomfort and immediate relaxation before resting with the needles. Some clients prefer to be less involved, and they will be more comfortable with the pulse techniques guiding their treatment. Other clients enjoy and appreciate participating in the testing process.

Some clients may be interested in learning to monitor their pulse and using pulse assessment with other family members. People with sensitive digestion can learn to test foods and check their digestive pulses after meals. Testing supplements before taking them can help ensure compatibility and indicate when rotation is needed. *Meramour's Guide to Supporting Your Acupuncture Meridian System* (2017) is the recommended resource for clients who would like to understand more about their health and the Body-Feedback treatment style.

CHAPTER 6

The Body-Feedback Testing Locations

The Body-Feedback testing locations guide the diagnosis and treatment processes through non-verbal communication with the client's body. Upon palpation, these testing locations experience discomfort when organ/meridian pathology is present. The testing process brings client and practitioner awareness of the root organ/meridian dysfunction and other compromised organs/meridians. Pre-checking acupoints, essential oils, herbs, or supplements using the testing locations indicates the body's probable response for the chosen treatment approach.

Clients report being surprised to feel their muscle tension and pain decrease or increase during the testing process. For many clients, this involuntary change in muscle tension and pain sensations seems fascinating, and some describe it as magical. Gathering information from the client's body through the Body-Feedback testing process provides insight, clarity, and focus. These testing sessions offer opportunities for both the client and practitioner to gain a deeper understanding of how to improve health.

The Body-Feedback testing locations include master alarm points, master regions, organ/meridian referral areas, and muscle associations. The Body-Feedback master alarm points and master regions identify systemic pathology affecting multiple body systems, organs, or meridians. The Body-Feedback organ/meridian referral areas and muscle associations assess the health of each organ and meridian individually. Depending on a client's needs, multiple combinations of testing locations can be utilized during each stage of the treatment process. During the pre-treatment and treatment stages, testing locations confirm the most effective essential oils and acupoints. During the post-treatment stage, these same testing locations can identify beneficial supplements, herbs, foods, and personal care products.

The Body-Feedback testing locations may overlap with other palpation-based techniques for assessing health because pathology is often identified through pain and discomfort. However, the Body-Feedback system integrates these testing locations with unique Body-Feedback testing techniques, specific acupoint prescriptions, and Meramour's Organ Supporting and Meridian Balancing essential oil blends. Additionally, the Body-Feedback system distinguishes between excess and deficient organ/meridian pathology, both of which can cause discomfort, muscle tightness, or muscle flaccidity at the testing locations.

6.1 Master Body-Feedback Alarm Points

The master alarm points become painful or tight when systemic pathology affects multiple meridians, organs, or body systems. Pathology affecting the entire body can include uncontrolled pathogenic heat, compromised brain function, or hormonal imbalances. Muscle knots can develop at the master alarm points due to chronic conditions. The longer the pathology is present, the larger, harder, and more painful the muscle knots become. The master alarm points are common testing locations throughout the entire treatment. The interconnectedness, along with the close proximity of these points, frequently causes them to be painful and tight at the same time.

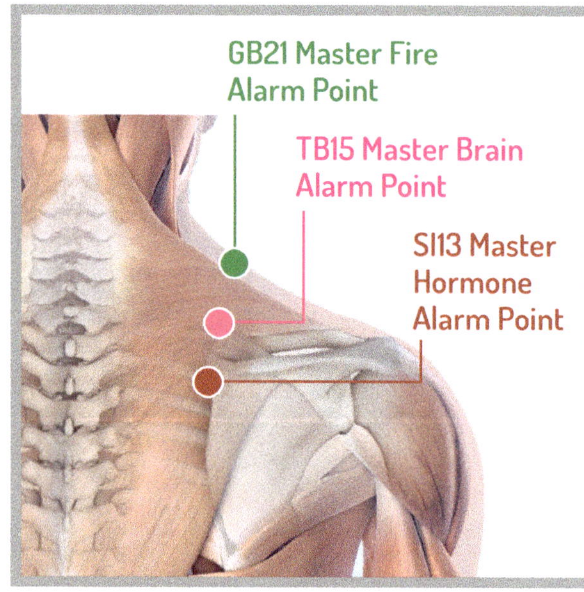

Master Alarm Points

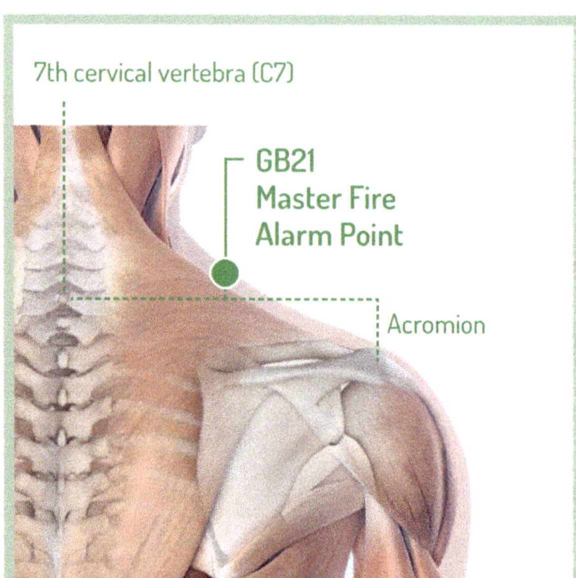

Midway between the seventh cervical vertebra and the tip of the acromion, at the crest of the trapezius muscle

GALLBLADDER 21:

The Master Fire Alarm Point becomes painful and tight with pathogenic heat or systemic inflammation. Excessive heat rises and accumulates at this point because it is the highest point on the torso (not including the neck). When this point is tight or painful, multiple meridians could be experiencing pathogenic heat. Pulse analysis and palpation of the meridian fire points can locate the individually affected organs/meridians. After inserting needles or using essential oils to resolve the pathogenic heat, GB21 will relax and become pain-free, indicating a successful treatment.

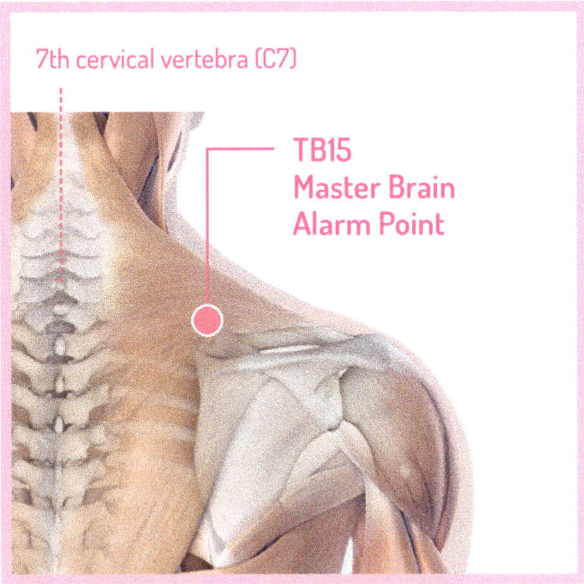

Midway between GB21 and SI13 above the superior angle of the scapula

TRIPLE BURNER 15:

The Master Brain Alarm Point becomes painful and tight with unhealthy brain activity or when the brain is managing dysfunction within the body. The brain has a central role in monitoring and maintaining homeostasis. Test involuntary functions, such as respiration, digestion, and heart rate, using TB15 as the brain is constantly monitoring these functions. Due to its convenient location, use TB15 to test acupoints on the face, scalp, ears, or other areas on the neck. This alarm point will relax and become pain-free after a beneficial treatment, which allows for efficient testing of herbs and supplements in the post-treatment stage. Beneficial herbs and supplements will further release remaining tension, and neutral ones will not induce additional muscle tension.

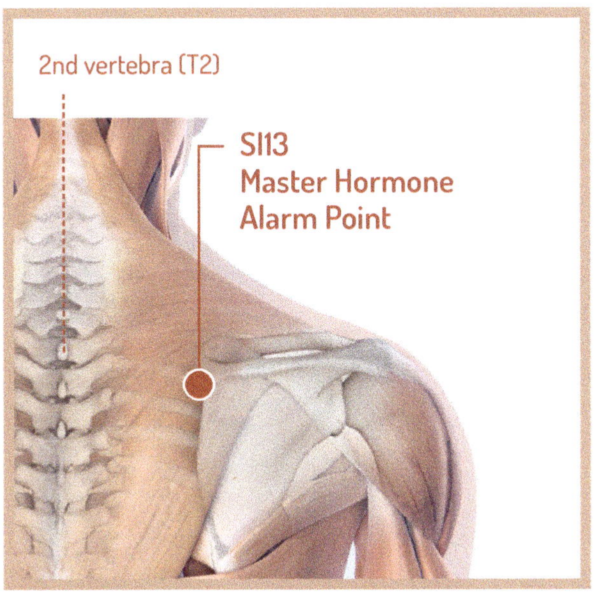

In the depression at the medial end of the scapular spine

SMALL INTESTINE 13:

The Master Hormone Alarm Point becomes painful with all hormonal imbalances and endocrine gland dysfunction. This point can identify the dysfunctional root gland, disrupting other glands below it in the endocrine funnel. The root gland dysfunction corresponds with the correct organ/meridian to treat. By addressing the appropriate gland, the entire system and hormonal balance optimizes.

The endocrine funnel hierarchy includes the hypothalamus, pituitary, adrenals, pancreas, thyroid, ovaries, and testes. Dysfunction in the hypothalamus, pituitary, or adrenals will impair the other glands' ability to work correctly. When multiple endocrine glands are affected, SI13 will radiate muscle tightness and pain at the rhomboid minor and major attachment sites on the medial border of the scapula. The tightness in both rhomboids can create a substantial muscle knot that encompasses a larger area than SI13. The muscle tightness and pain will diminish when the origin of the endocrine system dysfunction receives proper treatment, resulting in balanced hormones. Test acupoint prescriptions, essential oils, herbs, and supplements using SI13 to determine the individual gland causing dysfunction within the endocrine system. Then palpate the individual testing locations for corresponding glands to determine if the root treatment improves the subsequent glands below in the funnel.

Meramour's Endocrine Funnel

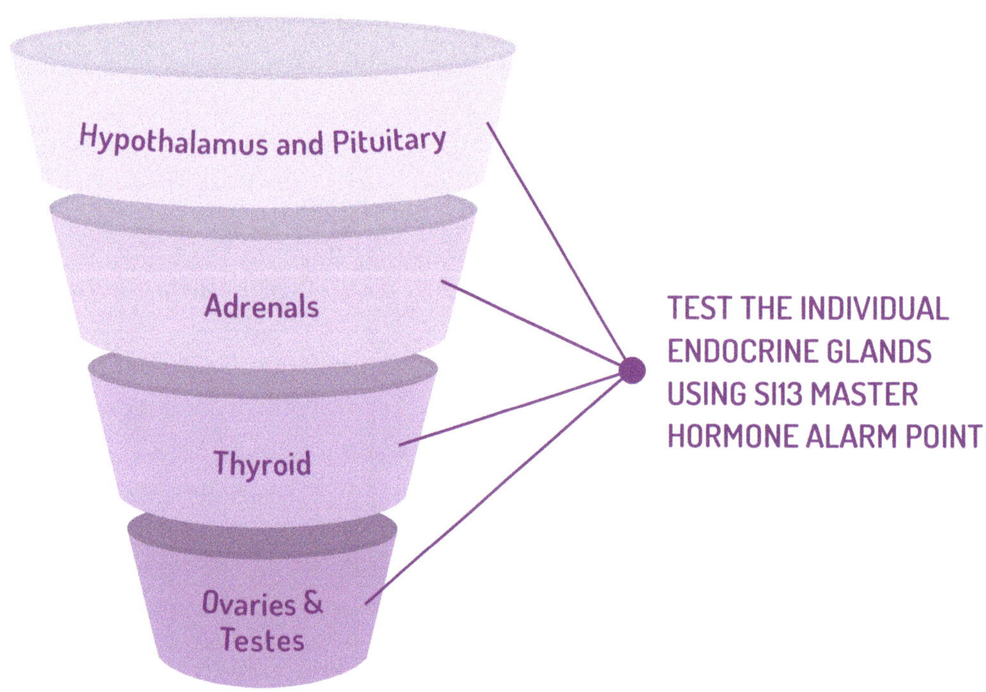

The muscles around the Master Hormone Alarm Point SI13 become tight and cause discomfort when any of the endocrine glands experience dysfunction. The dysfunctional root gland will cause the ones below it in the funnel also to experience dysfunction. Identifying and rectifying the origin of the endocrine dysfunction releases the discomfort at SI13 for all affected glands.

A typical example in determining the root dysfunctional endocrine gland occurs with hyperthyroid and hypothyroid symptoms. The neck muscles are the individual testing location for the thyroid. Check the balancing prescriptions for the hypothalamus (UB and SI), pituitary (PC and HT), adrenals (KD), and thyroid (ST) using SI13 first. If the hypothalamus is the root, SI13 and the neck flexors will release tension with the UB or SI balancing prescription. If the pituitary is the root, SI13 and the neck flexors will release tension with the PC or HT balancing prescription. If the adrenals are the root, SI13 and the neck flexors will release tension with the KD balancing prescription. Treatment of the dysfunctional root gland above the thyroid in the endocrine funnel indirectly restores proper function to the thyroid. When the thyroid is the root dysfunction, the ST balancing prescription reduces discomfort in SI13 and the neck flexors.

With Hashimoto's autoimmune thyroiditis, the root treatment to benefit the thyroid could be either a meridian associated with detoxification or immune function. Endocrine-disrupting chemicals in the environment can also cause thyroid symptoms. Test the LV, LU, and LI balancing prescriptions using SI13 to identify liver or immune system involvement for thyroid and other endocrine conditions.

6.2 Body-Feedback Master Regions

The five Body-Feedback master regions correspond with musculoskeletal pathology and asymmetry in the body. When these regions are painful or tight upon palpation, the alignment of the musculoskeletal system is negatively impacting a person's health and gait. Common causes include trauma, chronic inflammation, poor posture, scoliosis, repetitive use of specific muscle groups, stored toxins, dysfunctional organs, or imbalanced meridians. Use the master regions to assess for asymmetry during the pre-treatment planning stage.

MASTER REGIONS OF THE NECK: The neck flexor and extensor muscles will adapt to accommodate spinal misalignment and harmful posture to keep the eyes level. The brain requires visual equilibrium to properly function; otherwise, symptoms such as nausea, dizziness, and fatigue can occur. With scoliosis, the neck muscles will have different thickness and tautness from side to side. With lordosis or kyphosis, the anterior neck flexor muscles will have different thickness and tautness compared to the posterior neck extensor muscles. One set of neck muscles will feel tight and overdeveloped, while the opposing group of neck muscles will feel flaccid and underdeveloped.

An imbalanced trisection will cause multiple muscle groups to become tight and painful in the anterior, lateral, or posterior section of the neck. There are a total of 26 neck flexor and extensor muscles that work together and span multiple areas of the head, neck, and upper back. Many neck muscles span two trisection regions on the neck, and the affected muscles will be the tightest in the region that corresponds with the imbalanced trisection. For example, the sternocleidomastoid muscle originates on the anterior portion (first trisection region) and inserts on the lateral side (third trisection region). Each trisection refers to multiple muscles in the following regions of the neck:

Neck Region for the First Trisection

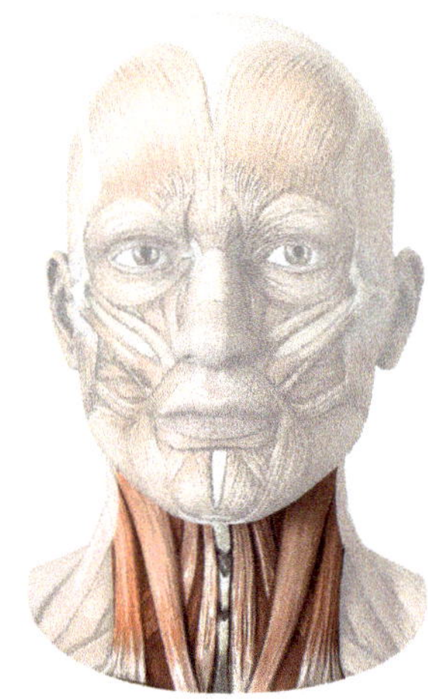

The front of the neck corresponds with the first trisection organs/meridians (lung, large intestine, stomach, and spleen).

Neck Region for the Second Trisection

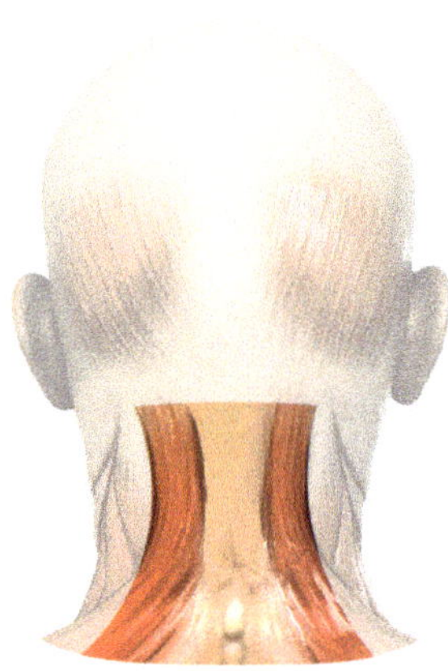

The back of the neck corresponds with the second trisection organs/meridians (heart, small intestine, urinary bladder, and kidney).

Neck Region for the Third Trisection

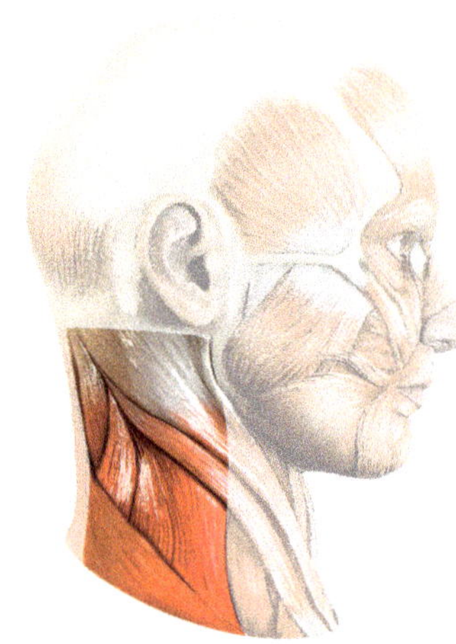

The sides of the neck correspond with the third trisection organs/meridians (pericardium, triple burner, gallbladder, and liver).

CONCEPTION VESSEL 15:

The Spinal Misalignment Region spans between the xiphoid process and CV15. This area becomes painful and can have a hollow, sharp, or burning sensation when lordosis, kyphosis, scoliosis, or organ/meridian pathology affect spinal alignment. Chapter 7, "Asymmetry and Health," has an expanded explanation about this region.

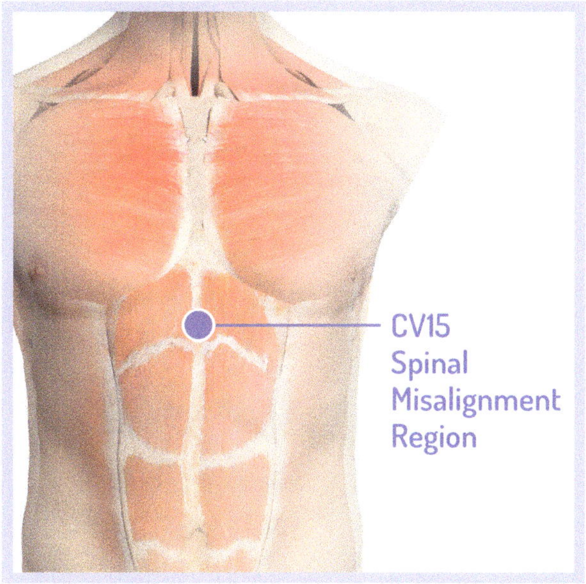

The region around the small cartilaginous extension of the lower part of the sternum

UPPER BORDER OF THE POSTERIOR ILIAC SPINE CREST:

In the lower back, the region above the border of the posterior iliac spine crest commonly stores phlegm nodules. The body encapsulates harmful substances and stores them here because it is the farthest away from vital organs and close to the colon. Stored phlegm nodules along the posterior iliac spine crest can cause lower back pain and immune system dysfunction. Check all clients for stored phlegm nodules along the posterior iliac spine crest to identify the need for extra detoxification support. Clients who are conscious of these nodules are usually unaware of the cause and potential impact on their health. Many clients unknowingly have phlegm nodules that are contributing to their health challenges.

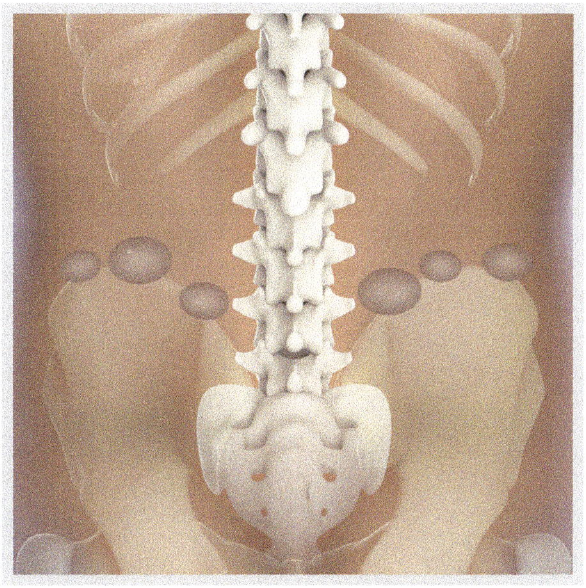

Phlegm nodules on the upper border of the PSIS

Section 3.7 contains additional information on pathogenic heat with phlegm nodules. Chapter 11 provides essential oil treatment options for phlegm nodules.

URINARY BLADDER 43-44 and 57-58 MUSCLE MEMORY REGIONS:

Two regions along the urinary bladder meridian can become tight and painful when the musculoskeletal system has adapted to misalignment in posture or gait. Sore or tight muscles in either of these regions indicate the body is remembering the long-standing structural imbalance. Beneficial treatment options will release the tightness and reduce the discomfort in these muscle memory regions and encourage the client's body to hold the new alignment.

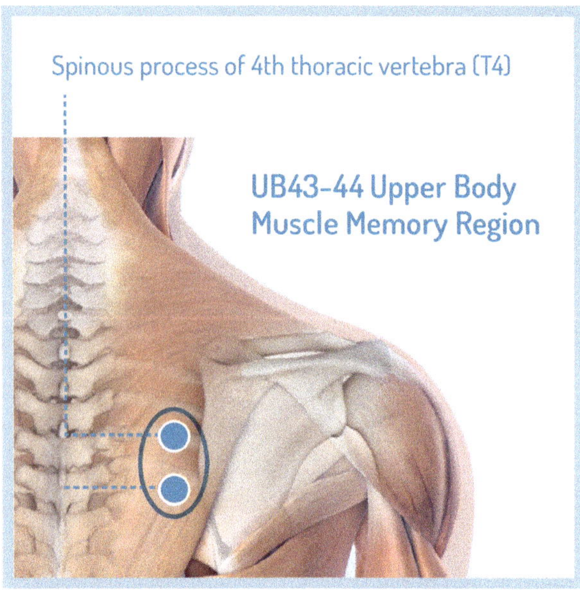

On the medial border of the scapula between the fourth and fifth thoracic vertebrae

The muscle memory region for misalignment affecting the upper body (above the level of the umbilicus) spans across the UB43-44 points. Use this region as a testing location for structural conditions involving the neck, shoulders, upper back, mid-back, rib cage, arms, and hands. Needle remaining muscle knots in this region as local ashi supporting acupoints in the last step in the treatment stage to erase the muscle memory. Use between two and four acupoints with transverse needle insertion directed towards the spine from the outer edge of the muscle knot.

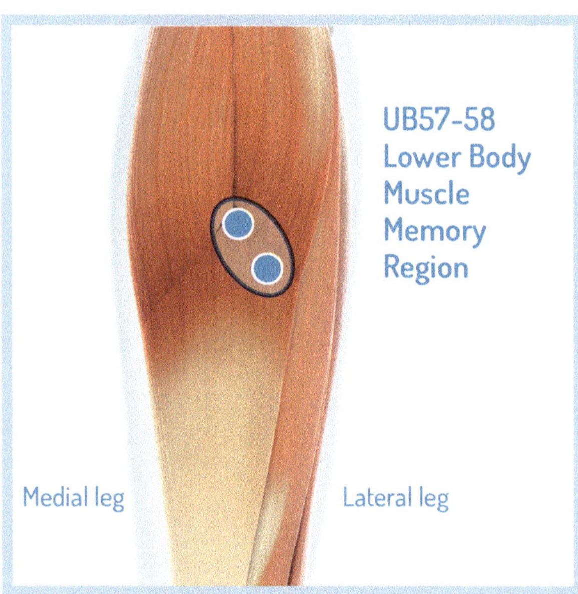

In the depression formed by the bellies of the gastrocnemius muscle that extends to the lateral edge

The muscle memory region for misalignment affecting the lower body (below the level of the umbilicus) spans across the UB57-58 points. Use this region as a testing location for structural conditions involving the lumbar area of the lower back, sacrum, hips, pelvis, legs, and feet. Needle the remaining muscle tightness in this region as local ashi supporting acupoints in the last step in the treatment stage to erase the muscle memory. Use between one and three acupoints with oblique needle insertion at the base of the gastrocnemius muscle into the Achilles tendon.

6.3 Assessing Individual Organs, Meridians, and Endocrine Glands

Classical TCM texts do not recognize the endocrine glands, nor do they include the ministerial-fire's pericardium and triple burner as organs. However, through clinical experience, the Body-Feedback system corresponds glands with specific organ associations, the lymph nodes with the triple burner organ, and certain functions of the pituitary gland (such as luteinizing hormone production) with the pericardium organ. The Body-Feedback system bridges standard TCM organ pathology with allopathic-type functional medicine pathology for the endocrine glands through the testing locations, related TCM organs, and extra-vessel associations.

Endocrine Gland	Testing Location	Organ and Extra-Vessel Association
HYPOTHALAMUS	Si Shen Cong	GV for hypothalamus-ovarian/testes axis
HYPOTHALAMUS	Occipital Area	UB for the adrenal axis
HYPOTHALAMUS	SI13	SI for the enteric nervous system
PITUITARY	UB2	CV for the pituitary-ovarian/testes axis
PITUITARY	Supraspinatus Muscle, CV8	HT for cortisol production and adrenal axis
PITUITARY	Supraspinatus Muscle, CV8	PC for hormones affected by blood sugar
ADRENALS	T11-T12 area on back, CV8	GV and CV for the adrenal glands
ADRENALS	KD27	KD for the adrenal glands
THYROID	Anterior Neck Muscles	ST for the thyroid gland
OVARIES/TESTES	KD10	KD for the reproductive glands
PANCREAS	CV8, SP9	SP for blood sugar regulation

The twelve main meridians and the eight extra-vessels continuously circulate qi and blood to influence all types of cellular function. The eight extra-vessels act as reservoirs to assist in draining excess or tonifying deficiency conditions in the twelve main meridians. When pathology affects one of the meridians or extra-vessels, their specific Body-Feedback associations will experience discomfort upon palpation. Meridian pathology may or may not cause organ dysfunction; however, organ dysfunction always creates an imbalance of qi or blood that affects its meridian. In summary, a meridian imbalance can stand alone, or it can lead to or result from its organ pair experiencing dysfunction.

Excess or deficiency affecting the meridians is often the first indication of compromised health. By monitoring meridian alarm points and muscle associations, early detection and correction can prevent symptoms and restore a healing vibration. Endocrine gland dysfunction, imbalanced immune system responses, exaggerated emotions, and physical trauma can cause meridian excess or deficiency that can compromise an organ.

Organ and meridian pathology often coincide because of the constant interaction between the two. In most cases, the individual organ/meridian referral areas and muscle associations are reflecting pathology for both. Therefore, the individual Body-Feedback testing locations can indicate pathology in an organ, meridian, or endocrine gland. The organ and meridian alarm points, along with the referral areas, can help differentiate pathology; however, in practice, they are often painful together.

Five-element theory identifies five (*zang*) yin and five (*fu*) yang organs. The zang organs (lungs, spleen, heart, kidneys, and liver) are solid, and they store and engender qi, blood, yin, yang, essence, and jing. The fu organs (large intestine, stomach, small intestine, urinary bladder, and gallbladder) are hollow, and they absorb nutrients, eliminate toxins, and excrete waste from the body. Together, the vitality of the zang and fu organs creates postnatal qi, governs the ability to self-heal, and influences the cellular aging process.

"Classical theory from the *Nei Jing* maintains that each of the channels has a particular proportion of qi and blood."[16] Each meridian requires a specific amount of qi and blood, which dictates its unique vibration when in a state of health and regeneration. Excess or deficient conditions occur when the amount of qi and blood differ from the meridian's optimal vibration. When the amount of qi and blood (vibratory energy) is not within the healthy range, pain and discomfort can occur at specific acupuncture points along the meridian pathway or surrounding the paired organ. Muscle tightness or flaccidity, which represents the loss of optimal vibration, can develop in the Body-Feedback muscle associations as a result of excess or deficient qi or blood.

The Body-Feedback approach integrates TCM organ/meridian pathology with functional medicine and the allopathic paradigm to incorporate current trends in healthcare. Laboratory testing or functional medicine questionnaires assessing body systems can indicate organ dysfunction before symptoms develop into a diagnosed disease. These tests and assessments provide insights for determining the organs, meridians, and endocrine glands for Body-Feedback testing of essential oils, acupoints, herbs, and supplements.

A complete blood chemistry (CBC) profile with differential provides information about red and white blood cells that corresponds to the referral areas and muscle associations for the first trisection organs. Use the lung and large intestine testing locations when a client has abnormal white blood cell counts, neutrophils, lymphocytes, eosinophils, or basophils. Use the spleen and stomach testing locations for abnormal red blood cells, blood sugar, and thyroid values. Fertility can be indirectly affected by any first trisection organ dysfunction.

Use the second trisection organ's testing locations to check laboratory values assessing hormones, along with adrenal and reproductive functions. Adrenal cortisol rhythms can detect dysfunction in the hypothalamus-pituitary-adrenal axis. Sperm analysis and ovarian reserve tests bring valuable information for fertility enhancement. Abnormal hormone values, including cortisol, DHEA, pregnenolone, progesterone, estrogen, and testosterone, may cause discomfort in the second trisection's testing sites. The interconnectedness of the endocrine system requires checking each gland's corresponding organ association to determine the root dysfunction according to the order of the endocrine funnel. For abnormal thyroid values, check the second trisection and stomach testing locations.

With laboratory values that involve hormone production, inflammation markers, vitamin A, vitamin D, and high or low cholesterol, use the liver and gallbladder testing locations. For abnormal lymphocytes or systemic infections, use the triple burner to assess the lymph system. Test the pericardium when abnormal levels of red blood cells are indicated. Check all of the third trisection organs for abnormal detoxification, as indicated on questionnaires or laboratory values. As functional medicine testing continues to expand, new information and testing methods related to the body systems can be integrated into the Body-Feedback testing techniques.

6.4 Body-Feedback Organ/Meridian Alarm Points

The Body-Feedback meridian, organ, and body-system alarm points become painful upon palpation to signal pathology is compromising health. Clients are often first made aware of the tenderness in the alarm points during a testing session. The he-sea and fire-element shu-point categories become painful to warn of organ dysfunction, meridian imbalance, or pathological heat. Additional special acupoints on the meridian will indicate pathology is affecting certain body systems or related organs. For example, the large intestine alarm points include the meridian alarm point (LI5), the organ alarm point (LI11), and the immune system alarm point (LI10).

The organ alarm point is the he-sea shu-point found around muscle attachment sites at the knees and elbows. The meridian alarm point is the fire-element point, which becomes tender when pathogenic heat (see Chapter 3) compromises the related meridian. Any of the five types of pathogenic heat (depressive, blood, damp, exterior-wind, and yin-deficiency) will cause discomfort at the fire points. If pathogenic heat is affecting both the meridian and the organ, the fire-element point and the he-sea shu-point will both be tender.

For the yin meridians, the fire element alarm points are the ying-spring shu-points, and for the yin organs, the water element alarm points are the he-sea shu-points:

	Yin Meridian Ying-spring	Yin Organ He-sea
	FIRE ELEMENT	WATER ELEMENT
LUNG	LU10	LU5
SPLEEN	SP2	SP9
HEART	HT8	HT3
KIDNEY	KD2	KD10
PERICARDIUM	PC8	PC3
LIVER	LV2	LV8

For the yang meridians, the fire element alarm points are the jing-river shu-points, and for the yang organs, the earth element alarm points are the he-sea shu-points:

	Yang Meridian Jing-river	Yang Organ He-sea
	FIRE ELEMENT	EARTH ELEMENT
LARGE INTESTINE	LI5	LI11
STOMACH	ST41	ST36
SMALL INTESTINE	SI5	SI8
URINARY BLADDER	UB60	UB40
TRIPLE BURNER	TB6	TB10
GALLBLADDER	GB38	GB34

6.5 Body-Feedback Referral Areas and Muscle Associations

When an organ is under distress, nerve fibers in the surrounding skin, muscle, connective tissue, and bone cause pain as a result of inflammation (pathogenic heat), fluid retention (dampness), or organ swelling (blood stasis). Any tenderness on the skin's surface, tightness in the muscle layer, or a bruised feeling along the bone in the general region of the organ or along its nerve pathways reflects organ pathology. The exact positioning of the organ varies by person, and therefore, the organ/meridian referral areas represent a general region to palpate looking for the apex of pain.

The Body-Feedback organ/meridian referral areas are similar to some of the organ-referred pain locations recognized by allopathic and chiropractic medicine; however, the Body-Feedback approach differentiates between distinct types of pain and their causes. An organ in a state of deficiency induces dull, empty, or deep pain. An organ in a state of excess generates sharp, distended, or severe surface pain. Some clients are able to distinguish pain sensations and evaluate changes in muscle tone, edema, and skin texture themselves. Carefully assess the skin, muscle, and circulation at the organ associations each session to monitor the treatment response.

The Body-Feedback muscle associations are a combination of the acupuncture sinew (collateral) channels and the meridian muscle associations used by Dr. George Goodheart and the Touch for Health organization. Through clinical experience, it is clear that organ pathology also reflects in the meridian muscle associations outlined by Dr. Goodheart and Touch for Health. Nerve pain, spinal conditions, and organ dysfunction commonly cause idiopathic muscle pain and tightness. Acute organ/meridian excess or deficiency will cause the associated muscle groups to become tight and tender. Long-term organ/meridian pathology can cause the muscle association to become flaccid and weak.

For pain conditions with inflamed and swollen areas, excessive palpation can aggravate the pain receptors. In this instance, avoid local palpation and utilize the related testing locations to check acupoints and essential oils. At the end of a session, test supplements and herbs to the master points or pulse first and then recheck them to the area of pain to ensure the best choice. Double-checking the beneficial treatment options to the area of pain will identify the ones with the most significant potential benefit. Clients are more likely to follow up with essential oils, herbs, and supplements when they can feel the reduction in pain during a Body-Feedback testing session.

Palpating and evaluating the Body-Feedback testing locations becomes an interactive physical dialogue between the body, the client, and the practitioner. The information gathered during this assessment provides intricate details to illuminate a superior path for long-term healing and optimizing health. Over time, clients become more aware of subtle changes in discomfort throughout the body, and they often remember to identify these for early detection at their maintenance acupuncture appointments.

When the same meridian and organ associations remain painful at multiple sessions, further investigation into heavy metals, low-grade infections, genetic factors, and exposure to environmental toxins may reveal causes of continued compromised health. Other hidden reasons for the Body-Feedback areas to remain painful include allergies, food intolerance, autoimmune conditions, toxic beauty products, electrical sensitivity, and low-quality food or water. Teaching a client how to monitor their most sensitive testing locations provides information on how long the acupuncture sessions are holding and when to rotate or change herbs and supplements.

Master Body-Feedback Alarm Points and Regions

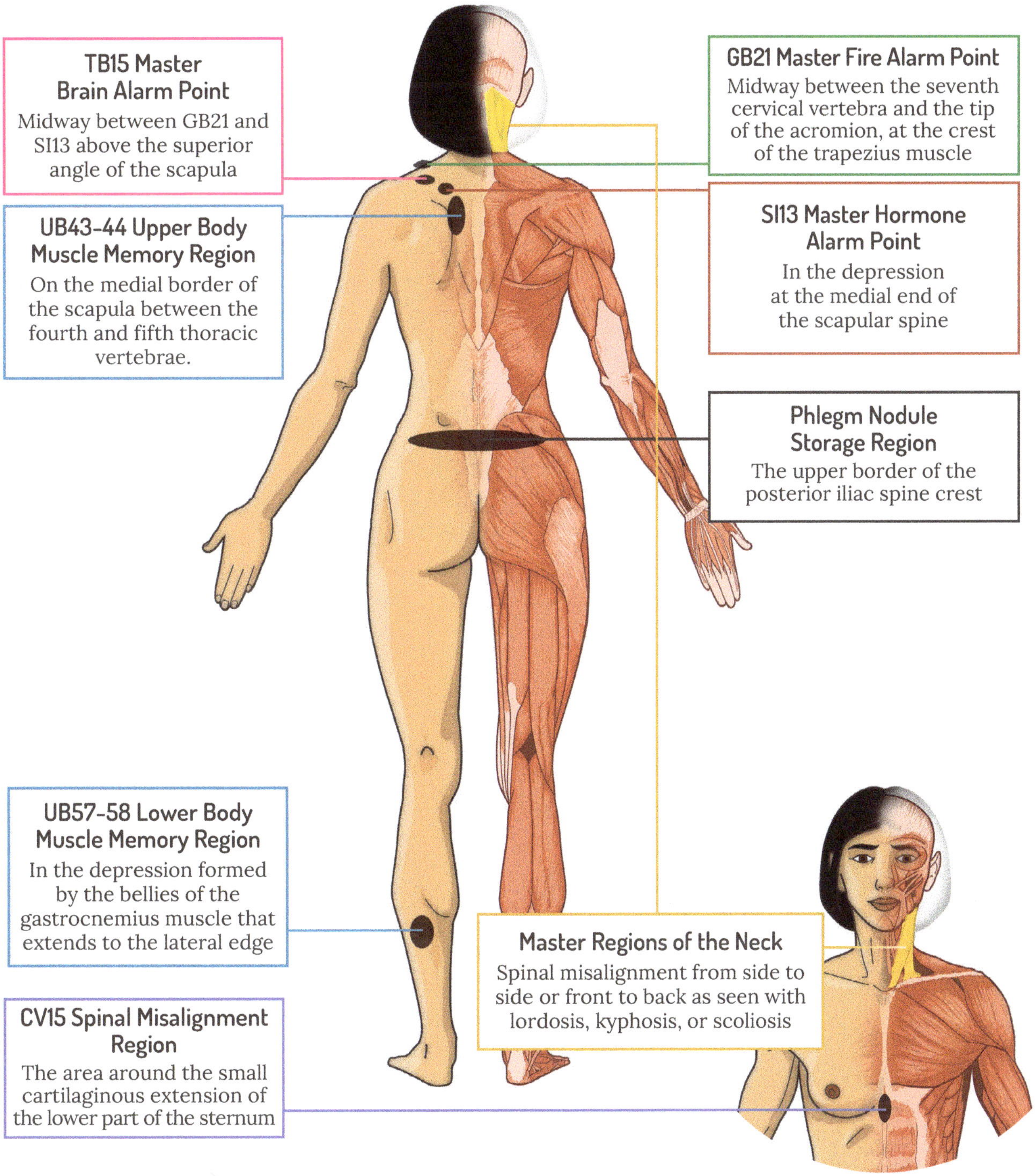

Lung Body-Feedback Testing Locations

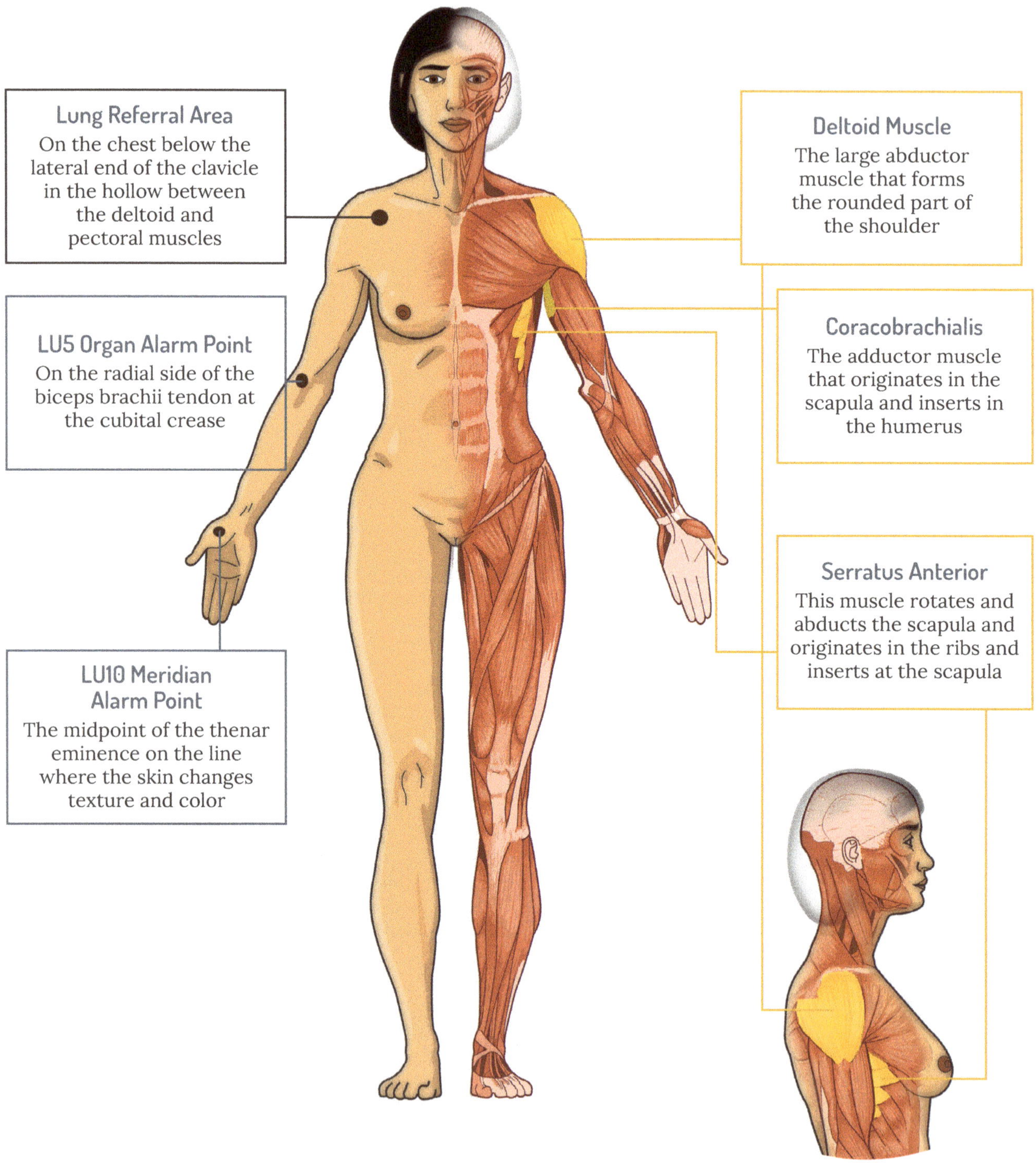

Lung Meridian and Organ Alarm Points

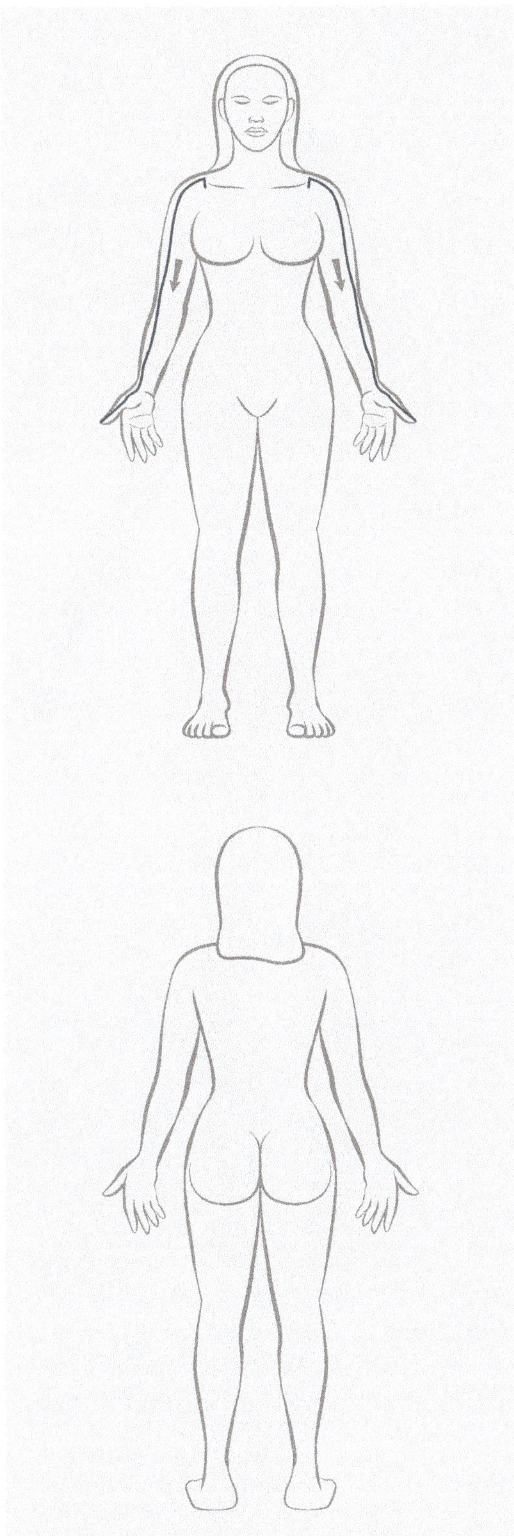

On the radial side of the biceps brachii tendon at the cubital crease

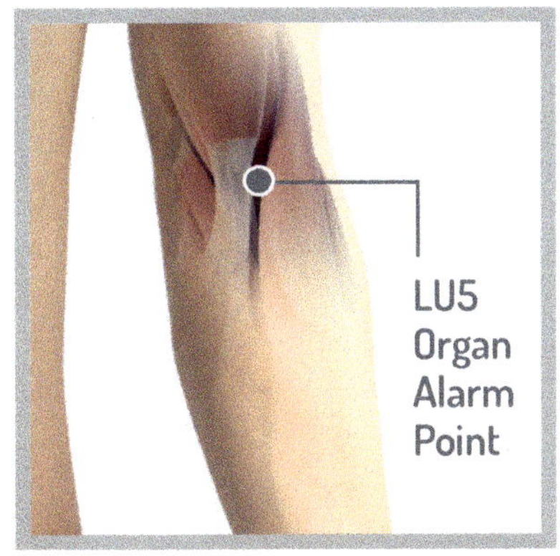

The midpoint of the thenar eminence on the line where the skin changes texture and color

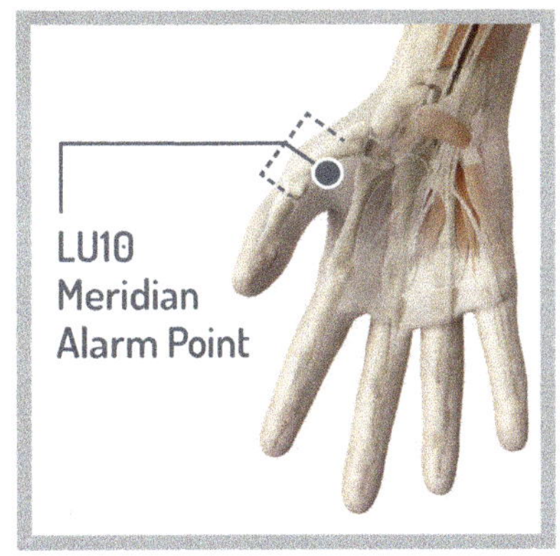

Large Intestine Body-Feedback Testing Locations

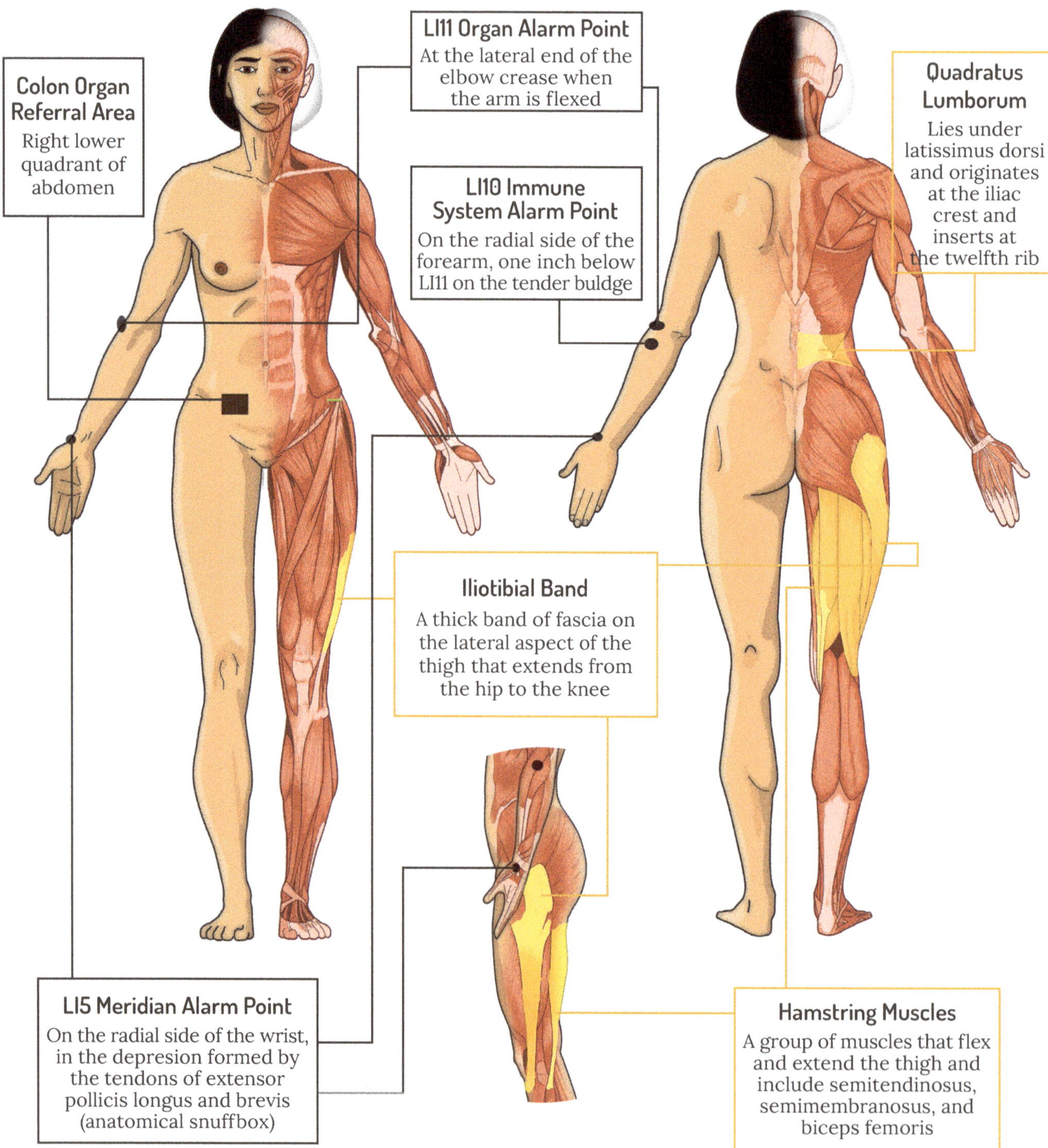

Large Intestine Meridian and Organ Alarm Points

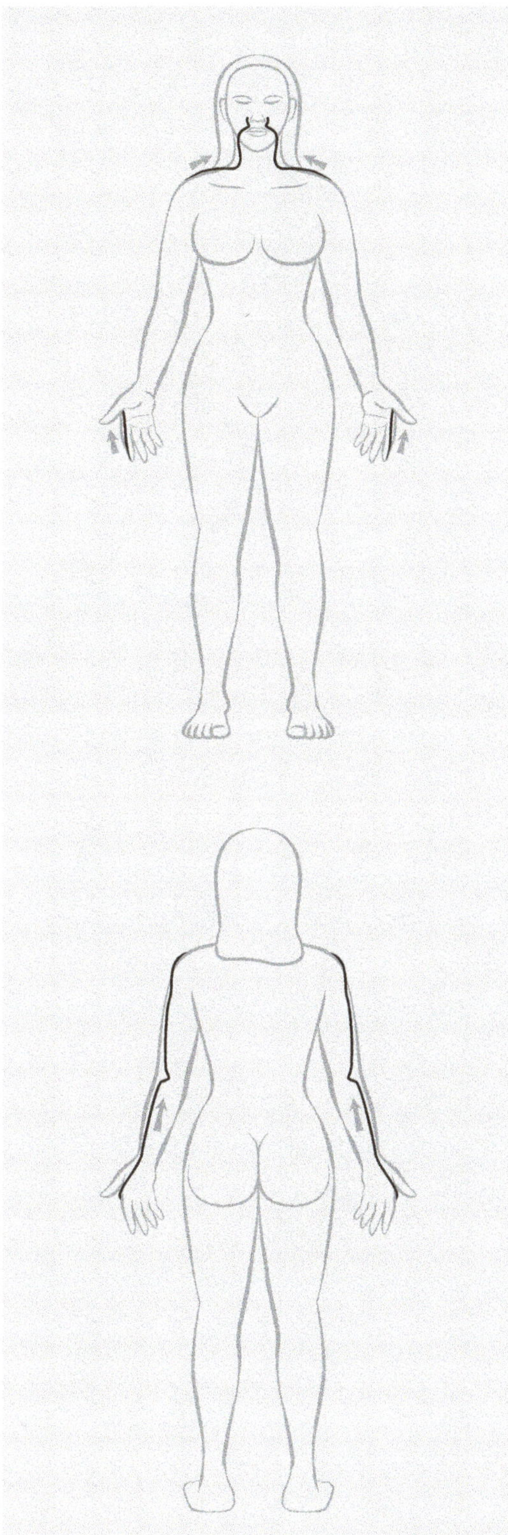

On the radial side of the wrist, in the depression formed by the tendons of extensor pollicis longus and brevis (anatomical snuffbox)

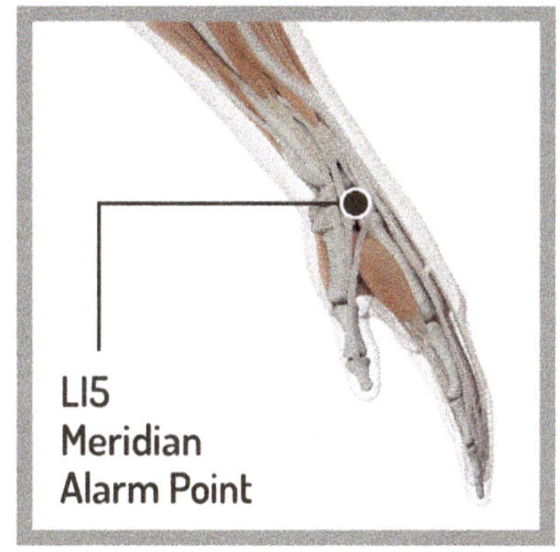

On the radial side of the forearm, one inch below LI11 on the tender bulge

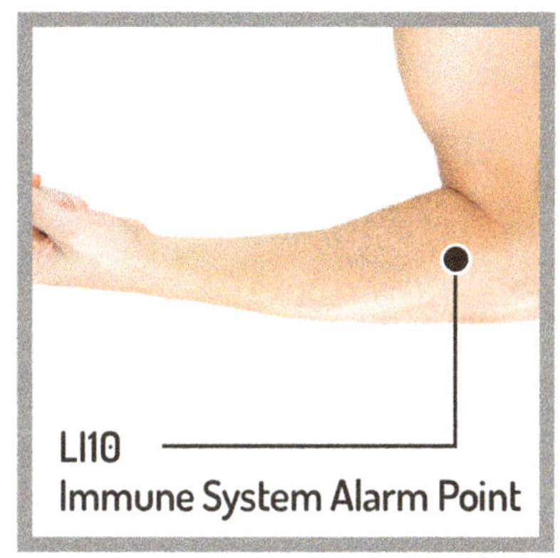

At the lateral end of the elbow crease when the arm is flexed

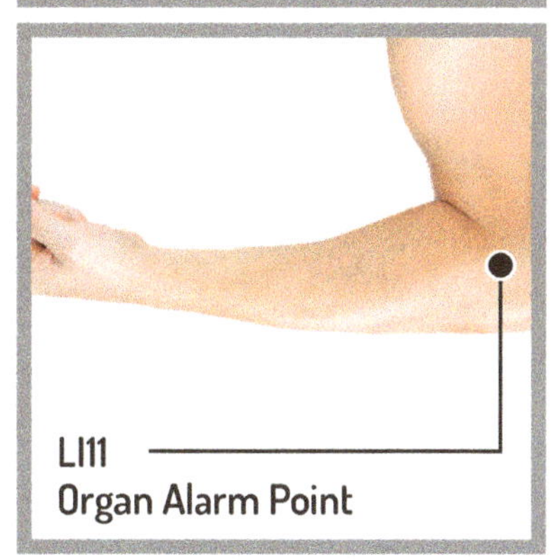

Stomach Body-Feedback Testing Locations

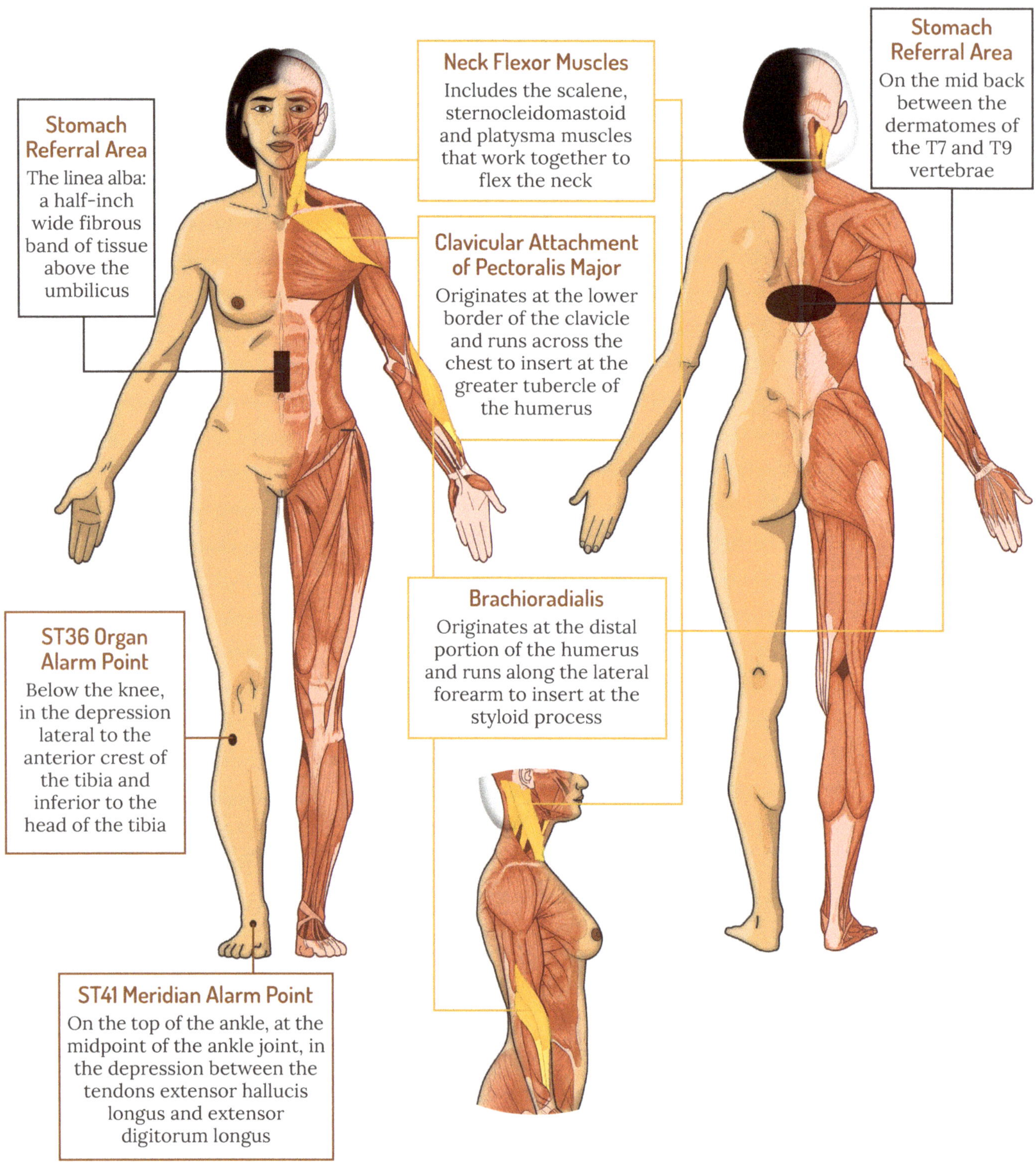

Stomach Meridian and Organ Alarm Points

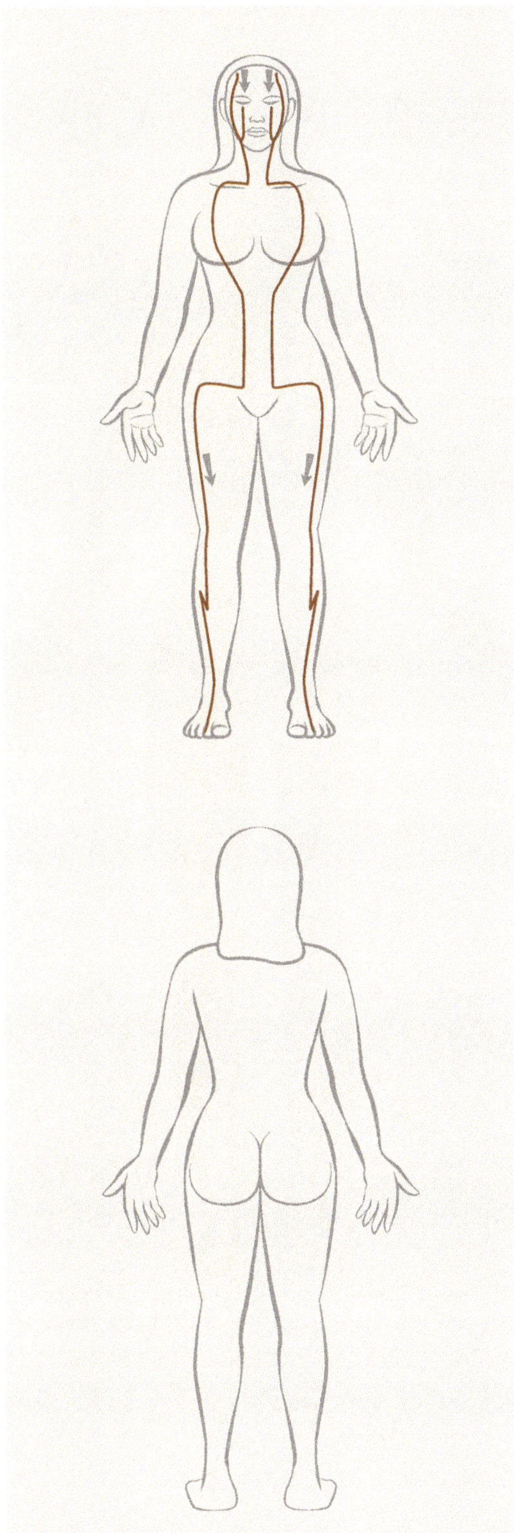

Below the knee, in the depression lateral to the anterior crest of the tibia and inferior to the head of the tibia

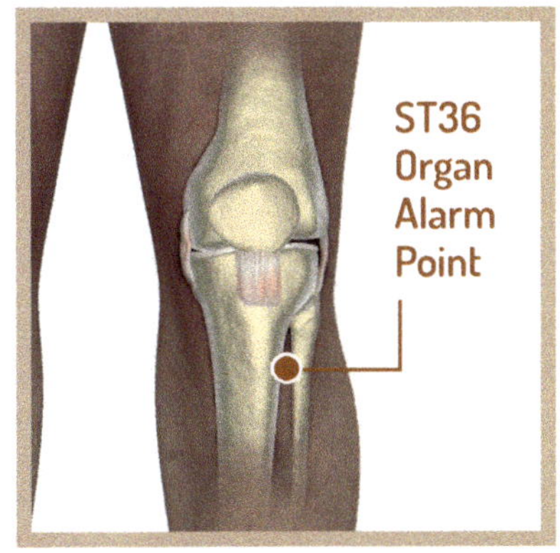

On the top of the ankle, at the midpoint of the ankle joint, in the depression between the tendons extensor hallucis longus and extensor digitorum longus

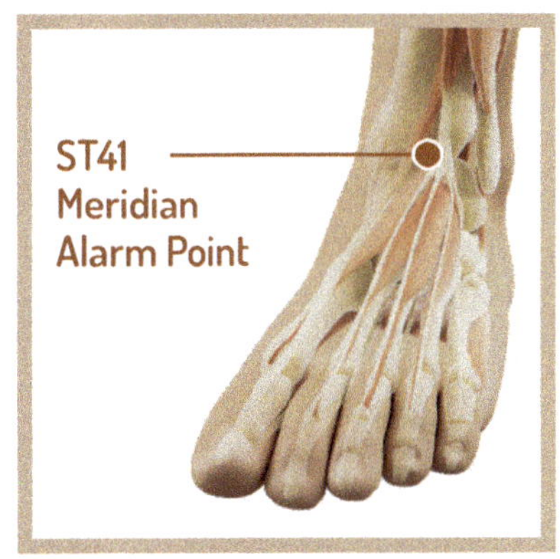

Spleen Body-Feedback Testing Locations

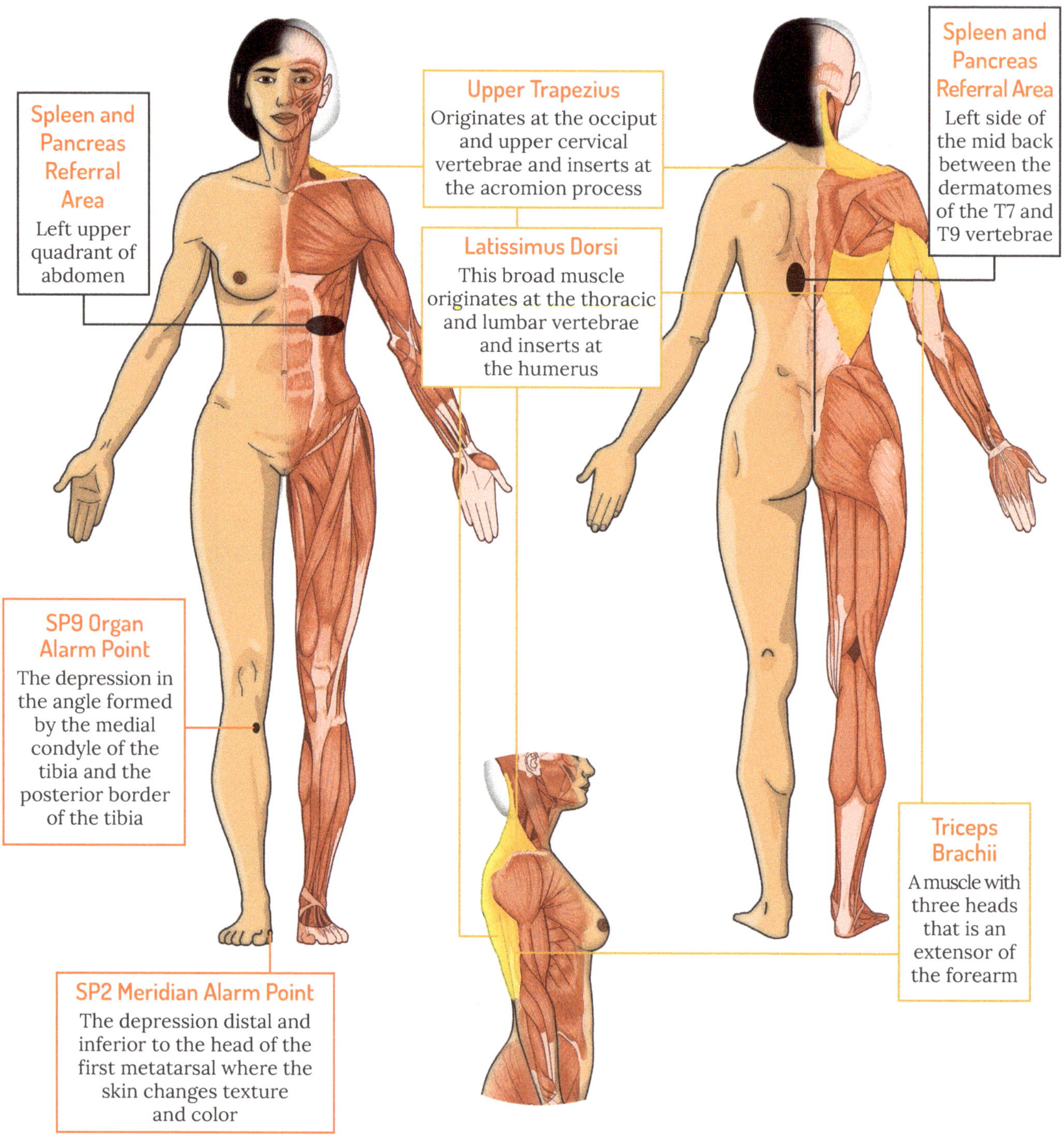

Spleen Meridian and Organ Alarm Points

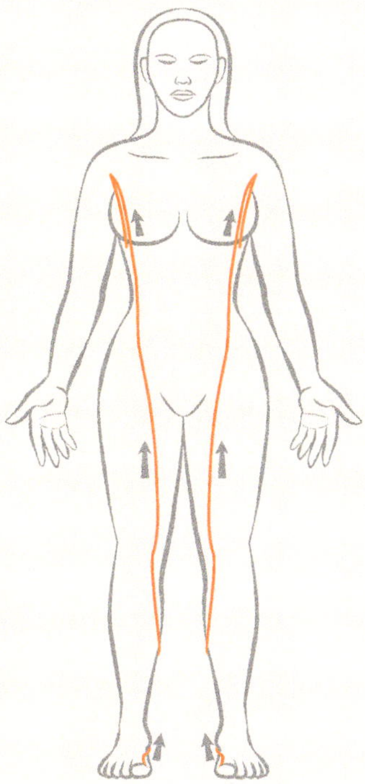

The depression distal and inferior to the head of the first metatarsal where the skin changes texture and color

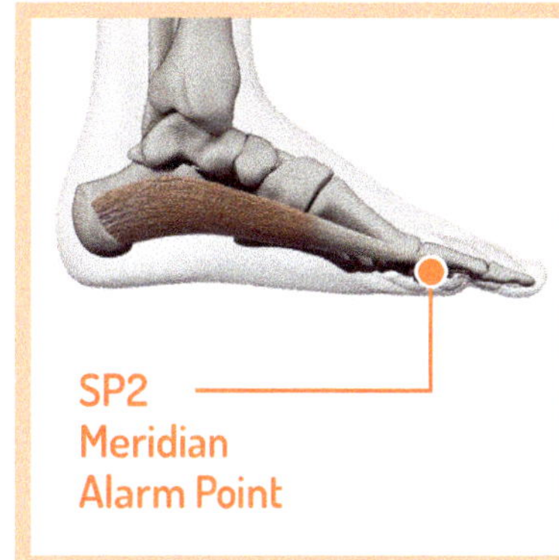

The depression in the angle formed by the medial condyle of the tibia and the posterior border of the tibia

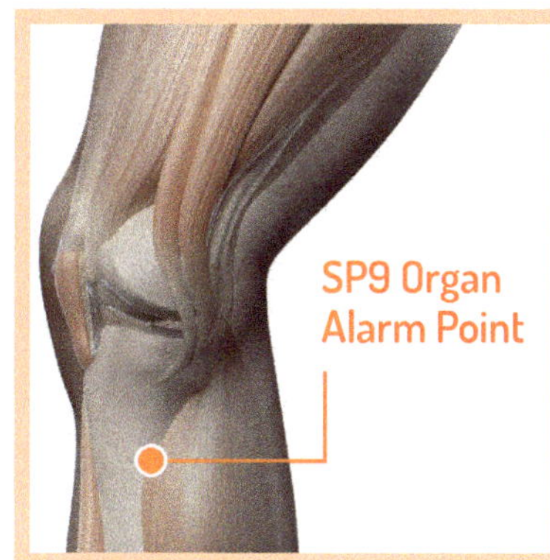

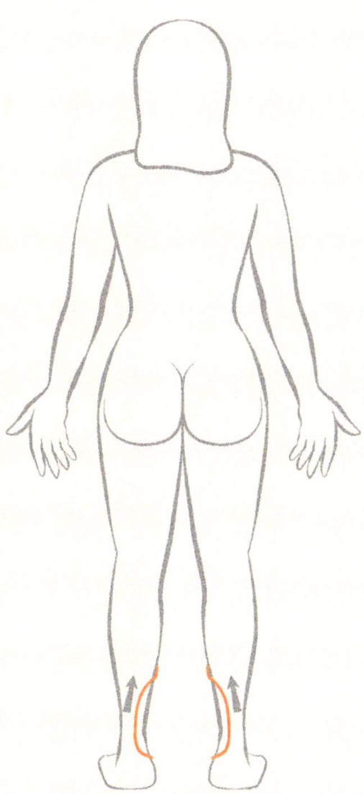

Heart Body-Feedback Testing Locations

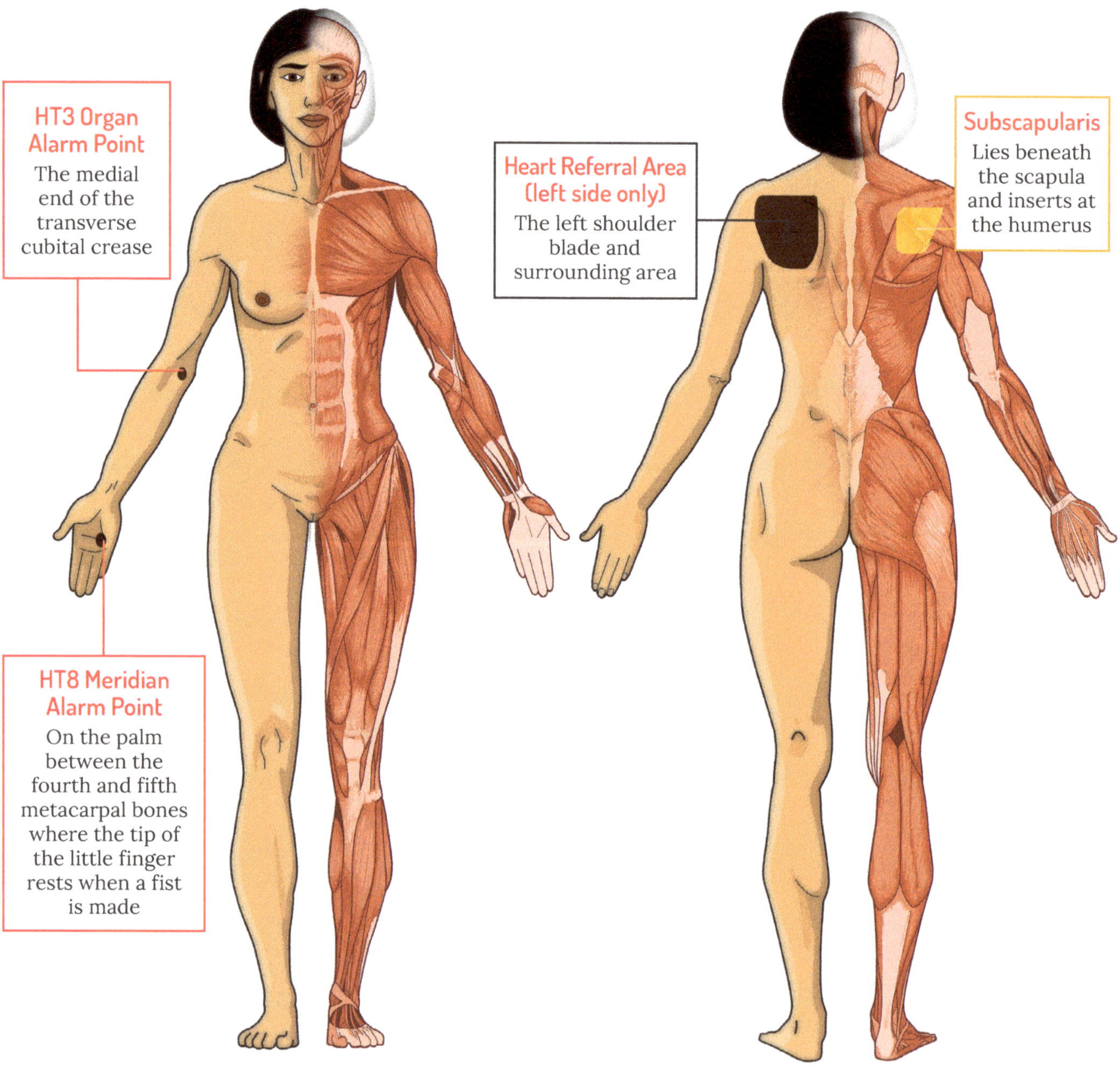

Heart Meridian and Organ Alarm Points

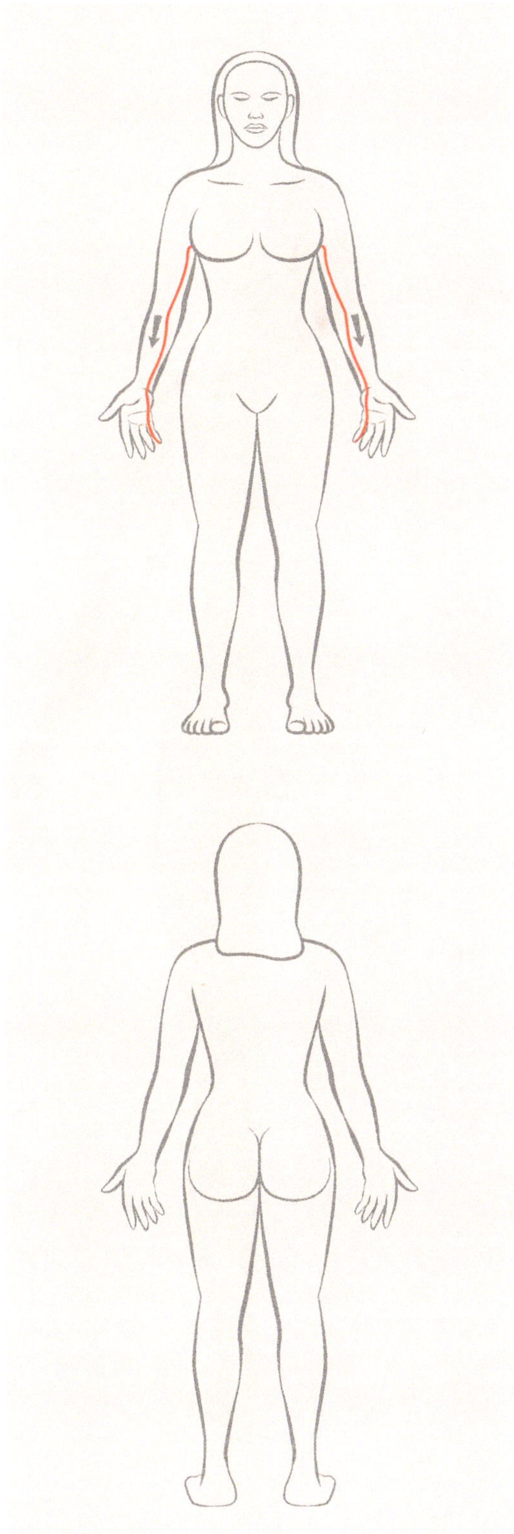

The medial end of the transverse cubital crease

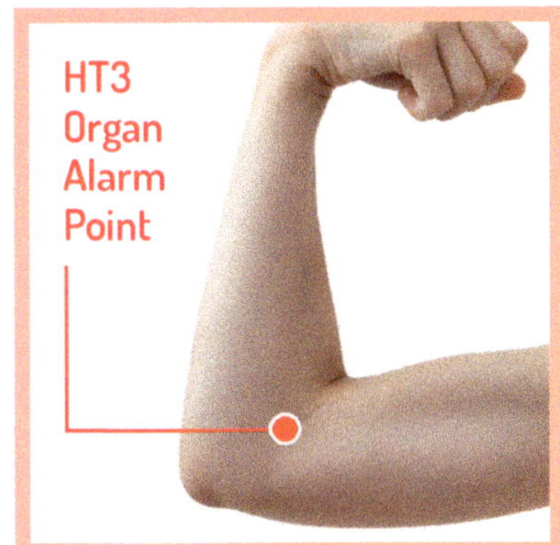

On the palm between the fourth and fifth metacarpal bones where the tip of the little finger rests when a fist is made

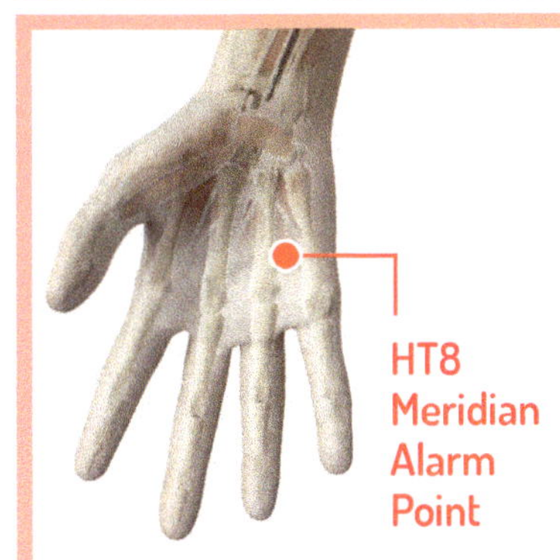

Small Intestine Body-Feedback Testing Locations

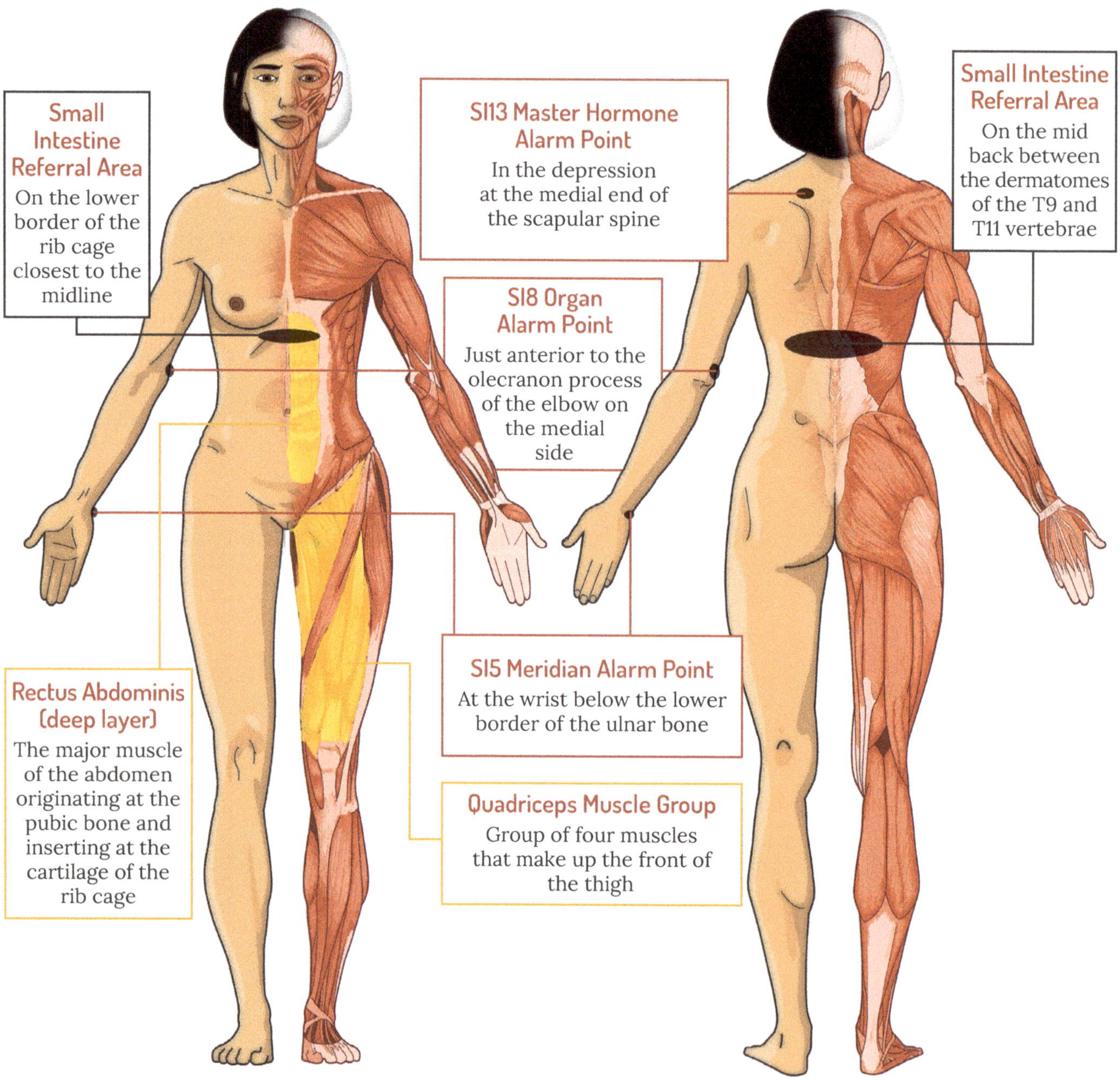

Small Intestine Meridian and Organ Alarm Points

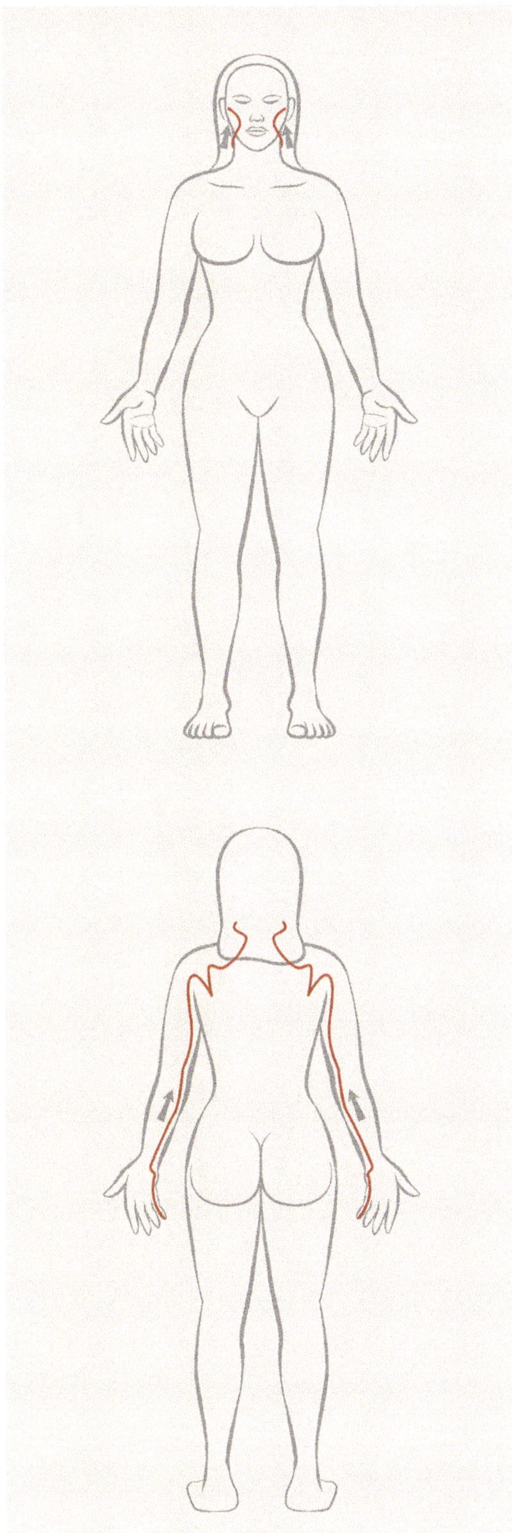

At the wrist below the lower border of the ulnar bone

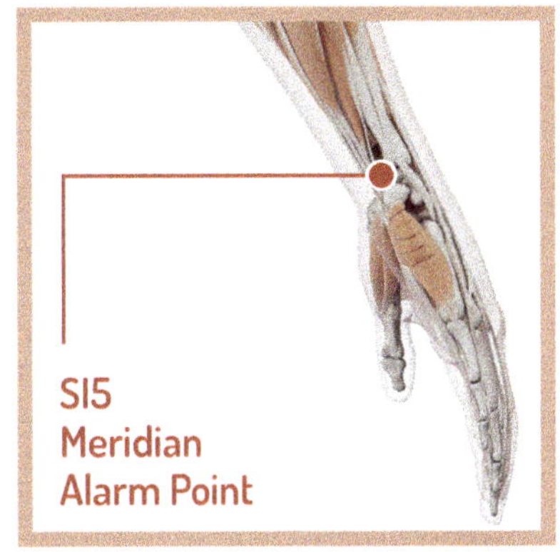

Just anterior to the olecranon process of the elbow on the medial side

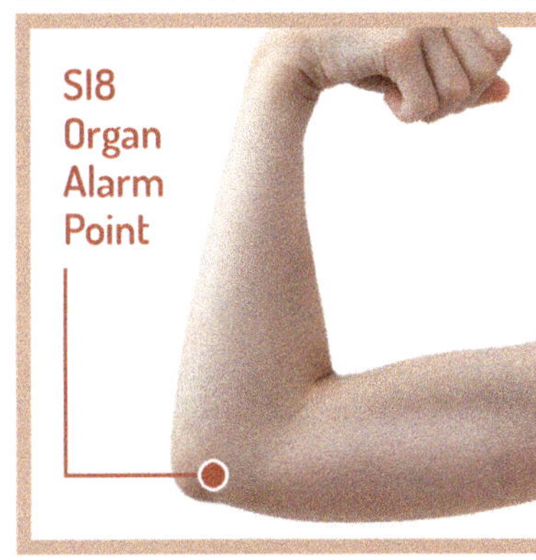

In the depression at the medial end of the scapular spine

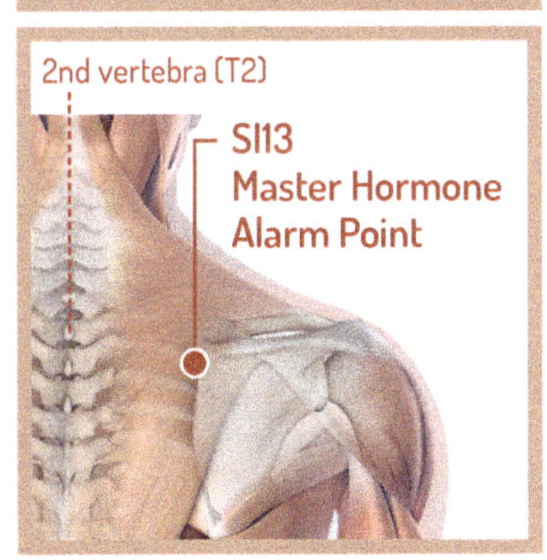

Urinary Bladder Body-Feedback Testing Locations

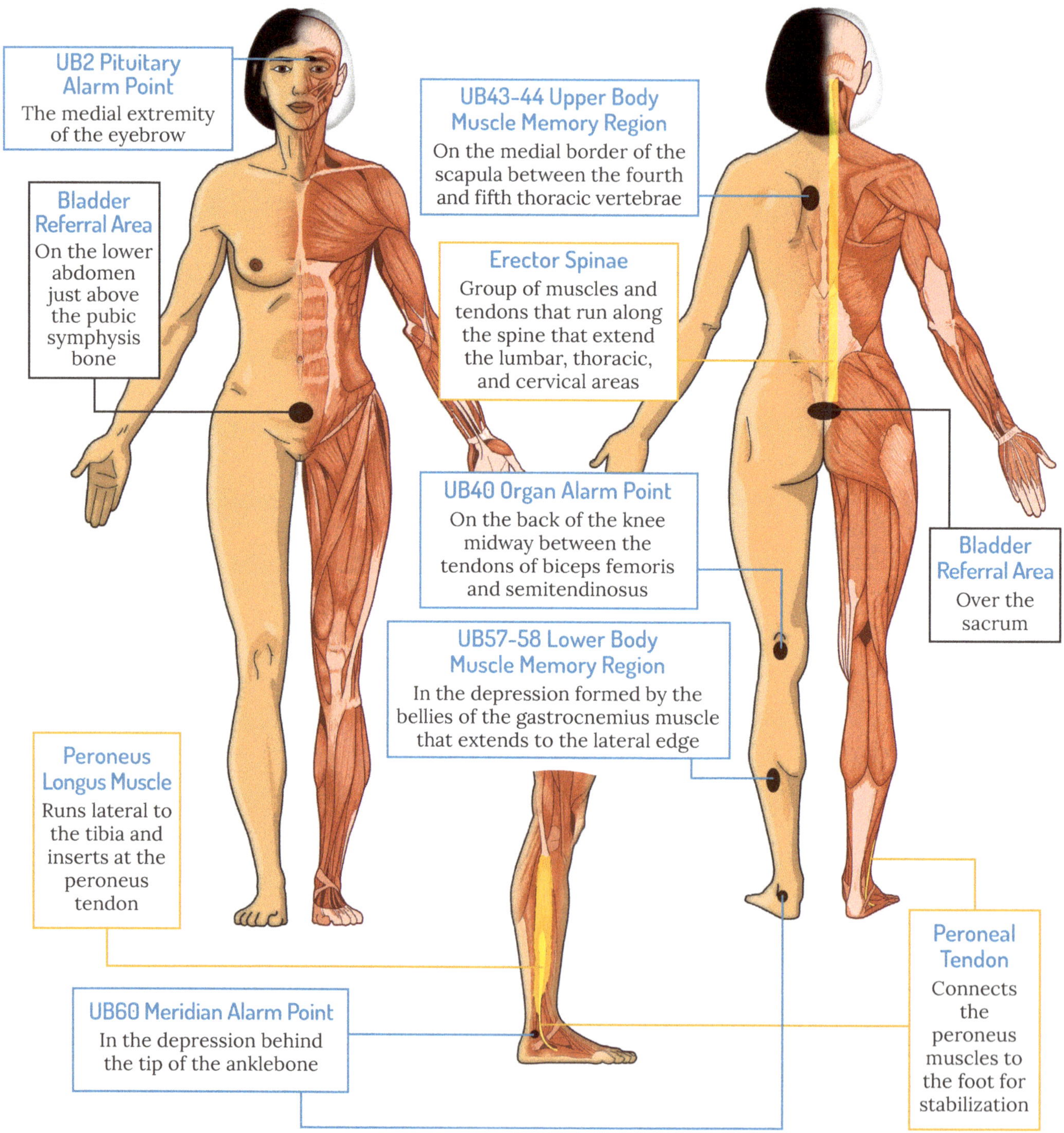

Urinary Bladder Meridian and Organ Alarm Points

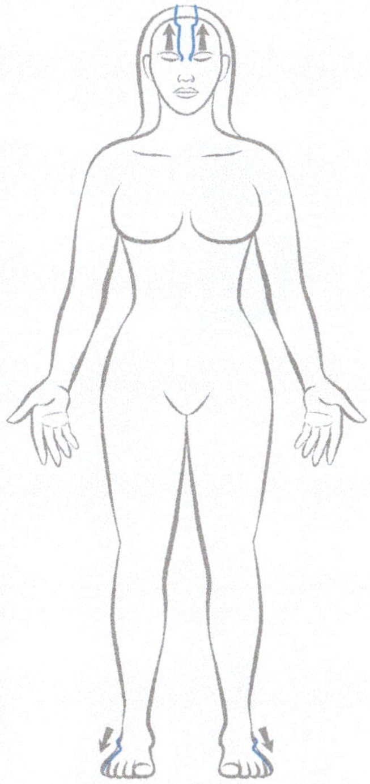

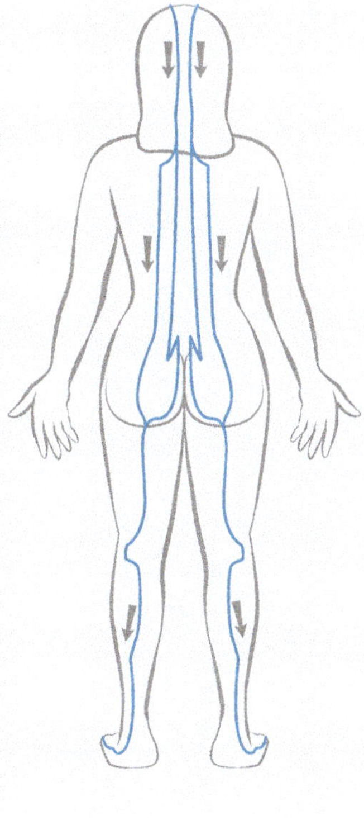

The medial extremity of the eyebrow

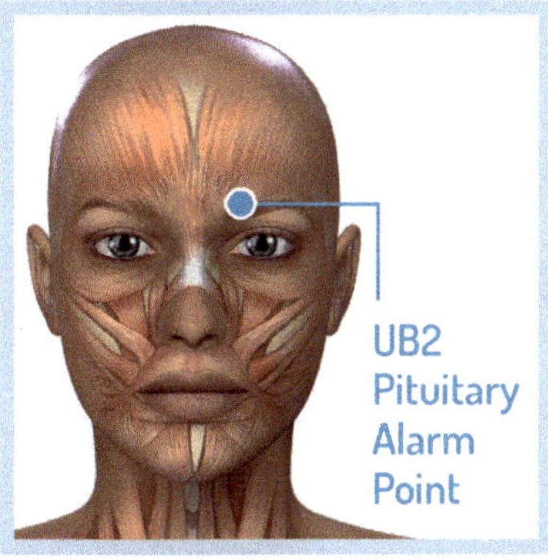

On the back of the knee midway between the tendons of biceps femoris and semitendinosus

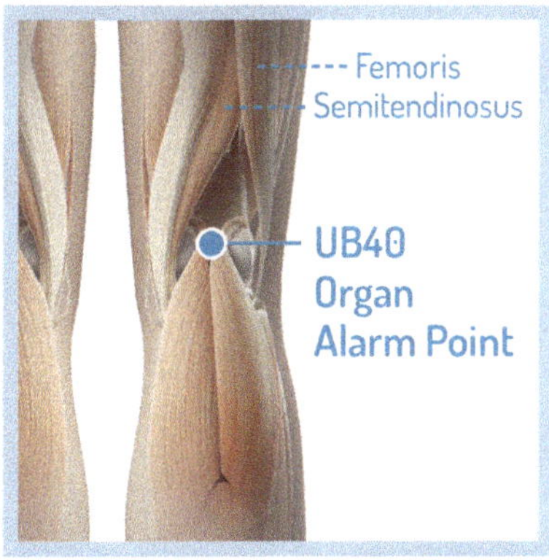

In the depression behind the tip of the anklebone

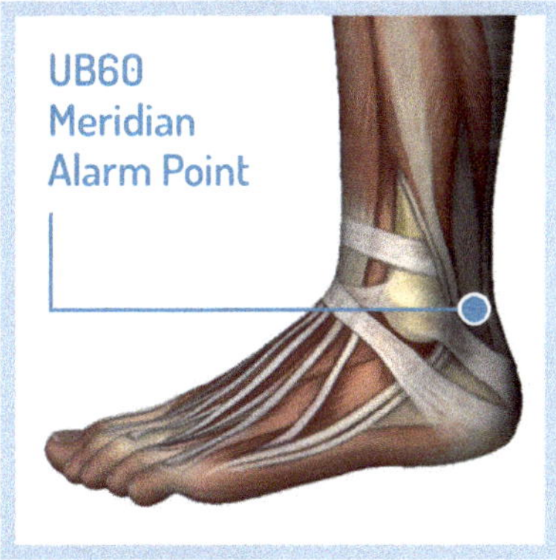

Kidney Body-Feedback Testing Locations

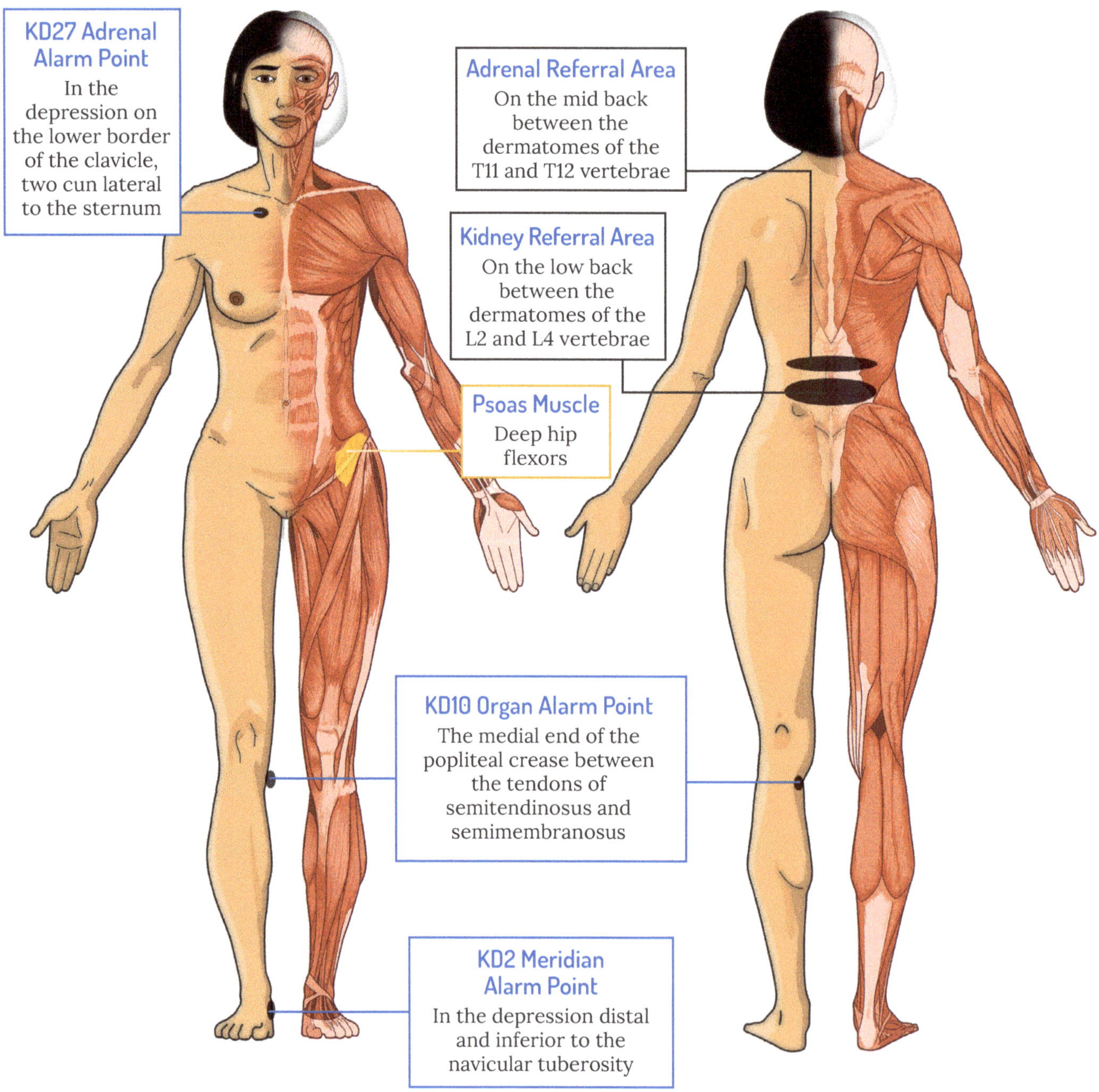

Kidney Meridian and Organ Alarm Points

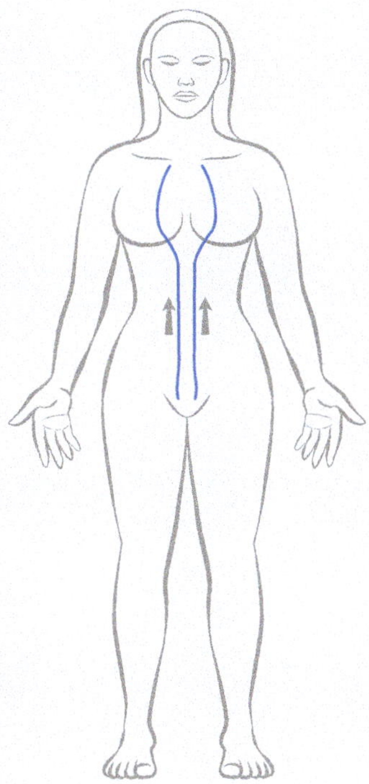

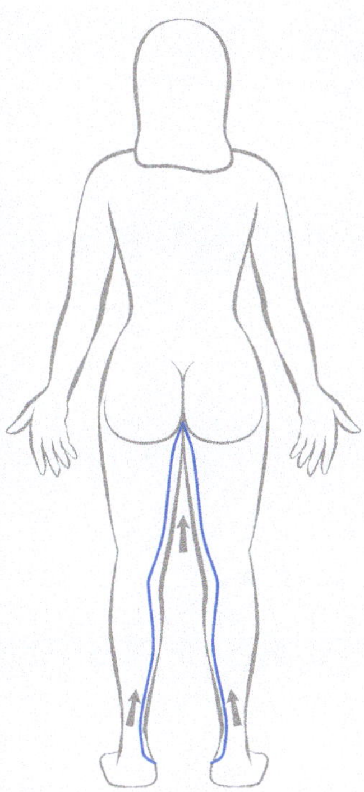

In the depression distal and inferior to the navicular tuberosity

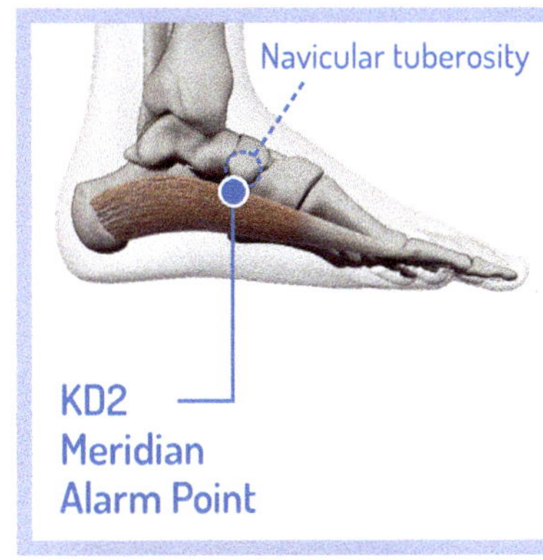

The medial end of the popliteal crease between the tendons of semitendinosus and semimembranosus

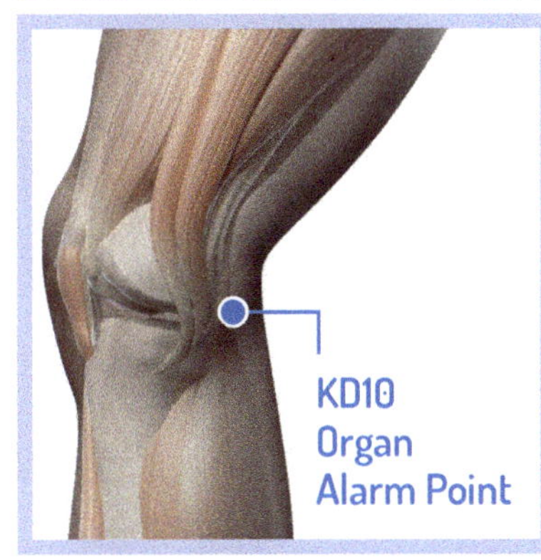

In the depression on the lower border of the clavicle, two cun lateral to the sternum

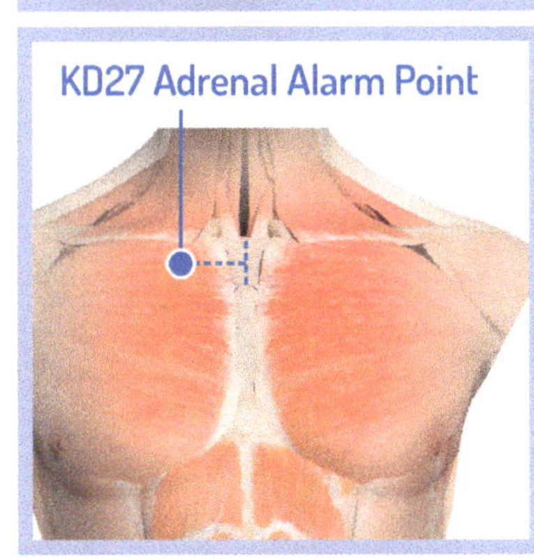

Pericardium Body-Feedback Testing Locations

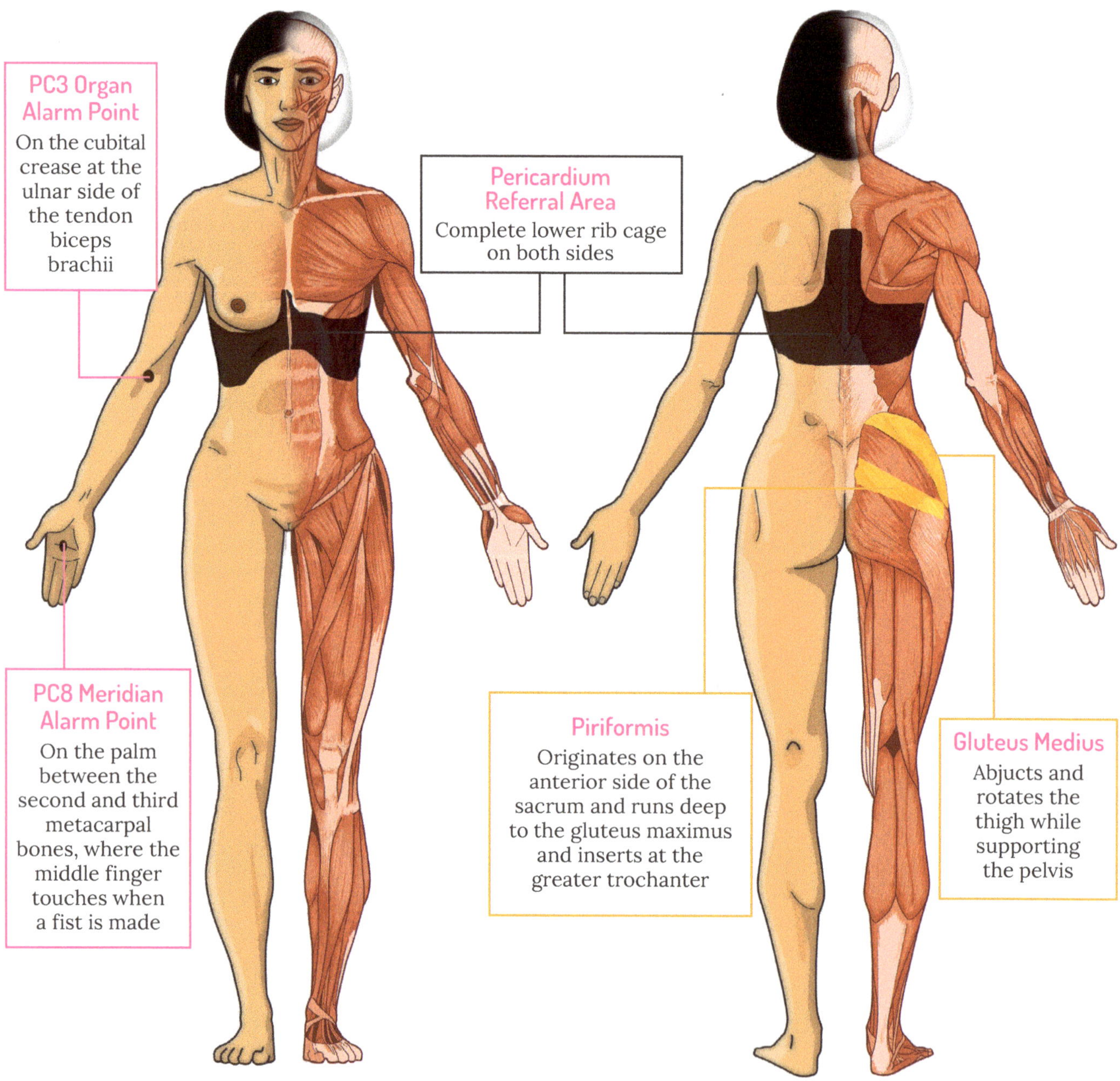

Pericardium Meridian and Organ Alarm Points

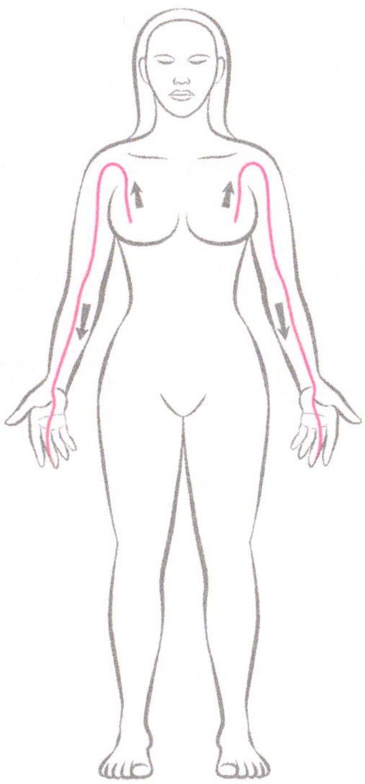

On the cubital crease at the ulnar side of the tendon biceps brachii

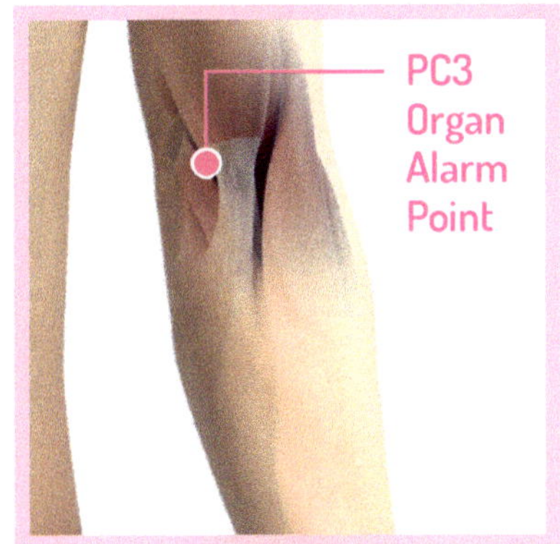

On the palm between the second and third metacarpal bones, where the middle finger touches when a fist is made

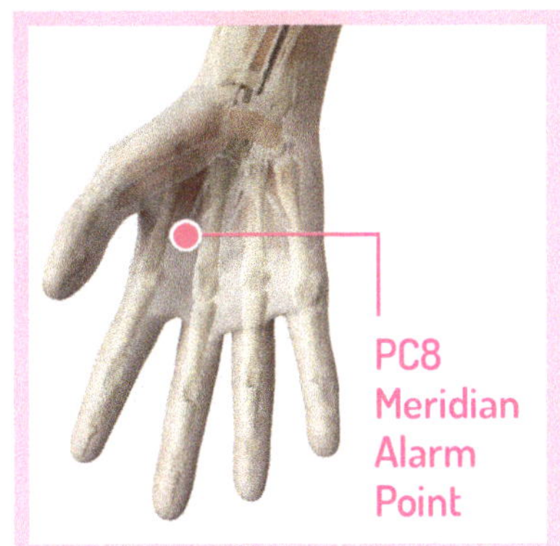

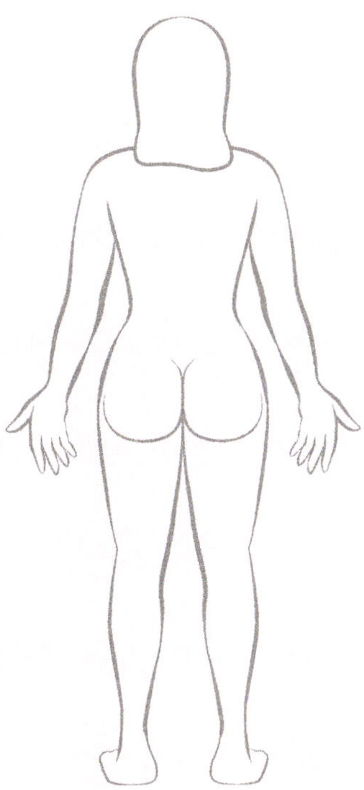

Triple Burner Body-Feedback Testing Locations

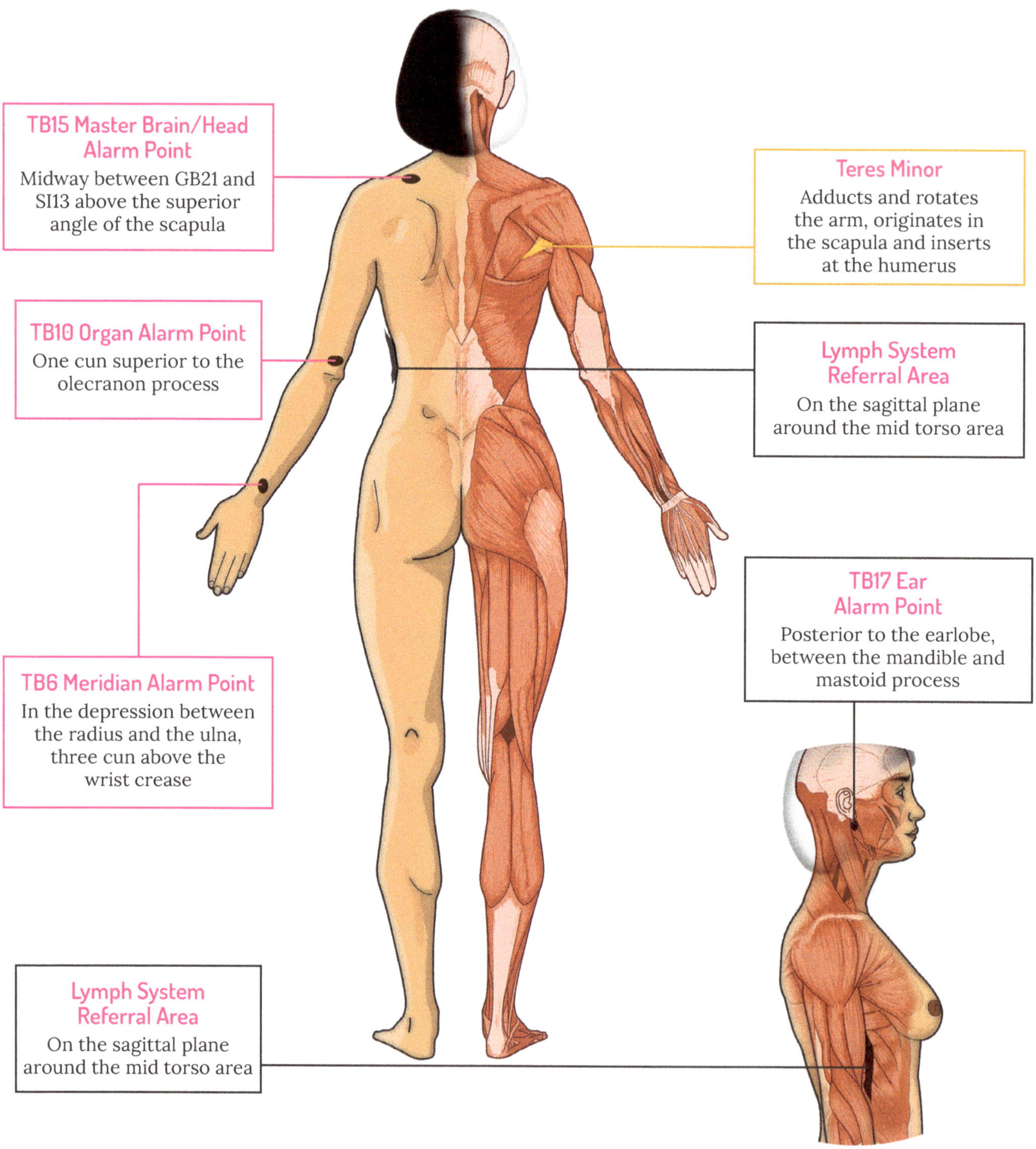

Triple Burner Meridian and Organ Alarm Points

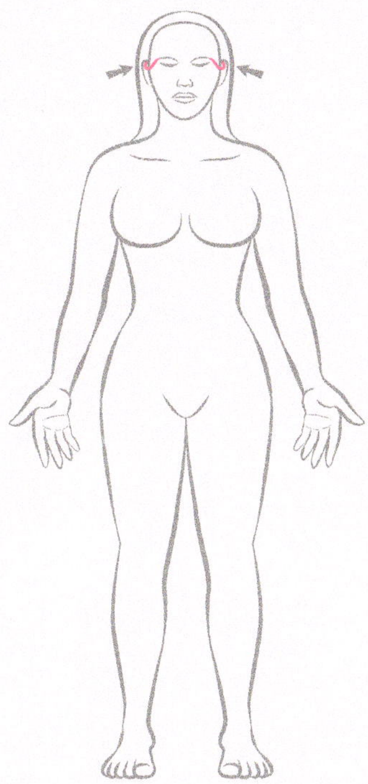

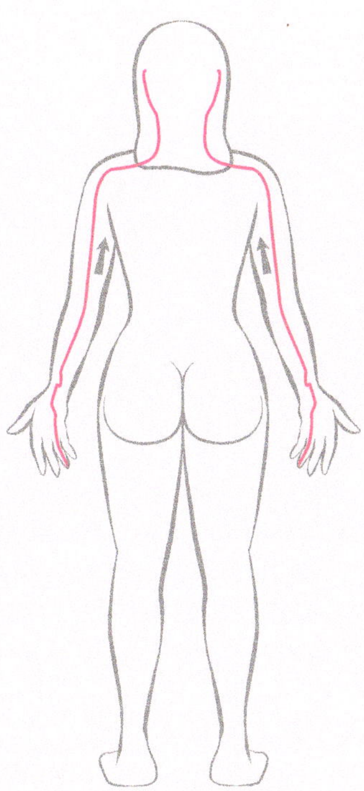

In the depression between the radius and the ulna, three cun above the wrist crease

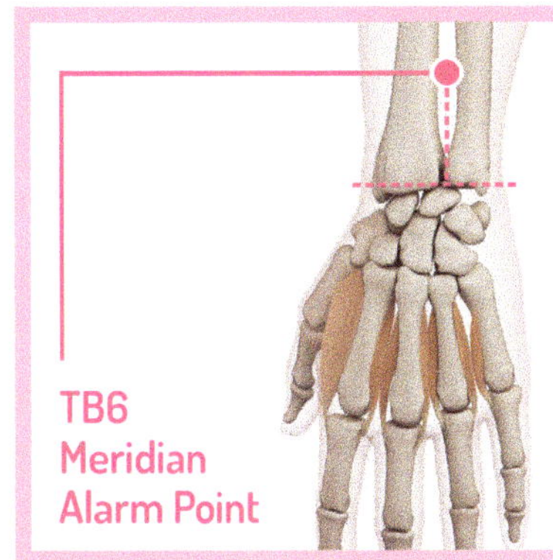

One cun superior to the olecranon process

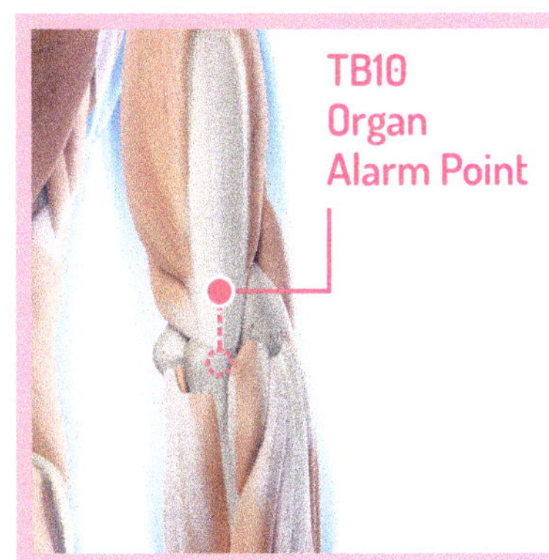

Midway between GB21 and SI13 above the superior angle of the scapula

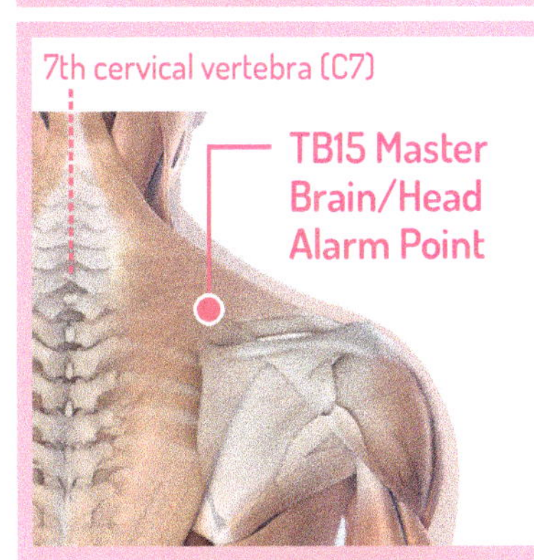

Posterior to the earlobe, between the mandible and mastoid process

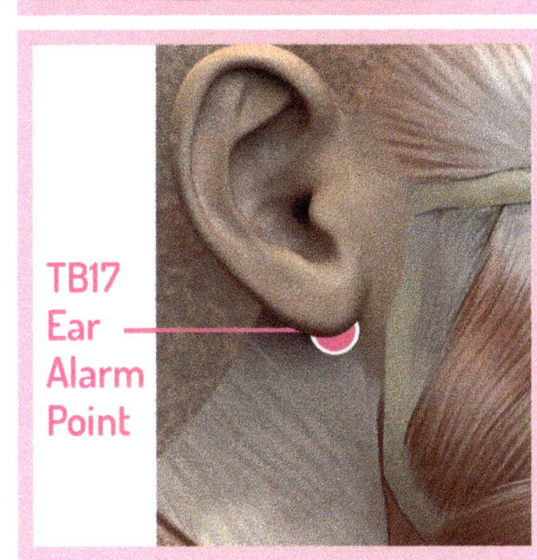

Gallbladder Body-Feedback Testing Locations

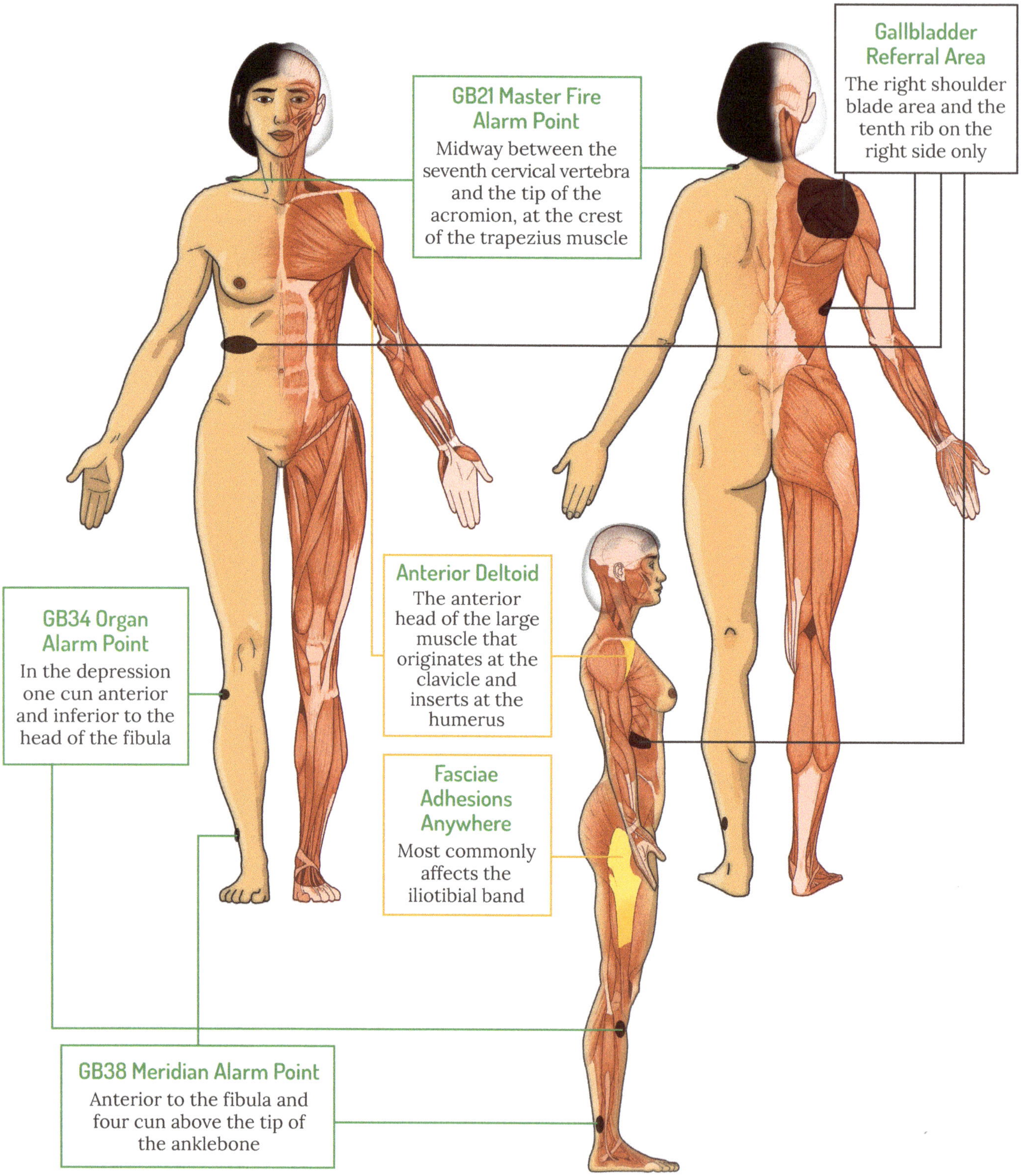

Gallbladder Meridian and Organ Alarm Points

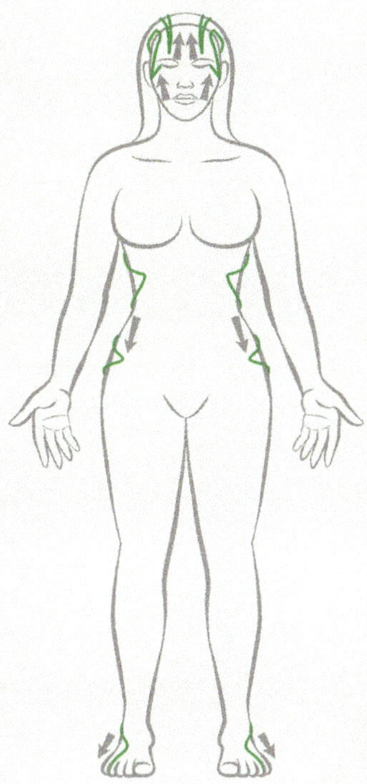

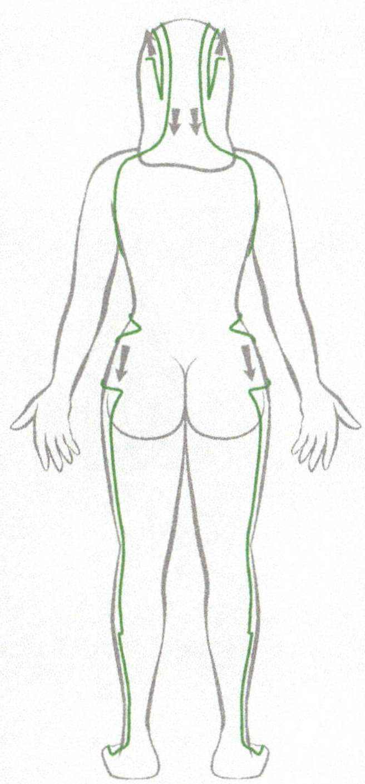

Midway between the seventh cervical vertebra and the tip of the acromion, at the crest of the trapezius muscle

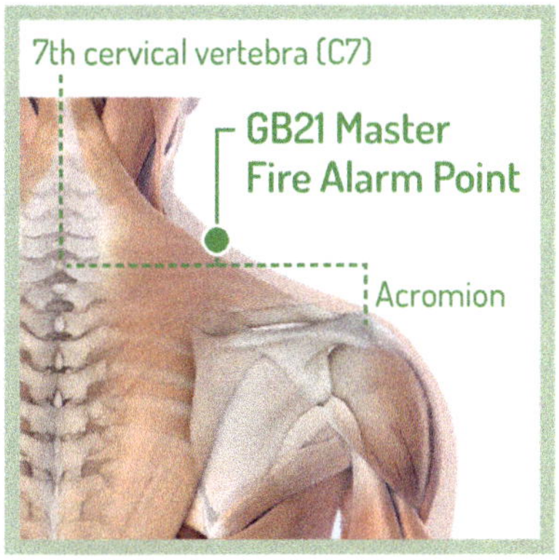

In the depression one cun anterior and inferior to the head of the fibula

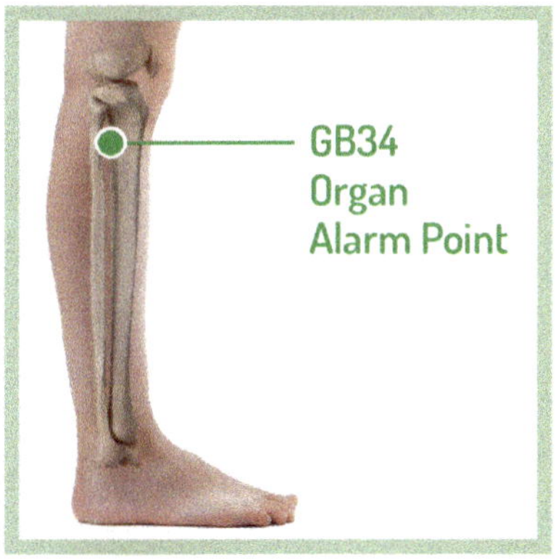

Anterior to the fibula and four cun above the tip of the anklebone

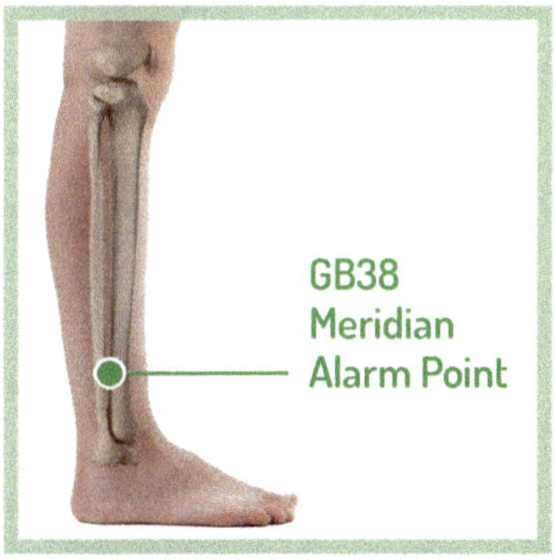

Liver Body-Feedback Testing Locations

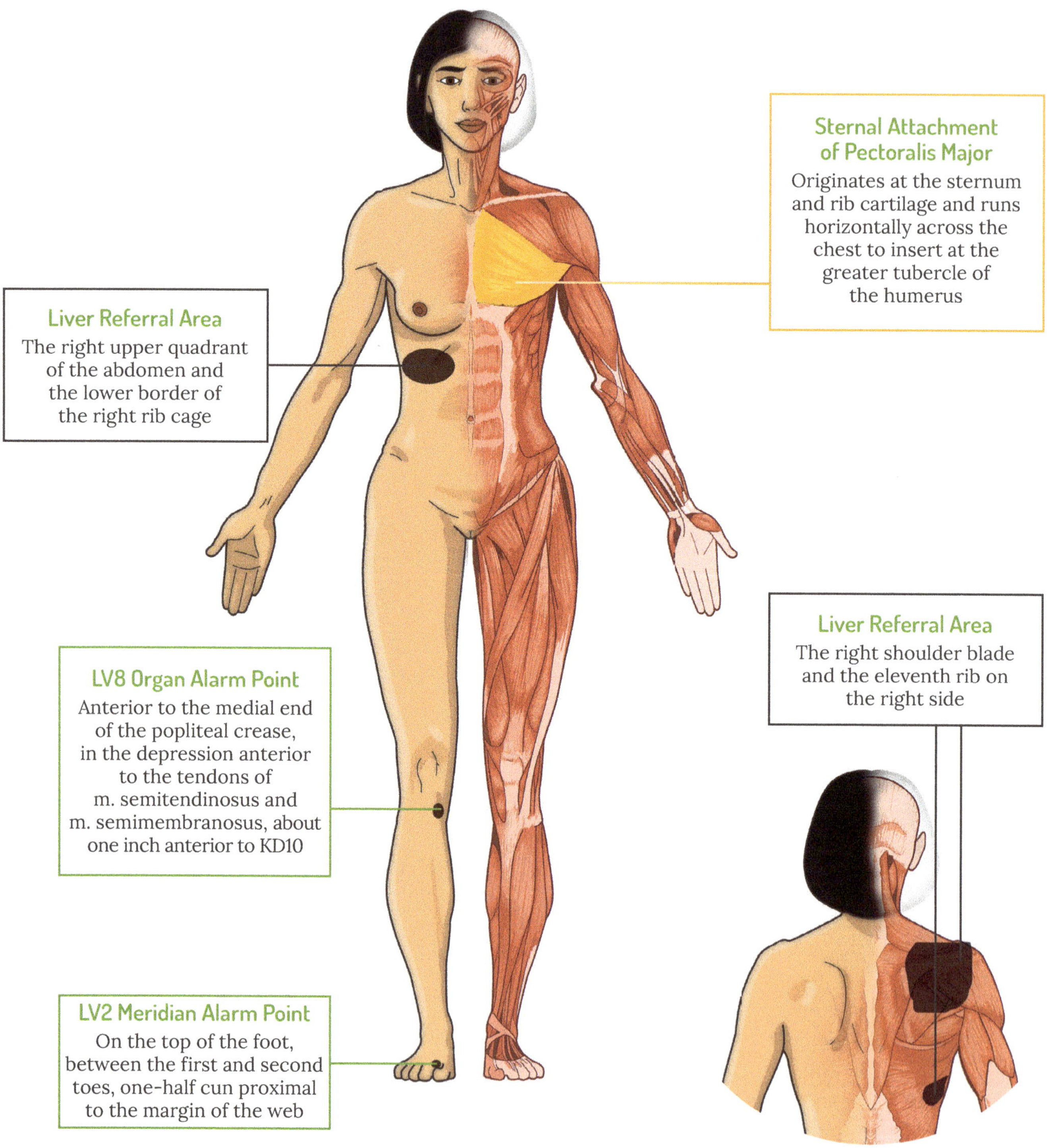

Liver Meridian and Organ Alarm Points

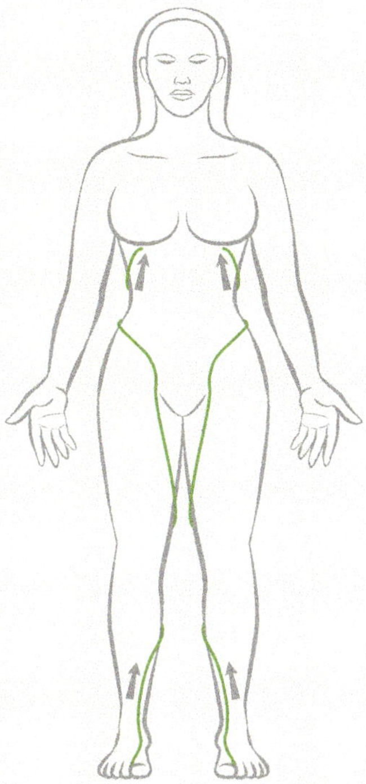

On the top of the foot, between the first and second toes, one-half cun proximal to the margin of the web

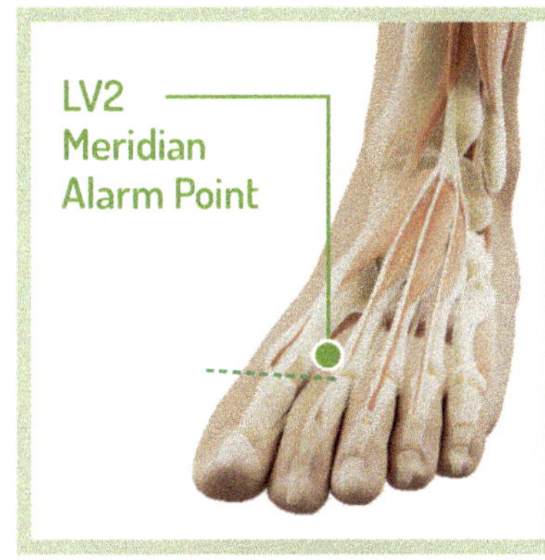

Anterior to the medial end of the popliteal crease, in the depression anterior to the tendons of m. semitendinosus and m. semimembranosus, about one inch anterior to KD-10

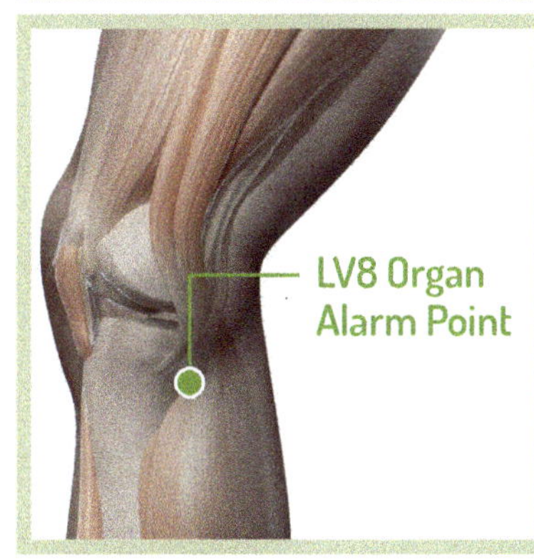

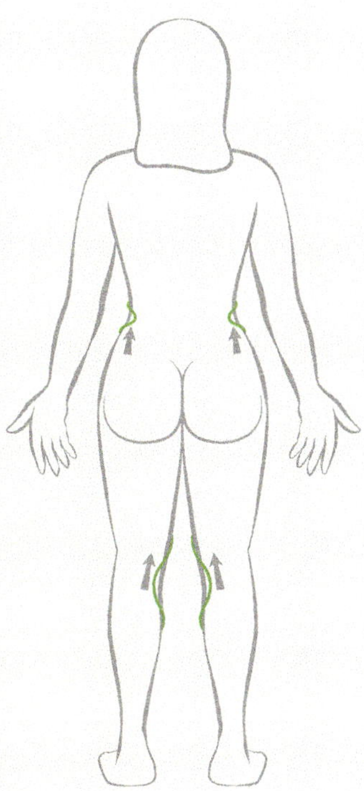

Conception Vessel Body-Feedback Testing Locations

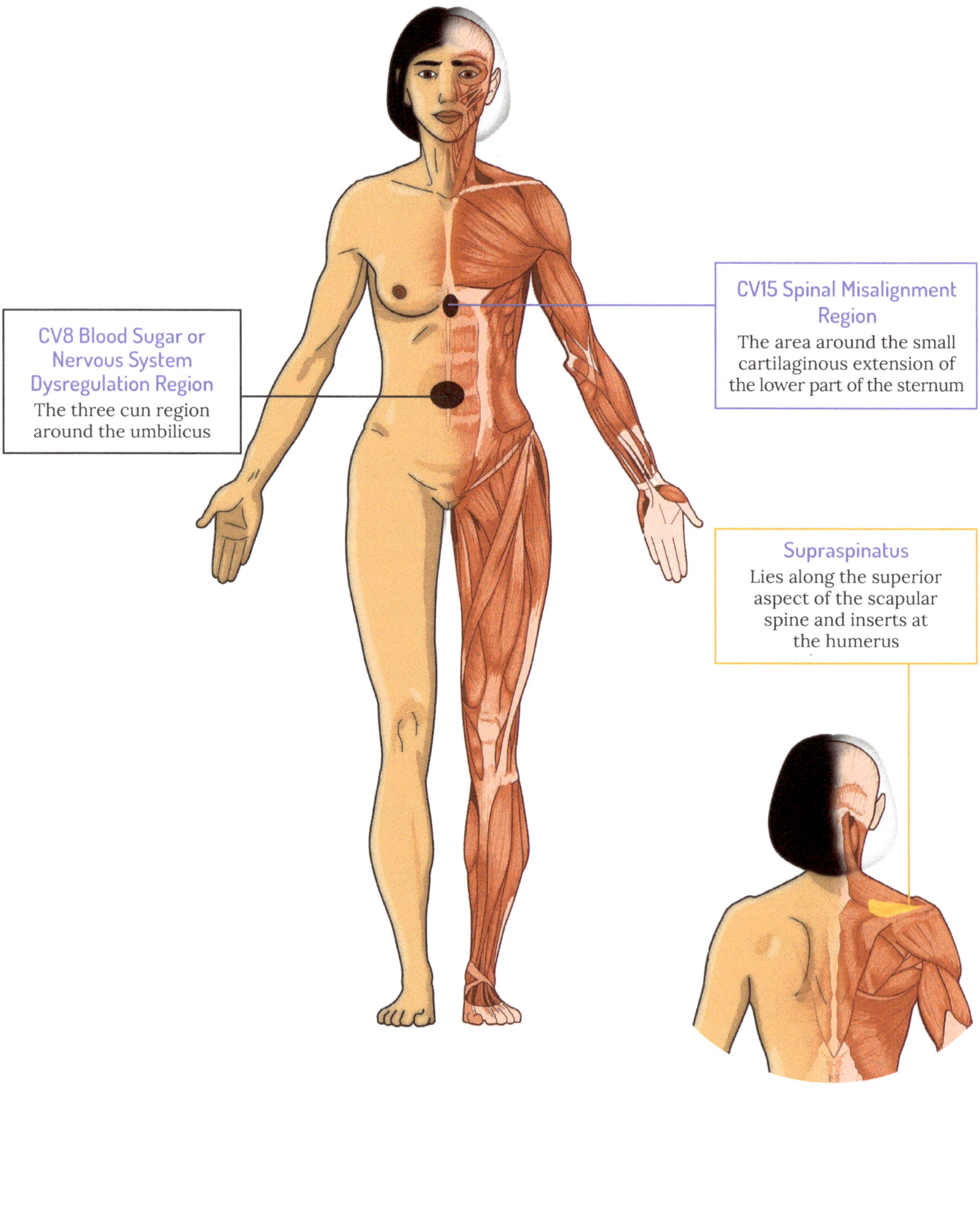

Conception Vessel Alarm Points

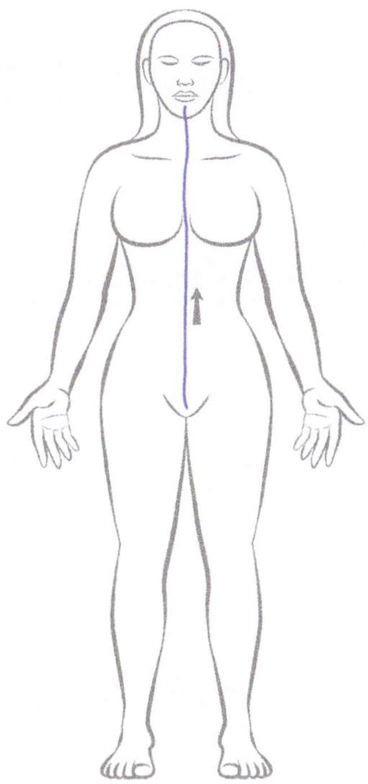

The small cartilaginous extension of the lower part of the sternum

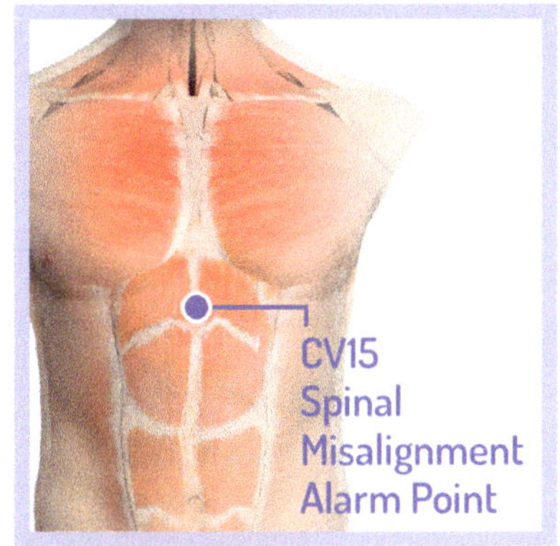

The three cun region around the umbilicus

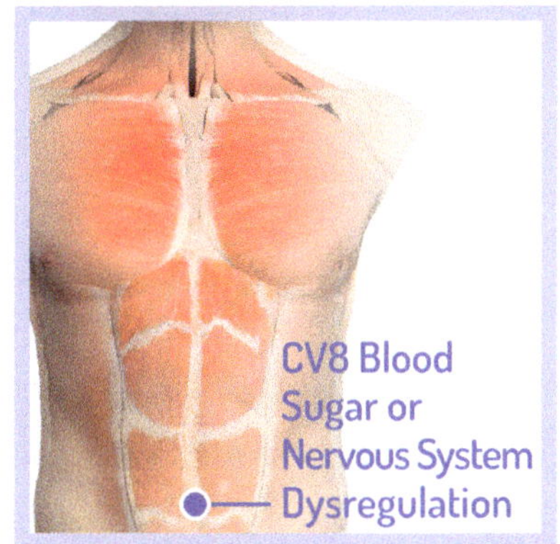

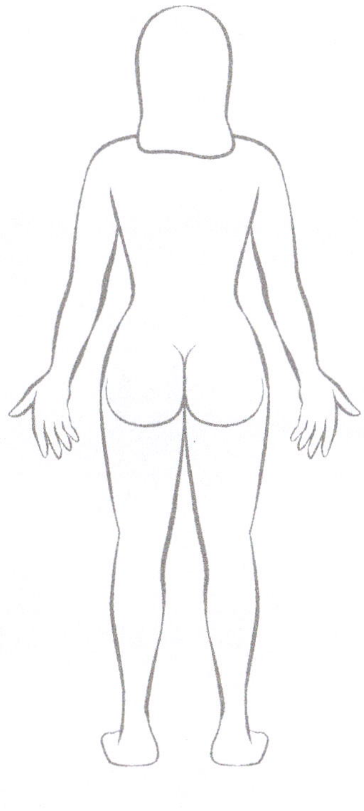

Governing Vessel Body-Feedback Testing Locations

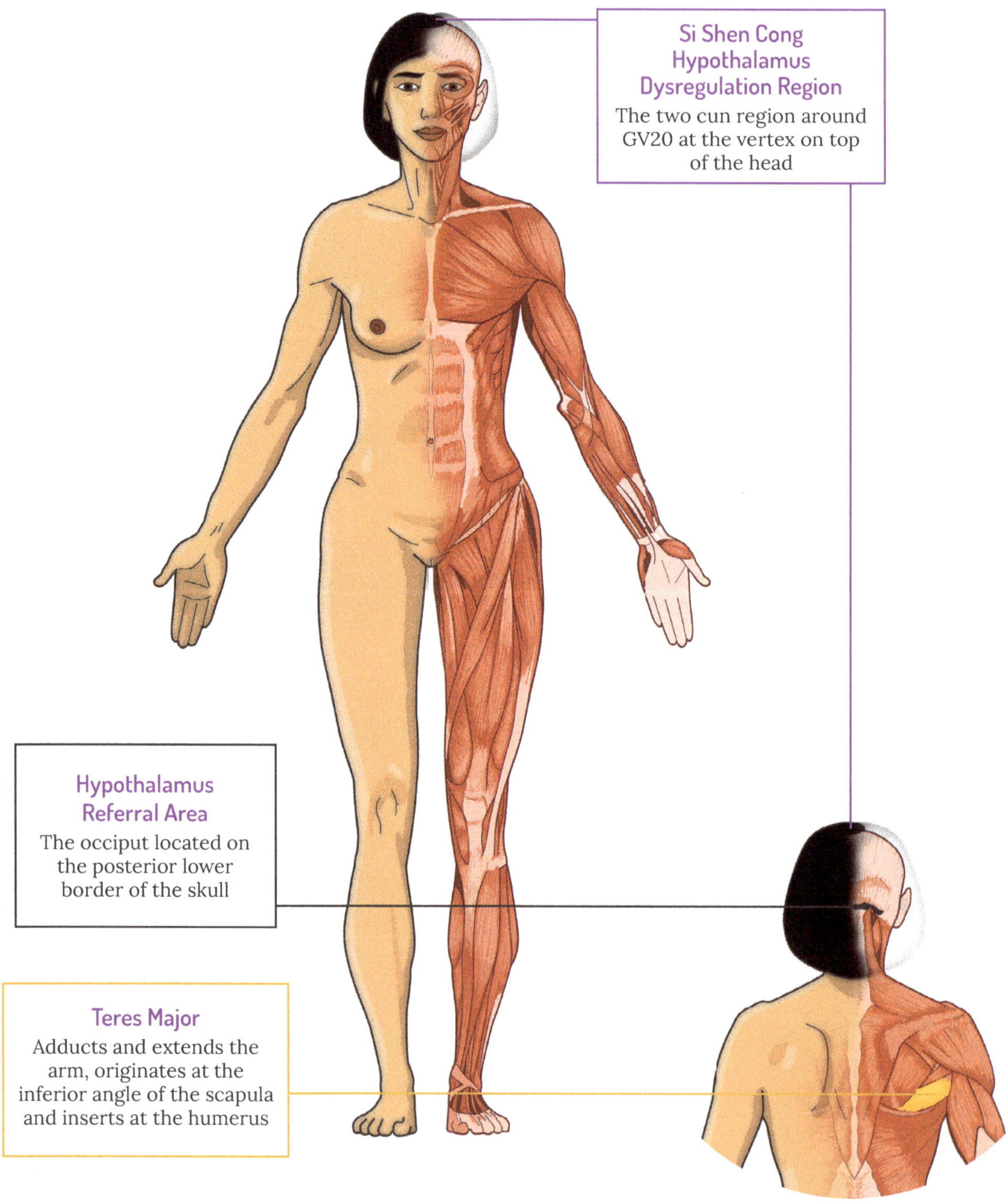

Governing Vessel Alarm Points

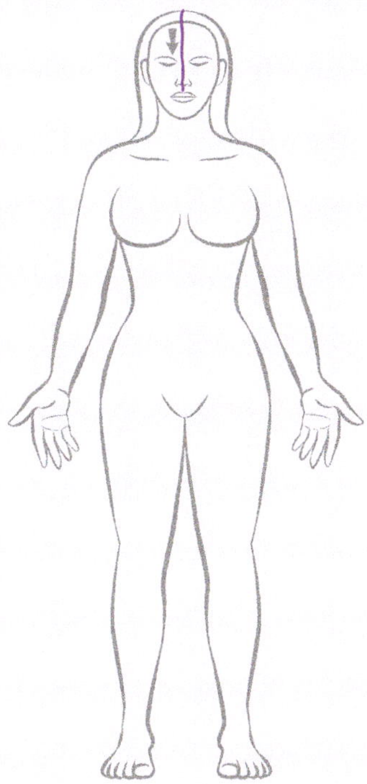

Approximately 1 cun lateral, posterior, and anterior to GV20

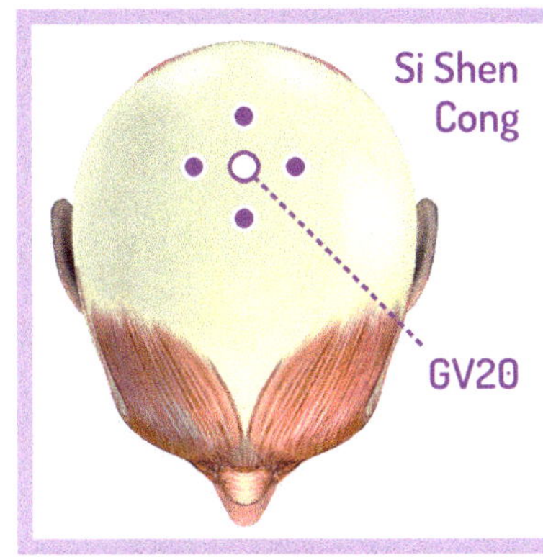

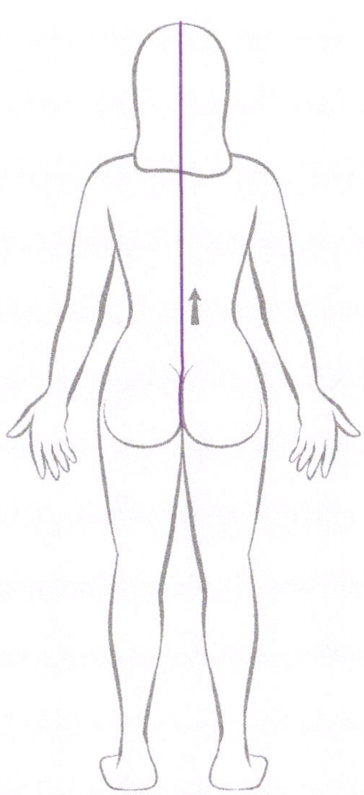

SECTION

2

The Pre-Treatment Planning Stage

CHAPTER 7

Asymmetry and Health

Growth in proportion to size and form is abundant in nature and results from optimal health and the synchronized flow of qi (energy). A plant's DNA programs its development for balanced growth, and this symmetry manifests in the structure of the flowers and leaves. Bumblebees have a preference for flowers with symmetrical patterns, which correspond with higher pollen rewards.[17] Flowers infected with viruses have distinctly different shapes than those not infected.[18]

Symmetry in Nature

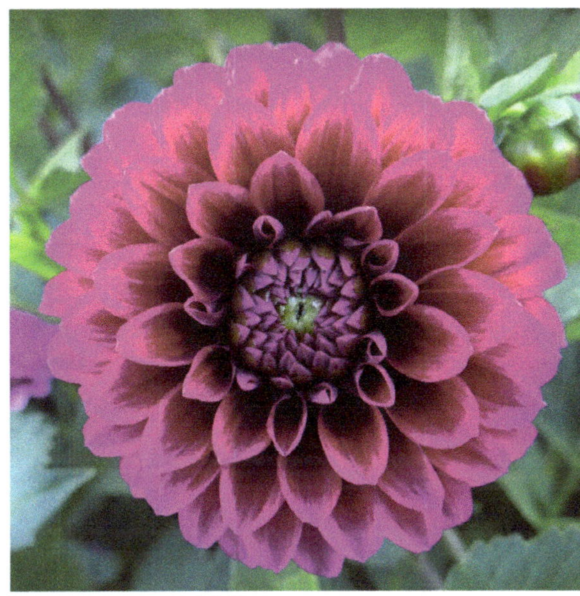

ID 77409299 © Luisa Vallon Fumi | Dreamstime.com

In the body, proportional growth occurs in many of its systems (skeletal, nervous, endocrine, lymphatic, and renal), as well as in the meridians, muscles, and connective tissue. Symmetrical development begins during pregnancy with healthy qi and blood, the mother's nourishing essence, optimal fetal positioning in the womb, and the free flow of the twelve main meridians and eight extra-vessels.

Health and vitality in plants, animals, and humans correspond with balanced structural alignment. When comparing one side to the other, symmetry is most noticeable in the face, head, neck, shoulders, hips, and feet. Most asymmetrical variations are a result of genetics, environmental factors, nutrient intake, or pathogenic infections. A group of studies[19] demonstrated that any deviation from perfect body symmetry is considered a sub-optimal situation, which will result in future performance issues. These studies found statistically significant differences in the states of health relating to optimal body symmetry.

- Male body symmetry corresponds with higher sperm counts and better sperm quality.
- Female breast symmetry corresponds with superior fertility.
- Growth rate, fertility, and survivability are positively associated with symmetry across a number of species.
- Facial symmetry correlates with fewer self-reported occurrences of respiratory diseases.
- Facial symmetry has a positive influence on attractiveness.
- Facial symmetry is positively related to physical health and immune response.

Symmetrical facial features

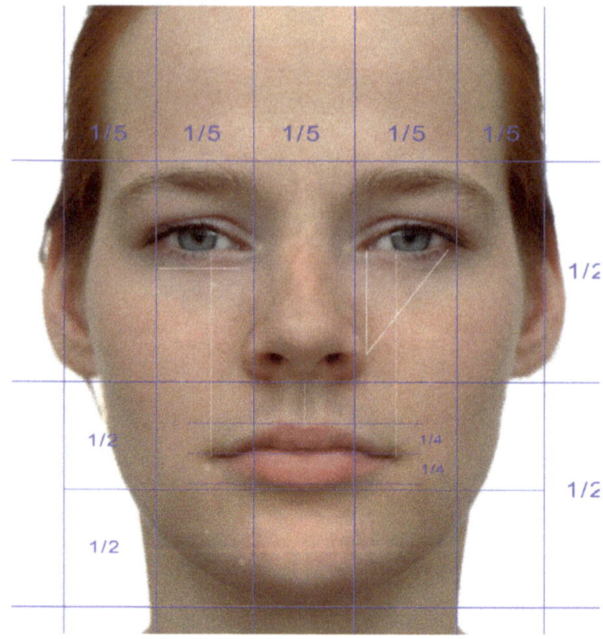

ID 1171612 © Lisavan | Dreamstime.com

Asymmetrical facial features

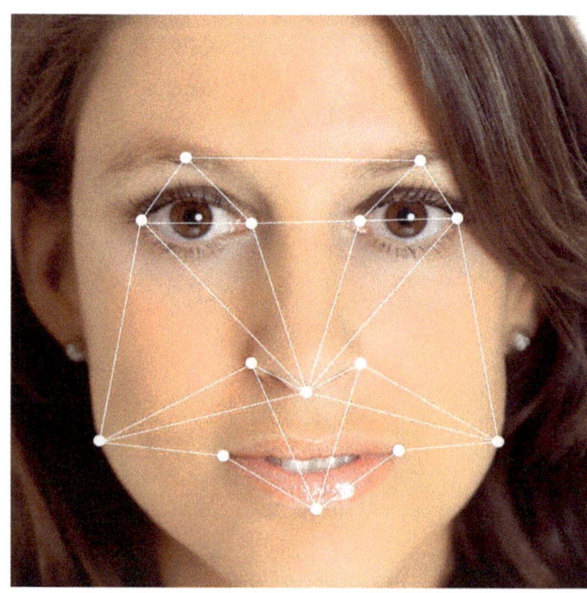

ID 46926132 © La Fabrika Pixel S.l. | Dreamstime.com

Studies show that asymmetry along the vertical axis (comparing the right side to the left side of the body) is more problematic than the horizontal axis (upper body to lower body).[20] Body-Feedback assessment and testing methods quickly identify this clinically significant asymmetry along the vertical axis. Differing acupoint prescriptions for each side of the body are necessary to restore optimal health. The Body-Feedback balancing, sedation, and tonification prescriptions accommodate this dual treatment approach by independently restoring balance for each side of the body, and then integrating the differing sides.

7.1 Causes of Asymmetry

Congenital scoliosis that develops in utero, and idiopathic scoliosis that occurs at any age due to unknown reasons, are the most common causes of asymmetry along the vertical axis. For certain people, long-term pathogenic heat in any organ or meridian can cause pain and tightness in the corresponding Body-Feedback muscle associations and pull on the spinal column resulting in scoliosis. The heart, spleen, pancreas, and stomach will refer discomfort to the left side of the body, and the liver, gallbladder, duodenum, and colon will refer to the right side of the body. Long-term organ dysfunction often corresponds with the most significant area of curvature in the spine.

Asymmetry from Scoliosis

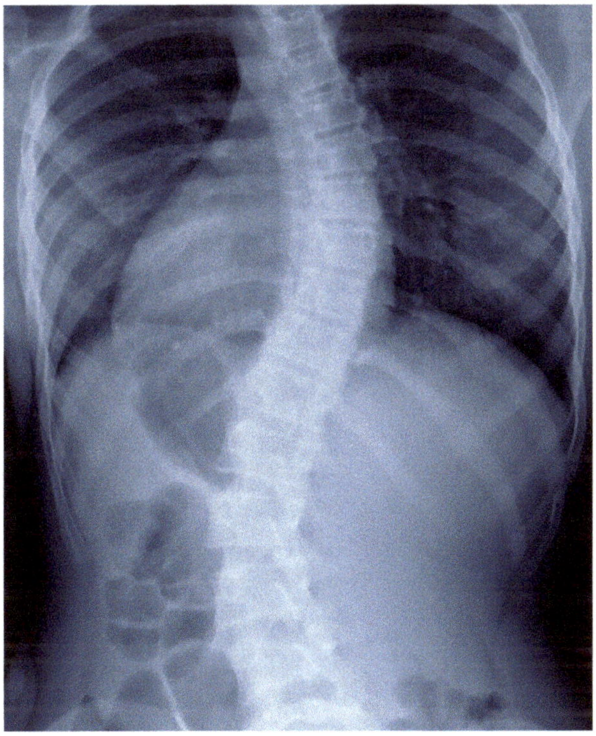

ID 63332341 © Draw05 | Dreamstime.com

Other causes of asymmetry along the vertical axis include:

- Viral and bacterial infections that live on spinal nerves and induce pathogenic heat at a specific location.
- Unresolved or severe trauma leading to structural imbalances if not correctly treated.
- Long-term pathogenic heat affecting multiple organs and meridians causing chronic tightness in different muscle groups and organ referral areas.
- Repetitive use and postural issues affecting one side of the body, such as sitting at a desk and leaning to one side, twisting, or carrying heavy objects on one side.
- Liver or gallbladder organ dysfunction, which can cause chronic muscle tightness in the right shoulder and side of the neck.
- Spleen organ dysfunction (including the pancreas), which can cause chronic muscle tightness in the left shoulder and side of the neck.
- Long-term dysfunction between paired five-element organs or paired six-level meridians, which may or may not affect the muscles and skeletal system.

Asymmetry in babies can form during pregnancy, due to restricted space, and frequently occurs in twins and triplets. When the position or size of an unborn baby restricts its movement, the baby's qi becomes stagnant and can develop depressive heat, leading to differences in development from side to side. Longstanding asymmetry in the mother caused by genetics can result in structural differences as the baby grows, due to organ dysfunction and unbalanced meridian flow. Asymmetry is easiest to detect in a baby's facial features and muscle development.

Asymmetry can develop at any age and commonly occurs with long-term posture issues, abnormal gait patterns, symptoms that affect only one side of the body, and headaches that are one-sided or change location. Health challenges with severe symptoms and migraines can cause deficiency on one side of the body and excess on the other. Inequality in muscle tone and size occur with long-term asymmetry and can affect a person's gait. Asymmetry from trauma, organ referral causing muscle tightness, and repetitive use movements can cause mild variations in muscle tension and discomfort.

A Baby Boy with Asymmetrical Facial Features

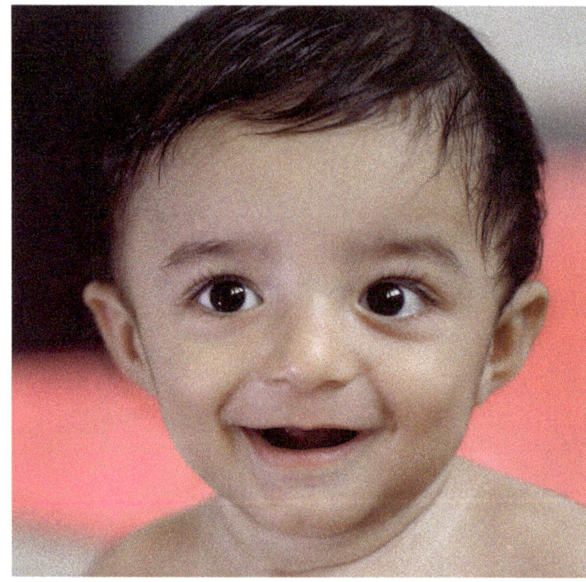

ID 137896016 © Matrixximages | Dreamstime.com

Clients with longstanding asymmetry accompanied by excess on one side of their body and deficiency on the other require frequent acupuncture sessions as the body transitions to symmetrical. The musculoskeletal system and brain need time and frequent treatments to adapt to and hold a new proportional structure. The meridians naturally strive for symmetry to harmonize and support organ function, and these clients will feel significant improvements with a balanced meridian system.

7.2 Identifying Asymmetry through Pre-Treatment Planning

A benefit of the Body-Feedback approach is the ability to separately distinguish organ/meridian dysfunctions affecting each side of the body. Identifying the need for an asymmetrical approach occurs throughout all six steps of the pre-treatment planning stage. Depending on the severity of the asymmetry, each of the six steps will have indications that the right and left sides of the body will require unique acupoint prescriptions. The treatment approach for asymmetry requires additional time during the pre-treatment planning stage. However, the treatment stage needs less supporting acupoints because of the inherent variety included with two different acupoint prescriptions and makes up for the additional time spent planning.

PLANNING STEP ONE: ASSESS FOR ASYMMETRY

The first step of the planning stage assesses for asymmetry by looking for differences between the right and left sides in muscle development, shoulder and hip alignment, and the natural resting position of the feet. With the client on the treatment table, visually assess these three areas by standing at the client's head or feet and looking down the centerline of their body to compare the right and left sides.

To find one-sided symptoms, palpate the surrounding muscle groups and compare side to side, looking for differences in tone, tension, and discomfort. The neck and shoulder muscles will compensate for a structural imbalance in the body to hold the eyes level. With scoliosis, there can be a significant difference in the thickness of the neck muscles from one side to the other. Because scoliosis is a common cause of asymmetry, identifying it on intake forms can be helpful.

Differences in alignment between the shoulders and hips can signal asymmetry. To assess the shoulders, visually compare the amount of space from the shoulder to the treatment table on each side. To check the hips, press on the anterior superior iliac spine and compare side to side for alignment. For people with shoulder and hip alignment issues, sitting with good posture, not crossing the legs, and placing a pillow between the knees when side-sleeping will improve the effectiveness of an asymmetrical treatment.

The xiphoid process is the cartilaginous section at the lower end of the sternum that tapers to a tip. The xiphoid process will adapt to accommodate rib cage misalignment, resulting in pain and discomfort at the lower border where it meets the rib cage. Palpate the CV15 Spinal Misalignment Region looking for tenderness as an indicator of rib cage misalignment.

The feet will naturally rest at the same angle to the treatment table when the body is symmetrical. When a client's feet appear to rest at different angles to the treatment table, an asymmetrical treatment approach is likely. This disparity in the slant of the feet at rest can occur due to scoliosis, hip misalignment, or unequal muscle tone from one leg to another. At the end of a Body-Feedback asymmetrical acupuncture session, the feet will often shift to a more balanced presentation.

PLANNING STEP TWO: REGULATE THE AUTONOMIC NERVOUS SYSTEM

The second step of the planning stage determines a supine (faceup) or prone (facedown) approach to regulate the Autonomic Nervous System (ANS). Chapter 8 explains how to check the abdomen to the master points in the shoulder area, the neck muscles, or the pulse to determine the optimal treatment position. When the abdominal acupoint combinations test favorably, a supine treatment is best. If the abdominal acupoint combinations test unfavorably, then a treatment to address the back, usually in a prone position, is best.

With a supine asymmetrical treatment, the abdominal acupoints may differ from one side to the other. Look for three diagonal acupoints along the upper abdomen on one side that test favorably, and continue the same trajectory checking for three acupoints along the lower abdomen on the other side. At times, the abdominal acupoints to balance the ANS will be the standard acupoint configurations discussed in Chapter 8.

Upper right to lower left asymmetry treatment

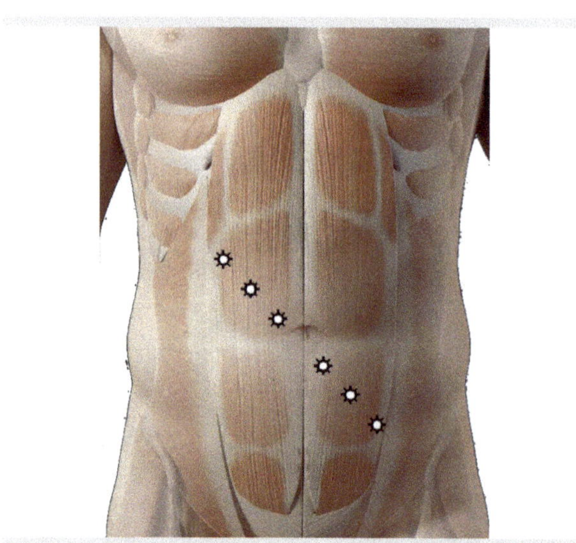

Upper left to lower right asymmetry treatment

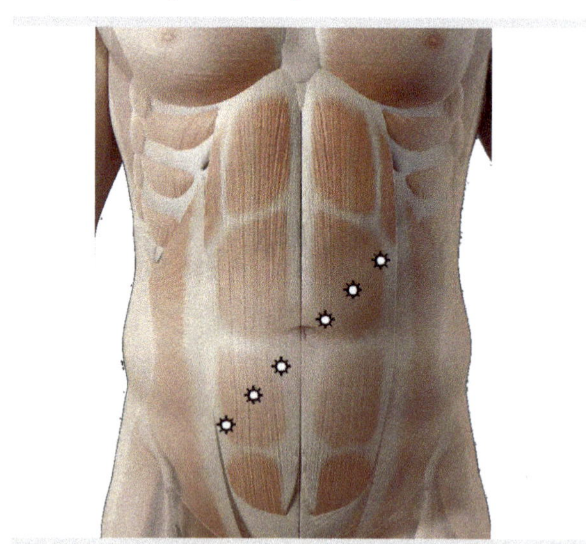

For a prone asymmetrical treatment, it is easier for the practitioner and more comfortable for the client to complete the planning stage in the faceup position. Testing and needling the back acupoints will occur during the treatment stage with the client in a prone position. These acupoints will differ from side to side except when needling the governing extra-vessel directly over the spine. Examples are provided later in the Rectifying Asymmetry section of this chapter and throughout this text.

PLANNING STEP THREE: DETERMINE BODY-FEEDBACK BALANCING PRESCRIPTIONS

Determining the balancing prescription for each side of the body is the third step of the planning stage. This step will confirm if a client needs an asymmetrical treatment. After deciding the balancing acupoints for one side of the body (see Chapter 9), check the same acupoints on the other side of the body. If the same acupoints on the second side cause an adverse response in the pulse or Body-Feedback testing locations, an asymmetrical treatment using a different balancing prescription is needed. Examples of a negative response include the pulse becoming wiry, thread-like, forceful, or confined, and an increase in muscle tension, discomfort, or pain in the Body-Feedback testing locations.

Check the following related organs/meridians to determine the second balancing prescription:

- five-element pair of the first balancing prescription
- six-level pair of the first balancing prescription
- non-paired organ/meridian in the same trisection as the first balancing prescription
- organ opposite the time of day of the first balancing prescription
- other organs/meridians based on the client's symptoms or pulse

For example, with a liver root dysfunction on the right, check the following options on the left:

- gallbladder as the five-element pair
- pericardium as the six-level pair
- triple burner as the non-paired organ/meridian in the trisection
- small intestine because it is the time of day opposite the liver

Longstanding asymmetry, recent trauma, or intense symptoms can induce two balancing prescriptions from unrelated organs or meridians. Within a few acupuncture sessions, the balancing prescriptions will occur between related organs and meridians as an indication of improving health.

PLANNING STEP FOUR: DETERMINE THE BODY-FEEDBACK SEDATION OR TONIFICATION PRESCRIPTIONS

Identifying the sedation or tonification acupoints for each side is the fourth step of the pre-treatment stage. With an asymmetrical treatment, both sides can be sedation or tonification prescriptions. In some cases, one side will need a sedation prescription while the other will require a tonification prescription. In this case, it is vital to needle the sedation acupoints first and the tonification acupoints second to accommodate the different optimal needle times (see Chapter 10). Removing the tonification acupoints first will give the sedation acupoints a little extra time for the body to process the differences between the two sides.

PLANNING STEP FIVE: ASSESS THE CORRESPONDING BODY-FEEDBACK TESTING LOCATIONS

Palpating and assessing the corresponding specific Body-Feedback organ referral areas and muscles associations (see Chapters 6 and 12) for the balancing prescriptions previously identified is step five in the pre-treatment stage. Carefully compare the muscle associations from one side to the other. The associated organ/meridian referral areas, the he-sea organ alarm point, and fire-element meridian alarm point may refer on the ipsilateral or contralateral side. For example, with a large intestine balancing prescription on the right and a lung balancing prescription on the left, palpate the following testing locations on both sides and chart any right, left, or bilateral tenderness, tightness, or flaccidity:

- lung referral area
- LU5 lung organ alarm point
- LU10 lung meridian alarm point
- deltoid muscle for the lung
- LI11 large intestine organ alarm point
- LI5 large intestine meridian alarm point
- iliotibial band for the large intestine
- quadratus lumborum for the large intestine

Acupoint prescriptions will often change from appointment to appointment, while the testing locations remain the same with steady improvements over the course of treatment. It is typical for the balancing prescription to alternate from side to side at each session to support the root dysfunction or constitutional weakness. However, the corresponding Body-Feedback testing locations, with pain and tightness identified for that specific root dysfunction, remain consistent. The discomfort and muscle tightness will diminish as the root dysfunction improves. When additional symptoms or health challenges arise, new testing locations will become painful or tight. In the previous example of the large intestine balancing root treatment on the right and lung balancing root treatment on the left, the testing locations stay the same during the course of treatment, and the acupoint prescriptions alternate as follows:

- The first treatment could be the lung tonification prescription on the left and large intestine sedation prescription on the right.
- The second treatment could be the large intestine tonification prescription on the left and lung sedation prescription on the right.
- The third treatment could be the lung tonification prescription on the left and large intestine tonification prescription on the right.
- The fourth treatment could be the large intestine tonification prescription bilaterally.

PLANNING STEP SIX: TEST ESSENTIAL OILS

The sixth and final step of the pre-treatment stage involves testing essential oils to the master points and corresponding Body-Feedback testing locations and then applying them. With an asymmetrical approach, check the meridian and organ blends for the two balancing prescriptions. Check any of the essential oil blends to the tight or painful Body-Feedback testing locations on either side of the body or to the master points. Depending on the blend and treatment position, apply the oils to the soles of the feet, tight muscles, or along the spine to encourage symmetry. See Chapter 11 on essential oils for more information.

7.3 Rectifying Asymmetry with Treatment

The treatment of asymmetry requires distinctly different acupoint prescriptions for the right and left sides of the body. For example, a person struggling with detoxification, digestion, and headaches can have a liver sedation prescription on the left side and a gallbladder tonification prescription on the right side. After determining the acupoint prescriptions in the pre-treatment stage, the three steps of the treatment stage are straightforward.

Examples of asymmetrical facial acupoints

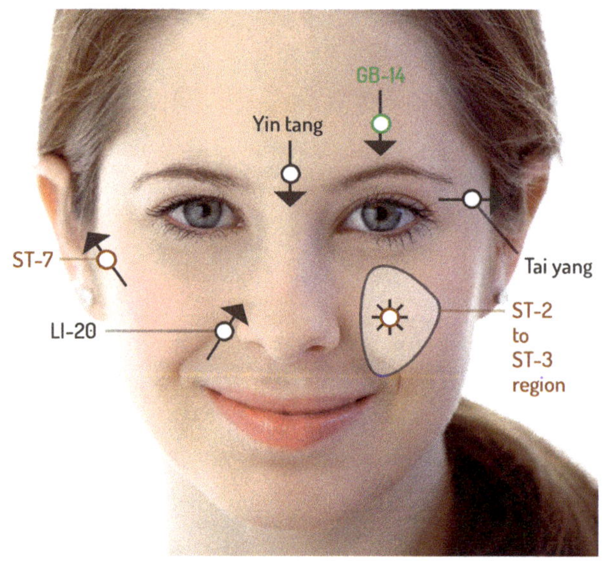

Asymmetrical Female Face

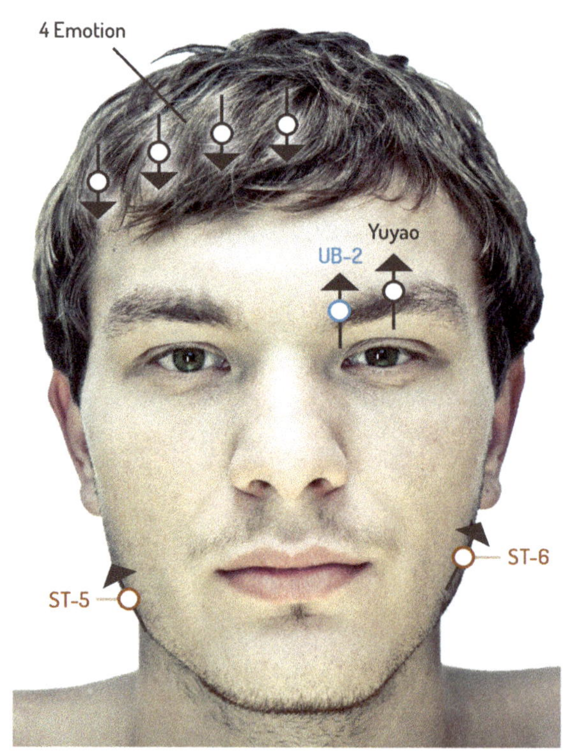

Asymmetrical Male Face

TREATMENT STEP ONE: BALANCE THE AUTONOMIC NERVOUS SYSTEM

The first step of the treatment stage is to identify the optimal treatment position and needle acupoints to balance the Autonomic Nervous System (see Chapter 8). Asymmetrical treatments usually require different acupoints on the left and right sides for the scalp, face, abdomen, ear, and back to harmonize the ANS.

There are four options for balancing the ANS: abdominal, facial/scalp, auricular, or back acupoints. Check one or more of the master points (GB21, TB15, or SI13), the neck muscles, or the pulse on the same side of the body to determine the treatment approach for the right and left sides to balance the ANS.

Scoliosis Treatment Approach

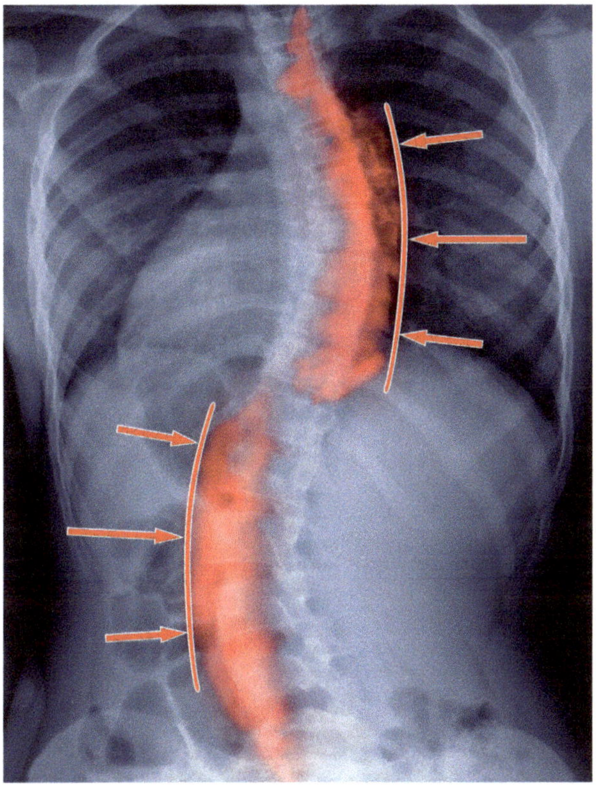

ID 77907636 © Draw05 | Dreamstime.com

In the prone position, rectifying the ANS when asymmetry is present treats the overdevelopment or tightness in different muscles located on the right and left sides of the back. With scoliosis, needling the outer edge of the erector spinae muscles towards the spine releases the muscle tightness and improves spinal alignment. Essential oils can strengthen the corresponding deficient areas of the spine.

TREATMENT STEP TWO: NEEDLE THE BALANCING, SEDATION, AND TONIFICATION PRESCRIPTIONS

The second step of the treatment stage is needling the balancing and sedation or tonification prescriptions previously identified during steps three and four of the pre-treatment stage. Severe asymmetry will cause one side of the body to be excess requiring sedation, and the other side to be deficient requiring tonification. Treating the sedation side first allows for the additional needle retention time needed on the excess side and less needle retention time on the deficient side, which also helps balance the meridian system. At the end of a session, remove the tonification acupoints first and the sedation acupoints last. Using larger needles on sedation points and magnetic pellets on tonification points can also help restore balance.

As the body's symmetry improves, or with mild cases of asymmetry, both sides of the body will require either sedation or tonification root treatments. In this case, you can insert and remove the needles in any order. In most cases of asymmetry, the meridian system will eventually attain balance and test best for symmetrical treatments even though the one-sided symptoms or curvature in the spine are still apparent. The goal for scoliosis is to continue treating the excess spinal curvature while needling the same balancing and sedation or tonification prescriptions on both sides. Depending on the age of the client and the severity of scoliosis, the time required to achieve symmetry in the meridian system and reduce the spinal curve can vary from a few months to a few years.

TREATMENT STEP THREE: CHOOSE SUPPORTING ACUPOINTS

The third step of the treatment stage is choosing supporting acupoints to test and needle. Check the supporting acupoints to the specific Body-Feedback testing locations associated with the balancing prescriptions, the master points, or the pulse. With the variety of different acupoints as the basis of an asymmetrical treatment, there is less need for additional supporting acupoints. However, checking for and clearing pathogenic heat is often necessary. First, look for any single metal or water acupoint included in the balancing, tonification, and sedation prescription. Then test its additional metal or water point to create the heat-clearing combination. For example, the liver tonification prescription includes KD10 (water point), and adding KD7 (metal point) creates the heat-clearing combination. Then test the metal + water combination for additional meridians affected by pathogenic heat not included in the balancing, tonification, or sedation prescription. In this same example, using the liver tonification prescription, pathogenic heat in the triple burner can be cleared by adding TB1 metal + TB2 water points for support.

For a facedown treatment, it is easier to check the metal + water combinations in the supine position while testing the balancing prescriptions during step three of the pre-treatment planning stage. Apply magnetic pellets or press tacks to treat metal + water combinations that rest on the table while the client is lying facedown. With a faceup treatment, test the additional metal + water combinations during either the pre-treatment or treatment stages.

Supporting scalp ashi acupoints can balance the different hemispheres of the brain for headaches, traumatic brain injury, or asymmetrical facial features. Using the tips of your four fingers to create a line, lightly massage the scalp looking for areas of swelling and fluid retention (indicating excess), or slight dips in the scalp and skull (indicating deficiency), known as the scalp ashi line. Find three or four ashi acupoints on each side of the head that test favorably to the master brain alarm point (TB15). Often with asymmetry, one side of the scalp ashi acupoints is posterior while the other side of the scalp is anterior. See Chapter 13 for more information on locating scalp and facial acupoints. Additional facial acupoints will differ on each side when the scalp ashi acupoints are asymmetrical. As the asymmetry improves, the scalp ashi acupoints on each side will meet to become more symmetrical. The client will eventually test best for symmetrical scalp ashi and facial acupoints when the root treatments become symmetrical.

Often with asymmetrical treatments, the supporting acupoints on each side of the body have a special relationship with each other to harmonize the other affected organs/ meridians within a trisection. For example, a client with sinus congestion and cold symptoms tested favorably for a lung sedation prescription on the right and a large intestine tonification prescription on the left. The supporting acupoint on the right was ST40 to sedate the resulting excess in the stomach. The supporting acupoint on the left was SP8 to move qi stagnation and blood stasis. Both supporting acupoints harmonized the first trisection.

ROOT LUNG EXCESS CAUSING DISCORD ON RIGHT

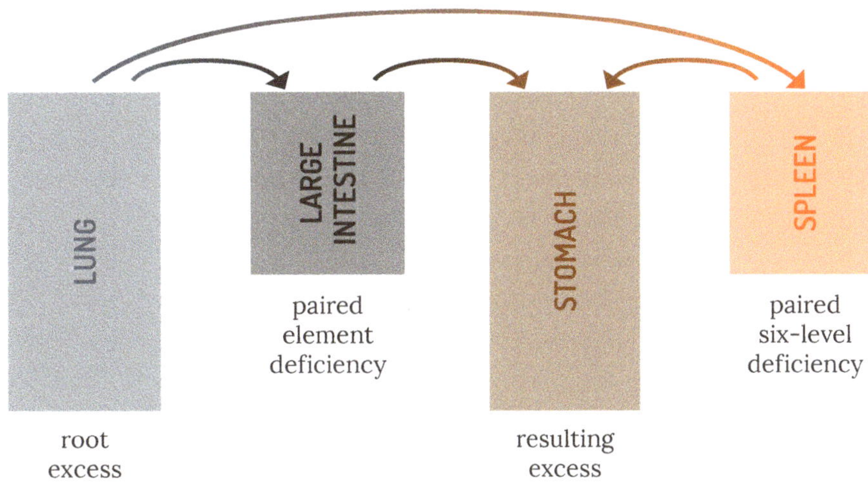

ROOT LARGE INTESTINE DEFICIENCY CAUSING DISCORD ON LEFT

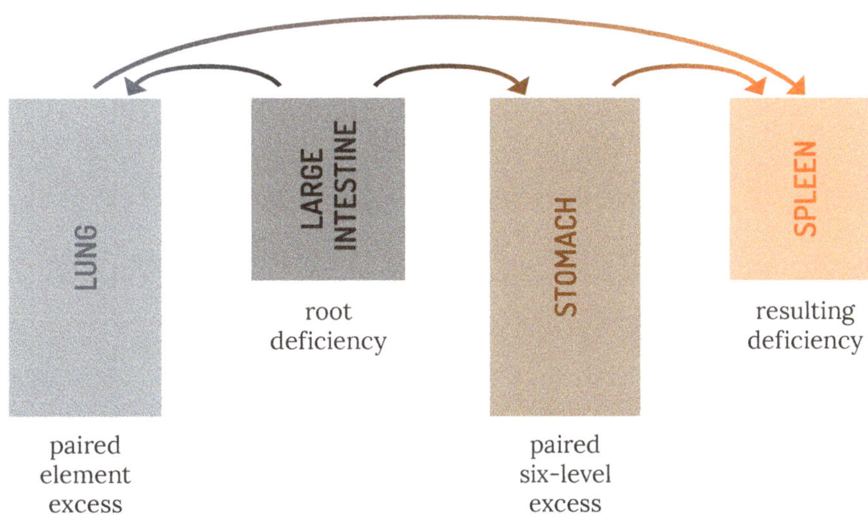

With longstanding asymmetry, the extra-vessel supporting acupoints (LU7, KD6, SP4, PC6, TB5, and UB62) are advantageous. For example, a liver tonification prescription on the left often includes the supporting acupoint PC6, and the gallbladder tonification prescription on the right often includes the supporting acupoint TB5. Both of these supporting acupoints harmonize the third trisection. An extra-vessel's controlling acupoint on the right or left side and its linking acupoints on the other side frequently test favorably with asymmetry. For example, the penetrating vessel (*chong mai*) controlling acupoint SP4 on the right side and the linking acupoint PC6 on the left side utilize the extra-vessel to help restore symmetry. See Chapter 15 for detailed information on the extra-vessel supporting acupoints.

7.4 The Asymmetrical Post-Treatment Stage

After removing the needles, test herbs, supplements, and foods using the pulse, neck muscles, or master points on either side. The items that test favorably will support the root dysfunctions affecting each side of the body and encourage symmetry. The asymmetrical master regions, individual organ/meridian referral areas, and muscle associations provide information on how an herb, supplement, or food affects each side's root dysfunction.

Educating clients about their specific symptoms of asymmetry and how, with acupuncture, their body can become more symmetrical over time encourages long-term commitment to the healing process. Discuss the differences identified during the session as they relate to their health concerns. Most clients will transition to symmetrical acupoint prescriptions indicating a dramatic advancement in health. Sharing this milestone with clients provides a sense of accomplishment and confirmation of improved health. If a client shifts from symmetry back to asymmetry, there will likely be an increase in symptoms. Encourage clients with recurring asymmetry to schedule an appointment as soon as they notice an increase in symptoms to reestablish symmetry.

A BODY-FEEDBACK SUCCESS STORY

At age 59, a client with severe scoliosis from birth came for acupuncture to address hip, back, neck, and shoulder pain due to her spinal curvature. Her initial assessment indicated the need for an asymmetrical treatment. With regular treatments, she transitioned from asymmetrical to symmetrical balancing prescriptions in four months. After receiving weekly acupuncture sessions for six weeks, she was able to transition to biweekly acupuncture for her hip, back, and neck pain. She changed her nutritional supplements and used essential oils daily at home. She has noticed significant improvement in her scoliosis curve due to the Body-Feedback style treatments improving her spinal alignment, and she now tests favorably for symmetrical balancing prescriptions most of the time. Through Body-Feedback testing, she understands how her progress and positive lifestyle choices result in symmetrical treatments. She now has little to no hip, back, or shoulder pain, her clothes fit her differently, and her shirts no longer fall off one shoulder. Above all else, she is elated with her renewed body image.

CHAPTER 8

Regulating the Autonomic Nervous System

The second step of the pre-treatment planning stage determines the optimal treatment position to balance the autonomic nervous system (ANS). By addressing the ANS first, clients immediately relax and feel safe during needle insertion. Body-Feedback testing techniques can determine if the client's nervous system will respond favorably to a supine or prone treatment. In certain situations, adjustments can occur to enable treatment in the non-optimal treatment position as necessary. A regulated ANS encourages the body, mind, and spirit to synchronize for accelerated self-healing. Body-Feedback utilizes acupoints on the scalp, face, ear, or abdomen in the supine position or specific regions of the spine in the prone position to balance the ANS.

8.1 Divisions of the Autonomic Nervous System

The three divisions of the ANS are the sympathetic, parasympathetic, and enteric systems. The sympathetic nervous system governs the fight-or-flight response and increases activity in the heart, lungs, and skeletal muscles. The parasympathetic nervous system promotes sleep, relaxation, digestion, and the absorption of nutrients. The enteric nervous system operates independently of the central nervous system and influences digestion and mental health.

8.1.1 The Sympathetic Nervous System

The sympathetic nervous system is more active during the day and corresponds with physical movement and mental alertness. The sympathetic nervous system response occurs through the nerves located between thoracic vertebrae one (T1) and lumbar vertebrae two (L2).[21] The governing vessel (*du mai*) and urinary bladder meridian from T1 to L2 directly influence the sympathetic response. The other yang meridians, which are also more active during the day, indirectly contribute to the sympathetic response.

The Sympathetic Nervous System

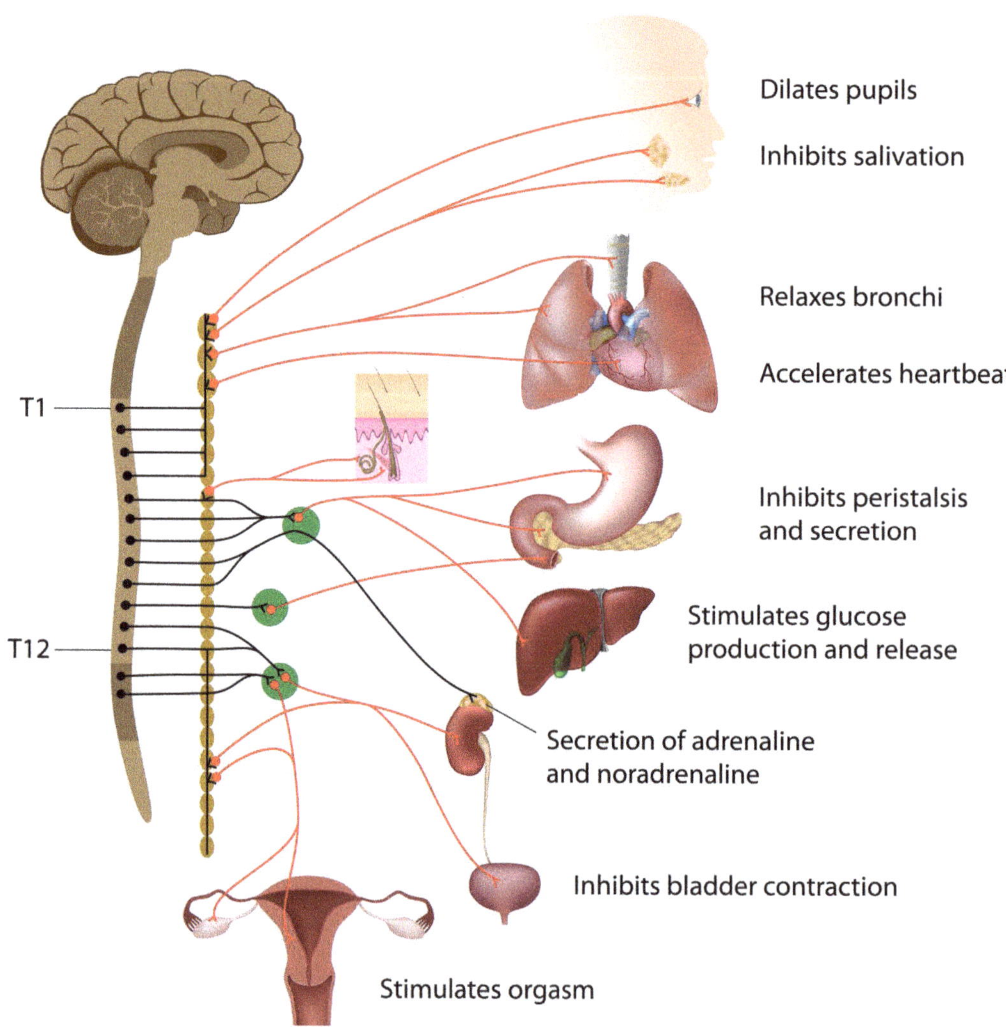

ID 25474175 © Alila07 | Dreamstime.com

8.1.2 The Parasympathetic Nervous System

The parasympathetic nervous system is more active during the night or after eating and corresponds with relaxation and sleep. The parasympathetic nervous system response occurs through the cranial nerves III, VII, IX, and X, and sacral nerves two through four (S2, S3, S4).[22] The front mu-alarm points on the conception vessel (*ren mai*) directly influence the parasympathetic activity in the internal organs via the vagus nerve (cranial nerve X). The points along the cervical vertebrae in the neck (DU14 through DU15), and the sacrum points along the urinary bladder meridian (UB28, UB29, UB30, UB32, UB33, and UB34), directly influence the parasympathetic response. The other yin meridians indirectly affect the parasympathetic response.

The Parasympathetic Nervous System

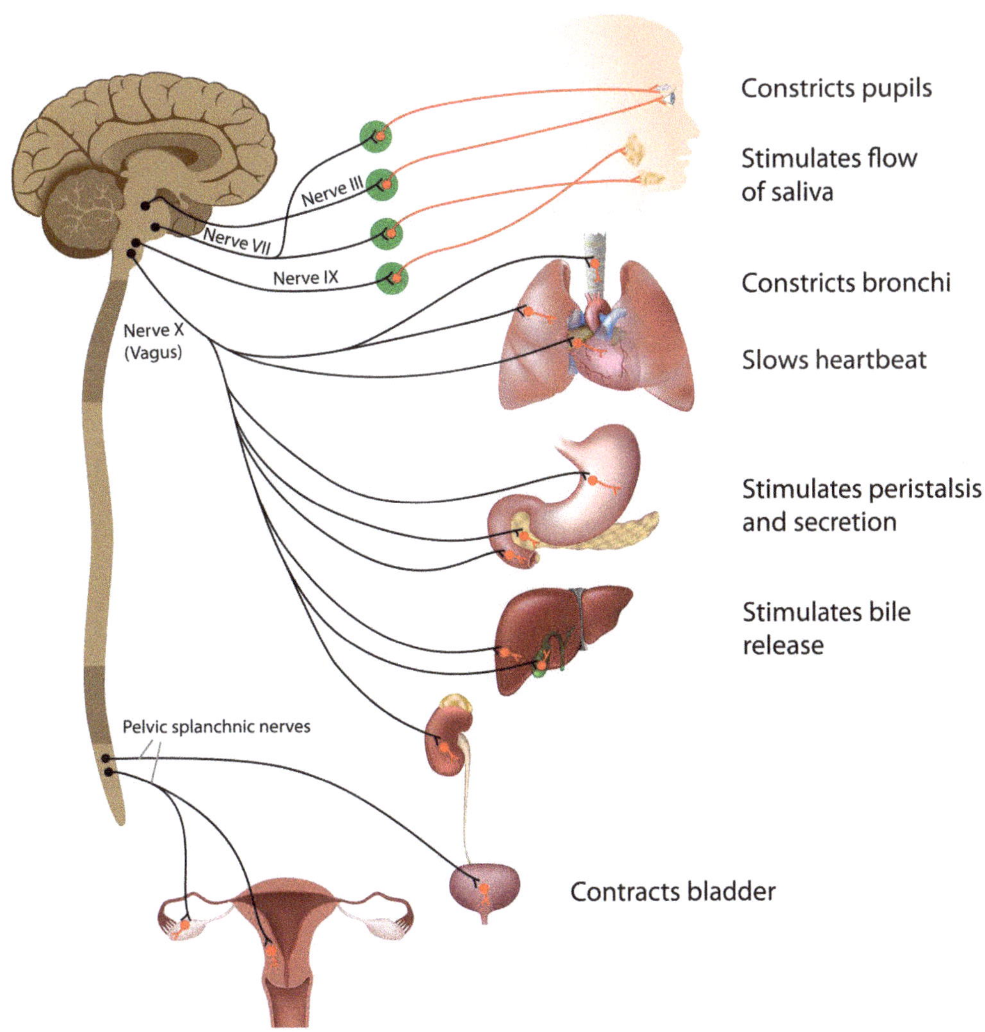

ID 25474169 © Alila07 | Dreamstime.com

Symptoms of ANS dysregulation caused by	
SYMPATHETIC DOMINANCE	PARASYMPATHETIC DOMINANCE
Dry mouth due to lack of saliva	Excessive saliva production
Chronic constipation with dry stools	Increased appetite and faster stool transit time
Resting heart rate of over 80 bpm	Resting heart rate below 70 bpm (not athletic)
Increased arterial blood pressure	Lower arterial blood pressure
Elevated body temperature	Lower body temperature
Elevated blood sugar levels or insulin resistance	Hypoglycemia or reactive hypoglycemia with insulin resistance
Excessive release of stress hormones	Falls asleep quickly and easily naps during the day
Long-term stress disrupting sleep	Prefers to sleep longer than eight hours
Low libido with infertility	Weight gain or difficulty losing weight
Adrenal fatigue with long-term stress	Depression and lack of motivation

Signs of dysregulation between the sympathetic and parasympathetic nervous responses include:

- a difference in pupil size between the right and left eyes
- irregular sleeping or breathing patterns
- alternating constipation and diarrhea
- digestive irregularities
- history of physical or emotional abuse
- long-term stress

8.1.3 The Enteric Nervous System

The enteric nervous system is made up of millions of neurons located in the digestive system. The enteric nerves communicate and travel along the myenteric plexus, which forms a continuous network from the upper esophagus to the internal anal sphincter. The small and large intestines contain submucosal ganglia and mesh fibers. The sympathetic pathways of the vagus and pelvic nerves create the connections between the enteric and central (sympathetic and parasympathetic) nervous systems.[23]

The enteric nervous system creates the "gut-brain axis" and regulates the gut flora. Gut flora has been found to not only be an essential component of immune and metabolic health, but also seems to influence development and diseases of the enteric and central nervous system. It affects neurodegenerative diseases, cerebrovascular accidents, behavioral disorders, and neuroimmune-mediated illnesses. Gut flora produces and consumes a wide range of mammalian neurotransmitters, including dopamine, norepinephrine, serotonin, or gamma-aminobutyric acid (GABA), which are identical to the ones found in the brain.[24]

The small and large intestine meridians, along with specific acupoints for treating the intestines, such as CV12, ST25, ST37, and ST39, impact gut flora and submucosal ganglia. Gut flora assists with detoxification of used hormone metabolites that affect neurotransmitters, the liver, and the gallbladder. The imperial-fire meridians (heart and small intestine) and ministerial-fire meridians (pericardium and triple burner) directly impact the neurotransmitters in the brain via the hypothalamus-pituitary axis.

The Enteric Nervous System

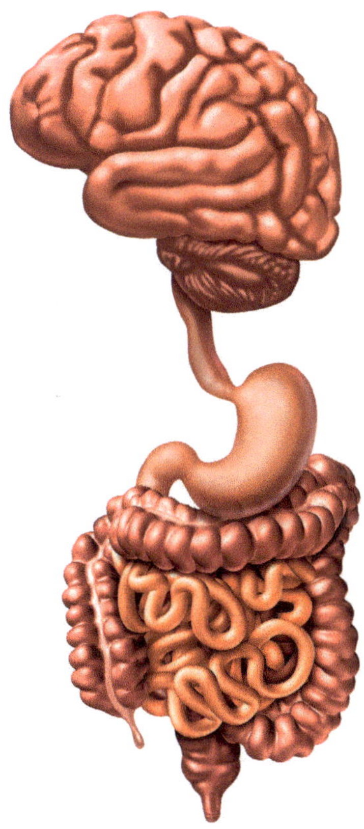

ID 156415386 © Skypixel | Dreamstime.com

8.1.4 Healing Potential and the ANS

Healing potential depends on a balanced autonomic nervous system to encourage cellular regeneration and regulate the immune system. The hypothalamus responds to unconscious and conscious stimuli that initiate changes in the autonomic nervous, somatic nervous (voluntary control of movement via the skeletal muscles), endocrine, and immune systems. The ANS response affects the internal organs, respiration rate, blood pressure, and the smooth muscles lining hollow organs and blood vessels. Emotions of fear and rage cause the hypothalamus to release stress hormones that trigger the ANS fight-or-flight response and disrupt the immune and endocrine systems and the circadian rhythm (sleep/wake cycle).[25]

Examples of scientific research linking the importance of a balanced ANS to promote healing and wellness include:

- Dysregulation of the ANS was significantly higher in rheumatoid arthritis patients and is related to disease activity, increased antibodies, and pro-inflammatory cytokines.[26]
- The ANS is responsible for the repair of injured and overused tendons, joints, bones, and muscles.[27]
- Elevated sympathetic nervous system activity levels at night, associated with post-traumatic stress syndrome, impair REM sleep.[28]
- Headaches may be related to dysregulated stress recovery, and mindfulness practice can promote effective heart-rate regulation.[29]

Acupuncture has a balancing effect on the ANS to enhance healing. One study demonstrated that acupuncture using UB20, UB23, CV6, CV12, CV4, ST36, SP6, and KD3 has an antihypertensive effect and can significantly halt deteriorating renal function by reducing renal sympathetic nerve activity.[30] Another study concluded that electro-magnetic acupuncture at BL15 successfully activates the parasympathetic nervous system as evidenced by decreased pupil size.[31]

Balancing the ANS first allows the gentle Body-Feedback approach to be highly effective and accommodate sensitive clients. One study demonstrated that the fear of acupuncture-induced pain can stimulate sympathetic activation of the fight-or-flight response. Significant increases in sympathetic response to acupuncture stimulation correlated with subjects that self-reported higher fear levels. This study concluded that the fear of pain could cause physiological changes and should be given consideration in acupuncture practice.[32]

8.2 Essential Oils and the ANS Connection

Both inhalation and topical application of essential oils activate olfactory receptor neurons located in the nasal cavity and the skin cells.[33] These neurons stimulate the olfactory cortex located within the cerebral cortex of the brain. The olfactory cortex connects with several other areas of the brain, including the frontal and temporal lobes, the limbic system, and the hypothalamus (see Section 8.4.2). The tiny molecular structure of essential oils allows them to swiftly circulate through the bloodstream and cross the blood-brain barrier. Inhalation and topical application of beneficial oils regulate brain activity, calm the limbic system, and balance ANS within minutes of application.

The limbic system develops early in the creation of the brain and includes several structures closely related to the olfactory cortex that initiate different bodily functions. The amygdala triggers emotional responses of anxiety, aggression, and fear, along with creating memories and processing social situations. The cingulate gyrus regulates heart rate and blood pressure, as well as cognitive, attentional, and emotional processing. The amygdala works with the nucleus accumbens to control motivation, addiction, and the reward circuit.[34] Inhaled beneficial essential oils pass through the olfactory cortex and into the limbic system to immediately deescalate the body's stress response and reset homeostasis for optimized healing.

Limbic System Structures

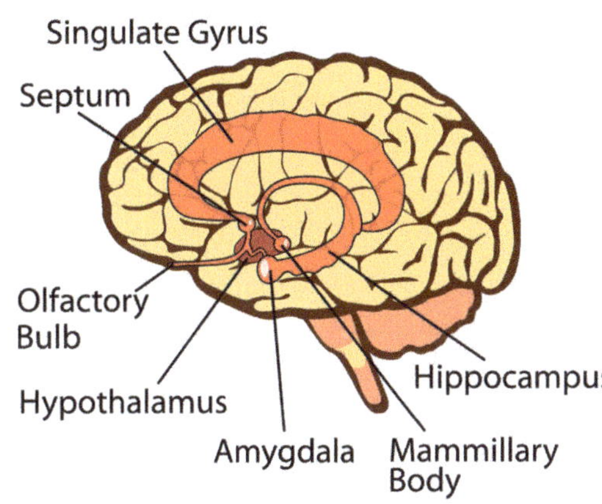

ID 31763752 © Nn555 | Dreamstime.com

Research on the use of essential oils to affect the brain and ANS include:

- In rats, basil essential oil alleviated depression, short-term memory impairment, and hippocampal neurodegenerative changes induced by exposure to chronic unpredictable stress. Basil essential oil should be studied further to test its effects on patients with Alzheimer disease.[35]
- Aromatherapy massage can significantly decrease stress and enhance immune function in pregnant women.[36]
- Lavender essential oil can effectively reduce blood pressure and heart rate in patients after open-heart surgery.[37]

Certain essential oils stimulate a sympathetic response while others encourage a parasympathetic response. Meramour's Organ Supporting and Meridian Balancing Blends are designed to balance the ANS while enhancing the Body-Feedback balancing prescriptions. Beginning acupuncture sessions by applying the essential oil blends that test favorably to the soles of the feet will calm the fight-or-flight response, reduce discomfort from needle insertion, and enhance treatment results. Topical application and inhalation of beneficial essential oils encourages healing by stimulating areas of the brain connected to the olfactory cortex.

Diffusing essential oils during the night and creating diluted topical facial blends can regulate the ANS, oxygenate the brain, and calm emotional responses. Using essential oils that test beneficial between appointments can enhance and lengthen the healing benefits from an acupuncture session. See Chapter 11 for information on essential oils and choosing the Organ Supporting and Meridian Balancing blends.

8.3 Treatment Position and the ANS

Body-Feedback testing techniques during the pre-treatment planning stage can quickly determine the optimal treatment position to encourage relaxation and balance the sympathetic, parasympathetic, and enteric components of the ANS. Some clients will always benefit from either a supine or prone treatment, while others may change from treatment to treatment. Testing for the optimal treatment position and acupoint combinations to balance the ANS occurs during each session to maximize healing potential. Research demonstrates that body position can directly affect the ANS. A sampling includes:

- When body position varies, several actions occur involving all parts of the cardiovascular system, as well as the ANS, which help to regulate their function.[38]
- Heart rate and blood pressure are measurably different in prone and supine positions, and these differences should be considered when autonomic regulation of cardiovascular function is studied in different postures.[39]

Specific treatment positions to regulate the ANS:

- Supine treatment position with abdominal, facial, scalp, or auricular acupoints.
- Supine treatment position with essential oils applied along the spine first.
- Prone treatment position with sacral, lumbar, thoracic, or cervical acupoints.

8.3.1 Determining the Optimal Treatment Position

Step two of the pre-treatment planning stage includes testing the abdomen to determine the optimal treatment position. After evaluating for asymmetry in step one, press on the abdomen in a clockwise motion while checking for an increase or decrease in discomfort or muscle tightness at one or more of the master alarm points (GB21, TB15, and SI13). Using Body-Feedback palpation techniques allows the client and the practitioner to feel the changes in muscle tightness and discomfort. Monitoring for changes in the pulse while checking the abdomen is acceptable; however, the client will not experience the difference.

Any release in muscle tension at the master alarm points from pressing on regions of the abdomen indicates a supine treatment is best. Any increase in tension or resistance in the abdominal muscles or at the master alarm points from pressing on regions of the abdomen means a prone treatment is best. At times, accommodating the less appropriate treatment position will be needed and is discussed in detail throughout the rest of the chapter.

The final decision on treatment position depends on multiple factors. Immediately after identifying the optimal treatment position (supine or prone) to balance the ANS, determine the location of the balancing prescription's acupoints (see Chapter 9). Some balancing acupoints are easier to access in a supine position while others are more accessible in a prone position. Next, consider the presenting complaint and acute symptoms to evaluate the use of local needling.

In summary, the following factors determine the treatment approach:

- the optimal position to balance the ANS
- the location of the balancing prescription's acupoints
- local needling to address the client's presenting complaint and acute symptoms

Steps to check the abdomen

1. Assess the master alarm points GB21, TB15, and SI13 for a baseline level of tension or tenderness.
2. Press the abdominal regions using three or four fingers in a row away from the umbilicus in a clockwise motion. Check, in this order:
   a. conception vessel (ren mai) line above the umbilicus
   b. upper diagonal left
   c. lateral left
   d. lower diagonal left
   e. lower conception vessel (ren mai) line below the umbilicus
   f. lower diagonal right
   g. lateral right
   h. upper diagonal right

Steps to check ANS

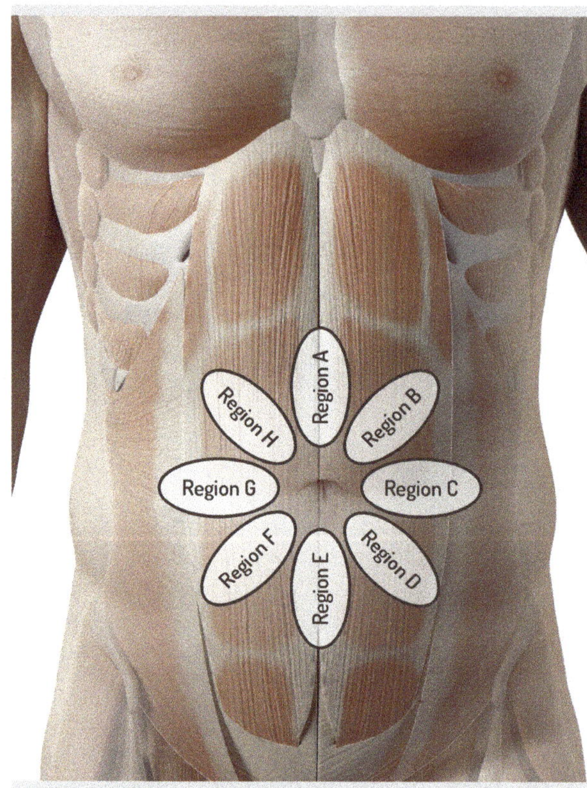

8.3.2 Supine Treatment Positions

The supine, or faceup, treatment position is ideal when the master alarm points soften while pressing on the abdomen. In this position, choose one category of acupoints (abdominal, facial and scalp, or auricular) to balance the ANS, depending on the client's needs.

Abdominal acupoint combinations are ideal for:

- improving the enteric nervous system
- strengthening organ function
- regulating the five-element system
- releasing the back muscles
- enhancing fertility and optimizing the endocrine system
- harmonizing the digestive and immune systems

Scalp and facial acupoint combinations are excellent for:

- jaw pain and misalignment
- concussions, headaches, Bell's Palsy, and trauma
- epilepsy and seizures
- brain-based neurological conditions, such as Parkinson's, multiple sclerosis, Alzheimer's, ADD, ADHD, and autism spectrum disorders
- tremors, memory weakness, and advanced symptoms of aging
- facial rejuvenation treatments

Auricular acupoint combinations are best for:

- emotional disorders and mental illness
- pain and musculoskeletal conditions
- addiction recovery
- post-traumatic stress disorders (PTSD)
- pre-surgical stress and anxiety
- post-surgical pain and recovery

If a client is uncomfortable lying flat in the faceup position, use wedges for their back and a higher bolster under their knees. Another option to increase comfort in the supine position is a zero-gravity chair like the ones utilized in community-style acupuncture clinics. In certain instances, a supine treatment will test best but the clients presenting complaint of back pain, infertility, or a neurological condition will require local needling on the posterior side. In these instances, essential oils can be applied to the outer ear, spine, abdomen, or soles of the feet to balance the ANS before treating in the non-optimal facedown position. See Section 8.5 for other options to adjust the supine optimal treatment position.

8.3.3 Prone Treatment Positions

The prone, or facedown, treatment position is preferred to balance the ANS when the master alarm points tense up or the abdomen tightens when checking the abdominal regions. In some instances, the abdominal muscles become taut and push back while pressing on them, indicating a facedown position is best. In this position, needling the sacrum, spine, along the sides of the spine, or neck can balance the ANS.

Prone acupoint combinations are ideal for:

- neck, shoulder, back, or coccyx (tailbone) pain
- scoliosis and other conditions of the spine
- calming the nervous system
- enhancing fertility
- increasing energy and boosting qi

In some instances, it is necessary to add a thin pillow or folded bath towel under the hips to support and elongate the lower back in the facedown position. Adding support under the hips is especially beneficial for lordosis (sway-back), compression of the spine, and misalignment of the sacrum, sacroiliac joint, and coccyx.

The ANS is a division of the peripheral nervous system, which conveys information using the central nervous system (CNS). The CNS is considered the control center for the entire body and influences other nervous system activities.

The brain and the spinal column work in unison to manage CNS activity. When the ANS tests favorably for back acupoints, this indicates that a nervous system imbalance is stemming from the spinal column. Therefore, treating the cervical, thoracic, lumbar, or sacral nerves is ideal for treating the CNS when the client is in a prone position. Furthermore, when needling the prone acupoint combinations to restore balance in the CNS, avoid the scalp or auricular acupoints, which would divert focus to the brain portion of the CNS.

With an asymmetrical treatment in the prone position, needling or cupping excessively tight muscle areas along the spine, as well as applying essential oils to deficient regions on the back and onto the soles of the feet will promote symmetry while balancing the ANS.

For people with cold or flu symptoms, allergies, sinus headaches, and rhinitis, the prone treatment position can increase sinus congestion and pressure. Adding stationary (dry) cupping to the upper back, base of the neck, and shoulder area can reduce the buildup of fluids that cause extra sinus pressure in the facedown position. See Section 8.5 for other options to balance the ANS when not in the optimal treatment position.

8.4 Optimal Treatment Position and Cupping

The Body-Feedback approach incorporates optional stationary and sliding cupping therapies with acupuncture sessions to address pain conditions and immune weakness. Depending on the client's individual needs, stationary and sliding cupping before, during, or after the acupuncture treatment can balance the ANS. One study found that cupping might be cardioprotective because it restored sympathetic-vagal imbalances by stimulating the peripheral nervous system.[40]

Benefits of sliding and stationary cupping include increased blood flow and stimulation of heme oxygenase to metabolize heme (iron-rich molecules). The heme molecules further produce carbon monoxide, biliverdin, bilirubin, and iron, which are shown to have anti-inflammatory, anti-tumor, neuromodulating, and immune system benefits.[41]

When integrating cupping with supine or prone treatment positions, it is important to coordinate it before, during, or after the insertion of acupuncture needles to balance the ANS based on the abdominal testing results.

- For a supine treatment position when cupping on the posterior side (neck, back, shoulders, glutes, hips, and hamstrings), it is best to apply cupping after removing the needles.
- For a supine treatment position when cupping on the anterior side (facial, abdominal, arms, and quadriceps), it is best to apply cupping before needle insertion or utilize a combination of cupping and needles during the acupuncture treatment.
- For a prone treatment position when cupping on the posterior side (neck, back, shoulders, glutes, hips, and hamstrings), it is best to apply cupping before needle insertion or utilize a combination of cupping and needles during the acupuncture treatment.
- For a prone treatment position when cupping on the anterior side (facial, abdominal, arms, and quadriceps), it is best to apply cupping after removing the needles.

Cupping alone is another option to balance the ANS. In certain instances, the prone or supine treatment position will test best, and yet the other position will be needed to access specific acupoints or for the client's comfort. The following section includes suggestions for using cupping alone to adjust the optimal treatment position.

8.5 Needling in a Non-Optimal Treatment Position

At times a client will need to be treated in a position that does not balance the ANS, and adjustments can be made to accommodate this. Essential oils and cupping can balance the ANS within minutes, allowing for needling acupoints in the non-optimal treatment position. After applying the essential oils and cupping, retest the abdomen using the steps in Section 8.3.1 to confirm that the master alarm points or neck muscles remain soft when palpating the abdomen, indicating a balanced ANS. If the master alarm points or neck muscles tighten when checking the abdomen, a two-sided treatment approach is best. The following examples illustrate changing the optimal treatment position.

A client has sinus congestion and pressure, along with a runny nose, and tests best for a prone treatment position. Sliding or stationary cupping on the back first for 5-10 minutes with essential oils applied to the spine and soles of the feet regulates the ANS, drains phlegm and dampness, and boosts the immune system. Afterward, acupuncture in the supine position with facial acupoints will be more effective.

A client is requesting facial rejuvenation acupuncture, yet tests best for a prone treatment. Sliding or stationary cupping on the back first for 5-10 minutes with essential oils applied to the spine and soles of the feet regulates the ANS. Afterward, acupuncture in the supine position with facial acupoints will be more effective.

A client has back pain, yet tests best for a supine treatment and only has time for a one-sided treatment. First, apply essential oils to the soles of the feet, outer ear, or abdomen. Afterward, a treatment in the prone position that includes local needling in the painful region will be more effective.

A client has back pain, yet tests best for a supine treatment. Needle the abdominal and auricular acupoints to balance the ANS first. Then needle the balancing and tonification or sedation prescriptions, along with supporting acupoints, to treat the back indirectly. After removing the first set of needles, in a prone position, use sliding cupping or a second set of needles in the local area to address the back pain directly.

With long-term ANS dysregulation, essential oils and cupping may not be powerful enough to adjust for the non-optimal treatment position. Some conditions respond best with two-sided treatments to achieve results and regulate the ANS. Allow extra time during the initial acupuncture session to address the anterior and posterior sides if necessary. Then explain to the client why the two-sided approach best addresses their needs, and how to schedule for two sides at future appointments. Some clients will be able to transition from two sides to one, while others will always respond best to including a second set of needles or cupping on their other side.

8.6 Indications the ANS is Remaining Dysregulated

In some cases, genetics, trauma, post-traumatic stress syndrome, hormonal imbalance, and prescription medications can create challenges in regulating the ANS. In addition to treatment in the optimal position, clients who have a heightened sensitivity to pain or feel increased discomfort with needle insertion require precise acupoint locations and less needle retention time to keep the ANS balanced. With a severely dysregulated ANS, the client can alternate between sympathetic and parasympathetic dominance during an acupuncture treatment and cause the optimal treatment position to change mid-session.

Indications that the ANS is remaining unbalanced include:

- difficulty relaxing during an acupuncture session
- feeling agitated or fidgeting during an acupuncture session
- struggling to fall or stay asleep at home
- low energy after a full night of sleep
- anxiety, depression, or excessive worry

When removing the needles, ask the client if they were able to relax during the treatment and how they feel. If they were unable to relax or experienced any muscle tension building during the session, reevaluate the ANS and check for pathogenic heat or inflammation (see Chapter 3). Recheck the abdomen using the steps in Section 8.3.1 to determine if the optimal treatment position was correct or changed during the acupuncture session. If the optimal treatment position changed, apply essential oils or add cupping therapy in the new position for 5-10 minutes, as time permits. Rebalancing the ANS at the end of the session will enhance the treatment results over the next couple of days.

If checking the abdomen confirms the optimal treatment position remains the same, pathogenic heat or inflammation is likely dysregulating the ANS. Check the metal + water combinations to the pulse or master fire alarm point (GB21) and apply magnetic pellets for a few days, as needed. Magnetic pellets on the metal + water combinations will release the pathogenic heat and improve the effectiveness of the treatment over the next few days. Make a note to check and use the metal + water combinations at future appointments to regulate the ANS in the optimal treatment position.

When a client relaxes through the majority of the session and then notices a shift to agitation or restlessness at the end, they will respond better with shorter needle retention time. In general, two-sided treatments, deficiency conditions, and Body-Feedback tonification prescriptions respond better to shorter treatment times: 20 minutes or less for one-sided treatments and 15 minutes or less for two-sided treatments.

As health improves, the ANS will remain regulated longer after each treatment session. With new clients or existing clients with recent trauma or new health challenges, monitor energy levels, sleep, and mood to determine how long the ANS remained balanced and schedule follow-up appointments around that length of time. With long-term clients and maintenance treatments, advise the client to call for follow-up appointments when their sleep, mood, or energy level is starting to decline. A regulated ANS encourages daily self-healing and longevity.

CHAPTER 9

Body-Feedback Balancing Prescriptions

The Body-Feedback balancing prescriptions combine four shu-points that augment a trisection and rectify organ/meridian dysfunction using the natural laws of the restraining cycle. The balancing acupoints create the foundation for the treatment approach. As symptoms diminish and health improves, the balancing prescriptions often change from session to session. When the balancing prescription remains the same for several consecutive sessions, a client's constitutional or genetic weakness becomes apparent. The balancing prescription identifies where to focus on herbs, supplements, and lifestyle changes that can have the most significant impact on healing.

> According to *The Yellow Emperor's Classic of Medicine*, Qi Bo continued, *"The principles of the five elements would help you understand all transformations in the universe. For example, metal can cut down wood; water can put out fire; wood can penetrate earth; fire can melt metal; earth can contain water. These transformations can be applied to the myriad of things in the universe. In acupuncture one applies the same principles. In this way, one can bestow benevolence upon all people."*[42]

The Five-Element Restraining Cycle

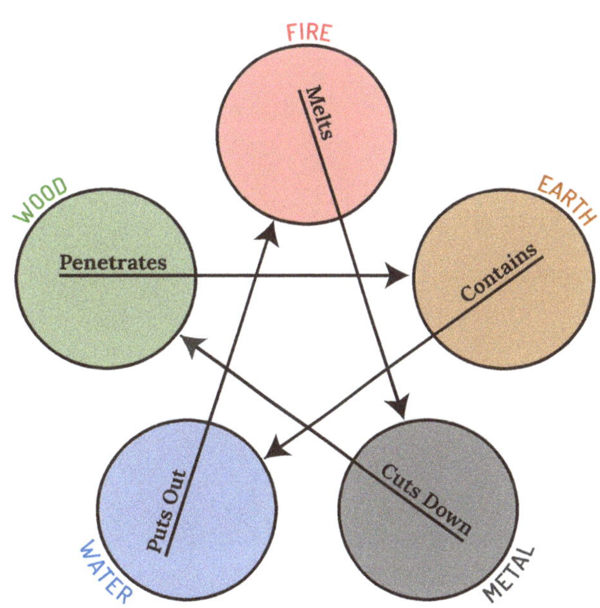

The Body-Feedback balancing prescriptions utilize specific acupoints with elemental properties to optimize the five elements according to the above restraining cycle. The ancient shu-transporting points, also known as antique points or shu-points, are a passageway to the five-elements through the meridians. These elemental shu-points are located between the elbows and fingertips or the knees and toes. Shu-points provide strong regulation of organ function and harmonize the meridian system when properly combined following the five-element rules.

Yin Meridian Shu-Points

Shu Category	Jing-well	Ying-spring	Shu-stream	Jing-river	He-sea
Element	WOOD	FIRE	EARTH	METAL	WATER
LUNG	LU11	LU10	LU9	LU8	LU5
SPLEEN	SP1	SP2	SP3	SP5	SP9
HEART	HT9	HT8	HT7	HT4	HT3
KIDNEY	KD1	KD2	KD3	KD7	KD10
PERICARDIUM	PC9	PC8	PC7	PC5	PC3
LIVER	LV1	LV2	LV3	LV4	LV8

Yang Meridian Shu-Points

Shu Category	Jing-well	Ying-spring	Shu-stream	Jing-river	He-sea
Element	METAL	WATER	WOOD	FIRE	EARTH
LARGE INTESTINE	LI1	LI2	LI3	LI5	LI11
STOMACH	ST45	ST44	ST43	ST41	ST36
SMALL INTESTINE	SI1	SI2	SI3	SI5	SI8
URINARY BLADDER	UB67	UB66	UB65	UB60	UB40
TRIPLE BURNER	TB1	TB2	TB3	TB6	TB10
GALLBLADDER	GB44	GB43	GB41	GB38	GB34

The Body-Feedback approach builds upon these powerful balancing point combinations to create a root treatment with lasting results. The balancing prescriptions indicate the individual Body-Feedback testing locations for checking essential oils, herbs, and supplements, along with monitoring the client's progress. The balancing prescriptions decide which sedation or tonification acupoints to test and use.

9.1 Origins of the Body-Feedback Balancing Prescriptions

The application of the five-element restraining cycle for choosing acupoints is credited to an unknown Korean Buddhist monk who published the Saam acupuncture manuscript sometime between 1644 and 1742; this approach is sometimes called "Saam" acupuncture.[43] Anonymous Chinese acupuncturists further expanded the five-element restraining cycle to create the Chinese six-point, five-element treatment approach. Within a Body-Feedback balancing acupoint prescription, two of the balancing points come from the Korean four-point theory, and the other two points come from the Chinese six-point method.

Saam acupuncture enhances the engendering cycle's mother-child treatment approach (see Chapter 10) by adding two shu-points from the restraining cycle's element (the grandmother-grandchild rule) based on the 50th and 75th chapters of the Nan-Jing.[44] The restraining element has a balancing effect for both excess and deficient pathology.

Modern Chinese acupuncturists discovered that the Korean four-point approach (Saam acupuncture) could be made more effective by adding two extra shu-points to support the restraining cycle. These additional supportive points are the restraining element's mother points following the engendering cycle.

The Body-Feedback balancing prescriptions come from reorganizing the steps of the Korean four-point and Chinese six-point treatment approaches. Two of the shu-points in the balancing prescriptions follow the grandmother-grandchild rule of the restraining cycle. The other two shu-points follow the mother-child rule of the engendering cycle to strengthen the restraining cycle. Together, these points optimize the root affected element. Each step for choosing the balancing acupoints is explained with diagrams below for all twelve meridians.

9.2 Balancing the Root-Affected Element

When an element is affected by internal or external pathogens, its paired organs/meridians become dysfunctional and create trisection discord. The balancing prescriptions consist of two primary points on the affected element's meridian and two secondary points on other related elements' meridians. These secondary balancing points are horary points (the same shu-point as the element), which strongly influence the five-element system. If the root-affected element's meridian is yin, then both of the other related meridians are yin. If the root-affected element's meridian is yang, then both of the other related meridians are yang. In the restraining cycle, the affected element is restrained by its grandmother and in turn restrains its grandchild, which also happens to be the mother to the grandmother element in the engendering cycle. Together, the three elements formulated from the restraining and engendering cycles create a triangular flow of energy to restore balance to the affected element.

The first balancing point is the shu-point from the element restraining the affected element (the grandmother) on the affected element's meridian. This shu-point restrains the affected element.

The second balancing point is the shu-point from the element restrained by the affected element (the grandchild) on the affected element's meridian. This shu-point strengthens the affected element's grandmother through the engendering cycle, thus completing the circuit for a triangular flow of energy.

Step One to Balance a Metal Element Excess or Deficiency Affecting the Lungs

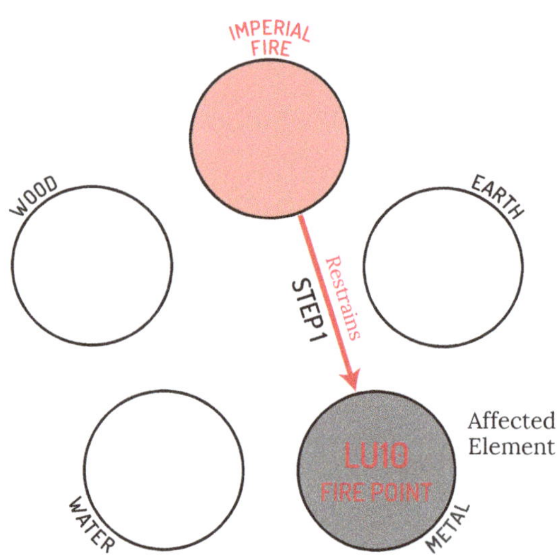

For example, an excess or deficiency affecting the lungs uses LU10 (the grandmother's element shu-point on the affected yin meridian) to restrain and balance metal.

Step Two to Balance a Metal Element Excess or Deficiency Affecting the Lungs

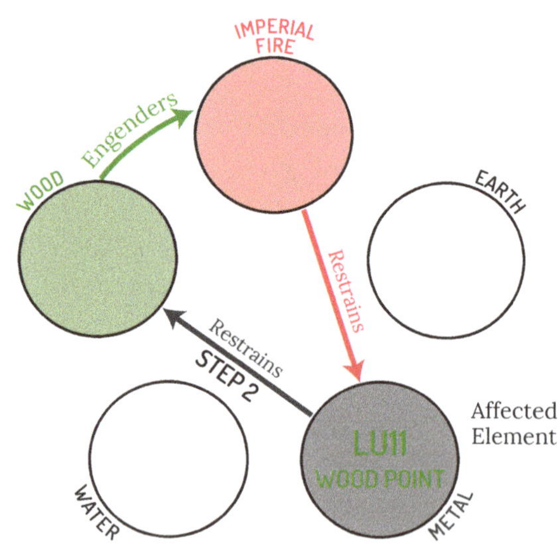

For example, an excess or deficiency affecting the lungs uses LU11 (the grandchild's element shu-point on the affected yin meridian) to strengthen the restraining element through the engendering cycle and balance metal.

The third balancing point is the horary shu-point from the element restrained by the affected element (the grandchild). This shu-point strengthens the affected element's grandmother through the engendering cycle.

The fourth balancing point is the horary shu-point from the element restraining the affected element (the grandmother). This shu-point restrains the affected element.

Step Three to Balance a Metal Element Excess or Deficiency Affecting the Lungs

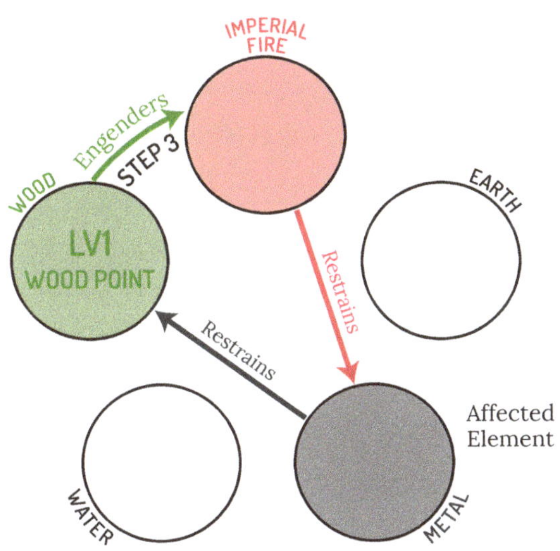

For example, an excess or deficiency affecting the lungs uses LV1 (the grandchild's horary shu-point) to strengthen the restraining element through the engendering cycle and balance metal.

Step Four to Balance a Metal Element Excess or Deficiency Affecting the Lungs

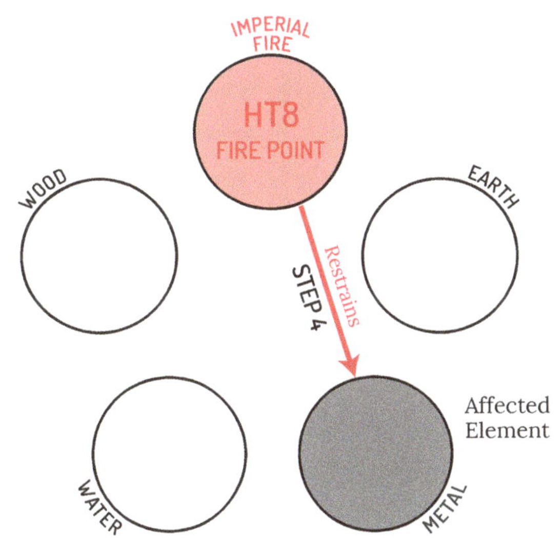

For example, an excess or deficiency affecting the lungs uses HT8 (the grandmother's horary shu-point) to restrain and balance metal.

Early in my practice, I treated the four points based on the restraining cycle first as the foundation for my treatments. With Body-Feedback palpation techniques, I confirmed that these points effectively harmonized the five-element system for both deficient and excess presentations. However, I quickly realized that adjustments were needed if pathogenic heat was present in specific organs/meridians.

Wood and earth are the two elements not involved in the restraining cycle (the grandmother-grandchild rule) with the fire element. Certain wood and earth shu-points will create additional heat that exacerbates pathogenic heat when needled or treated with magnetic pellets:

- A wood point on a wood meridian will engender additional pathogenic heat based on the mother-child rule unless it is a jing-well or ying-spring point category.
- An earth point on an earth meridian will be unable to disperse pathogenic heat from the fire element based on the mother-child rule, as it is not a jing-well or ying-spring point category.

There are three horary points (SP3, ST36, and GB41) in the balancing prescriptions that require modifications when pathogenic heat is detected, and one horary point (HT8) that can be overly draining for the heart. These points are bolded in the point prescriptions throughout this text for special attention. Chapter 3 provides a complete explanation of pathogenic heat and treatment options.

9.3 The Restraining Cycle and the Grandmother-Grandchild Relationship

In the early years of formulating the Body-Feedback System, I struggled to find a theory that resonated with my approach to the restraining cycle. Most of the information I found referenced the restraining cycle as destructive, controlling, and insulting on the affected meridian. My approach to the restraining cycle (grandmother-grandchild rule) is gentle, supportive, and harmonizing, which is nothing like the descriptions I read. After lengthy discussions, trusted colleague and fellow acupuncturist Gail Byrnes and I created a nurturing explanation for the reasoning behind choosing points from the restraining cycle and a simple analogy.

In ancient Chinese culture, the matriarch of the family had a significant impact on raising future generations. The grandmother ensured the grandchildren grew up with structure and supervision while the mother was busy. The restraining cycle uses this grandmother-grandchild structure and guidance to regulate the energy flow through the five elements. When a grandmother nurtures the grandchild, that grandchild in turn learns how to foster future generations and its grandchildren. Parents are more likely to do a better job raising their children when they have the reliable and supportive help of their parents. Through this system of supporting future generations, the children become contributing members of society. The children learn how to become good parents and grandparents, and this healthy family dynamic furthers the evolution of society.

Chinese medicine uses experiences in nature and society to describe physical and emotional health. The restraining cycle demonstrates the harmonizing and balancing nature of the grandmother-grandchild relationship within the family and the five-element system. With physically or emotionally unhealthy grandparents, the growth and development of future generations are more challenging, and the parents are overburdened. A genetically weak, injured, or compromised element disrupts organ function, and the body struggles to thrive and self-heal. Restoring balance and integrity to the engendering and restraining cycles is key to making lasting improvements in both physical and emotional health.

The mechanism behind the restraining cycle's ability to harmonize the five-elements occurs in a triangular exchange of energy between three elements that redistribute excesses and deficiencies in steps. The three elements and their balancing points are the same for both excess and deficient conditions. However, the movement of energy between the elements differs depending on if the affected element is excess or deficient.

Balancing A Root Metal Excess

For an element in a state of excess (e.g., metal element), the flow of energy through the retraining cycle is as follows:

STEP 1: The affected element (metal) releases its excess through the restraining cycle to the grandchild (wood).

STEP 2: The grandchild (wood) redistributes the affected element's excess to nourish the next element, or grandmother (imperial-fire), through the engendering cycle.

STEP 3: The grandmother (imperial-fire), strengthened through the engendering cycle, now has the capacity to restrain and balance the affected element (metal).

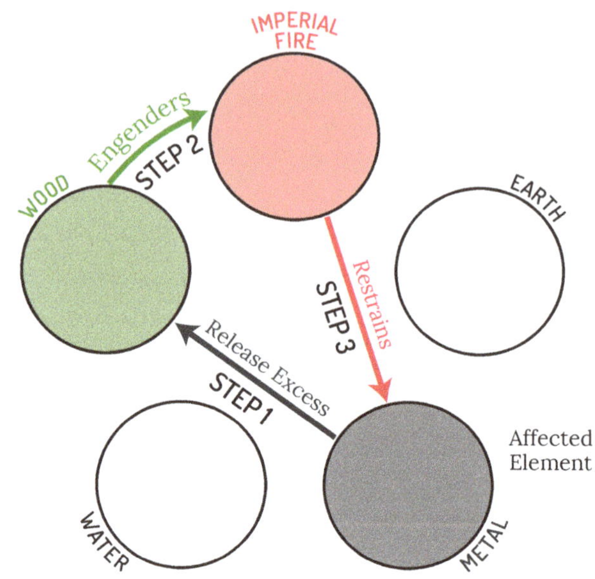

Balancing A Root Metal Deficiency

For an element in a state of deficiency (e.g., metal element), the flow of energy through the restraining cycle is as follows:

STEP 1: The affected element (metal) in a state of deficiency acquires energy from its grandmother (imperial-fire) through the restraining cycle.

STEP 2: The affected element (metal), now strengthened by its grandmother (imperial-fire), has the capacity to properly restrain and balance its grandchild (wood).

STEP 3: The grandchild (wood) of the affected element (metal) further strengthens the grandmother (imperial-fire) through the engendering cycle.

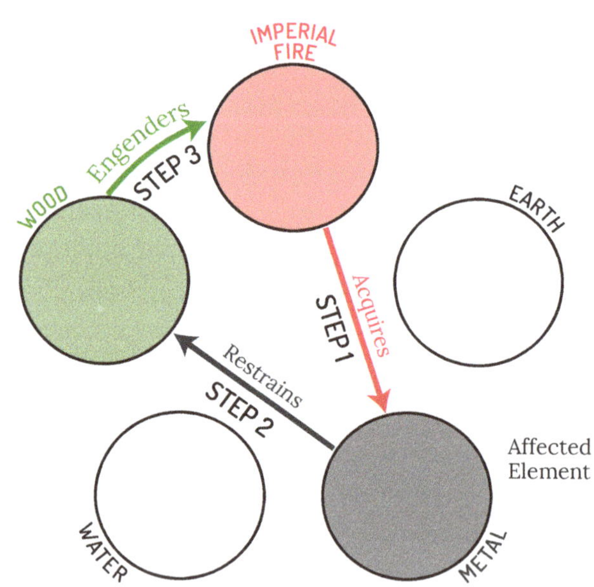

The three steps in both of the illustrations above create a continuous flow of energy between three elements that harmonize the entire five-element system. The balancing prescriptions use the grandmother-grandchild and mother-child relationships to efficiently balance the five elements and form the foundation to build upon for choosing additional acupoints.

9.4 First Trisection Balancing Prescriptions by Element

METAL RESTRAINS WOOD – WOOD ENGENDERS IMPERIAL-FIRE – IMPERIAL-FIRE RESTRAINS METAL

Balancing acupoints for lung excess or deficiency pathology:

STEP 1: LU10 is the restraining fire shu-point on the lung meridian.

STEP 2: LU11 is the restraining wood shu-point on the lung meridian.

STEP 3: LV1 is the yin wood horary shu-point that engenders fire.

STEP 4: **HT8** is the yin imperial-fire horary shu-point that restrains metal (compare **HT8** to HT4 metal + HT3 water combination).

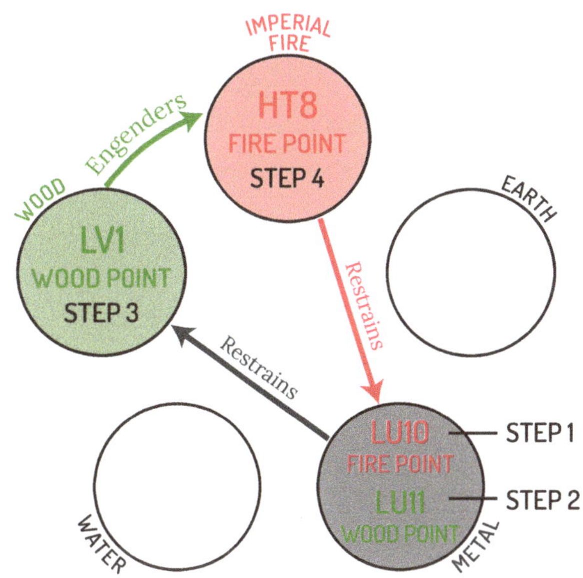

Affected Element

Balancing acupoints for large intestine excess or deficiency pathology:

STEP 1: LI5 is the restraining fire shu-point on the large intestine meridian.

STEP 2: LI3 is the restraining wood shu-point on the large intestine meridian.

STEP 3: **GB41** is the yang wood horary shu-point that engenders fire (compare **GB41** to GB44 metal + GB43 water combination for pathogenic heat).

STEP 4: SI5 is the yang imperial-fire horary shu-point that restrains metal.

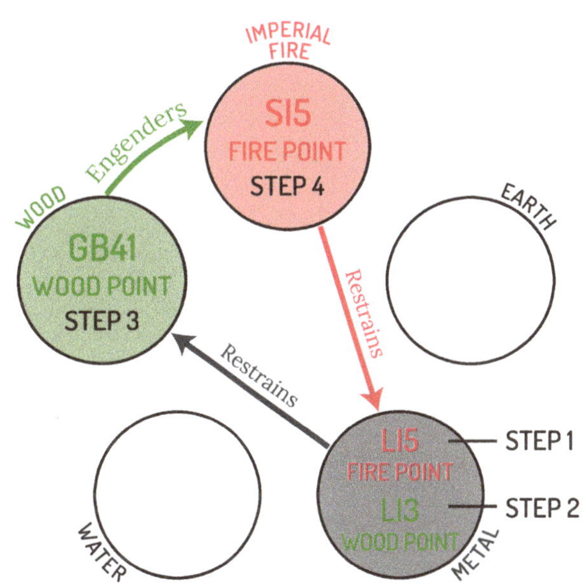

Affected Element

EARTH RESTRAINS WATER - WATER ENGENDERS WOOD - WOOD RESTRAINS EARTH

Balancing acupoints for stomach excess or deficiency pathology:

STEP 1: ST43 is the restraining wood shu-point on the stomach meridian.

STEP 2: ST44 is the restraining water shu-point on the stomach meridian.

STEP 3: UB66 is the yang water horary shu-point that engenders wood.

STEP 4: **GB41** is the yang wood horary shu-point that restrains earth (compare **GB41** to GB44 metal + GB43 water combination for pathogenic heat).

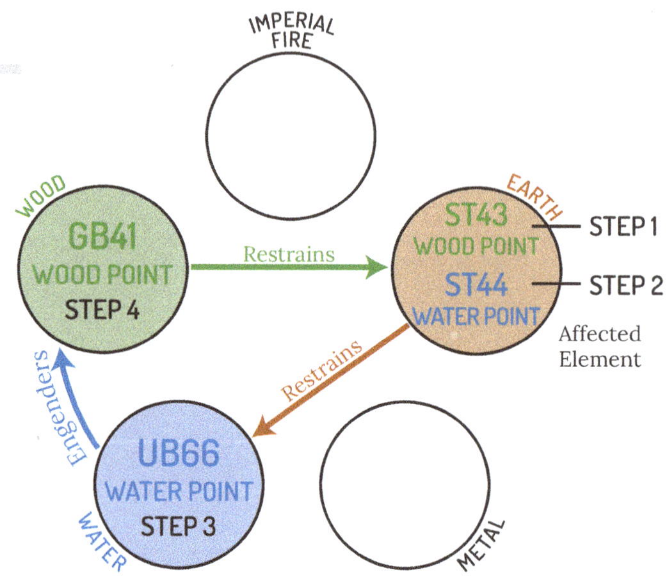

Balancing acupoints for spleen excess or deficiency pathology:

STEP 1: SP1 is the restraining wood shu-point on the spleen meridian.

STEP 2: SP9 is the restraining water shu-point on the spleen meridian.

STEP 3: KD10 is the yin water horary shu-point that engenders wood.

STEP 4: LV1 is the yin wood horary shu-point that restrains earth.

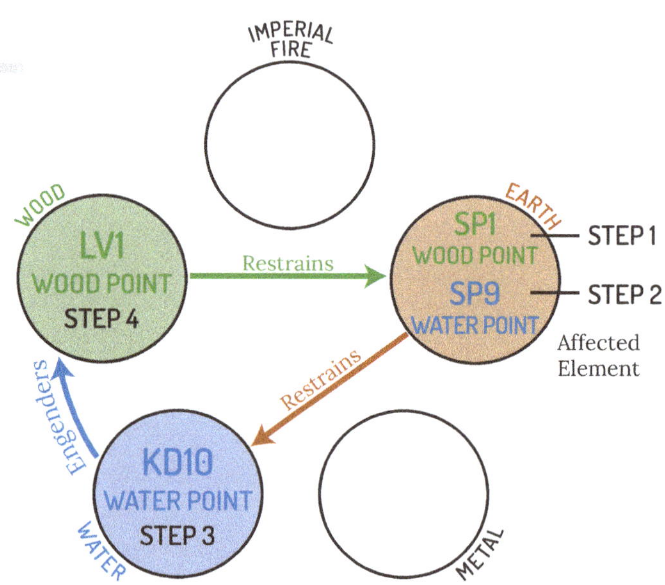

9.5 Second Trisection Balancing Prescriptions by Element

IMPERIAL-FIRE RESTRAINS METAL – METAL ENGENDERS WATER – WATER RESTRAINS IMPERIAL-FIRE

Balancing acupoints for heart excess or deficiency pathology:

STEP 1: HT3 is the restraining water shu-point on the heart meridian.

STEP 2: HT4 is the restraining metal shu-point on the heart meridian.

STEP 3: LU8 is the yin metal horary shu-point that engenders water.

STEP 4: KD10 is the yin water horary shu-point that restrains imperial-fire.

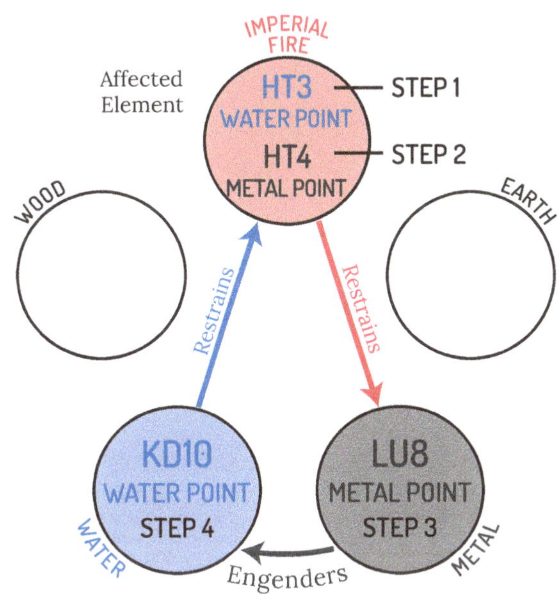

Balancing acupoints for small intestine excess or deficiency pathology:

STEP 1: SI2 is the restraining water shu-point on the small intestine meridian.

STEP 2: SI1 is the restraining metal shu-point on the small intestine meridian.

STEP 3: LI1 is the yang metal horary shu-point that engenders water.

STEP 4: UB66 is the yang water horary shu-point that restrains imperial-fire.

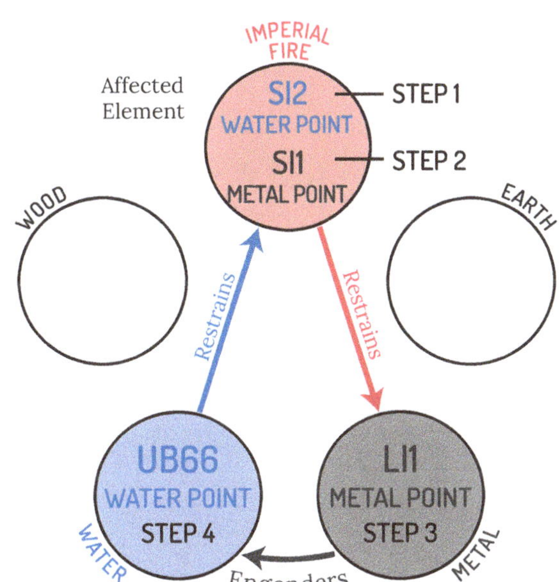

WATER RESTRAINS IMPERIAL-FIRE – IMPERIAL-FIRE ENGENDERS EARTH – EARTH RESTRAINS WATER

Balancing acupoints for urinary bladder excess or deficiency pathology:

STEP 1: UB40 is the restraining earth shu-point on the urinary bladder meridian.

STEP 2: UB60 is the restraining fire shu-point on the urinary bladder meridian.

STEP 3: SI5 is the yang fire horary shu-point that engenders earth.

STEP 4: **ST36** is the yang earth horary shu-point that restrains water (compare **ST36** to ST45 metal + ST44 water combination for pathogenic heat).

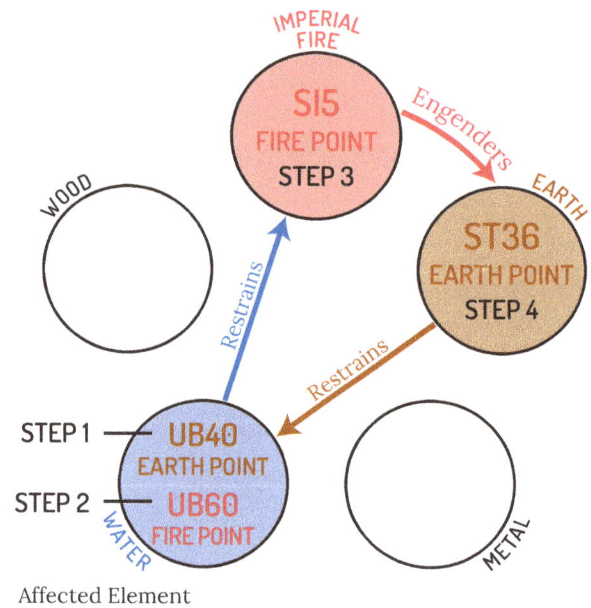

Balancing acupoints for kidney excess or deficiency pathology:

STEP 1: KD3 is the restraining earth shu-point on the kidney meridian.

STEP 2: KD2 is the restraining fire shu-point on the kidney meridian.

STEP 3: **HT8** is the yin imperial-fire horary shu-point that engenders earth (compare **HT8** to HT4 metal + HT3 water combination).

STEP 4: **SP3** is the yin earth horary shu-point that restrains water (compare **SP3** to SP5 metal + SP9 water combination for pathogenic heat).

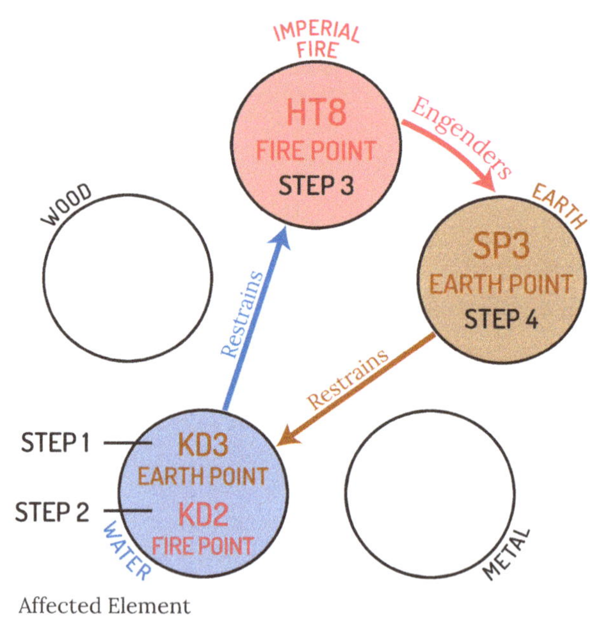

9.6 Third Trisection Balancing Prescriptions by Element

MINISTERIAL-FIRE RESTRAINS METAL – METAL ENGENDERS WATER – WATER RESTRAINS MINISTERIAL-FIRE

Balancing acupoints for pericardium excess or deficiency pathology:

STEP 1: PC3 is the restraining water shu-point on the pericardium meridian.

STEP 2: PC5 is the restraining metal shu-point on the pericardium meridian.

STEP 3: LU8 is the yin metal horary shu-point that engenders water.

STEP 4: KD10 is the yin water horary shu-point that restrains ministerial-fire.

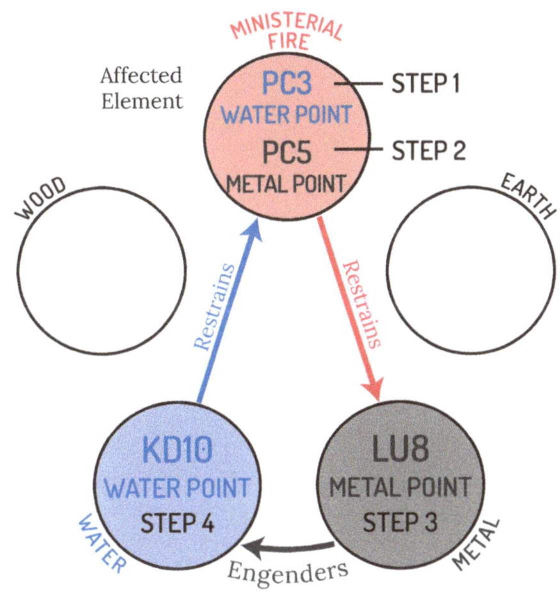

Balancing acupoints for triple burner excess or deficiency pathology:

STEP 1: TB2 is the restraining water shu-point on the triple burner meridian.

STEP 2: TB1 is the restraining metal shu-point on the triple burner meridian.

STEP 3: ST45 is the yang metal-point on the yang earth meridian*.

STEP 4: UB66 is the yang water horary shu-point that restrains the ministerial-fire element.

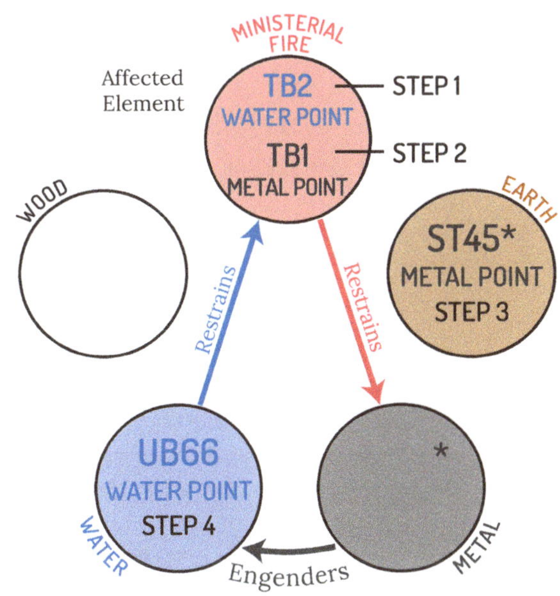

*The triple burner uses the metal point on the earth meridian instead of the metal point on the metal meridian from the Chinese six-point approach, and Body-Feedback testing confirms this is the correct acupoint for this prescription.

WOOD RESTRAINS EARTH - EARTH ENGENDERS METAL - METAL RESTRAINS WOOD

Balancing acupoints for gallbladder excess or deficiency pathology:

STEP 1: GB44 is the restraining metal shu-point on the gallbladder meridian.

STEP 2: GB34 is the restraining earth shu-point on the gallbladder meridian.

STEP 3: **ST36** is the yang earth horary shu-point that engenders metal (compare **ST36** to ST45 metal + ST44 water combination for pathogenic heat).

STEP 4: LI1 is the yang metal horary shu-point that restrains the wood element.

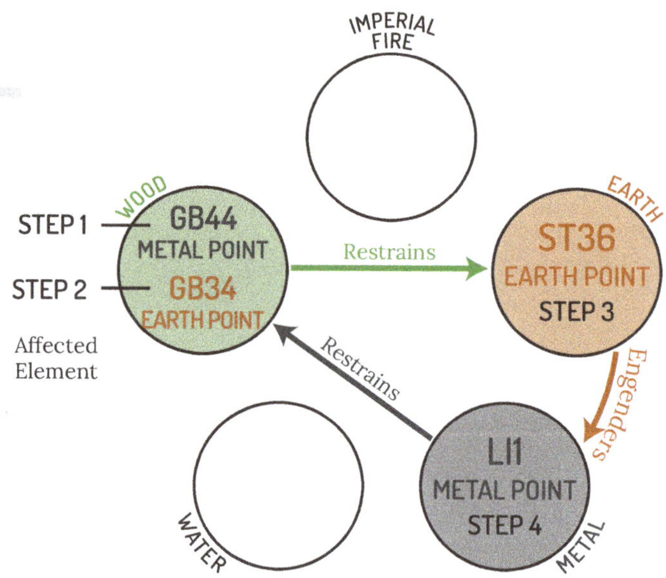

Balancing acupoints for liver excess or deficiency pathology:

STEP 1: LV4 is the restraining metal shu-point on the liver meridian.

STEP 2: LV3 is the restraining earth shu-point on the liver meridian.

STEP 3: **SP3** is the yin earth horary shu-point that engenders metal (compare **SP3** to SP5 metal + SP9 water combination for pathogenic heat).

STEP 4: LU8 is the yin metal horary shu-point that restrains wood.

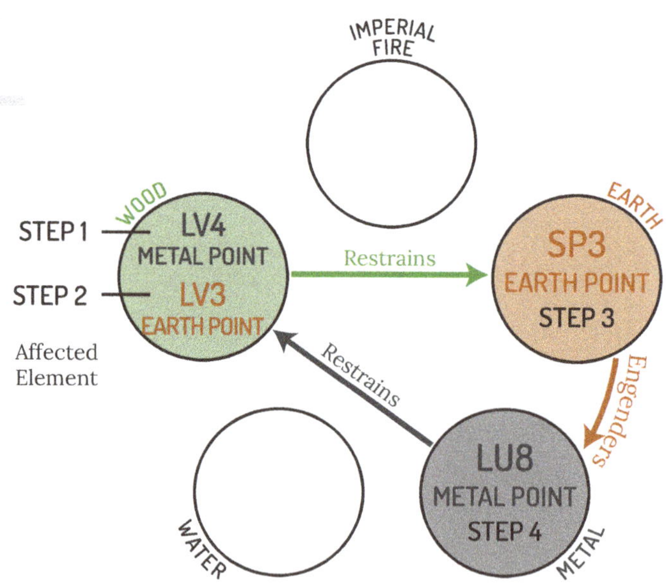

9.7 The Body-Feedback Pregnancy Balancing Prescription

Early pregnancy is a unique time in a woman's life when her immune system identifies the newly fertilized embryo as non-self yet safe to nourish. The first trisection modulates the immune system's ability to accept the pregnancy and allow for implantation after fertilization occurs. Within a few days after ovulation, a unique combination of hand and foot yang-ming balancing points will test favorably to the pulse, master points, and Body-Feedback areas when the immune system needs support to accept a pregnancy. Other standard Body-Feedback balancing prescriptions can test favorably when the immune system is properly accepting a pregnancy. The Body-Feedback pregnancy prescription can indicate conception has occurred even before the client has reached the end of her menstrual cycle or taken a pregnancy test.

The Body-Feedback Pregnancy Balancing Prescription (ST43, ST44, **GB41**, SI5, LI5) integrates the hand and foot yang-ming restraining cycles to balance all five elements. The wood phase (**GB41**) links together the earth (ST43 and ST44) and metal (SI5 and LI5) phases of the yang-ming level and provides the unifying point in this special combination. This pregnancy balancing prescription harmonizes the five elements through the immune system's relationship with the affected earth and metal elements.

EARTH RESTRAINS WATER – WATER ENGENDERS WOOD – WOOD RESTRAINS EARTH
METAL RESTRAINS WOOD – WOOD ENGENDERS IMPERIAL-FIRE – IMPERIAL-FIRE RESTRAINS METAL

Balancing acupoints to support the immune system during the early stages of pregnancy:

STEP 1: ST43 is the restraining wood shu-point on the stomach meridian.

STEP 2: ST44 is the restraining water shu-point on the stomach meridian.

STEP 3: **GB41** is the yang wood horary shu-point that engenders fire (compare **GB41** to GB44 metal + GB43 water combination for pathogenic heat).

STEP 4: SI5 is the yang imperial-fire horary shu-point that restrains metal.

STEP 5: LI5 is the restraining fire shu-point on the large intestine meridian.

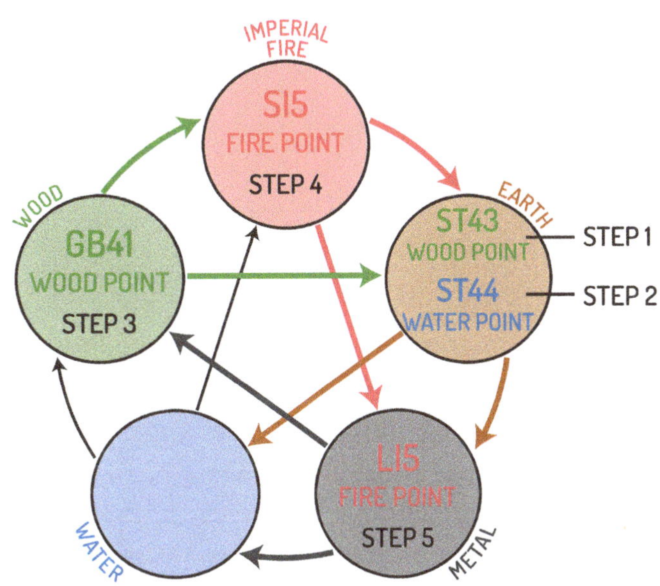

Improving egg and sperm quality responds best to weekly acupuncture, herbs, and supplements for three or more months before conception occurs to achieve a healthy pregnancy. Some women who are trying to conceive may still test favorably for the pregnancy prescription when they have a chemical pregnancy (a delayed menstrual period with pregnancy hormone levels too low to detect on a home pregnancy test) or a regular period while the other factors that influence fertility are improving. Because this unique point selection only happens in response to conception, knowing that conception has occurred with or without implantation can provide valuable information on a case-by-case basis.

9.8 Practical Application of the Balancing Prescriptions

"The principles of healing and medicine in general are difficult to grasp because many changes occur in illness, and the healing process must adapt to that. It becomes difficult to know the root. The origin of illness can be so small and vague, in fact, so elusive, but the illness can still become substantial over time."[45]

9.8.1 Identifying and Rectifying the Root Imbalance

Step three of the pre-treatment planning stage begins with determining the Body-Feedback balancing prescription by testing key shu-points to the pulse, master points (GB21, TB15, or SI13), or neck muscles. The balancing prescription that normalizes the pulse to slightly slippery and releases tension or discomfort in the neck muscles or master points identifies the organ/meridian dysfunction at the root of the current trisection imbalance.

Remember to compare the four shu-points that may require the metal + water combination to address pathogenic heat when they are part of any of the Body-Feedback prescriptions. The three horary points **(SP3, ST36,** and **GB41)** can increase existing pathogenic heat, and the horary point **(HT8)** on the heart meridian may be excessively draining for some clients. Immediately after identifying the root balancing treatment, check the tonification and sedation points to the pulse or Body-Feedback testing locations (see Chapter 10).

Start with gently pressing one of the balancing points with the direction of the meridian in the same angle as the potential needle insertion for 5-10 seconds while monitoring the pulse or checking the Body-Feedback testing locations. The balancing prescriptions respond best to needling either with the flow of the meridian or perpendicular to it (the direction of needle insertion is provided in the point location illustrations in Chapter 14). When testing the balancing points, compare pressing the point with the flow of the meridian to pressing perpendicularly while monitoring the pulse. After finding one balancing point that tests favorably, check all of the prescription's balancing points and identify any points that need the metal + water combination to release pathogenic heat.

If all of the balancing prescriptions acupoints are not tested, the metal + water combinations to clear pathogenic heat for supporting meridians can cause confusion when choosing the correct root treatment. For example, the LU8 metal + LU5 water combination can be supporting acupoints for any root treatment when pathogenic heat affects the lung organ/meridian. LU8 (the metal horary acupoint) is part of the heart, pericardium, and liver balancing prescriptions, and may also include LU5 when pathogenic heat is present. Using the recommended shu-points below can help identify the root balancing prescription for meridians already containing one metal or water shu-point, such as the heart, pericardium, and liver.

The correct root balancing prescription will restore the pulse to slightly slippery or release discomfort and tightness in master alarm points. Remember to check both the left and right sides of the body to identify and verify asymmetry. Certain acupoints (exclusive shu-points) only occur in the balancing prescription for their element, and these points can confirm or reject the potential root treatment. Memorizing the exclusive shu-points listed below allows for quick determination of the root balancing treatment, as these acupoints only appear in their respective balancing prescriptions.

FIRST TRISECTION:
Lung: LU10
Large Intestine: LI5
Stomach: ST43
Spleen: SP1

SECOND TRISECTION:
Heart: HT3*
Small Intestine: SI2**
Urinary Bladder: UB60
Kidney: KD3

THIRD TRISECTION:
Pericardium: PC3**
Triple Burner: TB2**
Gallbladder: GB34
Liver: LV3

*HT3 can be part of the metal + water substitution for **HT8** in the lung and kidney prescriptions. Check all acupoints in the heart prescription to identify the correct balancing prescription.

**SI2, TB2, and PC5 are part of the metal + water combination to release pathogenic heat. Check all acupoints in these prescriptions to confirm that they are the correct root balancing prescription or supporting acupoints.

9.8.2 Assessing the Corresponding Body-Feedback Areas

After determining the balancing prescription, which identifies the root dysfunction, palpate looking for the most tender corresponding individual Body-Feedback testing locations (organ and meridian alarm points, muscle associations, and referrals areas). Chapter 6 contains the charts, and Chapter 12 summarizes the steps for checking the Body-Feedback testing locations. Many clients are unaware of discomfort at these regions until it is brought to their attention. Explain that discomfort at the Body-Feedback testing locations corresponds with the organs/meridians that need the most support. Then demonstrate how essential oils, herbs, and supplements impact these testing locations by using the Body-Feedback palpation methods. When clients feel the positive impact of acupuncture, essential oils, herbs, or supplements in their bodies, compliance and follow-through are dramatically increased.

Confirmation of a masterful treatment happens when the tender or tight Body-Feedback testing locations improve by at least 75%. Supportive lifestyle choices can improve the acupuncture's effectiveness and extend the relief of discomfort at the related testing locations. Basic Body-Feedback palpation methods can be taught to clients so they can monitor their testing locations. When clients observe changes in these areas between appointments, they can learn how to identify the lifestyle choices and supplements that support their health. Clients often describe the release of pain and tenderness from the application of essential oils and acupuncture treatments as tangible confirmation that indicates improvements in their health.

9.8.3 Steps for Recognizing the Balancing Prescriptions

Depending on your learning style, you may find memorizing the balancing prescriptions works best, or you may apply the formula below to select the balancing points by element (except for the triple burner meridian, which requires an adjustment to the rule):

STEP 1: Choose the restraining element's (grandmother) shu-point on the affected meridian.

STEP 2: Choose the mother shu-point for the restraining element on the affected meridian (also the grandchild point on the affected meridian).

***STEP 3:** Choose the horary point on the meridian of the restrained element (grandchild).

***STEP 4:** Choose the horary point on the meridian of the restraining element (grandmother).

*Test and compare the metal + water combinations for the four special horary points **(SP3, ST36, GB41,** and **HT8).**

SUMMARY OF THE BODY-FEEDBACK BALANCING PRESCRIPTIONS

Exclusive testing points are italicized

Horary points to check for substitution are in bold

FIRST TRISECTION:

Lung: LU10, LU11, LV1, **HT8** (HT4+HT3)

Large Intestine: LI5, LI3, **GB41** (GB44+GB43), SI5

Stomach: ST43, ST44, UB66, **GB41** (GB44+GB43)

Spleen: SP1, SP9, LV1, KD10

Pregnancy Immune Support: ST43, ST44, **GB41** (GB44+GB43), SI5, LI5

SECOND TRISECTION:

Heart: HT3, HT4, LU8, KD10

Small Intestine: SI2, SI1, LI1, UB66

Urinary Bladder: UB40, UB60, SI5, **ST36** (ST45+ST44)

Kidney: KD3, KD2, **HT8** (HT4+HT3), **SP3** (SP5+SP9)

THIRD TRISECTION:

Pericardium: PC3, PC5, LU8, KD10

Triple Burner: TB2, TB1, ST45, UB66

Gallbladder: GB44, GB34, **ST36** (ST45+ST44), LI1

Liver: LV4, LV3, **SP3** (SP5+SP9), LU8

The ability to quickly recall the balancing prescriptions will improve the efficiency of the planning and treatment stages. Having a chart or wall poster to refer to during the session is also helpful. Committing these unique combinations to memory increases productivity and confidence.

CHAPTER 10

Body-Feedback Sedation and Tonification Prescriptions

The Body-Feedback system simplifies pathology by identifying a dysfunctional organ or meridian imbalance as either excess or deficient at the time of treatment. Organ/meridian pathology regularly fluctuates between excess and deficiency depending on supplements, lifestyle, weather patterns, and emotions. A dysfunctional organ or meridian imbalance in a state of excess requires the Body-Feedback sedation acupoint prescription. When in a state of deficiency, it requires the Body-Feedback tonification acupoint prescription.

The Body-Feedback sedation and tonification prescriptions come from the first two steps of the Korean four-point and Chinese six-point approaches. The acupuncturist Gao-Wu of the Ming Dynasty (1519 AD) created these practical steps to tonify or sedate an affected element based on the *Nan-Jing*.[46] "According to five-phase theory when a particular phase is depleted, the phase preceding it in the engendering cycle (the 'mother' phase) must be supplemented. Likewise, when a particular phase is replete, the phase following it in the engendering cycle (the 'child' phase) must be drained."[47] This mother-child treatment approach is fairly simple and uses two shu-points from the engendering cycle to address an affected element's deficiency or excess.

10.1 Sedating Excess and Tonifying Deficiency

The Body-Feedback sedation and tonification prescriptions apply the engendering cycle (mother-child rule) to treat excess and deficient organ/meridian pathologies. This step adds two shu-points from either the affected element's child to sedate the excess, or the affected element's mother to tonify the deficiency. Combining the appropriate two shu-points with Body-Feedback balancing acupoints creates a highly effective root treatment to promote accelerated self-healing that can last for up to three weeks with a supportive lifestyle.

To sedate an excess organ/meridian pathology affecting an element, choose points on the next (child) phase of the engendering cycle to assist in the redistribution of the excess:

STEP 5: Choose the shu-point from the child's phase on the affected meridian.

STEP 6: Choose the horary shu-point from the child's phase on the corresponding yin or yang meridian.

To tonify a deficient organ/meridian pathology affecting an element, choose points on the previous (mother) phase of the engendering cycle to assist in strengthening the deficiency:

STEP 5: Choose the horary shu-point from the mother's phase on the corresponding yin or yang meridian.

STEP 6: Choose the shu-point from the mother's phase on the affected meridian.

Steps five and six add a fourth element to the Body-Feedback treatment that further supports and harmonizes the five-element system. Again, it is critical to check the four shu-points that may require the metal + water substitutions to the pulse or other Body-Feedback testing locations. The three horary points **SP3**, **ST36**, and **GB41** can increase existing pathogenic heat, and the horary point **HT8** on the heart meridian may be excessively draining for some clients (see Chapter 3).

10.1.1 Sedation and Tonification Points for the First Trisection

WATER SEDATES METAL AND EARTH TONIFIES METAL

Sedation points for lung excess pathology:

STEP 5: LU5 is the water shu-point on the lung meridian that sedates metal.

STEP 6: KD10 is the yin water horary shu-point that sedates metal.

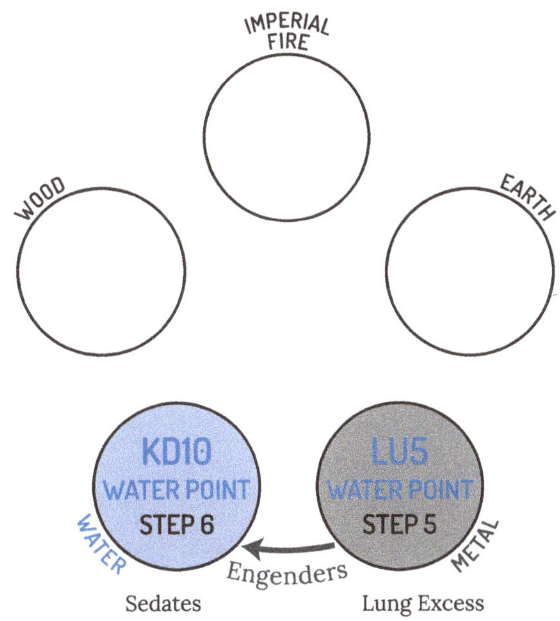

Tonification points for lung deficiency pathology:

STEP 5: **SP3** is the yin earth horary shu-point that tonifies metal (compare **SP3** to SP5 metal + SP9 water combination for pathogenic heat).

STEP 6: LU9 is the earth shu-point on the lung meridian that tonifies metal.

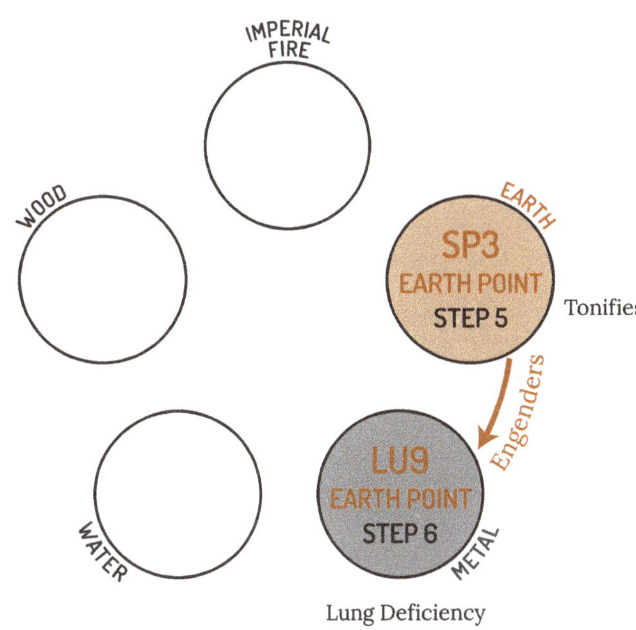

Sedation points for large intestine excess pathology:

STEP 5: LI2 is the water shu-point on the large intestine meridian that sedates metal.

STEP 6: UB66 is the yang water horary shu-point that sedates metal.

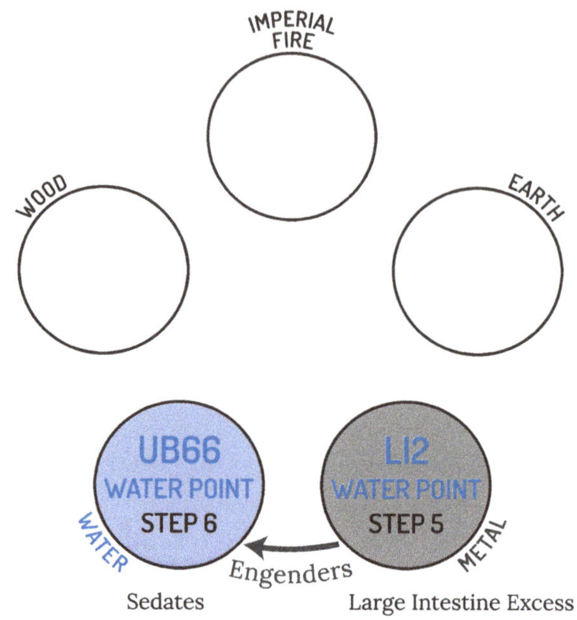

Tonification points for large intestine deficiency pathology:

STEP 5: **ST36** is the yang earth horary shu-point that tonifies metal (compare **ST36** to ST45 metal + ST44 water combination for pathogenic heat).

STEP 6: LI11 is the earth shu-point on the large intestine meridian that tonifies metal.

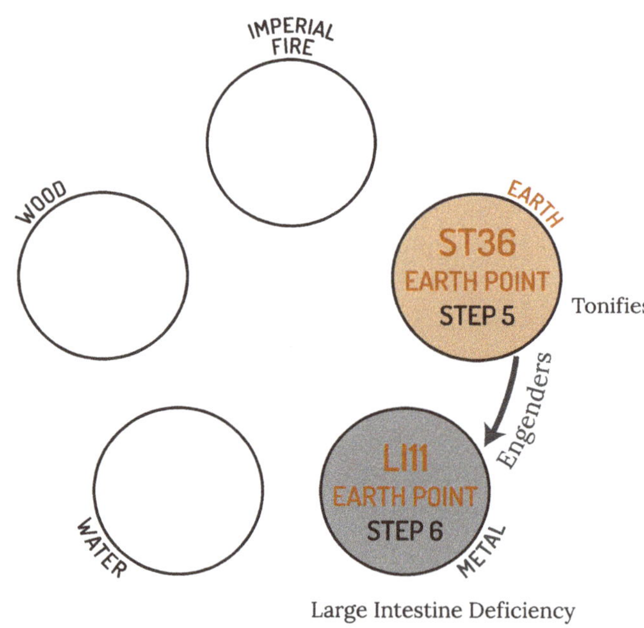

METAL SEDATES EARTH AND IMPERIAL-FIRE TONIFIES EARTH

Sedation points for stomach excess pathology:

STEP 5: ST45 is the metal shu-point on the stomach meridian that sedates earth.

STEP 6: LI1 is the yang metal horary shu-point that sedates earth.

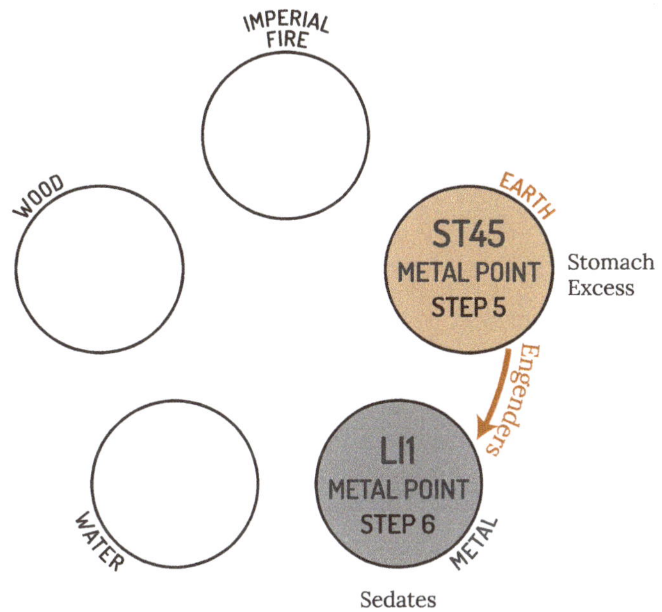

Tonification points for stomach deficiency pathology:

STEP 5: SI5 is the yang imperial-fire horary shu-point that tonifies earth.

STEP 6: ST41 is the fire shu-point on the stomach meridian that tonifies earth.

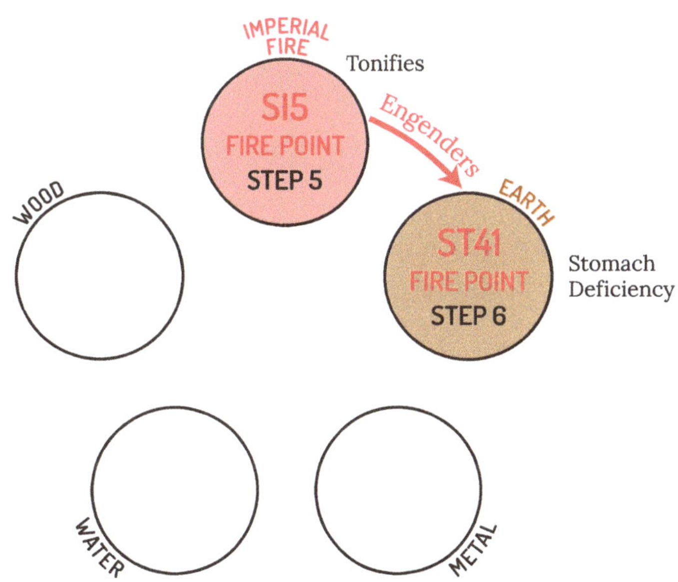

Sedation points for spleen excess pathology:

STEP 5: SP5 is the metal shu-point on the spleen meridian that sedates earth.

STEP 6: LU8 is the yin metal horary shu-point that sedates earth.

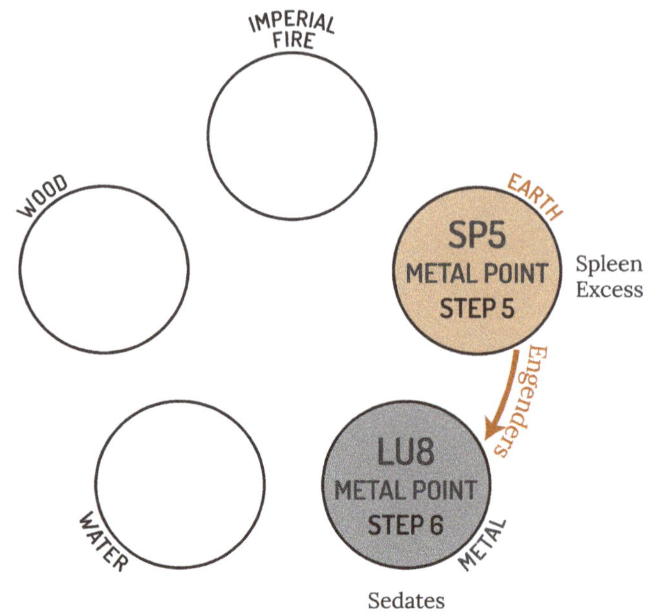

Tonification points for spleen deficiency pathology:

STEP 5: **HT8** is the yin imperial-fire horary shu-point that tonifies earth (compare **HT8** to HT4 metal + HT3 water combination).

STEP 6: SP2 is the fire shu-point on the spleen meridian that tonifies earth.

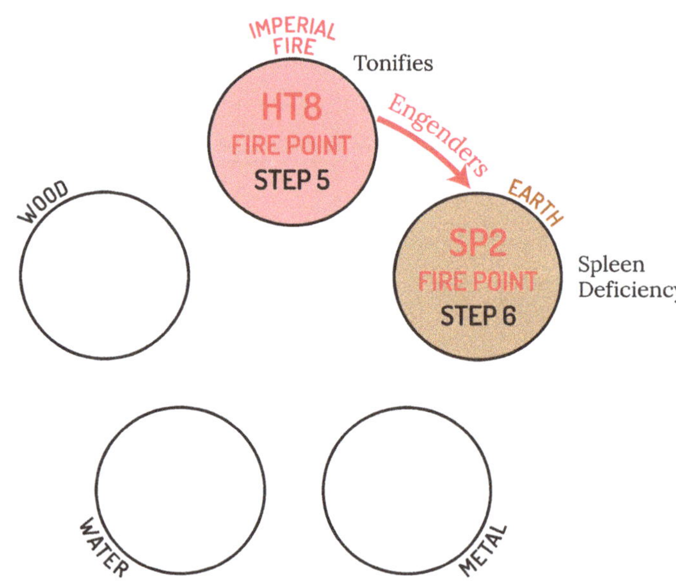

10.1.2 Sedation and Tonification Points for the Second Trisection

EARTH SEDATES IMPERIAL-FIRE AND WOOD TONIFIES IMPERIAL-FIRE

Sedation points for heart excess pathology:

STEP 5: HT7 is the earth shu-point on the heart meridian that sedates imperial-fire.

STEP 6: **SP3** is the yin earth horary shu-point that sedates imperial-fire (compare **SP3** to SP5 metal + SP9 water combination for pathogenic heat).

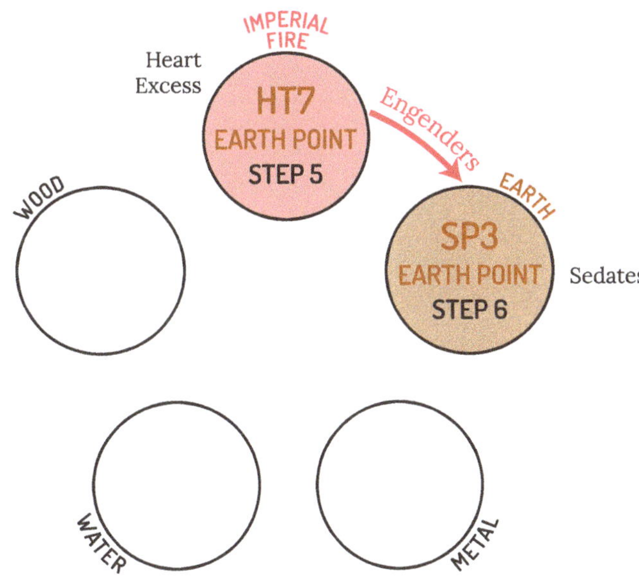

Tonification points for heart deficiency pathology:

STEP 5: LV1 is the yin wood horary shu-point that tonifies imperial-fire.

STEP 6: HT9 is the wood shu-point on the heart meridian tonifies imperial-fire.

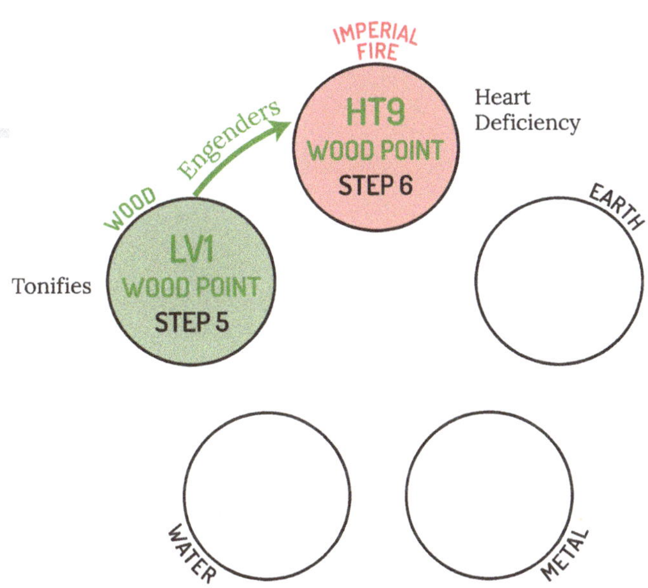

Sedation points for small intestine excess pathology:

STEP 5: SI8 is the earth shu-point on the small intestine meridian that sedates imperial-fire.

STEP 6: **ST36** is the yang earth horary shu-point that sedates imperial-fire (compare **ST36** to ST45 metal + ST44 water combination for pathogenic heat).

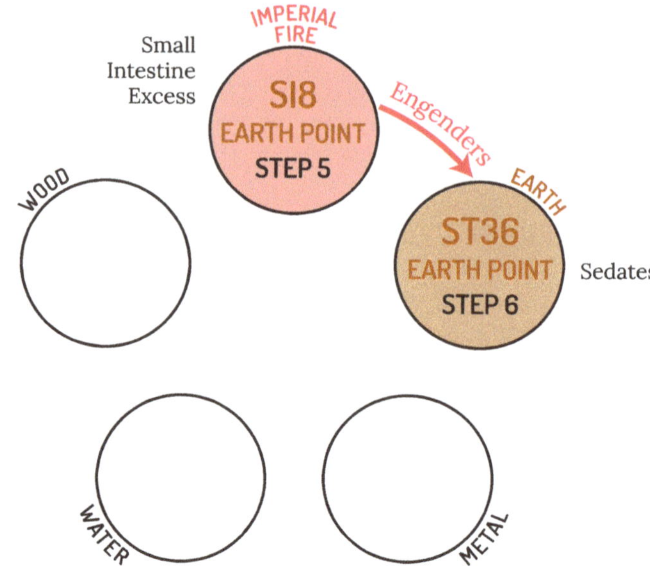

Tonification points for small intestine deficiency pathology:

STEP 5: **GB41** is the yang wood horary shu-point that tonifies imperial-fire (compare **GB41** to GB44 metal + GB43 water combination for pathogenic heat).

STEP 6: SI3 is the wood shu-point on the small intestine meridian that tonifies imperial-fire.

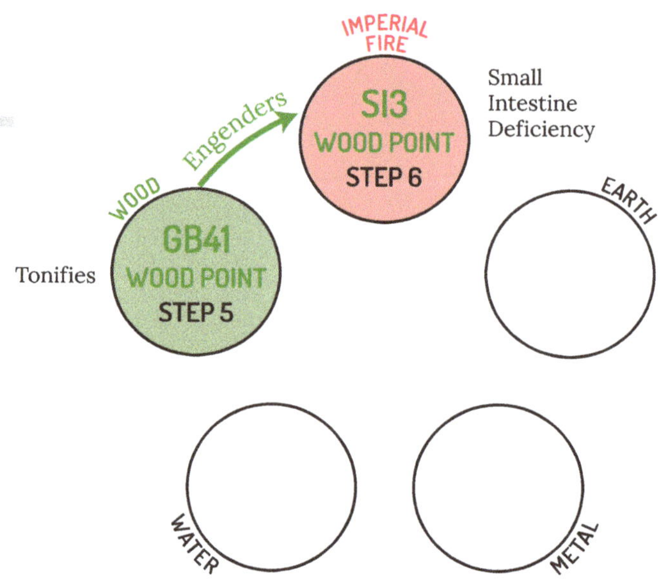

WOOD SEDATES WATER AND METAL TONIFIES WATER

Sedation points for urinary bladder excess pathology:

STEP 5: UB65 is the wood shu-point on the urinary bladder meridian that sedates water.

STEP 6: **GB41** is the yang wood horary shu-point that sedates water (compare **GB41** to GB44 metal + GB43 water combination for pathogenic heat).

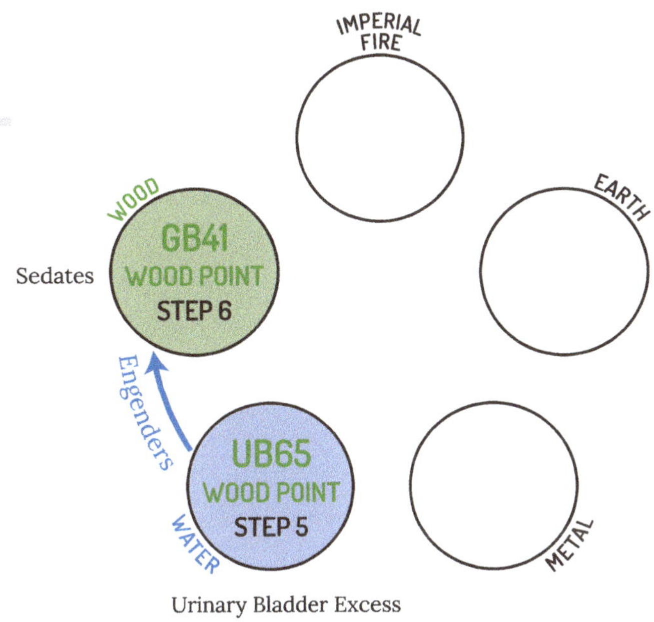

Tonification points for urinary bladder deficiency pathology:

STEP 5: LI1 is the yang metal horary shu-point that tonifies water.

STEP 6: UB67 is the metal shu-point on the urinary bladder meridian that tonifies water.

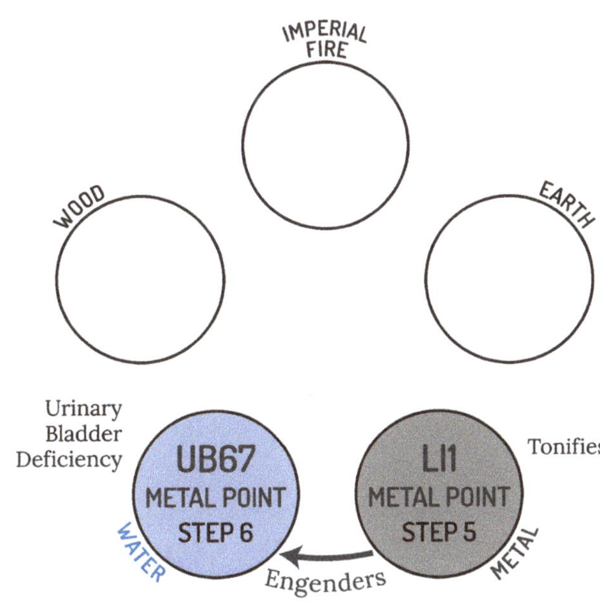

Sedation points for kidney excess pathology:

STEP 5: KD1 is the wood shu-point on the kidney meridian that sedates water.

STEP 6: LV1 is the yin wood horary shu-point that sedates water.

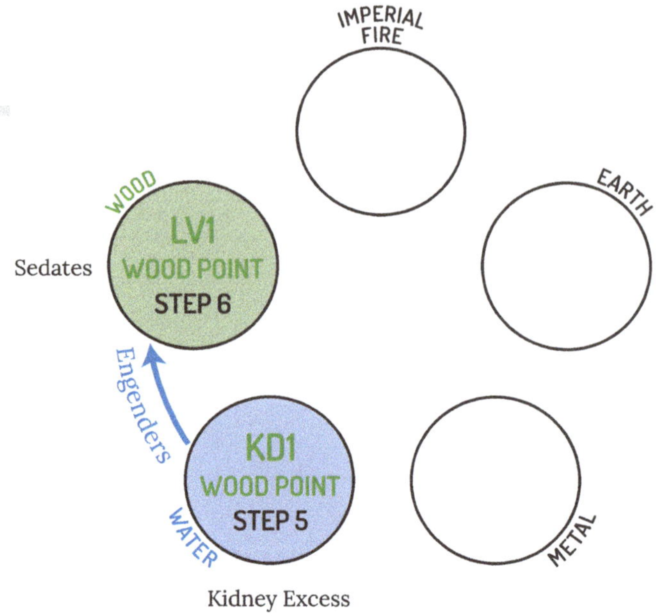

Tonification points for kidney deficiency pathology:

STEP 5: LU8 is the yin metal horary shu-point that tonifies water.

STEP 6: KD7 is the metal shu-point on the kidney meridian that tonifies water.

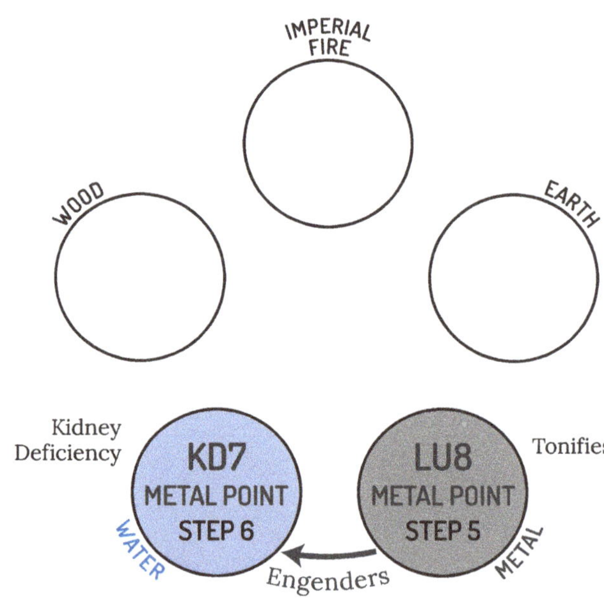

10.1.3 Sedation and Tonification Points for the Third Trisection

EARTH SEDATES MINISTERIAL-FIRE AND WOOD TONIFIES MINISTERIAL-FIRE

Sedation points for pericardium excess pathology:

STEP 5: PC7 is the earth shu-point on the pericardium meridian that sedates ministerial-fire.

STEP 6: **SP3** is the yin earth horary shu-point that sedates ministerial-fire (compare **SP3** to SP5 metal + SP9 water combination for pathogenic heat).

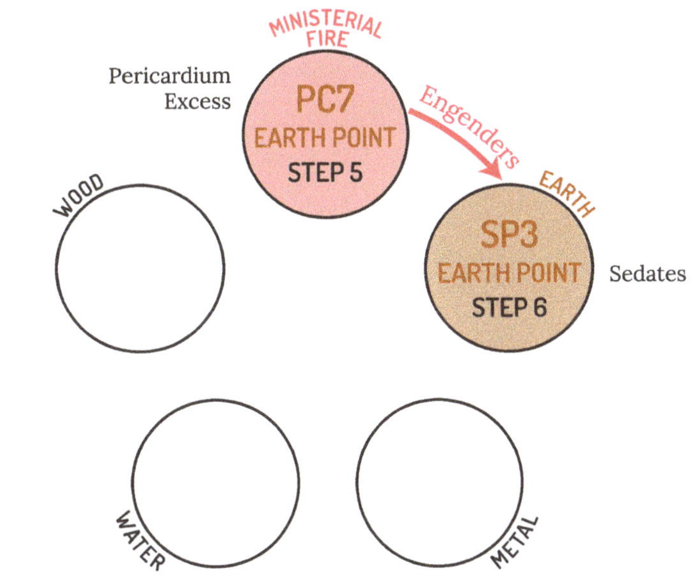

Tonification points for pericardium deficiency pathology:

STEP 5: LV1 is the yin wood horary shu-point that tonifies ministerial-fire.

STEP 6: PC9 is the wood shu-point on the pericardium meridian that tonifies ministerial-fire.

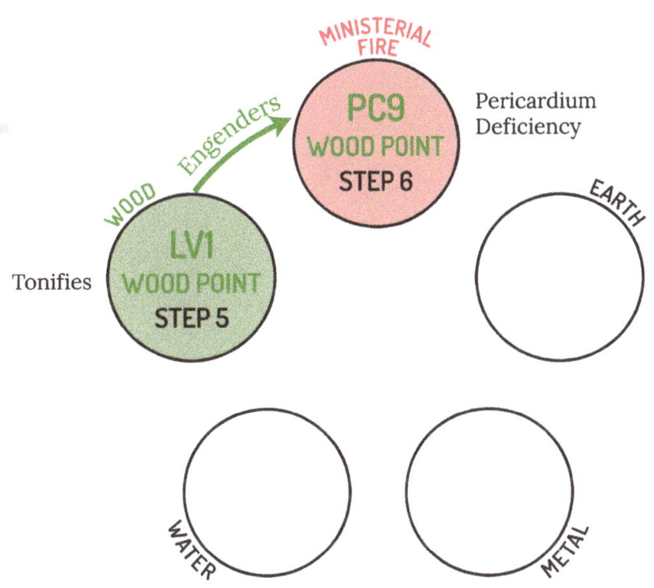

Sedation points for triple burner excess pathology:

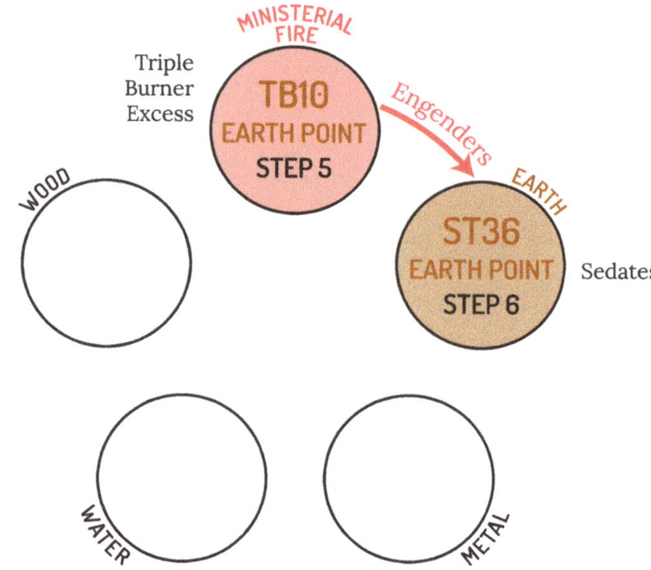

STEP 5: TB10 is the earth shu-point on the triple burner meridian that sedates ministerial-fire.

STEP 6: **ST36** is the yang earth horary shu-point that sedates ministerial-fire (compare **ST36** to ST45 metal + ST44 water combination for pathogenic heat).

Tonification points for triple burner deficiency pathology:

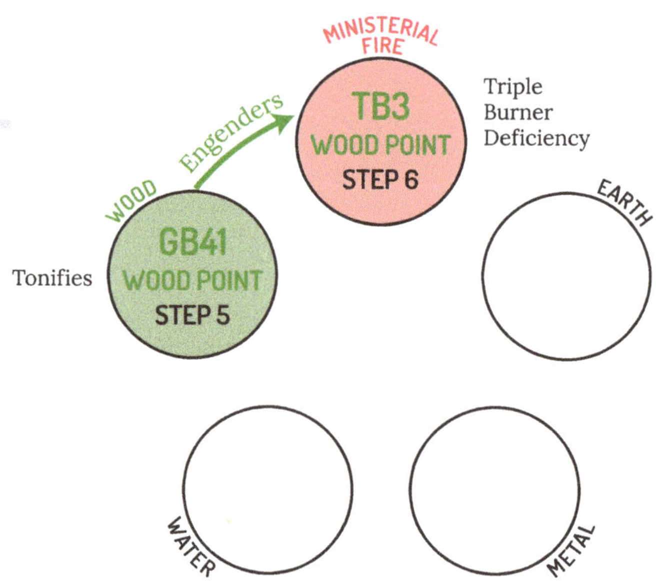

STEP 5: **GB41** is the yang wood horary shu-point that tonifies ministerial-fire (compare **GB41** to GB44 metal + GB43 water combination for pathogenic heat).

STEP 6: TB3 is the wood shu-point on the triple burner meridian that tonifies ministerial-fire.

IMPERIAL-FIRE SEDATES WOOD AND WATER TONIFIES WOOD

Sedation points for gallbladder excess pathology:

STEP 5: GB38 is the fire shu-point on the gallbladder meridian that sedates wood.

STEP 6: SI5 is the yang imperial-fire horary shu-point that sedates wood.

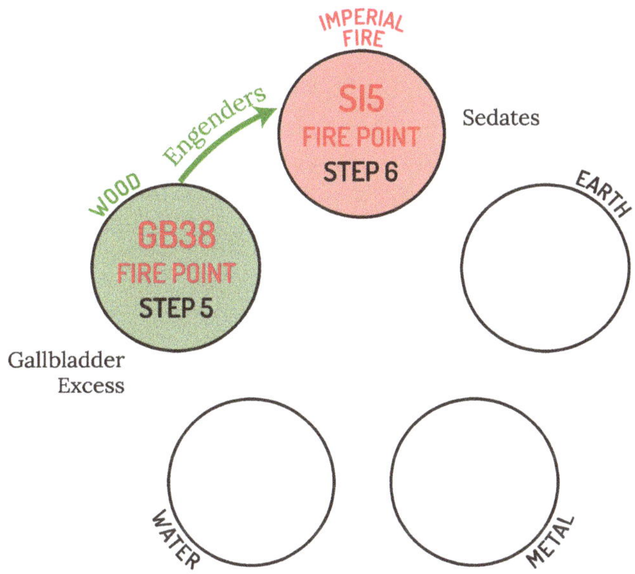

Tonification points for gallbladder deficiency pathology:

STEP 5: UB66 is the yang water horary shu-point that tonifies wood.

STEP 6: GB43 is the water shu-point on the gallbladder meridian that tonifies wood.

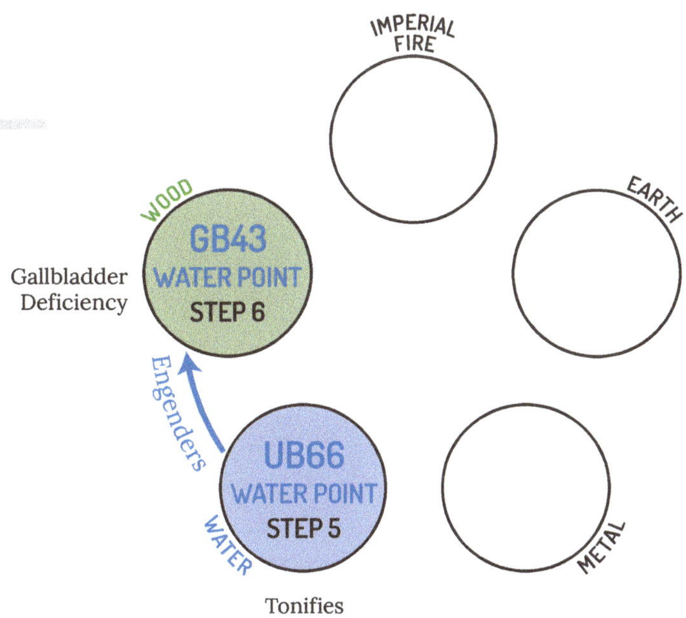

The sedation points for liver excess pathology:

STEP 5: LV2 is the fire shu-point on the liver meridian that sedates wood.

STEP 6: **HT8** is the yin imperial-fire horary shu-point that sedates wood (compare **HT8** to HT4 metal + HT3 water combination).

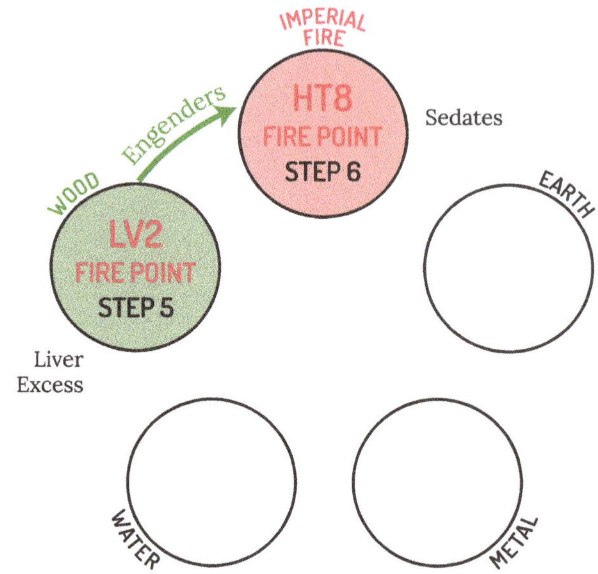

The tonification points for liver deficiency pathology:

STEP 5: KD10 is the yin water horary shu-point that tonifies wood.

STEP 6: LV8 is the water shu-point on the liver meridian that tonifies wood.

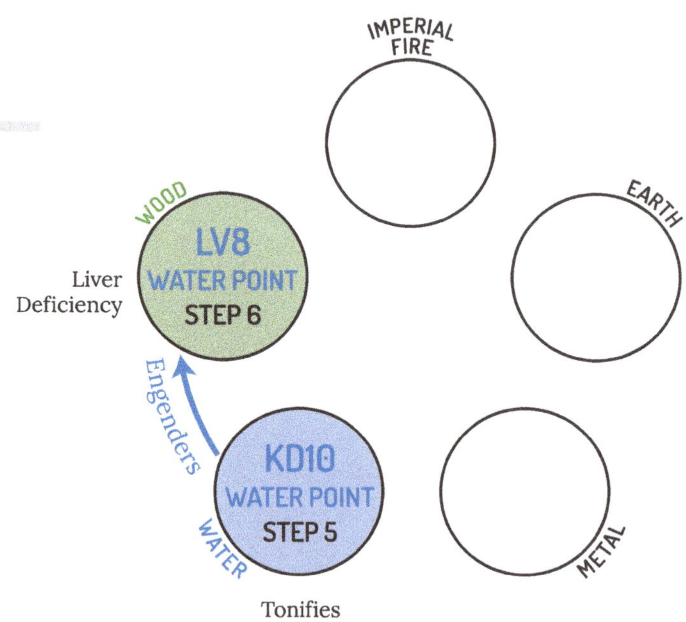

10.2 Identifying and Rectifying Excess or Deficiency

"The key to acupuncture is first of all to concentrate and focus. You must perceive the deficiencies and excesses of the organs, the variations of the three divisions of the body, and the nine pulses. Then you can administer acupuncture... Patients themselves must be categorized into excess and deficiency. When one encounters the five deficiencies, one must not be careless in the treatment. When one encounters the five excesses, one must not give up easily."[48]

Choosing the Body-Feedback sedation or tonification shu-points comprise the fifth and sixth steps in determining the root treatment. After identifying the affected element using the balancing prescriptions, immediately test that meridian's sedation and tonification acupoints to the pulse, master alarm points, or related Body-Feedback testing locations.

When comparing the tonification acupoints to the sedation acupoints, the effect on the pulse and testing locations will be the opposite from one set to the other. The correct set of acupoints normalizes the pulse to slightly slippery and balanced, releases tension in the master alarm points, and relaxes the muscles in the upper back and neck. The incorrect set of acupoints causes the pulse to become tight, wiry, forceful, or confined, increases discomfort in the master alarm points, and causes the muscles in the upper back and neck to become tense. Because the root dysfunction can alternate between excess or deficiency, it is imperative to check these points at every session.

A sedation prescription indicates the body is trying to remove something that should not be there. Acute bouts of inflammation and organ swelling can trigger excess conditions that require sedation acupoint prescriptions. When a client continually needs a sedating treatment, look into food choices, lifestyle, pathogenic infections, and environmental toxins.

A tonification prescription indicates the organ requires additional support due to genetics, lifestyle factors, trauma, or age. The body's ability to produce enzymes, hormones, blood, and bone naturally reduces with age. Long-term support with supplements, herbs, and essential oils are highly beneficial and minimize cellular aging. When a client continually needs a tonification treatment, look into food choices and organ support.

Organ/Meridian	Possible Causes of Excess Pathology
LUNG	bronchitis, skin infections, exposure to viruses, allergens, toxins, or irritants
LARGE INTESTINE	inflammatory large bowel (colon), food allergies, colon polyps or blockages, sinus congestion, or pathogenic infections
STOMACH	gastritis, ulcers, food allergies, sinus congestion, or bacterial infections
SPLEEN	pancreatitis, enlarged spleen, excessive carbohydrates or sugar intake, obesity, diabetes, or insulin resistance
HEART	myocarditis, excessive stress, high cortisol at night, or blockages in the cardiovascular system
SMALL INTESTINE	inflammatory small bowel, food allergies or intolerance, bacterial flora overgrowth, or pathogenic infections
URINARY BLADDER	cystitis, excessive stress, elevated cortisol, urine retention, or bladder infection
KIDNEY	nephritis, ovarian cysts, or kidney crystals, stones, or cysts
PERICARDIUM	pericarditis, thickening of the esophagus, elevated testosterone in women, elevated estrogen in men, or excessive cortisol
TRIPLE BURNER	lymphadenitis, encephalitis, acute infections, enlarged lymph nodes, or fluid retention
GALLBLADDER	cholecystitis, gallstones, thick bile, or bacterial infection in the gallbladder
LIVER	hepatitis, enlarged liver, fatty liver, elevated cholesterol, or cysts on the liver

In general, clients respond best to longer needle retention time for sedation treatments and shorter needle retention time for tonification treatments. The optimal needle retention time for an excess condition is between 20-30 minutes, and for a deficient condition is between 15-25 minutes. With asymmetrical treatments, needle the sedation prescription first and the tonification prescription second to account for the difference in needle retention time. If the tonification prescription is inadvertently needled first, remove the tonification points after 15 minutes and allow the client to rest an additional 5-10 minutes with the sedation points.

Organ/Meridian	Possible Causes of Deficient Pathology
LUNG	depressed immune system or lung function, or loss of elasticity in the blood vessels or skin
LARGE INTESTINE	chronic sinus irritation or infection, poor vitamin absorption, or lack of healthy bacterial flora in colon
STOMACH	chronic sinus irritation or infection, thin stomach lining, or thyroid dysfunction
SPLEEN	hypoglycemia with or without insulin resistance, prolonged fasting, or organ prolapse
HEART	depressed cortisol or weakness in the heart muscle
SMALL INTESTINE	chronic inflammation, leaky gut, or depressed enzyme or neurotransmitter production
URINARY BLADDER	chronic cystitis, bladder prolapse or weakness, or degenerative neurological conditions
KIDNEY	adrenal fatigue, depressed kidney function, diminished ovarian reserve, or accelerated cellular aging
PERICARDIUM	chronic pericarditis, low testosterone in men and women, or amenorrhea in women
TRIPLE BURNER	lymph node or brain deterioration, or chronic low-grade infections
GALLBLADDER	insufficient bile, weak gallbladder contractions, or post cholecystectomy
LIVER	chronic hepatitis, depressed liver enzyme production, or compromised detoxification

The balancing, sedation, and tonification acupoint prescriptions automatically address the most important organ/meridian to treat at that session. Add additional supporting points (see Chapter 15) to address the client's presenting complaints and other health concerns. When a client tests best for the same sedation and tonification acupoint prescriptions at multiple appointments after their general symptoms have improved, their constitutional or genetic weakness is the root dysfunction compromising health.

10.3 Interplay of Excess and Deficiency Pathology

When a healthy person experiences organ/meridian pathology, he or she can recover quickly, and the ability to self-heal restores. For example, a client with food allergies but a strong constitution can experience mild symptoms when ingesting food allergens. Shortly after eating the food allergen, this client's small or large intestine becomes excess, triggering the overreaction to the food that cannot be processed. During the acute stage, this client requires a sedation prescription to help discharge the allergen. After the food allergen leaves the body, the immune system response normalizes, and the small or large intestine experiences deficiency, requiring a tonification prescription. Depending on food choices, this client can alternate between small and large intestine sedation or tonification prescriptions to support the constitutional weakness of food allergies.

Clients experiencing multiple health concerns such as fibromyalgia, autoimmune diseases, neuropathy, migraines, or obesity often struggle to self-heal after ingesting food allergens. These clients experience prolonged unhealthy immune responses in the small or large intestine, creating a root excess dysfunction. High amounts of inflammation and histamine can damage the digestive tract lining and allow small food particles to escape the digestive system, creating leaky gut syndrome. The resulting damage from the food allergen becomes more severe as health deteriorates. After eliminating food allergens, the excessive immune response can normalize, and these clients often experience significant deficiency requiring long-term tonification. Clients with prolonged immune and digestive system dysfunction can experience symptoms of excess and deficiency that constantly fluctuate and restrict the body's ability to self-heal.

Genetics, food choices, weather patterns, exercise, quality of sleep, stress, nutritional supplementation, western treatments, and holistic therapies can influence a client's organ/meridian dysfunction. These influences can shift the root dysfunction from excess to deficiency daily for some people and less frequently for others. Furthermore, according to the laws of yin and yang, when an organ or meridian becomes deficient or excess, its corresponding five-element and six-level pair instantly results in the opposite. Depending on the severity of the root dysfunction, pathology can quickly spread to other meridians, organs, and trisections. The root dysfunction can alternate in multiple ways, such as between excess and deficiency, between the five-element or six-level pairs, or between trisections.

One of the six pathogenic influences (fire, dampness, summer-heat, dryness, cold, and wind) or one of the five types of pathogenic heat (blood heat, damp heat, exterior-wind heat, yin-deficiency heat, and depressive heat) can quickly cause a client with deficiency to shift into excess pathology. After resolving the excess pathogen, the client reverts to the underlying deficiency. For example, a client experiencing thick, yellow sinus congestion and diarrhea with damp heat requires a large intestine sedation treatment. After resolving the phlegm and dampness, the client requires a large intestine tonification treatment to strengthen the immune system (*wei qi*).

A client with immune system dysfunction may require the following root treatments at different appointments:

- A lung excess root treatment during an acute respiratory infection.
- A large intestine deficiency root treatment with seasonal allergies.
- A large intestine excess root treatment with food allergies.
- A lung deficiency root treatment with wheezing due to cold-induced asthma.

Menstruating women who are not using hormone-based birth control can transition between sedation and tonification acupoint prescriptions throughout a monthly menstrual cycle. Sedation acupoint prescriptions commonly occur during menstruation when the body is expelling the uterine lining, and during ovulation when the body is releasing a mature egg. Tonification acupoint prescriptions commonly occur during the preovulation phase because hormone levels are at their lowest for the month. After ovulation, women with excessive stress or anxiety usually require sedation acupoint prescriptions, and women with low progesterone usually require tonification acupoint prescriptions. The Body-Feedback Pregnancy Balancing Prescription (see Section 9.7) is an alternative option for women at conception and in the first trimester to support the immune system.

Menopausal and postmenopausal women can struggle with a combination of damp heat excess with liver and kidney yin deficiency, causing hot flashes during the day and night. High-fat foods can increase damp heat and worsen the daytime hot flashes. Yin decreases with age as a result of low hormones, inflammation, and stress, leading to hot flashes at night. Liver sedation treatments reduce the damp heat while liver and kidney tonification treatments nourish the yin. Depending on diet, stress, activity level, and age, treatments for menopausal women often fluctuate between liver sedation, liver tonification, and kidney tonification prescriptions.

A multitude of factors can cause pathology to alternate between excess and deficiency. It is crucial to compare the tonification and sedation acupoint prescriptions at each session to confirm the correct treatment approach. In the Body-Feedback system, which differs from typical TCM point protocols, the root treatment approach frequently changes from one appointment to another, based on how a client's body presents each time. By following the Body-Feedback system, each session ensures that the organ/meridian most in need of aid receives a precise treatment.

CHAPTER 11

The Meramour Organ Supporting and Meridian Balancing Blends

Essential oils can be used to enhance and simplify the acupuncture treatment process, provide no-needle treatment options, and extend treatment benefits with continued use at home. By incorporating the oil blends that support particular organs and balance specific meridians, the root acupoint prescriptions are more effective with less supporting acupoints, and treatment results last longer. The Meramour Organ Supporting and Meridian Balancing Blends address both excess and deficient organ pathology.

Isoprenes are the tiny, volatile molecules within essential oils that produce their healing attributes and physiological effects. Each isoprene consists of five carbon molecules and eight hydrogen molecules. When essential oils are applied topically or diffused, the isoprenes absorb directly into the skin, fat cells, brain matter, and bloodstream. Essential oil isoprenes are the only botanical supplements known to easily pass through the blood-brain barrier to address health concerns affecting brain functions. Essential oils can immediately trigger a healing response and bypass the usual digestive route required for supplements, herbs, and medications.

Isoprene Molecule

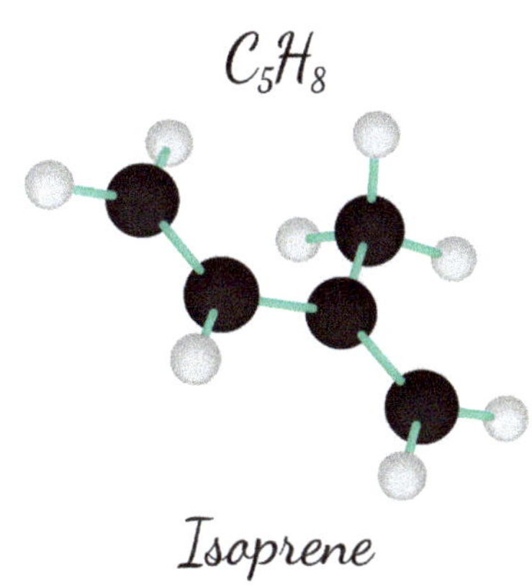

Illustration 68582594 © Schmitt Maria - Dreamstime.com

The characteristics of specific isoprene groups became the foundation for the Meramour Organ Supporting and Meridian Balancing Blends. The focus of a blend's isoprene structure determines its most beneficial therapeutic use and application methods. Some blends are best applied around the hairline or the back of the neck to quickly cross the blood-brain barrier and enhance facial or scalp acupoints. Other blends are best applied to the soles of feet or diffused due to cleansing properties that can be irritating on the skin. Blends designed to enhance digestion are best taken internally by either adding a few drops to a glass of water or diluting with an organic vegetable oil in a capsule.

11.1 Origins of the Meramour Organ Supporting and Meridian Balancing Blends

In 2009, I began incorporating essential oils into my acupuncture treatments. I found peer-reviewed research on the National Institutes of Health's PubMed website and read desk reference guides to learn the basic characteristics of therapeutic-grade essential oils. Essential oils contain enzymes and oxygen, which allows them to absorb into the body through topical application or diffusion and immediately release their therapeutic properties. Essential oils consist of small molecules called terpenes, which are found in plant-based natural remedies. Upon inhalation, these terpenes pass through the sinuses and olfactory bulb to cross the blood-brain barrier and affect emotions and brain functions. With topical application, these terpenes pass through and cleanse cellular receptor sites to provide enzymes and oxygen for the cells to immediately uptake.

Essential oils have immediate effects that last for a few hours when applied topically, which I found could increase the efficiency and effectiveness of acupuncture sessions. The essential oils that tested favorably for a client released superficial meridian imbalances and organ dysfunctions, allowing for easier identification of the root acupoint prescription. Fewer supporting points were needed to achieve superior treatment results when using essential oils that tested favorably. Many clients reported that their acupuncture treatment benefits were stronger and lasted longer when I incorporated essential oils at the beginning of a treatment. Clients began requesting that I use essential oils before inserting the needles because they found the treatment process more relaxing.

Essential Oil Inhalation

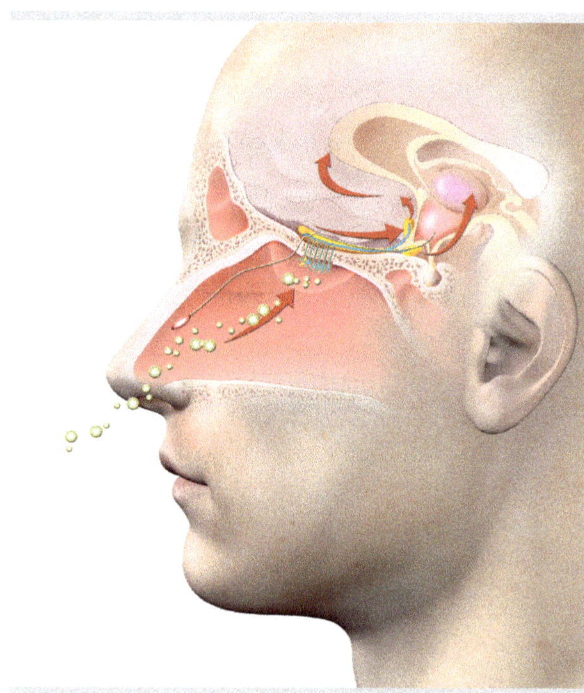

Illustration 156235957 © Axel Kock - Dreamstime.com

As I studied the chemical properties of the oils and their isoprenes, I organized them based on the TCM parameters for classifying herbs: exterior releasing, harmonizing, consolidating, up-bearing, down-bearing, warming, or cooling. I also noted the meridians and organs affected, as evidenced by changes in the Body-Feedback testing locations. Essential oils contain a combination of single-terpene (*phenol*), double-terpene (*monoterpene*), and triple-terpene (*sesquiterpene*) bonds. The single-terpene bonds have yang qualities. The triple-terpene bonds have yin qualities. The double-terpene bonds have harmonizing properties. Using these criteria, I determined the essential oils to test for each root treatment. For the next five years, I used Body-Feedback testing methods on an average of 50 clients a week to check the accuracy of my classifications.

From five years of testing individual oils, I realized that as the meridian imbalance and organ dysfunction fluctuated from excess to deficiency, the essential oils that tested best also changed. I next identified which oils within a meridian grouping were more sedating, tonifying, and harmonizing. When I combined these oils, the blends better supported the root organ dysfunction with less rotation. From here, I created the Meramour's Meridian Balancing and Organ Supporting Blends.

The Meramour Meridian Balancing Blends consist of three essential oils, an odd or yang number that represents their active nature. One oil is sedating, one is tonifying, and the third is harmonizing. These blends adapt to the constant fluctuation of excess and deficiency that normally occurs within a meridian. Therefore, when treating the same meridian, these blends require less rotation.

The Meramour Organ Supporting Blends consist of four essential oils, an even or yin number that represents their stability and predictability. Each of the four oils supports a different aspect of a particular organ's function and common pathology. In some instances, using the organ and meridian blends together will test the best.

Essential oil substitutions for the meridian and organ blends cover the basic safety precautions for high blood pressure and pregnancy. At times, certain oils may become unavailable because they come from natural resources with a limited crop yield. For oils that can be difficult to procure, recommended substitutions are available on the body-feedback.com website. Always remember to check with an essential oil manufacturer for acceptable uses and application methods.

11.2 Therapeutic and Other Grades of Essential Oils

Therapeutic-grade essential oils vary in quality and fragrance from one manufacturer to another. An essential oil's aroma and healing properties differ depending on the distillation process, farming practices, and geographical location. Most therapeutic-grade essential oil manufacturers use a steam distillation extraction process with conventionally grown, organic, or wild-harvested plants. Harvesting practices and the exact timing of distillation significantly impact the healing properties of essential oils. Some manufacturers will distill the plant matter multiple times to increase yields. In some cases, lower-quality therapeutic-grade essential oils can further disturb a client's root meridian or organ imbalance, causing unwanted side effects.

Three grades of essential oils are available for consumers: food, perfume, and therapeutic. Food-grade and perfume-grade oils use the cheapest manufacturing methods available. Chemicals used in the food- and perfume-grade manufacturing processes include pesticides and fertilizers applied during the plants' growing stages, as well as toxic solvents used for extracting their oils. Diluted food-grade oils contain only a small percentage of the essential oil to keep costs down and often contain preservatives. Avoid all food- and perfume-grade oils for diffusing, internal use, or topical application.

When incorporating essential oils in acupuncture treatments, it is recommended to investigate the manufacturing process to ensure quality. The distributors of essential oils can provide information on manufacturing processes, types of harvest (conventional, organic, or wild), and origins of their plants. Inquire where the distilleries are located and if they use a single distillation process or multiple distillations of the same plant materials. For example, in some instances, wild-harvested plants from South America are shipped to China for distillation. The shipping time causes the plant matter to deteriorate, which results in lower-quality therapeutic-grade oils.

The Body-Feedback testing methods can help evaluate therapeutic-grade essential oils from different manufacturers. Compare the same plant oil from multiple manufacturers by testing them to the master points and the liver and lung Body-Feedback testing locations. Place a bottle from one manufacturer on the client's upper abdomen and wait 30 seconds to test. The GB21 master point and the liver organ referral area (anterior right side of the rib cage) may become tender or painful if pesticides, fertilizers, chemical solvents, or cleaning agents were involved in the manufacturing process that can compromise health. The TB15 master point and the lung referral areas (deltoid muscle, serratus anterior muscle, LU5, LU10, or LU2) can become tight or tender due to the distillation of inferior quality plant matter. Some clients are more sensitive than others to the quality of essential oils in the same way some people are negatively affected by non-organic foods and preservatives.

11.3 Meramour Blend Formulations

The descriptions of the Meramour Organ Supporting and Meridian Balancing Blends include their recipes with percentages for each ingredient, common substitutions, supported allopathic body systems, TCM treatment actions, general attributes, standard application methods, and safety information. A narrative including the synergistic effects of the blend, related facts on the individual oils, and pertinent information on Body-Feedback theory are also provided.

Many essential oils influence hormonal balance for men and women by cleansing the cellular receptor sites and providing small amounts of *phyto* (plant-based) hormones that the body can readily use. For women, it is crucial to use the correct essential oils at the appropriate times to properly support the ebb and flow of hormones throughout the menstrual cycle. Essential oils contain phytohormones that activate and cleanse the cellular receptor sites, which improves how the body uses its own hormones. For cycling women and especially fertility clients, test essential oils at each phase of the cycle: menstrual, follicular, ovulation, and luteal. The following sections in this chapter indicate the most appropriate time for cycling women to use the Meramour blends that contain phytohormones.

The formulation of the organ and meridian blends allows them to be used individually or together, depending on the client's needs. At each session, a single blend or a combination of two, three, or four meridian or organ blends can test best. After identifying the root acupoint prescription, check those organ and meridian blends, along with the five-element or six-level pair's organ and meridian blends. Always use the Body-Feedback testing or pulse methods to determine the most effective blend or combination of blends at each session. The practical application section at the end of this chapter discusses in detail the steps for testing the blends.

11.4 First Trisection Blends

THE MERAMOUR LUNG ORGAN SUPPORTING BLEND

40% lemon *(Citrus limon)*
40% lemon myrtle *(Backhousia citriodora)*
10% basil *(Ocimum basilicum)*
10% peppermint *(Mentha piperita)*

Benefits the circulatory, digestive, endocrine, immune, lymph, musculoskeletal, and respiratory systems.

Releases the exterior, clears heat, regulates the qi, drains dampness, and transforms phlegm.

Increases cortisol, promotes clarity, and releases tension from the head, neck, and shoulders.

Cleanses the cellular receptor sites in the sinuses, head, and lungs.

The Lung Organ Supporting Blend contains a high percentage of phenols and citrus oil, which can irritate the skin with long-term use, but are perfect for detoxifying cells and cleansing the air. Basil oil directs this blend to the lungs, upper back, neck, and shoulders, while the other oils clear congestion and pathogenic heat. This blend is stimulating and best to apply or diffuse during the day, before physical activity, or to boost the immune system against external pathogens. For cycling women, this blend is appropriate to use all month.

Application and safety tips for the Lung Organ Supporting Blend

- contains a citrus oil, which increases photosensitivity in the applied area, and is best diffused or applied to areas not exposed to the sun
- apply undiluted to the soles of the feet during treatment sessions
- diffuse at home during the day between treatment sessions
- dilute 50/50 with an organic carrier oil and apply to the soles of the feet before exercise
- add a few drops to organic lotion and apply over sore muscles in the neck, shoulder, and upper back
- substitute spearmint for peppermint with high blood pressure or a family history of hypertension
- avoid during pregnancy and postpartum, and with epilepsy

THE MERAMOUR LUNG MERIDIAN BALANCING BLEND

50% lavender *(Lavandula angustifolia)*
25% tea tree *(Melaleuca alternifolia)*
25% niaouli *(Melaleuca quinquenervia)*

Benefits the endocrine, exocrine (skin, hair, and nails), immune, nervous, and respiratory systems.

Releases the exterior, clears heat, regulates the qi, drains dampness, and transforms phlegm.

Supports a balanced histamine response for people with seasonal allergies and environmental sensitivities.

Cleanses the skin and cellular receptor sites.

Promotes a balanced immune response for both immune weakness or autoimmune tendencies.

While the two Melaleuca species are from the same family, their healing properties differ. Tea tree is stronger against pathogenic infections and cleansing the skin and air. Niaouli contains phytotestosterone hormones for tissue regeneration and is stronger against fungus and radiation. Lavender harmonizes the blend and provides adaptogenic properties to accommodate the changing needs of the immune system. Lavender contains phytoestrogens, which are cooling and soothing for the skin. For cycling women, this blend tests best during the menstrual period, follicular phase, and when combined with progesterone supporting blends for the luteal phase.

Application and safety tips for the Lung Meridian Balancing Blend

- apply undiluted to the soles of the feet during treatment sessions
- diffuse at home during the day or night between treatment sessions
- dilute 50/50 with an organic carrier oil for sensitive skin, long-term use, or application over a large area
- add a few drops to an organic lotion and apply over scars and mild skin irritation
- for cycling women, apply a few drops diluted with an organic carrier oil or lotion to the lower abdomen during the menstrual period and the follicular phase to cleanse the estrogen receptor sites
- diffuse or apply to the soles of the feet during pregnancy and apply topically postpartum

THE MERAMOUR LARGE INTESTINE ORGAN SUPPORTING BLEND

40% lemon (*Citrus limon*)
40% cypress (*Cupressus sempervirens*)
10% lemon myrtle (*Backhousia citriodora*)
10% spearmint (*Mentha spicata*)

Benefits the cardiovascular, circulatory, digestive, endocrine, excretory, immune, lymph, musculoskeletal, renal, and respiratory systems.

Releases the exterior, clears heat, regulates the qi, drains dampness, and transforms phlegm.

Increases cortisol and stimulates metabolism.

Cleanses the cellular receptor sites in the sinuses, head, and colon.

Benefits people with leaf mold allergies and mold sensitivity.

The Large Intestine Organ Supporting Blend regulates stool transit time, enhances absorption and synthesis of specific vitamins in the colon, and detoxifies and discharges used hormone metabolites. All four of the oils in this blend balance the flow of qi and can be used with diarrhea or constipation. This blend is slightly stimulating, and using it in the morning enhances the peak colon organ activity time from 7 a.m. to 9 a.m. Check this blend for added detoxification support when addressing phlegm nodules. For cycling women, this blend tests best during the menstrual period and follicular phase, and when combined with progesterone supporting blends for the luteal phase.

Application and safety tips for the Large Intestine Organ Supporting Blend

- contains a citrus oil, which increases photosensitivity in the applied area, and is best diffused or applied to areas not exposed to the sun
- apply undiluted to the soles of the feet during treatment sessions
- diffuse at home during the day between treatment sessions
- dilute 50/50 with an organic carrier oil for sensitive skin, long-term use, or application over the lower abdomen or lower back
- apply undiluted to the soles of the feet prior to exercise
- for phlegm nodules in the lower back, add a few drops to an organic carrier oil or lotion and apply to the lower back before bed
- for cycling women, apply a few drops diluted with an organic carrier oil or lotion to the lower abdomen during the menstrual period and the follicular phase to cleanse the estrogen receptor sites and balance estrogen levels
- avoid during pregnancy and with epilepsy
- considered safe to use topically postpartum

THE MERAMOUR LARGE INTESTINE MERIDIAN BALANCING BLEND

50% palmarosa (*Cymbopogon martinii*)
25% lemongrass (*Cymbopogon citratus*)
25% citronella (*Cymbopogon nardus*)

Benefits the digestive, endocrine, excretory, immune, lymph, musculoskeletal, and respiratory systems.

Releases the exterior, drains dampness, transforms phlegm, and warms the interior.

Supports healthy bacterial flora in the colon and the synthesis of specific vitamins.

Promotes detoxification of used hormone metabolites.

Strengthens the ligaments (bone-to-bone connections).

Reduces yeast and candida overgrowth.

Benefits people with leaf mold allergies and mold sensitivity.

The three oils in the Large Intestine Meridian Balancing Blend come from grasses that are commonly used to remove odors and keep insects away. This blend provides nutrients that support the beneficial bacteria in the colon and offset diets high in sugar and carbohydrates. Palmarosa, known as Turkish rose, benefits the skin and helps to reduce the irritating properties of citronella and lemongrass. However, always dilute this blend for sensitive skin or repeated use. For cycling women, this blend can be used at any time of the month if testing favorably.

Application and safety tips for the Large Intestine Meridian Balancing Blend

- apply undiluted to the soles of the feet during treatment sessions and dilute 50/50 with an organic carrier oil for sensitive skin
- diffuse at home during the day or night between treatment sessions
- add a few drops to organic lotion and apply over strained ligaments
- discontinue use if signs of skin irritation occur, and avoid long-term topical use
- avoid during pregnancy and postpartum

THE MERAMOUR STOMACH ORGAN SUPPORTING BLEND

30% lemon (*Citrus limon*)

30% copaiba (copal: *Copaifera reticulate* or *Copaifera L. genus*)

30% patchouli (*Pogostemon cablin*)

10% peppermint (*Mentha piperita*)

Benefits the cardiovascular, circulatory, digestive, endocrine, excretory, immune, musculoskeletal, nervous, and respiratory systems.

Drains dampness, transforms phlegm, regulates qi, harmonizes, and calms the spirit.

Promotes mental stimulation and focus while calming the nervous system.

Supports the detoxification of pesticides, herbicides, food additives, and preservatives.

The Stomach Organ Supporting Blend is ideal for long-term daily use due to its balancing and harmonizing properties. The sweet honey-like aroma of copaiba, the cleansing fragrance of lemon, and the minty smell of peppermint balance patchouli's intense aroma and create a blend appealing to most people. The stomach organ, which controls the initial stages of digestion, works directly with the large intestine, spleen, gallbladder, and small intestine to ensure proper absorption of nutrients. This blend is ideal when emotional stress and poor-quality foods challenge the stomach organ and impair the entire digestive system. For cycling women, this blend can be used at any time of the month if testing favorably.

Application and safety tips for the Stomach Organ Supporting Blend

- contains a citrus oil, which increases photosensitivity in the applied area, and is best diffused or applied to areas not exposed to the sun
- apply undiluted to the soles of the feet during treatment sessions
- diffuse at home during the day or night between treatment sessions
- dilute 50/50 with an organic carrier oil for sensitive skin, long-term use, or application over a large area
- for phlegm nodules in the lower back, add a few drops to an organic carrier oil or lotion and apply to the lower back before bed
- substitute spearmint for peppermint with high blood pressure or family history of hypertension
- for cycling women, dilute with an organic carrier oil or lotion and apply to the lower abdomen during the menstrual period to reduce discomfort and support detoxification of hormones
- considered safe to use during the first and second trimesters of pregnancy
- substitute spearmint for peppermint in the third trimester of pregnancy

THE MERAMOUR STOMACH MERIDIAN BALANCING BLEND

50% grapefruit *(Citrus x paradisi)*
25% lime *(Citrus aurantifolia)*
25% spearmint *(Mentha spicata)*

Benefits the cardiovascular, digestive, immune, lymph, musculoskeletal, and renal systems.

Clears heat, drains dampness, transforms phlegm, invigorates blood, and reduces food stagnation.

Stimulates the mind and body to boost metabolism and help put ideas into action.

Soothes and benefits the lining of the upper digestive tract.

Relaxes the muscles in the jaw, neck, and upper back.

The Stomach Meridian Balancing Blend is designed for internal use; however, always confirm that the oils are approved for internal use by the manufacturer and the FDA. All three of the oils in this blend down-bear stomach qi to promote continuous movement of food through the digestive system. Adding a few drops to a glass of water first thing in the morning with breakfast, and again with lunch, will boost metabolism and support healthy digestion. The slight blood-thickening properties of lime balance the blood-thinning properties of grapefruit, thereby harmonizing blood flow and circulation. For cycling women, this blend can be used at any time of the month if testing favorably.

Application and safety tips for the Stomach Meridian Balancing Blend

- contains two citrus oils, which increases photosensitivity in the applied area, and is best taken internally or used in areas that are not exposed to the sun
- apply undiluted to the soles of the feet during treatment sessions
- if approved for internal use by the manufacturer and the FDA, add a few drops to eight to twelve ounces of water in a glass or ceramic cup
- apply undiluted to the soles of the feet prior to exercise
- avoid during the first trimester of pregnancy
- considered safe to apply this blend to the soles of the feet during the second and third trimesters of pregnancy and postpartum
- substitute peppermint for spearmint during the first trimester of pregnancy

THE MERAMOUR SPLEEN ORGAN SUPPORTING BLEND

40% tangerine (*Citrus nobilis* or *Citrus reticulata* var. *tangerine*)

40% fennel (*Foeniculum vulgare*)

10% clove (*syzygium aromaticum*)

10% coriander (*Coriandrum sativum L.*)

Benefits the circulatory, digestive, endocrine, excretory, immune, lymph, renal, and reproductive systems.

Drains dampness, transforms phlegm, warms the interior, boosts the qi, harmonizes, and reduces food stagnation.

Supports digestion of carbohydrates, fats, and sugars.

Reduces sugar cravings and calms emotional eating.

Enhances fertility in men and women.

In the Body-Feedback system, the spleen organ includes the pancreas, and when these organs are functioning optimally, energy is stable, and the muscles are strong. The Spleen Organ Supporting Blend is beneficial for people who struggle with emotional eating, hypoglycemia, elevated glucose, insulin resistance, weight gain due to stress, and excessive sugar or carbohydrate consumption. The tangerine oil is up-bearing to support the spleen's lifting and organ-securing functions. The synergistic effects of the fennel, clove, and coriander oils enhance sperm production in men and egg development in women by optimizing hormone receptor sites.

Application and safety tips for the Spleen Organ Supporting Blend

- contains one citrus oil, which increases photosensitivity in the applied area, and is best diffused, taken internally, or applied to areas not exposed to the sun
- apply undiluted to the soles of the feet during treatment sessions
- if approved for internal use by the manufacturer and the FDA, dilute 50/50 with a healthy cooking oil (olive, avocado, or coconut) and take six to nine drops in a capsule with meals
- apply undiluted to the soles of the feet in the morning to boost energy
- for cycling women, apply diluted with an organic carrier oil or lotion to the lower abdomen during the follicular phase of the menstrual cycle to support egg quality
- for men, apply undiluted to the soles of the feet daily to support sperm quality
- avoid during pregnancy and postpartum

THE MERAMOUR SPLEEN MERIDIAN BALANCING BLEND

50% orange (*Citrus sinensis*)
25% clove (*Syzygium aromaticum*)
25% copaiba (copal: *Copaifera reticulate* or *Copaifera L. genus*)

Benefits the circulatory, digestive, endocrine, excretory, immune, lymph, musculoskeletal, and nervous systems.

Drains dampness, warms the interior, boosts qi, harmonizes, and invigorates the blood.

Supports digestion, blood sugar regulation, the assimilation of carbohydrates, and reduces pathogenic heat caused by sugar.

Cleanses the cellular receptor sites, including insulin receptor sites.

The Spleen Meridian Balancing Blend is designed for internal use; however, always confirm that the oils are approved for internal use by the manufacturer and the FDA. Add a few drops to a glass of water with meals and before workouts to support stable energy, blood, and sugar levels. This blend benefits the brain when it is affected by blood sugar highs and lows, and it can help stabilize energy and mood when skipping meals or waiting too long to eat.

Application and safety tips for the Spleen Meridian Balancing Blend

- contains one citrus oil, which increases photosensitivity in the applied area, and is best diffused or used in areas that are not exposed to the sun
- apply undiluted to the soles of the feet during treatment sessions
- dilute 50/50 with an organic carrier oil and apply to the soles of the feet between treatment sessions and with long-term use
- if approved for internal use by the manufacturer and the FDA, add a few drops to eight to twelve ounces of water in a glass or ceramic cup or add to coffee in a ceramic cup to enhance coffee's flavor and positive effects
- apply undiluted to the soles of the feet when craving sugar
- avoid during pregnancy and postpartum

11.5 Second Trisection Blends

THE MERAMOUR HEART ORGAN SUPPORTING BLEND

30% marjoram (*Origanum majorana*)
30% cypress (*Cupressus sempervirens*)
30% orange (*Citrus sinensis*)
10% helichrysum (*Helichrysum angustifolia* var. *italicum*)

Benefits the cardiovascular, circulatory, digestive, endocrine, immune, lymph, musculoskeletal, nervous, and renal systems.

Clears heat, drains dampness, transforms phlegm, harmonizes, tonifies, regulates the qi, invigorates the blood, stops bleeding, and calms the spirit.

Supports multiple aspects of heart function, including muscle tone, nerve connection, blood viscosity, and oxygenation.

The Heart Organ Supporting Blend addresses the physical aspects of heart function, including the nervous system connections that regulate the heart rate, the cardiac muscle that pumps the heart, the strength of vessel walls, and circulation and oxygenation of the blood. To address the TCM emotional aspects of heart function, combine this blend with the Heart Meridian Balancing Blend. Substitute ylang ylang or copaiba for the orange oil when applying this blend to the chest to reduce possible skin irritation to sun-damaged skin.

Application and safety tips for the Heart Organ Supporting Blend

- contains one citrus oil, which increases photosensitivity in the applied area, and is best diffused or used in areas that are not exposed to the sun
- apply undiluted to the soles of the feet during treatment sessions
- apply undiluted to the soles of the feet in the morning and before bed between acupuncture sessions
- diffuse at home during the night between treatment sessions
- avoid during pregnancy
- considered safe to use postpartum

THE MERAMOUR HEART MERIDIAN BALANCING BLEND

50% ylang ylang (*Cananga odorata*)
25% sacred frankincense (*Boswellia sacra*)
25% frankincense (*Boswellia carterii*)

Benefits the cardiovascular, circulatory, endocrine, exocrine, immune, musculoskeletal, nervous, and reproductive systems.

Harmonizes, tonifies, regulates the qi, and calms the spirit.

Calms stress response, optimizes melatonin and cortisol, and regulates the circadian rhythm (sleep-wake cycle).

Enhances the hypothalamus and pituitary functions with the adrenals, thyroid, ovaries, and testes.

Uplifts mood for people affected by reduced sunlight.

The Heart Meridian Balancing Blend includes two types of frankincense that come from different trees. Sacred frankincense supports more yin, feminine, calming, and harmonizing functions in the body. Frankincense supports more yang, masculine, energizing, and warming functions in the body. Ylang ylang harmonizes the two types of frankincense and allows the blend to adapt its yin or yang qualities as needed. This blend contains the three oils with the strongest adaptogenic and harmonizing properties.

Application and safety tips for the Heart Meridian Balancing Blend

- dilute 50/50 with an organic carrier oil and apply to the forehead, back of neck, hairline, or spine during treatment sessions
- apply undiluted to the soles of the feet during treatment sessions
- dilute 50/50 with an organic carrier oil and apply to the face, scars, and age spots between treatment sessions
- diffuse at home during the night between treatment sessions
- wear as perfume or cologne or apply over the heart area to support emotional health
- add a few drops to an organic moisturizer
- considered safe during pregnancy for all of the above application methods

THE MERAMOUR SMALL INTESTINE ORGAN SUPPORTING BLEND

30% marjoram (*Origanum majorana*)
30% copaiba (copal: *Copaifera reticulate* or *Copaifera L. genus*)
20% lavender (*Lavandula angustifolia*)
20% lemon (*Citrus limon*)

Benefits the cardiovascular, circulatory, digestive, immune, musculoskeletal, and nervous systems.

Clears heat, drains dampness, harmonizes, regulates the qi, calms the spirit, and reduces food stagnation.

Relaxes and strengthens the muscles and tendons (bone-to-muscle connections).

Enhances nutrient absorption and promotes a balanced immune response to foods.

The Small Intestine Organ Supporting Blend boosts energy and concentration while relaxing the muscles and calming the mind. This blend helps bring clarity to emotional stressors and calms digestive irritability. With two energizing oils, copaiba and lemon, and two calming oils, marjoram and lavender, this blend adapts for use any time of day. This blend can enhance exercise routines by simultaneously strengthening and relaxing the muscles to improve muscle tone and flexibility. If the manufacturer and the FDA have approved the oils for internal use, dilute this blend with vegetable oil to take internally.

Application and safety tips for the Small Intestine Organ Supporting Blend

- contains one citrus oil, which increases photosensitivity in the applied area, and is best diffused or used in areas not exposed to the sun
- apply undiluted to the soles of the feet during treatment sessions
- if approved by the manufacturer and the FDA for internal use, dilute 50/50 with a healthy cooking oil (olive, avocado, or coconut) and take six to nine drops in a capsule with meals
- dilute 50/50 with an organic carrier oil and apply to sore or tight muscles
- apply undiluted to the soles of the feet before or after exercise
- add a few drops to an organic moisturizer and apply to the abdomen between treatment sessions
- avoid during pregnancy and postpartum

THE MERAMOUR SMALL INTESTINE MERIDIAN BALANCING BLEND

50% ylang ylang (*Cananga odorata*)
25% vetiver (*Vetiveria zizanoides*)
25% copaiba (copal: *Copaifera reticulate* or *Copaifera L. genus*)

Benefits the digestive, endocrine, exocrine, immune, lymph, musculoskeletal, and nervous systems.

Harmonizes, tonifies, regulates the qi, calms the spirit, and reduces food stagnation.

Supports the hypothalamus and pituitary functions with the adrenals and the enteric nervous system.

Calms the stress response and balances melatonin and cortisol to regulate the circadian rhythm.

Releases cellular memories of emotional and physical trauma.

The Small Intestine Meridian Balancing Blend benefits scars in the skin, muscle, and connective tissue, along with emotional scarring. This blend addresses different causes of scarring, such as acne, physical injury, and emotional trauma. Pain or discomfort when palpating a scar indicates that qi stagnation and blood stasis are currently negatively impacting health. Treating scars with a combination of acupuncture and this blend encourages the release of hidden factors compromising health. Ylang ylang adapts the energizing qualities of copaiba and the sedating properties of vetiver to support a healthy circadian rhythm. Copaiba addresses pathogenic heat and inflammation caused by diet, while vetiver supports the beneficial bacteria in the small intestine. This blend enhances the digestive and nervous system connections through the enteric nervous system.

Application and safety tips for the Small Intestine Meridian Balancing Blend

- dilute 50/50 with an organic carrier oil and apply to the forehead, back of neck, hairline, or spine during treatment sessions
- apply undiluted to the soles of the feet during treatment sessions
- dilute 50/50 with an organic carrier oil and apply over painful scars
- diffuse at home during the day or night between treatment sessions to release emotional blockages
- dilute 50/50 with an organic carrier oil and wear as perfume or cologne to support emotional health
- add a few drops to an organic moisturizer
- avoid during pregnancy and postpartum

THE MERAMOUR URINARY BLADDER ORGAN SUPPORTING BLEND

25% vetiver (*Vetiveria zizanoides*)
25% geranium (*Pelargonium graveolens*)
25% clary sage (*Salvia sclarea*)
25% black spruce (*Picea mariana*)

Benefits the circulatory, digestive, endocrine, exocrine, musculoskeletal, nervous, reproductive, and urinary systems.

Clears yin-deficiency heat, harmonizes, tonifies, and calms the spirit.

Supports balanced hormones and emotional health for both men and women.

Provides the raw materials to remyelinate nerves, strengthen connective tissue, and enhance bones.

The urinary bladder is the farthest organ from the brain along the spinal column. Frequent urination or incontinence can be an early indication of a compromised nervous system due to age or pathogenic heat. The Urinary Bladder Organ Supporting Blend promotes regeneration of the nervous system and the release of pathogenic heat. This blend contains small amounts of plant-based hormones with harmonizing oils to encourage healthy, balanced cortisol, progesterone, estrogen, and testosterone levels for men and women.

Application and safety tips for the Urinary Bladder Organ Supporting Blend

- apply undiluted to the soles of the feet during treatment sessions
- dilute 50/50 with an organic carrier oil and apply to the spine, lower back, or lower abdomen during treatment sessions or between sessions
- dilute 50/50 with an organic carrier oil and apply to the face at night as a moisturizer
- diffuse at night between treatment sessions to support brain function
- add a few drops to an organic moisturizer and apply to the lower abdomen or sore and stiff joints between treatment sessions
- avoid during pregnancy and postpartum

THE MERAMOUR URINARY BLADDER MERIDIAN BALANCING BLEND

50% marjoram (*Origanum majorana*)

25% cedarwood (*Cedrus atlantica*)

25% copaiba (copal: *Copaifera reticulate* or *Copaifera L. genus*)

Benefits the cardiovascular, circulatory, endocrine, immune, lymph, musculoskeletal, nervous, and urinary systems.

Drains dampness, transforms phlegm, harmonizes, regulates the qi, and calms the spirit.

Promotes physical and emotional flexibility.

Regulates the autonomic nervous system for clients with hypersensitive sensory perception.

The Urinary Bladder Meridian Balancing Blend has adaptogenic properties, which encourages the nervous system to adjust to different situations. This blend contains stimulating, relaxing, and harmonizing oils that support healthy cortisol levels for energy and focus during the day and healthy melatonin levels for sleep and relaxation during the night. The urinary bladder meridian runs alongside the spine, and combining the Organ Supporting and Meridian Balancing blends enhances the central nervous system benefits.

Application and safety tips for the Urinary Bladder Meridian Balancing Blend

- dilute 50/50 with an organic carrier oil and apply to the forehead, back of neck, hairline, or spine during treatment sessions
- apply undiluted to the soles of the feet during treatment sessions
- diffuse at home during the day or night between treatment sessions
- add a few drops to an organic moisturizer and apply to sore or tight muscles
- considered safe to apply to the soles of the feet postpartum for recovery of the pelvic floor and adapting to the demands of a new baby
- avoid during pregnancy

THE MERAMOUR KIDNEY ORGAN SUPPORTING BLEND

30% copaiba (copal: *Copaifera reticulate* or *Copaifera L. genus*)

30% cypress (*Cupressus sempervirens*)

30% black spruce (*Picea mariana*)

10% jasmine (*Jasminum officinale*)

Benefits the cardiovascular, circulatory, endocrine, exocrine, musculoskeletal, nervous, renal, and reproductive systems.

Drains dampness, harmonizes, tonifies, regulates the qi, and calms the spirit.

Nourishes the conception vessel to encourage regeneration of the endocrine glands and enhance fertility.

In the Body-Feedback system, the kidney organ includes the adrenals, ovaries, testes, bone marrow, and the brain, all of which store a person's life force known as jing or essence. The Kidney Organ Supporting Blend contains oils from two evergreens that promote longevity and cellular renewal because they remain green and retain their leaves all year. Cypress is a fast-growing evergreen, and black spruce is one of the tallest conifers. Jasmine enhances fertility for both men and women. Copaiba is made from the tree's resin that responds to injury. The copaiba amplifies and harmonizes the blend to reach the deepest shao-yin level. This blend promotes longevity by providing nutrients for cellular regeneration and acquired essence.

Application and safety tips for the Kidney Organ Supporting Blend

- dilute 50/50 with an organic carrier oil and apply to the forehead, neck, lower abdomen, back, or spine during treatment sessions
- dilute 50/50 with an organic carrier oil and apply as a moisturizer and to scars and age spots
- apply undiluted to the soles of the feet during treatment sessions
- add a few drops to an organic moisturizer
- for women, add a few drops to an organic carrier oil or lotion and apply to the lower abdomen during the follicular phase of the menstrual cycle to support egg quality
- for men, add a few drops to an organic carrier oil or lotion and apply to the lower abdomen to support sperm quality
- avoid during pregnancy and postpartum

THE MERAMOUR KIDNEY MERIDIAN BALANCING BLEND

50% cedarwood (*Cedrus atlantica*)
25% sandalwood (*Santalum album*)
25% carrot seed (*Daucus carota*)

Benefits the cardiovascular, circulatory, endocrine, exocrine, lymph, musculoskeletal, nervous, renal, and reproductive systems.

Clears heat, drains dampness, transforms phlegm, harmonizes, warms the interior, tonifies, regulates the qi, and calms the spirit.

Benefits people with hormonal acne and sun-damaged skin.

Tonifies the governing vessel to encourage regeneration of the endocrine glands and enhance fertility.

The Kidney Meridian Balancing Blend contains the essential oils with the highest amounts of sesquiterpene alcohols that promote regeneration of the endocrine system, brain, and internal organs. This blend enhances fertility by supporting all of the endocrine glands and quickly passes through the blood-brain barrier for the hypothalamus, pineal, and pituitary. This blend harmonizes the adrenal glands, which sit atop the kidneys, and the limbic system to reduce the adverse effects of stress on cellular aging.

Application and safety tips for the Kidney Meridian Balancing Blend

- dilute 50/50 with an organic carrier oil and apply to the forehead, neck, hairline, lower abdomen, back, or spine during treatment sessions
- dilute 50/50 with an organic carrier oil and apply as a moisturizer and to scars and age spots
- apply undiluted to the soles of the feet during treatment sessions
- dilute 50/50 with an organic carrier oil and wear as perfume or cologne for emotional support during times of stress
- add a few drops to an organic moisturizer
- for women, add a few drops to an organic carrier oil or lotion and apply to the lower abdomen during the follicular phase of the menstrual cycle to support egg quality
- for men, add a few drops to an organic carrier oil or lotion and apply to the lower abdomen to support sperm quality
- avoid during pregnancy and postpartum

11.6 Third Trisection Blends

THE MERAMOUR PERICARDIUM ORGAN SUPPORTING BLEND

30% cedarwood (*Cedrus atlantica*)

30% copaiba (copal: *Copaifera reticulate* or *Copaifera L. genus*)

20% geranium (*Pelargonium graveolens*)

20% cardamom (*Elettaria cardamomum*)

Benefits the cardiovascular, circulatory, endocrine, lymph, and nervous systems.

Drains dampness, transforms phlegm, harmonizes, regulates the qi, invigorates the blood, stops bleeding, and calms the spirit.

Protects the heart organ from pathogenic heat and stagnant fluids.

The Pericardium Organ Supporting Blend contains three adaptogenic oils that allow the properties of this blend to address different needs of the body. This blend regulates the viscosity of blood and lymph to support the triple burner (five-element pair) and the liver (six-level pair). Cedarwood and geranium together protect the body from pathogens that target the blood. This blend protects the heart organ by promoting a healthy inflammatory cycle and cleansing the blood.

Application and safety tips for the Pericardium Organ Supporting Blend

- dilute 50/50 with an organic carrier oil and apply to the neck, back, or spine during treatment sessions
- apply undiluted to the soles of the feet during treatment sessions
- diffuse this blend during the evening between treatment sessions
- add a few drops to an organic moisturizer
- for women, add a few drops to an organic carrier oil or lotion and apply to the lower abdomen anytime during the menstrual cycle to enhance blood and lymph flow to the reproductive organs
- considered safe during all trimesters of pregnancy and postpartum

THE MERAMOUR PERICARDIUM MERIDIAN BALANCING BLEND

50% lavender (*Lavandula angustifolia*)
25% marjoram (*Origanum majorana*)
25% patchouli (*Pogostemon cablin*)

Benefits the cardiovascular, circulatory, endocrine, exocrine, musculoskeletal, and nervous systems.

Clears heat, regulates the qi, and calms the spirit.

Relaxes the muscles, calms nervous energy, reduces cravings, and benefits sleep.

The Pericardium Meridian Balancing Blend calms physical restlessness, anxiousness, and heightened stress responses. The combination of patchouli and lavender encourages healthy estrogen and progesterone levels. They cleanse xenoestrogens from estrogen receptor sites and reduce excess cortisol that can lower progesterone and contribute to premenstrual symptoms. Using this blend in the evening reduces excess cortisol levels and promotes restful sleep. If available, substitute balsam fir for marjoram in this blend to enhance cellular regeneration by providing plant-based hormones for accelerated growth. Balsam fir is ideal for people over the age of 50.

Application and safety tips for the Pericardium Meridian Balancing Blend

- dilute 50/50 with an organic carrier oil and apply to the neck, back, or spine during treatment sessions
- apply undiluted to the soles of the feet during treatment sessions
- diffuse this blend in the evening between treatment sessions
- add a few drops to bath salts for a relaxing bath in the evenings
- add a few drops to an organic moisturizer and apply to sore muscles
- for cycling women, add a few drops to an organic carrier oil or lotion and apply to the lower abdomen during the menstrual period to moderate discomfort and detoxify xenoestrogens
- avoid during pregnancy and postpartum

THE MERAMOUR TRIPLE BURNER ORGAN SUPPORTING BLEND

40% cedarwood (*Cedrus atlantica*)

40% cypress (*Cupressus sempervirens*)

10% helichrysum (*Helichrysum angustifolia var. italicum*)

10% ledum (*Ledum groenlandicum*)

Benefits the cardiovascular, circulatory, endocrine, exocrine, immune, lymph, musculoskeletal, nervous, renal, and reproductive systems.

Drains dampness, transforms phlegm, harmonizes, warms the interior, tonifies, regulates the qi, invigorates the blood, stops bleeding, and calms the spirit.

Supports cellular regeneration and cleanses the lymph nodes.

In TCM, the triple burner includes the upper burner (chest, heart, and lungs), the middle burner (spleen, stomach, liver, and small intestine), and the lower burner (kidneys, urinary bladder, and large intestine). In the Body-Feedback system, the lymph nodes are the triple burner organ. Between 500-700 lymph nodes are found throughout the torso alone, with more throughout the rest of the body. The lymph vessels connect with the lymph nodes to filter toxins and infections out of the blood. The Triple Burner Organ Blend includes ledum and helichrysum, which influence regeneration. The cedarwood and cypress cleanse lymph fluids and direct this blend to the lymph system.

Application and safety tips for the Triple Burner Organ Supporting Blend

- dilute 50/50 with an organic carrier oil and apply to the neck, back, or spine during treatment sessions
- apply undiluted to the soles of the feet during treatment sessions
- dilute 50/50 with an organic carrier oil and apply to the neck, face, groin, and other regions with concentrated lymph nodes between sessions
- add a few drops to an organic moisturizer and apply to swollen or painful lymph nodes between treatment sessions
- avoid during pregnancy and postpartum

THE MERAMOUR TRIPLE BURNER MERIDIAN BALANCING BLEND

50% cypress (*Cupressus sempervirens*)

25% tangerine (*Citrus nobilis* or *Citrus reticulata* var. *tangerine*)

25% grapefruit (*Citrus x paradisi*)

Benefits the circulatory, digestive, immune, lymph, musculoskeletal, and renal systems.

Drains dampness, transforms phlegm, harmonizes, regulates the qi, invigorates the blood, and reduces food stagnation.

Connects the three burners of the body through the lymph system.

In the Body-Feedback system, the triple burner meridian corresponds with the lymph system, which connects the upper, middle, and lower burners. The lymph system generates a small number of adult stem cells called hematopoietic stem cells, which hold the potential for extensive regeneration and the ability to differentiate into all blood cell types. The Triple Burner Meridian Balancing Blend supports the cleansing, immune, and anti-pathogenic functions of the lymph system. The tangerine oil up-bears the qi, the grapefruit oil down-bears the qi, and the cypress oil circulates and harmonizes the two; together, they promote continual flow in the body.

Application and safety tips for the Triple Burner Meridian Balancing Blend

- contains two citrus oils, which increases photosensitivity in the applied area, and is best used in areas that are not exposed to the sun
- apply undiluted to the soles of the feet during treatment sessions
- diffuse this blend during the day or night between treatment sessions
- add a few drops to an organic moisturizer and apply to areas with excessive fluid retention
- avoid during pregnancy

THE MERAMOUR GALLBLADDER ORGAN SUPPORTING BLEND

30% lavender (*Lavandula angustifolia*)
30% marjoram (*Origanum majorana*)
20% rosemary (*Rosmarinus officianalis*)
20% wintergreen (*Gaultheria procumbens*)

Benefits the circulatory, digestive, endocrine, immune, lymph, musculoskeletal, and nervous systems.

Clears heat, invigorates the blood, and calms the spirit.

Encourages the release of congested bile from the gallbladder.

Supports the regeneration of tendons, ligaments, and cartilage.

The gallbladder organ augments and stores the liver bile for the proper digestion of fats. It is prone to dysfunction and congested bile due to partially hydrogenated fats, genetically modified foods, and elevated hormone levels seen during pregnancy. The Gallbladder Organ Supporting Blend enhances the digestion of fats, promotes the release of congested bile, and improves the detoxification of used hormone metabolites. This blend balances the stimulating properties of rosemary and wintergreen with the relaxing qualities of lavender and marjoram for use anytime. Lavender and wintergreen reduce high blood pressure, rosemary increases blood pressure, and marjoram can help regulate blood pressure. Used together, these oils can help balance normal blood pressure fluctuations due to stress. Substitute nutmeg essential oil in place of rosemary oil for clients with hypertension and a family history of hypertension for long-term blend use. Avoid nutmeg with epilepsy.

Application and safety tips for the Gallbladder Organ Supporting Blend

- dilute 50/50 with an organic carrier oil and apply over the gallbladder on the right anterior side of the rib cage, or to the neck, back, or spine during treatment sessions
- apply undiluted to the soles of the feet during treatment sessions
- dilute 50/50 with an organic carrier oil and apply over the right anterior side of the rib cage before meals to improve gallbladder function between sessions
- diffuse this blend during the day or night between treatment sessions
- add a few drops to an organic moisturizer and apply to sore muscles
- for cycling women, add a few drops to an organic carrier oil or lotion and apply to the lower abdomen during the menstrual period to reduce discomfort and detoxify xenoestrogens
- avoid during pregnancy and postpartum

THE MERAMOUR GALLBLADDER MERIDIAN BALANCING BLEND

50% marjoram (*Origanum majorana*)
25% rosemary (*Rosmarinus officianalis*)
25% tangerine (*Citrus nobilis* or *Citrus reticulata* var. *tangerine*)

Benefits the digestive, endocrine, immune, musculoskeletal, and nervous systems.

Drains dampness, transforms phlegm, tonifies, and calms the spirit.

Supports the digestion of fats into cholesterol that provides the raw materials to make hormones and collagen.

Detoxifies used hormone metabolites.

The Gallbladder Meridian Balancing Blend strengthens and relaxes the muscles and tendons (muscle-to-bone connective tissue), provides the raw materials to enhance connective tissue regeneration, and benefits the temporal lobe of the brain. This blend is physically and emotionally uplifting and beneficial for any long-term or chronic health challenges. Rosemary is stimulating and can increase blood pressure with a history of hypertension. Marjoram's relaxing qualities balance the rosemary in this blend for people with normal or lower blood pressure. Substitute lavender essential oil in place of rosemary oil for clients with hypertension and a family history of hypertension for long-term blend use.

Application and safety tips for the Gallbladder Meridian Balancing Blend

- contains one citrus oil, which increases photosensitivity in the applied area, and is best diffused, taken internally, or applied to areas not exposed to the sun
- apply undiluted to the soles of the feet during treatment sessions
- if approved by the manufacturer and the FDA for internal use, dilute 50/50 with healthy cooking oil (olive, avocado, or coconut) and take six to nine drops in a capsule with meals
- apply undiluted to the soles of the feet in the morning to boost energy
- considered safe to apply to the soles of the feet postpartum for breastfeeding and recovery of the pelvic floor
- avoid during pregnancy

THE MERAMOUR LIVER ORGAN SUPPORTING BLEND

40% fennel (*Foeniculum vulgare*)
40% orange (*Citrus sinensis*)
10% rosemary (*Rosmarinus officianalis*)
10% celery seed (*Apium graveolens*)

Benefits the digestive, endocrine, excretory, immune, lymph, renal, and reproductive systems.

Drains dampness, transforms phlegm, tonifies, and reduces food stagnation.

Cleanses the blood and cellular receptor sites.

Enhances the absorption of healthy fats.

Nourishes the conception vessel to encourage regeneration of the endocrine glands and enhance fertility.

The Liver Organ Supporting Blend includes safe and effective detoxifying oils to assist with transporting toxins, including xenoestrogens, out of the body. This blend strengthens the digestive tract lining and eases the burden of detoxification on the kidneys. It is appropriate for clients with compromised liver function, environmental sensitivities, genetic issues, exposure to heavy metals, chronic low-grade infections, allergies, food intolerances, or overuse of prescription medications. When used in large amounts or long-term, rosemary essential oil can increase blood pressure with preexisting hypertension or a family history of hypertension. Substitute lemon essential oil for the rosemary in this blend for clients with hypertension, a family history of hypertension, or epilepsy. If the manufacturer and the FDA approve the oils for internal use, dilute this blend with vegetable oil and take in a capsule with meals.

Application and safety tips for the Liver Organ Supporting Blend

- contains one citrus oil, which increases photosensitivity in the applied area, and is best diffused, taken internally, or applied to areas not exposed to the sun
- apply undiluted to the soles of the feet during treatment sessions
- if approved by the manufacturer and the FDA for internal use, dilute 50/50 with a healthy cooking oil (olive, avocado, or coconut) and take six to nine drops in a capsule with meals
- apply undiluted to the soles of the feet before bed to support detoxification during peak liver organ activity time
- for cycling women, apply diluted with an organic carrier oil or lotion to the lower abdomen during the follicular phase of the menstrual cycle to support egg quality
- for men, apply undiluted to the soles of the feet daily to support sperm quality
- considered safe to apply to the soles of the feet postpartum for breastfeeding and recovery of the pelvic floor
- avoid during pregnancy

THE MERAMOUR LIVER MERIDIAN BALANCING BLEND

50% bergamot (*Citrus bergamia*)
25% geranium (*Pelargonium graveolens*)
25% cardamom (*Elettaria cardamomum*)

Benefits the circulatory, digestive, endocrine, immune, lymph, nervous, and reproductive systems.

Drains dampness, transforms phlegm, harmonizes, regulates the qi, invigorates the blood, stops bleeding, calms the spirit, and reduces food stagnation.

Calms the nervous system and the mind to release stress.

Promotes feelings of tranquility, peace, and satisfaction.

The Liver Meridian Balancing Blend moves stagnant liver qi with accompanying blood stasis to release feelings of frustration, irritability, and anger. This blend supports a restful night's sleep by calming the mind and lowering excess stress hormones. All three of the oils in this blend cleanse xenoestrogens and other environmental toxins from the blood. For cycling women, this blend enhances the uterine lining by balancing estrogens and promoting progesterone. This blend can be used during the entire menstrual cycle and often tests beneficial in the luteal phase and the first trimester of pregnancy.

Application and safety tips for the Liver Meridian Balancing Blend

- contains one citrus oil, which increases photosensitivity in the applied area, and is best diffused or applied to areas not exposed to the sun
- dilute 50/50 with an organic carrier oil and apply over the liver area on the right anterior side of the rib cage, lower abdomen, or lower back during treatment sessions
- apply undiluted to the soles of the feet during treatment sessions
- diffuse this blend during the night between treatment sessions
- for cycling women, add a few drops to an organic carrier oil or lotion and apply to the lower abdomen during the entire month and during pregnancy
- the above application methods are considered safe to use during pregnancy and postpartum

11.7 Extra-Vessel Blends

THE MERAMOUR GOVERNING VESSEL MERIDIAN BALANCING BLEND

50% sacred frankincense (*Boswellia sacra*)
25% sandalwood (*Santalum album*)
25% blue spruce (*Picea pungens*)

Benefits the cardiovascular, endocrine, lymph, musculoskeletal, nervous, renal, and reproductive systems.

Harmonizes, warms the interior, tonifies, regulates the qi, and calms the spirit.

Tonifies the governing vessel to encourage regeneration of the brain and endocrine glands.

The Governing Vessel Meridian Balancing Blend contains the essential oils with the highest amounts of phytotestosterone that promote regeneration of the endocrine system and brain. This blend activates the hypothalamus, pituitary, and pineal glands to enhance meditation, focus, and sex drive. Testosterone balances estrogen dominance for men. As men age, their ratio of estrogen to testosterone becomes unbalanced as testosterone naturally declines and estrogen increases due to the widespread xenoestrogens in our environment that linger in cellular receptor sites. For women, low levels of testosterone can also cause estrogen dominance in the uterus. This blend supports healthy testosterone levels for both men and women by cleansing and activating the hormone receptor sites. If blue spruce or sacred frankincense is unavailable, then substituting with black spruce (*picea mariana*) and regular frankincense (*boswellia carterii*) is best. Black spruce combines better with regular frankincense, while blue spruce combines better with sacred frankincense.

Application and safety tips for the Governing Vessel Meridian Balancing Blend

- dilute 50/50 with an organic carrier oil and apply to the forehead, neck, hairline, lower abdomen, back, or spine during treatment sessions
- dilute 50/50 with an organic carrier oil and apply as a moisturizer and to scars and age spots
- apply undiluted to the soles of the feet during treatment sessions
- dilute 50/50 with an organic carrier oil and wear as perfume or cologne to enhance natural pheromones
- add a few drops to an organic moisturizer
- for cycling women, add a few drops to an organic carrier oil or lotion and apply to the lower back just before and during ovulation to increase sex drive and support a strong luteinizing hormone (LH) surge to release a mature egg
- for men, combine this blend with the Kidney Organ or Liver Organ blends by adding a few drops to an organic carrier oil or lotion and apply to the lower back to enhance sperm quality
- avoid during pregnancy and postpartum

THE MERAMOUR CONCEPTION VESSEL MERIDIAN BALANCING BLEND

50% lavender (*Lavandula angustifolia*)
25% black pepper (*Piper nigrum*)
25% myrrh (*Commiphora myrrha*)

Benefits the endocrine, exocrine, musculoskeletal, nervous, and reproductive systems.

Clears heat, harmonizes, tonifies, regulates the qi, and calms the spirit.

Nourishes the conception vessel to encourage regeneration of the endocrine glands and enhance fertility.

The Conception Vessel Meridian Balancing Blend combines exceptionally well with other oils and blends. Lavender oil cleanses the estrogen hormone receptor sites, calms the nervous system, and harmonizes with other essential oils. Myrrh essential oil amplifies the effects of other oils mixed with it. Black pepper essential oil supplies oxygen to the cells and stimulates the brain, which balances the calming effects of lavender and myrrh. Black pepper oil connects the endocrine glands in the brain with the reproductive organs to promote healthy sexual expression. To enhance fertility, this blend can be used in conjunction with the Governing Vessel Meridian Balancing Blend, the Kidney Organ Supporting and Meridian Balancing Blends, or the Liver Organ Supporting and Meridian Balancing Blends.

Application and safety tips for the Conception Vessel Meridian Balancing Blend

- dilute 50/50 with an organic carrier oil and apply to the forehead, neck, lower abdomen, back, or spine during treatment sessions
- dilute 50/50 with an organic carrier oil and apply as a moisturizer and to scars and age spots
- apply undiluted to the soles of the feet during treatment sessions
- add a few drops to an organic moisturizer
- for women, add a few drops to an organic carrier oil or lotion and apply to the lower abdomen during the follicular phase of the menstrual cycle to enhance egg quality
- for men, add a few drops to an organic carrier oil or lotion and apply to the lower abdomen to support sperm quality
- avoid during pregnancy and postpartum

11.8 Pregnancy Support Blends

Pregnant women can benefit from the supportive and gentle nature of therapeutic-grade essential oils. During pregnancy, careful attention to the quality of the essential oils used is required. Please check with the manufacturer to ensure their products are approved for use with pregnant women. Always test the essential oils to the master points in the neck and shoulders and the pulse to confirm the proper selection. The following Organ Supporting, Meridian Balancing, and Pregnancy Support Blends can support women throughout their pregnancy.

THE MERAMOUR PEACEFUL ESSENCE BLEND

25% tangerine (*Citrus nobilis* or *Citrus reticulata* var. *tangerine*)
25% orange (*Citrus sinensis*)
25% patchouli (*Pogostemon cablin*)
25% ylang ylang (*Cananga odorata*)

Benefits the circulatory, digestive, endocrine, and immune systems.

Drains dampness, transforms phlegm, boosts the qi, and harmonizes.

Supports progesterone by lowering the stress hormone cortisol that depletes it.

Encourages healthy development and positioning of the placenta.

The Peaceful Essence Blend is ideal for the first and second trimesters when tangerine's uplifting effects, combined with the harmonizing attributes of orange, patchouli, and ylang ylang, secure the pituitary's connection with the womb. This blend encourages the smooth flow of qi, which can become stagnant with the increased blood volume and fluids during pregnancy. All four of these oils carry the vibration of peace and happiness that lowers the everyday response to stress, which allows the progesterone reserves to focus on the needs of the pregnancy. Discontinue this blend by 34 weeks of pregnancy to encourage the baby to engage down into the birth canal and prepare for labor and delivery.

Application and safety tips for the Meramour Peaceful Essence Blend

- contains two citrus oils, which increases photosensitivity in the applied area, and is best diffused or applied to areas not exposed to the sun
- apply undiluted to the soles of the feet during treatment sessions
- apply undiluted to the soles of the feet in the morning to boost energy and in the evening to release stress
- considered safe to apply to the soles of the feet postpartum for breastfeeding and recovery of the pelvic floor
- considered safe during pregnancy through week 33

THE MERAMOUR PREGNANCY IMMUNE HARMONIZING BLEND

50% palmarosa *(Cymbopogon martinii)*
25% bergamot *(Citrus bergamia)*
25% cardamom *(Elettaria cardamomum)*

Benefits the circulatory, digestive, endocrine, and immune systems.

Drains dampness, transforms phlegm, regulates the qi, and harmonizes.

Supports progesterone by lowering the stress response that depletes it to make cortisol.

Harmonizes the immune system to protect the baby and mother.

The Immune Pregnancy Harmonizing Blend is especially beneficial for the first trimester, when the immune system is adapting to the needs of the pregnancy. Palmarosa and bergamot enhance the regulating function of the immune system and support the pituitary and womb connection. In TCM, cardamom in herb form (*sha ren*), stabilizes the fetus and aids digestion. This blend can be used as needed and long-term during all trimesters of pregnancy, labor and delivery, and postpartum to assist the immune system in adapting to the changing needs of the different stages of pregnancy.

Application and safety tips for the Immune Pregnancy Harmonizing Blend

- contains one citrus oil, which increases photosensitivity in the applied area, and is best diffused or applied to areas not exposed to the sun
- apply undiluted to the soles of the feet during treatment sessions
- apply undiluted to the soles of the feet in the morning to harmonize the immune system
- considered safe during all stages of pregnancy and postpartum

THE MERAMOUR PREGNANCY SKIN BEAUTIFYING BLEND

30% ylang ylang (*Cananga odorata*)
30% geranium (*Pelargonium graveolens*)
30% palmarosa (*Cymbopogon martinii*)
10% cardamom (*Elettaria cardamomum*)

Benefits the exocrine, digestive, and immune systems.

Drains dampness, transforms phlegm, regulates the qi, and harmonizes.

Supports progesterone by lowering the stress response that depletes it to make cortisol.

Harmonizes the immune and digestive systems while supporting skin elasticity.

The Pregnancy Skin Beautifying Blend addresses the special needs of the skin during pregnancy to help accommodate the growing womb and baby. Ylang ylang and geranium have adaptogenic properties that help the skin expand during pregnancy and contract postpartum. Palmarosa and cardamom support the immune component of the skin while enhancing digestion during pregnancy. This blend is best diluted and applied to the skin during all trimesters of pregnancy, labor and delivery, and postpartum.

Application and safety tips for the Pregnancy Skin Beautifying Blend

- apply undiluted to the soles of the feet during treatment sessions
- add a few drops to an organic moisturizer and apply to skin daily
- considered safe during all stages of pregnancy and postpartum

The following Meramour Organ Supporting and Meridian Balancing Blends are safe to use during pregnancy as recommended:

LUNG MERIDIAN BALANCING BLEND supports a balanced immune system during all trimesters and postpartum.

STOMACH ORGAN SUPPORTING BLEND supports digestion with substitutions during the second and third trimesters.

STOMACH MERIDIAN BALANCING BLEND supports digestion during the second and third trimesters.

HEART MERIDIAN BALANCING BLEND supports the hypothalamus and pituitary axis during all trimesters and postpartum.

PERICARDIUM ORGAN SUPPORTING BLEND supports blood and lymph flow during all trimesters of pregnancy and postpartum.

LIVER MERIDIAN BALANCING BLEND supports progesterone and the uterus during all trimesters and postpartum.

11.9 Safety Precautions for Essential Oils

Essential oil substitutions included in this book for the oils contained in the Meramour blends cover the necessary safety precautions for pregnancy, photosensitivity, and high blood pressure. The individual blend descriptions include the applicable essential oil substitutions for high blood pressure. To better understand the chemical properties and healing actions of individual oils, please look to an essential oil desk reference guide.

There are several essential oils to avoid or use with caution during pregnancy that are included in the organ supporting and meridian balancing blends. In general, essential oils to avoid during pregnancy can raise blood pressure, stimulate the uterus, cause vasoconstriction, or contain phytohormone properties.

ESSENTIAL OILS TO AVOID DURING PREGNANCY

Basil
included in the Lung Organ Supporting Blend

Celery seed
included in the Liver Organ Supporting Blend

Clary sage
included in the Urinary Bladder Organ Supporting Blend

Clove
included in the Spleen Organ and Meridian Balancing Blends

Cypress
included in the Large Intestine, Heart, Kidney, and Triple Burner Organ Supporting, and the Triple Burner Meridian Balancing Blends

Fennel
included in the Spleen and Liver Organ Supporting Blends

Lemongrass
included in the Large Intestine Meridian Balancing Blend

Marjoram
included in the Heart, Small Intestine, and Gallbladder Organ Supporting, and the Urinary Bladder, Pericardium, and Gallbladder Meridian Balancing Blends

Myrrh
included in the Conception Vessel Meridian Balancing Blend

Rosemary
included in the Gallbladder and Liver Organ Supporting and Gallbladder Meridian Balancing Blends

Vetiver
included in the Urinary Organ and Small Intestine Meridian Balancing Blends

Wintergreen
included in the Gallbladder Organ Supporting Blend

ESSENTIAL OILS TO USE WITH CAUTION DURING PREGNANCY:

Citronella
included in the Large Intestine Meridian Balancing Blend

Nutmeg
included as a substitute in the Gallbladder Organ Supporting Blend

Peppermint
included in the Lung and Stomach Organ Supporting Blends (use with caution in the second and third trimesters)

Spearmint
included in the Large Intestine Organ Supporting and Stomach Meridian Balancing Blends, and as a substitute for peppermint in the Lung and Stomach Organ Supporting Blends (use with caution in the first and second trimesters)

ESSENTIAL OILS THAT INCREASE PHOTOSENSITIVITY

Bergamot
included in the Liver Meridian Balancing Blend

Grapefruit
included in the Stomach and Triple Burner Meridian Balancing Blends

Lemon
included in the Lung, Large Intestine, Stomach, and Small Intestine Organ Supporting Blends, and as a substitute in the Liver Organ Supporting Blend

Lime
included in the Stomach Meridian Balancing Blend

Orange
included in the Spleen Meridian Balancing and Heart and Liver Organ Supporting Blends

Tangerine
included in the Gallbladder and Triple Burner Meridian Balancing Blends, the Spleen Organ Supporting Blend, and the Peaceful Essence Blend

In general, rotating the application site for essential oils reduces the risk of skin irritation with long-term use. If an essential oil causes irritation, dilute it with vegetable oil or organic lotion and the discomfort should subside within minutes. If immediate relief of irritation is needed, dilute the essential oil with a carrier oil, then wash it with soap, and apply carrier oil again. Rinsing with water first can increase the irritation. To wash essential oils off of the hands, use a liberal amount of soap before rinsing your hands with water.

The application of essential oils should avoid the eyes, the area surrounding the eyes, and ear canals. If an essential oil gets too close to the eye and causes irritation, apply vegetable oil to the bony socket surrounding the eye. If an essential oil touches the eye, use a Q-tip or a clean finger to dab a few drops of vegetable oil into the corner of the eye and blink to spread it around the eye. If an essential oil is too close to the ear canal, dip a Q-tip in vegetable oil and gently apply it to the outer edge of your ear canal, allowing it to drip inside the ear. Rinsing the eyes or ear canals with water will only increase and spread the irritation.

Therapeutic-grade essential oils can lose their healing properties if stored in direct sunlight or by heat sources. Avoid storing oils in the car in warmer weather or by other heat sources such as a radiator. Store essential oils in a cool and dark location to preserve their healing potential. Blends mixed with a carrier oil can become rancid after a few years of storage. Pure oils, if stored properly, will last for multiple years.

11.10 Practical Application for Choosing Essential Oils

The Meramour blends provide a simple way to integrate sophisticated knowledge of therapeutic-grade oils into practice. Pre-packaged blends from a manufacturer are convenient; however, when a client is experiencing multiple organ/meridian pathologies, the Meramour blends often test favorably for a longer time. The pre-packaged blends that test beneficial frequently change as the client's root dysfunction alternates between excess and deficiency and different organ/meridian pathologies. The Meramour blends adapt to sedate or tonify a root dysfunction and optimize the trisection for a longer duration while a client's health is regenerating. Essential oil blends require less rotation when treatments focus on constitutional support. The Body-Feedback approach gives straightforward instructions on how to utilize essential oils and aromatherapy to accommodate a variety of clients. For practitioners who are already incorporating essential oils into their practice, the Body-Feedback testing techniques will confidently guide the oil selection for each client and advance the use of therapeutic-grade oils.

Choosing essential oils that focus on the root dysfunction is the most effective way to improve the acupuncture treatment results. During a session, the ideal time to test essential oils is in the planning stage after identifying the root imbalance and before inserting the needles. There are two ways to approach selecting essential oils to use during a session. The first approach tests the Meramour blends based on the balancing acupoint prescriptions identified in Chapter 10. The second approach tests single oils or manufactured blends to the master alarm points, pulse, or root dysfunction's individual testing locations.

Check the Meramour blends for those that support the treatment of the root imbalance identified in Chapter 10. Use any one of the master alarm points or the neck muscles to test the blends separately. If more than one blend tests well, recheck the beneficial blends together and find the combination that tests the best. Check the organ and meridian blends for the root imbalance and the five-element and six-level pairs. It is typical for the root imbalance to rotate between the five-element and six-level pairs at treatment sessions, along with alternating the organ and meridian blends.

The following are examples of how to choose the Meramour blends:

For symmetrical treatment with one root dysfunction, check the organ and meridian blends for the root and its five-element and six-level pairs. For example, with a liver root imbalance, test the Liver, Gallbladder, and Pericardium Organ Supporting and Meridian Balancing Blends.

For an asymmetrical treatment with two root dysfunctions within one element, check the Organ Supporting and Meridian Balancing blends for that elemental pair. If needed, check the organ and meridian blends for the second element within the trisection. For instance, with asymmetry affecting the wood element, test the Liver and Gallbladder Organ Supporting and Meridian Balancing Blends, along with the Pericardium and Triple Burner blends.

For an asymmetry treatment with two root dysfunctions in different elements, check the Organ Supporting and Meridian Balancing blends for both root treatments. In the case of a spleen root dysfunction on one side and a kidney root dysfunction on the other side, test the Spleen and Kidney Organ Supporting and Meridian Balancing Blends.

In some cases, using pre-made blends from a manufacturer or creating custom blends from individual oils may test best. There are four scenarios that typically respond well to pre-made manufactured and custom blends: managing pain, during pregnancy, with physical and emotional trauma, and at the initial stages of an exterior pathogen, such as a virus during cold and flu season.

Test the pre-made manufactured and custom blends to the specific Body-Feedback areas associated with the root imbalance to ensure they will enhance the treatment. For example, a standard pre-made blend among different manufacturers to boost the immune system at the first sign of a cold or flu includes clove, cinnamon, eucalyptus, rosemary, and either orange or lemon. When a client presents with a lung root imbalance at the initial stages of a cold or flu, compare a manufactured immune-boosting blend to the Lung and Large Intestine Organ Supporting and Meridian Balancing Blends, and test using the individual lung alarm points (LU5 and LU10) and Body-Feedback areas (deltoid muscles) to find the most effective option at that treatment session.

Testing oil blends to the pulse is helpful in pre-checking combinations and evaluating the subtle differences between blends. Checking the oils to the specific Body-Feedback areas allows the client to feel the difference the oils can make and confirm they are benefiting the root imbalance. Testing oils only to the pulse is necessary for some circumstances, such as with sensory disorders and paralysis, but lacks the client's participation and confirmation in the testing process. Using a combination of the master points, individual Body-Feedback areas, and pulse provides multiple testing options and methods to double-check the results.

Summary of essential oils testing steps:

- Determine the root balancing point prescription (or prescriptions for asymmetry).
- Test the organ supporting and meridian balancing blends for the:
  - Root dysfunction (or dysfunctions for an asymmetrical treatment);
  - Five-element pair of the root dysfunction(s); and
  - Six-level pair of the root dysfunction(s).
- Place one blend at a time (the closed bottle of essential oils) on the upper abdomen (or spine if in the prone position) and allow 10-15 seconds for the meridian system to respond.
- Monitor the pulse for changes or palpate the master points or neck muscles to identify the most beneficial blends.
- If multiple blends test positively, recheck possible combinations and palpate the testing locations that correspond with the root balancing prescription to determine the most effective combination.

Test and apply the essential oils before inserting any needles. Oils encourage the qi and blood to flow, diminish surface blockages, balance the ANS, and change the pulse presentation immediately. The use of essential oils allows for fewer supporting acupoints to achieve desired treatment results. Also, the number of tight, tender, or flaccid Body-Feedback testing locations will reduce after using oils, leaving the most significant testing areas for confirming the effectiveness of the treatment session after removing the needles.

BODY-FEEDBACK CLINICAL PEARLS

When the meridian alarm (fire) points are tender, the meridian balancing blends will often test most favorably. When the organ alarm (he-sea) points are tender, the Organ Supporting blends will often test most favorably. During pregnancy, test the Meramour Pregnancy blends using the pulse, master points, and neck muscles.

11.11 Practical Application for Applying Essential Oils in Treatment

In acupuncture sessions, applying oils topically to the soles of the feet or the spine is most common. The skin on the bottom of the feet is thicker and is the body part that best tolerates undiluted oils. Essential oils applied to the soles of the feet absorb quickly into the bloodstream due to the high number of capillaries that end there. Oils used on the feet can also activate the foot reflexology points to benefit the entire body. Oils applied over the spine immediately harmonize the autonomic nervous system. Avoid applying essential oils topically over sun-damaged skin on the neck of people with short hair.

In general, use a total of four to six drops of essential oils on the sole of each foot and a total of nine to twelve drops of essential oils on the spine. When using multiple blends, apply two to three drops of each blend. If the client feels the oils are too hot, burning, or prickling, use vegetable oil (such as olive, almond, jojoba, coconut, or avocado) to safely dilute. Water actually drives essential oils deeper into the skin tissue, making them feel more intense.

Skin reactions may occur with people who have used or are currently using topically applied products containing toxic chemicals. Skin irritation can happen when essential oils break down the toxic residue left in the skin layer. Avoid using essential oils topically with clients who have autoimmune skin conditions to avoid further irritation of the skin and immune system. Clients with autoimmune skin conditions benefit from diffusing essential oils at home between acupuncture treatments. Chemicals that can create skin reactions when mixed with essential oils include:

- synthetic fragrances (phthalates)
- synthetic colors
- parabens
- ureas
- propylene and polyethylene glycols
- sodium lauryl sulfate made from petroleum
- MEA (monoethanolamine)
- DEA (diethanolamine)
- TEA (triethanolamine)

If the acupuncturist has a skin sensitivity or autoimmune skin condition, ask the patient to apply the essential oils to their feet before inserting the needles. Remind the client to wash their hands after the treatment to avoid accidentally rubbing the essential oils into the eyes. With severe skin sensitivity, it may be best to avoid using essential oils altogether.

11.12 Practical Application for Using Essential Oils at Home

Many clients enjoy diffusing or applying essential oils at home. Diffusing essential oils is beneficial for immune, brain, and nervous system conditions. Topical use of diluted essential oils is helpful for endocrine disorders, hormonal imbalances, phlegm nodules, and dysfunctional organs.

Diffusing essential oils releases tiny molecules that activate olfactory receptor sites in the brain and on the skin.[49] Essential oils contain oxygen and enzymes that instantly support organ function and meridian balance. With clients new to essential oils or with highly sensitive nervous systems, diffuse oils for 20 minutes every couple of hours. Robust clients can usually benefit from diffusing essential oils for up to several hours at a time. Non-diluted essential oils are best for diffusing as the essential oil molecule easily disperses into the water vapor that is released into the air. Blends diluted with a carrier oil create particles too dense to vaporize, and the oily residue coats the diffuser.

Cold air and cold water diffusers atomize essential oils into tiny molecules that remain in the air for hours after being diffused. Avoid diffusion methods that use heat, as it can destroy the beneficial properties of essential oils. Cold air diffusers atomize the oils without diluting them in water and work best in humid climates or where there are issues with mold. Cold water diffusers mix the oils with water first and are beneficial in dry climates and with children.

When essential oils are applied topically, they absorb into the skin and bloodstream to circulate quickly throughout the body. Diluting a blend will slow down the absorption rate and allow the blend to better target specific tissues, organs, or phlegm nodules at the site of application. Always dilute essential oils that will be applied repeatedly or long-term. It is a good practice to rotate the application sites when using essential oils long-term. For example, rotate applying the kidney blends between the low to mid-back, the lower abdomen, and the spine. In general, dilute oils to:

- benefit the skin with 50% carrier oil
- apply to the face with 70% carrier oil
- apply over phlegm nodules with 50-75% carrier oil
- prevent skin irritation with 50-80% carrier oil
- use with chemical residue left in the skin with 90% organic carrier oil or lotion

Essential oils approved for internal use by a manufacturer and the FDA can be taken in a capsule or added to liquids like water, coffee, or tea. Always check on the sourcing (location and method) of the essential oils and manufacturing process when recommending oils internally. Advise the client to only add essential oils in glass, ceramic, or stainless-steel containers because the oils will break down plastics. When adding essential oils to a capsule, always dilute with 50% organic cooking oil, such as olive oil, and take them with a meal for easy digestion. To improve the absorption and effectiveness of herbs and supplements, take them with a few drops of citrus or one drop of mint essential oil added to the water.

CHAPTER 12

Pre-Treatment Planning Stage

The pre-treatment planning stage follows a specific testing sequence to determine if the treatment is supine-symmetrical, prone-symmetrical, supine-asymmetrical, or prone-asymmetrical. Assessing the client for asymmetry during the pre-treatment stage determines if one root Body-Feedback acupoint prescription is best, or if the right and left sides of the body need different acupoint prescriptions. Allow 3-5 minutes at the beginning of each appointment to design a powerful healing strategy using the pre-treatment planning stage sequence.

12.1 Pre-Treatment Planning Steps

Begin the planning stage with the client in a supine position. Each planning step recommends specific testing methods to provide opportunities for client participation and efficiency. When needed, the testing methods can be interchanged based on the client's needs or physical limitations.

Planning step one: Assess for asymmetry

Inspect the alignment of the feet, hips, shoulders, and facial features. Palpate feeling for differences in muscle tightness and discomfort between the right and left sides at the master alarm points, neck muscles, and CV15.

Planning step two: Regulate the autonomic nervous system

Test the tautness of the abdomen to the master alarm points. A decrease in muscle tightness and discomfort at the testing locations indicates a supine treatment position to regulate the ANS. An increase in muscle tightness and discomfort at the testing locations indicates a prone treatment position to regulate the ANS.

Planning step three: Determine the Body-Feedback balancing prescriptions

Test the root Body-Feedback balancing prescription or prescriptions by pressing on the shu-points while monitoring the pulse for the right and left sides of the body to establish if the treatment approach is symmetrical or asymmetrical.

Planning step four: Determine the Body-Feedback sedation or tonification prescriptions
Test the Body-Feedback sedation and tonification prescriptions associated with the balancing prescriptions by checking the shu-points to the pulse for the right and left sides of the body. The sedation or tonification acupoints identify the root dysfunction as excess or deficient.

Planning step five: Assess the corresponding Body-Feedback testing locations
Palpate and assess the individual corresponding root testing locations (meridian and organ alarm points, referral areas, and muscle associations) for pain and muscle tightness.

Planning step six: Test essential oils
Test the root's and the five-element pair's corresponding Meridian Balancing and Organ Supporting Blends.

Planning step seven: Check for phlegm nodules
Check the upper border of the Posterior Superior Iliac Spine (PSIS) crest for phlegm nodules.

To prepare for Body-Feedback testing, fully support the client's back and neck to disengage their muscles. Contour pillows support the head and neck while allowing for easy access to the master alarm points in the upper back, neck, and shoulder areas. Traditional pillows require careful positioning to properly support the head and neck while allowing access to the master alarm points. To confirm that the client's head is resting in a supportive position, check for disengagement of the upper trapezius and neck muscles.

Use a bolster or pillow under the client's knees to relax the back and erector spinae muscles. For clients with spinal pain, use a wedge for their upper torso and additional pillows to support their legs and arms, if needed, to reduce pressure and increase relaxation. In some instances, a client may relax better in a reclining chair with a pillow to support the head. Clients with severe neck and back pain often respond best to two-sided treatments with the first set of needles in a reclining or zero-gravity position and the second set of needles in a prone position to directly treat the spine. If it is challenging to release muscle tension during the planning stage testing, recheck head, neck, and back support.

To determine the ideal amount of pressure to use when palpating muscles, monitor the client's body language. Ask the client if they can feel a release in muscle resistance when comparing essential oils or acupoints that test favorably. For sensitive clients, adjustments can be made to make the testing process more enjoyable. First, reduce the amount of pressure applied and slowly palpate the points and areas. Second, identify two or three testing locations to rotate between to avoid over-stimulating one area. Third, palpate any painful muscles or points at the beginning and the end of the session for reference, and test the acupoints, essential oils, supplements, and herbs to the pulse. For overweight and overly muscular clients, increase the amount of pressure to assess the testing locations accurately.

12.2 General Overview of Body-Feedback Testing

When testing essential oils, acupoints, herbs, supplements, or other items, it takes between 10-30 seconds to register a change in the testing locations or pulse. The acupoint or object usually tests neutral for the first 5-10 seconds while the body is registering the change, and then the response shifts to beneficial or adverse. Allow the client's body enough time to respond before re-pressing the testing location or deciding if the pulse is improving or not. Always re-press the testing location with the same pressure as before and let the client know this. Otherwise, the client may perceive the increase or decrease in discomfort as a change in the amount of force applied while checking the testing location.

If a client is having difficulty identifying changes in muscle tension or discomfort during the testing process, recheck the acupoints, essential oils, supplements, and herbs using the pulse (see Chapter 5). Then palpate the testing locations to compare items that balance and normalize the pulse with those that cause the pulse to become the most forceful and wiry. Clients can often discern the difference between the two extremes.

In certain situations, some clients may respond best to testing using the pulse only. Examples include people with paralysis, sensory integration issues, or those who feel ticklish during the testing process. Some clients prefer less physical contact, and babies can find it difficult to remain still during the testing process.

The general steps for checking Body-Feedback testing locations are as follows:

- Assess baseline muscle tension or discomfort at a testing location (master alarm point/region, neck muscles, organ/meridian referral area, or muscle association).
- Keeping your hand in the same place, release the pressure and gently rest your hand at the skin's surface.
- Test an acupoint by pressing it for five seconds, then continue holding the acupoint while re-pressing the testing location with the other hand, looking for an increase or decrease in muscle tension or discomfort.
- Test an essential oil, supplement, or herb by placing it on the upper abdomen and waiting a minimum of ten seconds, and then re-press the testing location looking for an increase or decrease in muscle tension or discomfort.
- A beneficial acupoint, essential oil, herb, or supplement will reduce the muscle tension or pain and support healing of the root dysfunction.
- A non-beneficial acupoint, essential oil, herb, or supplement will increase muscle tension or pain, and further hinders healing of the root dysfunction.
- A neutral acupoint, essential oil, herb, or supplement will cause the muscle tension or discomfort to remain the same and does not affect the root dysfunction; however, it may still be beneficial for other concerns.

12.3 Test the Master Alarm Points and Regions

Palpate the master alarm points and regions by pressing the area around the point perpendicularly with two to three pounds of pressure. Check a *cun** (body-inch) diameter around the traditional point location to find the most tender spot to use for testing. When checking the master alarm points and regions, the client usually feels point-specific pain, while the provider can notice subtle changes in muscle knots and tautness at these points during the testing process. With each beneficial treatment option (application of essential oils, balancing the ANS, and Body-Feedback point prescriptions), the master points will relax and become less painful. If any treatment options are not beneficial, the master alarm points and regions will immediately become tense and sore again.

The positioning of the scapula can cause deviations in the locations of GB21, TB15, and SI13. Start with finding GB21 on the top of the trapezius muscle and SI13 at the medial end of the scapular spine. TB15 is about midway between GB21 and SI13. The master points are all located on the upper trapezius muscle, which is also a muscle association for the spleen. When the spleen is not the root dysfunction, clients usually feel pain at these specific master alarm points greater than general tension in the upper trapezius muscle. When the spleen is the root dysfunction, muscle tension in the upper trapezius is more intense than the pain at the specific master points. Check for tension and pain in the upper trapezius at locations different from GB21, TB15, and SI13 to rule out a root spleen dysfunction.

BODY-FEEDBACK CLINICAL PEARLS

When checking acupoints, the testing locations and the pulse positions on the same side of the body will respond faster than on the opposite side of the body. For example, when standing on the client's right side of the body, re-press the right master alarm points (GB21, TB15, and SI13) after pressing LV3 on the right for five seconds and LV3 on the left for ten seconds. Assess the pulse positions on the right wrist after five seconds of holding LV3 on the right and then after ten seconds of holding LV3 on the left. A delay in the response time occurs when checking points on the opposite side of the testing location or pulse positions.

* Cun has several meanings in Chinese medicine and in this case is referring to a body-inch, which is different than the cun pulse position in Chapter 5.

When testing the meridian alarm points (fire shu-points), the client can sense pain or discomfort, and the provider can notice changes in the bone and muscle structure with long-term inflammation or pathogenic heat.

When testing the organ alarm points (he-sea shu-points), the client can sense pain and discomfort, and the provider can notice swelling or an indentation in the muscle, cartilage, fat, or bone in the region.

When testing the organ/meridian referral areas, the client can sense pain and discomfort, and the provider may notice swelling, phlegm nodules, or small broken blood vessels (spider veins).

When testing the muscle associations and the neck muscle regions, the client can sense general muscle tension and discomfort, and the provider can notice more subtle changes in the muscle's tautness during the testing process.

Clients with heightened sensitivity can feel the changes in muscle tightness as much as, or better than, the provider. These clients usually enjoy helping to choose acupoints, essential oils, supplements, and herbs because the testing process validates their extraordinary sensory skills.

12.4 Evaluate for Asymmetry

The first step of the planning stage investigates for asymmetry by palpating the neck muscles and visually inspecting the facial features, hips, and feet for alignment as early as possible. Different organ/meridian pathologies affecting the left and right sides of the body cause a significant difference from side to side in the tautness and thickness of the neck muscles. Restoring symmetry synchronizes the different hemispheres of the brain to accelerate healing. For clients with complex health concerns, this approach brings clarity to intricate organ/meridian pathology.

Asymmetrical features and posture may or may not affect a client's organs and meridian system. When asymmetry compromises health, the body recognizes it as a pathology affecting the left and right sides of the body independently, requiring two root treatments. In some instances, the brain allows for and adapts to the asymmetrical structural symptoms, as evidenced by the same root balancing prescription on both sides of the body. Asymmetry can also occur when trisection discord requires two different root treatments before manifesting in visually detectable symptoms. Therefore, visual inspection for asymmetry is helpful; however, testing the balancing prescriptions on the left and right sides of the body provides final confirmation of the need for a symmetrical or asymmetrical treatment approach.

Neck Regions of the Trisections

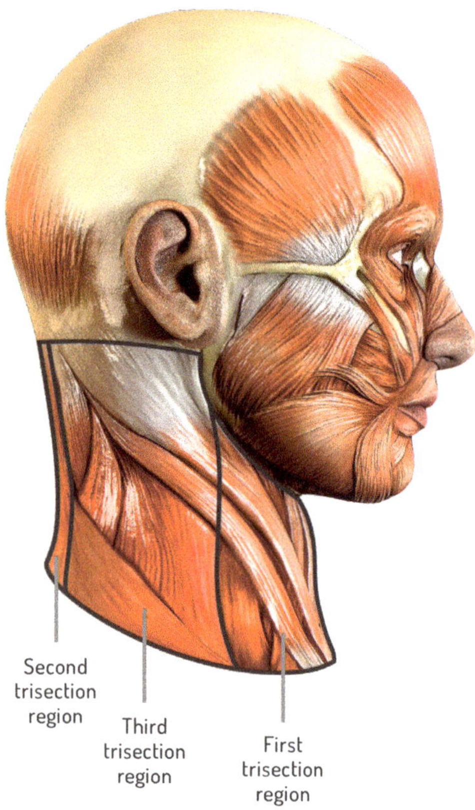

Test the anterior neck muscles by palpating the sternocleidomastoid between ST9 and LI18.

Test the lateral neck muscles by palpating the sternocleidomastoid just below the insertion at the second and third cervical vertebrae and the muscles posterior to this area.

Test the posterior neck muscles by palpating just below the insertion of the muscles along the occiput.

Stand at the midpoint of the client's head or between their feet and visually compare the alignment of the feet, hips, and shoulders on the left and right sides. Assess hip alignment by locating the peak of the right and left anterior superior iliac spine crests. Pressing on the hip bones in the same location highlights structural differences. Visually assess the client's facial features for symmetrical eyes, eyebrows, lips, ears, and cheekbones.

Palpate and compare the thickness and tautness of the anterior, lateral, and posterior neck muscles that correspond with the trisections on the left and right sides. Before checking the neck muscles, confirm that they are disengaged, and the head is fully supported. Start palpating the anterior muscles next to the thyroid and work around laterally to the posterior neck muscles, comparing one side to the other side, looking for differences in tension and size. Assess the level of muscle tension in the neck by using one or two fingers to roll perpendicularly over the muscle body against the natural direction of the individual fibers. Often, one side of the neck muscles are thicker and tighter, and the muscles on the opposite side of the neck are thinner and looser.

With asymmetry, use the neck muscles with the most tension for testing during the planning, treatment, and post-treatment stages. Check essential oils to the neck muscles in the planning stage. Check the location of an acupoint's *aperture* (the precise point of insertion) before needling in the treatment stage. An acupoint's aperture creates a slight palpable separation or indentation in the muscle layer where the needle penetrates the skin easily and with minimal sensation. Check herbs and supplements to the neck muscles in the post-treatment stage.

Palpate the Conception Vessel 15 Spinal Misalignment Region looking for tenderness as an indicator of rib cage misalignment. Check CV15 with new clients to help identify asymmetry and use this point to monitor existing clients with asymmetry. Palpate the CV15 region by pressing inward towards the xiphoid process with two to three pounds of pressure. For some clients with asymmetry, the xiphoid process will slightly deviate and protrude at the tip or one side causing pain. Needling different root treatments on the left and right sides can realign the tip of the xiphoid process and reduce discomfort in the CV15 area, indicating an effective treatment.

Palpate and compare any muscle tightness and discomfort in the master alarm points GB21, TB15, or SI13 on the left and right sides. An asymmetrical treatment approach is likely needed when there is uneven muscle tightness or discomfort at GB21, TB15, or SI13. With asymmetry, use the master alarm points on the same side of the body when checking essential oils in the planning stage, checking the acupoint prescriptions, and locating the acupoint's *aperture* before needling in the treatment stage. Check herbs and supplements to master alarm points on the side with the most residual discomfort in the post-treatment stage.

12.5 Regulate the Autonomic Nervous System

Step two of the planning stage determines the optimal treatment position to regulate the ANS by pressing on the abdomen while testing the master alarm points with significant muscle tightness and discomfort already identified. The state of health of the ANS is directly related to Triple Burner 15 Master Brain Alarm Point and Small Intestine 13 Master Hormone Alarm Point, and it is indirectly related to Gallbladder 21 Master Fire Alarm Point. The master alarm points respond within three to five seconds to any stimulus that affects the ANS because of their close relationship. See Chapter 8 for illustrations regarding ANS testing.

- Press the belly using three or four fingers in a row out from the umbilicus in a clockwise motion.
- Hold the pressure on the abdomen at each angle outward from the umbilicus for three to five seconds and then re-press GB21, TB15, or SI13, looking for an increase or decrease in muscle tightness.
- Note any angles that decrease muscle tightness at GB21, TB15, or SI13 because they are the areas to needle during the treatment stage to balance the ANS in a supine treatment position.
- If all angles of the abdomen increase muscle tightness at GB21, TB15, or SI13, use a prone treatment position to balance the ANS.

The combination of the optimal treatment position determined by testing the abdomen, the client's presenting complaints, and the location of acupoints included in root Body-Feedback prescription (step three) determines the final supine or prone treatment position. Chapter 8 provides instructions for balancing the ANS in the non-optimal treatment position when needed.

12.6 Determine the Root Body-Feedback Balancing Prescriptions

The third step of the planning stage identifies one root balancing prescription for symmetrical treatments or two root balancing prescriptions for asymmetrical treatments. In general, the pulse quickly responds to changes in the meridian system initiated by pressing individual acupoints. Checking the exclusive shu-points in the balancing prescriptions to the pulse is the most efficient testing method for this step. However, testing the exclusive shu-points to the master alarm points and neck muscles is acceptable by allowing a few additional seconds before re-pressing the testing locations. See Chapter 9 for the balancing shu-points.

First, identify the most forceful and wiry or deep and confined individual pulse position on either the right or left wrist. Use this pulse position to monitor the changes that result from pressing and holding the select acupoints. Individually check the exclusive shu-points on the same side of the body associated with this pulse position by pressing and holding each acupoint for 5-10 seconds. If these exclusive shu-points do not normalize the pulse to slightly slippery and more balanced, then test the exclusive shu-points for other organs/meridians associated with the client's symptoms. The correct exclusive shu-point from the root balancing prescription will cause the pulse to transition to slightly slippery and more balanced. All other balancing prescription's shu-points will cause the pulse to become more forceful and wiry or deep and confined.

After identifying the correct root balancing exclusive shu-point, check the other acupoints in that balancing prescription. If **SP3**, **ST36**, **GB41**, or **HT8** are included, test their metal + water combination for a possible substitution. Check the same points from the first side's root balancing prescription to the opposite side of the body. Remember that acupoints on the opposite side of the body will take a few extra seconds to register a change in the pulse.

Symmetry is confirmed by the pulse transitioning to slightly slippery and balanced when pressing all of the shu-points from the first root prescription on the second side. Asymmetry is confirmed when any of the shu-points from the first root prescription on the opposite side causes the pulse to become more forceful and wiry. Because of the time delay with testing points on the opposite side of the body, it may be easier to move and check an imbalanced pulse position on the corresponding side.

With asymmetry, the second root balancing treatment may or may not be related to the first side's root balancing organ/meridian:

- Test the exclusive shu-points for the five-element, six-level, and resulting trisection pairs associated with the first side. For example, if the first side is a liver treatment, test the exclusive shu-points for the gallbladder, pericardium, and triple burner.
- Test the exclusive shu-points for the organs/meridian associated with the same pulse position on the opposite side. For example, if the first side is a liver treatment (middle left pulse position), test the spleen and stomach exclusive shu-points (middle right pulse positions).
- Test the exclusive shu-points for the organ opposite the first side on the twenty-four-hour clock. For example, if the first side is a liver treatment (1 a.m. to 3 a.m.), test the small intestine exclusive shu-point (1 p.m. to 3 p.m.).
- Test any remaining organ/meridian exclusive shu-points to identify the second side's root balancing prescription.
- After identifying the second side's correct root balancing exclusive shu-point, check the other acupoints in that balancing prescription. If **SP3**, **ST36**, **GB41**, or **HT8** are included, test their metal + water combination for a possible substitution.

12.7 Determine the Body-Feedback Sedation or Tonification Prescriptions

Check the two sedation and two tonification acupoints to add to the root balancing prescription or multiple prescriptions with asymmetry and determine if the root treatment is excess or deficient. Another factor to consider when determining a client's treatment position is the needle retention time for sedation versus tonification point prescriptions. Clients are usually more comfortable in the supine position for sedation treatments and can tolerate the shorter needle retention time for tonification treatments in the prone position.

Once the root prescriptions are known, determine if they are accessible with the client in the optimal treatment position (supine or prone) identified in step two above. If the acupoints are not accessible in the optimal treatment positions, either adjust the treatment to balance the ANS that allows for needling in the non-optimal treatment positions or apply magnetic pellets or press tacks to the inaccessible acupoints. Chapter 8 provides different options for needling in the non-optimal treatment position.

Examples of adapting acupoint prescriptions to accommodate needling in the optimal treatment positions include:

- For a root spleen sedation or tonification prescription with a prone optimal treatment position, lift the foot and apply magnetic pellets or press tacks to LV1 and SP1 first.
- For a root stomach sedation or tonification prescription with a prone optimal treatment position, either apply a combination of press tacks and magnetic pellets to ST43, ST44, ST45 (sedation) or ST41 (tonification), and GB41 (or GB44 metal + GB43 water substitution), or apply essential oils to the spine first and then recheck the abdomen to confirm that needling in a supine position is acceptable.
- For a root urinary bladder sedation or tonification prescription with a supine optimal treatment position, slightly bend the client's knee and apply a press tack on UB40.
- For a root liver sedation prescription with a prone optimal treatment position, lift the foot and apply press tacks to LV2 and LV3. For a root liver tonification prescription with a prone optimal treatment position, lift the foot and apply a press tack or magnetic pellet to LV3.

At this point in the pre-treatment planning stage, determine this session's treatment approach: **supine-symmetrical**, **prone-symmetrical**, **supine-asymmetrical**, or **prone-asymmetrical**.

12.8 Assess the Corresponding Root Testing Locations

Step five of the planning stage includes palpating the individual balancing prescription's corresponding testing locations for pain or muscle tightness. Check the meridian and organ alarm points, referral areas, and muscle associations to find the one or two testing locations with the most discomfort or muscle tightness to use throughout the treatment and post-treatment stages. Often, clients are unaware of discomfort at the individual testing locations; bringing awareness to resolving the discomfort provides tangible results.

The individual testing location is used in multiple treatment stages. In the planning stage, use the individual testing location to identify the essential oils with potential to address specific meridian or organ pathology. During the treatment stage, check other meridians that transverse these testing locations for pathogenic heat requiring the metal + water combinations. After removing the needles, use these same locations to validate the effectiveness of the root acupoint prescription and check for beneficial herbs and supplements.

Palpate the testing locations for the root balancing prescriptions and their five-element pairs, because the root treatments often rotate from appointment to appointment. Evaluating individual testing location associations provides a comprehensive understanding of how each treatment option (acupoint, essential oil, herb, or supplement) impacts a specific organ or meridian. After resolving or managing the client's symptoms, the remaining painful, tight, or flaccid individual testing locations indicate constitutional or genetic weaknesses. Between appointments, clients can check for discomfort in their testing locations to evaluate their food, water, and personal care choices, along with monitoring their healing progress.

12.9 Test the Essential Oil Blends

The sixth step of the planning stage tests the root and five-element pair corresponding Meramour's Organ Supporting and Meridian Balancing Blends. Using the essential oil blends first to reduce the severity of root organ/meridian pathology enhances the effectiveness of acupuncture treatments.

- Palpate a tender or tight master alarm point or neck region to use as the initial testing location for the essential oils.
- Place the essential oil blend on the upper abdomen, around CV12, and wait 5-10 seconds for the client's meridian system to register a change. Re-press the master alarm point or neck region with the same amount of force and determine if the essential oil is beneficial or not.
- Check between two and eight blends (one at a time) to identify the ones that best release the muscle tightness and discomfort. To test for compatibility, start with one essential oil blend on the upper abdomen and place a second blend next to it. After waiting 5-10 seconds, re-press the master alarm point or neck region with the same amount of force and determine if the oils are beneficial together or not.
- If the combined blends test more favorably together, then add another blend to the upper abdomen to check for compatibility again. If the combined blends do not test favorably together, add a different blend with each of the first two blends and continue checking for compatibility using various combinations of the blends.
- To determine which of the beneficial essential oils are benefiting specific organs/meridians, test each blend to the root treatment's individual Body-Feedback testing locations (meridian and organ alarm points, referral areas, and muscle associations).

Pulse analysis is another option for testing the essential oil blends. Place the essential oil blend on the upper abdomen and wait 10-20 seconds for the client's meridian system to register a change. For the first few seconds, the essential oil blend may disrupt the pulse as the meridian system adapts. The pulse will represent an accurate response to the essential oil blend after ten or more seconds. The longer the blend or blends rest on the upper abdomen, the more precise the pulse response is.

12.10 Check for Phlegm Nodules

The final step of the planning stage is to inspect for phlegm nodules in the lower back on the upper border of the PSIS. If phlegm nodules are present, extra detoxification support using essential oils, herbs, or nutritional supplements is necessary. If the optimal treatment position is supine, palpate under the lower back and press upward against the client's body weight. If the optimal treatment position is prone, palpate for phlegm nodules after the client rotates to a facedown position before applying essential oils or inserting needles. Make sure to follow the entire edge of the PSIS and the lumbar vertebrae to find these nodules.

BODY-FEEDBACK CLINICAL PEARLS

Muscle tightness and discomfort at any of the master alarm points or regions can encompass multiple organ/meridian pathology. The master alarm points and regions are ideal for choosing essential oils, determining the root Body-Feedback balancing prescription, confirming the accuracy of the acupoint locations for needling, and testing oils, supplements, and herbs. Body-Feedback testing for the entire treatment can occur using only the master alarm points and regions. However, identifying and testing the individual organ/meridian referral areas and muscle associations imparts a deeper understanding of how the essential oils, acupoint prescriptions, supplements, and herbs affect each organ/meridian.

For example, a client with metabolic syndrome, polycystic ovarian disease, and elevated blood sugar has an imbalanced third trisection (pericardium, triple burner, gallbladder, and liver) with dampness and spleen and liver organ dysfunction. This client has pain and tightness in GB21, TB15, and SI13 master alarm points signifying systemic inflammation, brain involvement, and unbalanced hormones. Further testing of the individual Body-Feedback associations identifies spleen and liver organ dysfunctions. The beneficial essential oils and acupoint prescriptions identified during the pre-treatment planning stage affect each of the master points in the same way, while effects on the spleen and liver organ referral areas and muscle associations differ. The supplements, herbs, and diet changes also affect the spleen and liver differently. Testing to the individual liver and spleen referral areas and muscle associations can clarify which treatment options are benefiting each organ individually.

BODY-FEEDBACK CLINICAL PEARLS

When a severe form of pathogenic heat affects the entire body, all of the fire-element and he-sea points are tender. Exposure to environmental toxins, acute infections, high fever, trauma, vaccines, autoimmune diseases, and other causes of immune dysfunction can trigger systemic pathogenic heat. In this situation, a combined treatment approach with acupuncture, essential oils, and herbs delivers maximum effectiveness. At the first appointment, needle all the metal + water combinations on either yin or yang meridians. At the next appointment, needle all the metal + water combinations on the other set of meridians. As the heat pathogens dissipate, the essential oil and herbal blends require frequent retesting. After a few sessions, the trisection imbalance, root organ dysfunction, and meridians with lingering pathogenic heat will become apparent.

The wisdom of the body is unrivaled even by the intelligence of the brain; listening to each client's unique needs through the Body-Feedback approach yields a wealth of knowledge. The Body-Feedback testing locations reveal health challenges while providing access to the body's wisdom to identify treatment approaches that restore the ability to self-heal. Body-Feedback style treatments are highly specific and client-driven, which yield results and loyalty. Body-Feedback style palpation skills require practice to attain proficiency. Mastering the Body-Feedback approach results in a rich unfolding of your ability as a practitioner to recognize, understand, and treat intricate patterns with a multi-factorial, yet laser-focused, approach.

SECTION

3

The Treatment Stage

Needle Angle, Depth, and Aperture Size

The degree of needle insertion is in relationship to the skin's surface.

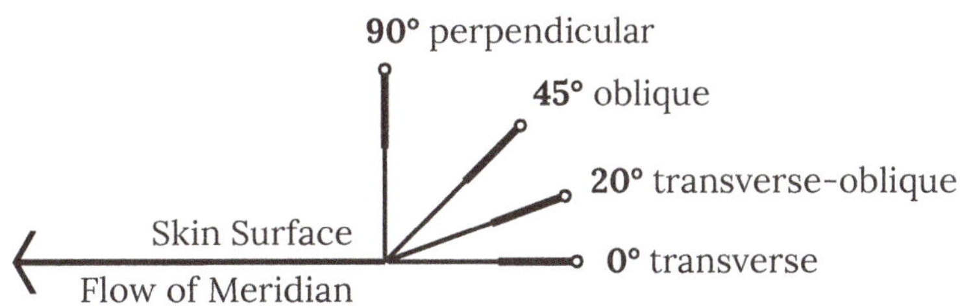

NEEDLE ANGLE AND DEPTH

90°  .10 – .25 **cun** needle depth

90° 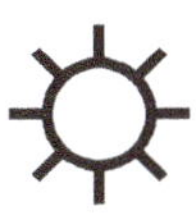 .25 – .75 **cun** needle depth

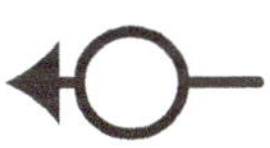 .5 – 1.0 **cun** needle depth

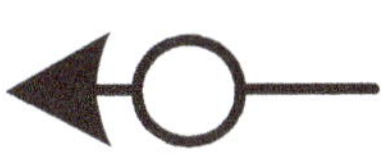 .75 – 1.5 cun needle depth

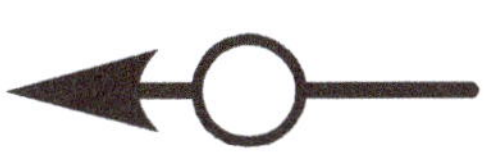 1.0 – 2.0 cun needle depth

Jing-well points:	**90°**
Ying-spring points:	**45°**
Shu-stream points:	**45°**
Jing-river points:	**45° - 90°**
He-sea points:	**20° - 45°**

ACUPOINT APERTURE SIZE

An acupoint's aperture size is larger around the knees and elbows and becomes smaller at the fingers and toes. The acupoint's location reflects this approximate aperture size independent of the needle insertion depth. Below is an example of a shallow .5 – 1.0 cun needle insertion depth with three different acupoint sizes from below the knee to the toes on the liver meridian.

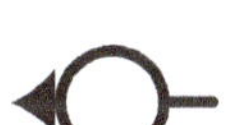 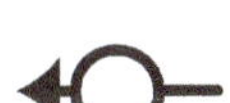 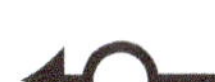

CHAPTER 13

Acupoint Combinations to Regulate the Autonomic Nervous System

The first group of acupoints to needle relaxes the client and harmonizes the parasympathetic, sympathetic, and enteric nervous systems. The optimal treatment position identified in step two of the pre-treatment planning stage indicates the regions of the body ideal for needling to balance the ANS. In the supine position, choose either abdominal, scalp, facial, or auricular acupoint combinations. In the prone position, choose a combination of acupoints along the spine, sacrum, or scapula.

The Body-Feedback treatment approach requires following set rules for specific acupoint combinations, such as the metal + water substitutions for **SP3, ST36,** and **GB41** when pathogenic heat affects an organ or meridian. However, balancing the ANS provides opportunities for creating unique acupoint combinations based on each client's needs. The combinations in this chapter can be customized by choosing additional acupoints and determining their exact locations. Acupoint locations on the abdomen and back can vary significantly for each client. Check for the precise location of each acupoint within the general regions or quadrants indicated on the following illustrations. Utilizing multiple combinations from different areas of the body or other acupoint combinations not contained in this chapter are acceptable to use as long as they test favorably to the pulse or master alarm points.

When balancing the ANS, it is imperative to test each acupoint's precise aperture location to the master alarm points, neck muscles, or pulse at every session. Check and immediately needle each acupoint within a combination before moving on to test the next one. With practice, testing and needling each acupoint will become an intuitive routine.

Some of the acupoint combinations correspond with a trisection, while others support specific body systems (detoxification, digestive, endocrine, musculoskeletal, immune, reproductive, and nervous). The acupoints that test favorably to balance the ANS may or may not correspond with the trisection's root balancing prescriptions. For example, a root balancing prescription in the third trisection (LV/GB/PC/TB) can have a scalp or facial combination that corresponds with the first, second, or third trisections. Start with testing the acupoint combinations that relate to the root dysfunction's trisection or body system. If needed, check acupoints based on the client's symptoms. The acupoint combinations to harmonize the ANS often relate to the root dysfunction's trisection or body system.

When needling with the client in the non-optimal treatment position, follow the steps in Chapter 8 to adjust the treatment position with essential oils or cupping first. Then retest the abdomen and confirm that the master alarm points, neck muscles, or abdominal muscles remain soft, indicating the adjustments successfully harmonized the ANS. If the master alarm points or neck muscles tighten when checking the abdomen after applying essential oils or cupping, a two-sided treatment approach is best.

13.1 Body-Feedback Abdominal Acupoint Combinations

The Body-Feedback abdominal acupoint combinations harmonize the five elements, along with the body systems. Superimposing the five-element system onto the belly with the umbilicus as the center creates treatment regions by element on the abdomen. These five-element abdominal combinations represent the restraining cycle that is the basis for the Body-Feedback balancing prescriptions. The other abdominal combinations use traditional TCM acupoints to address immune, digestive, detoxification, and reproductive symptoms.

Unbalanced elements respond best to three or four acupoints in a line radiating from the umbilicus. Each line's trajectory is unique, depending on the precise aperture location that releases the muscle tightness in the master alarm points or neck muscles, or improves the pulse. With light pressure, palpate the regions identified in step two of the pre-treatment planning stage (see Chapter 12) to find each acupoint's aperture and needle the locations that test best. Add an additional single acupoint from either the element included in the balancing acupoint prescriptions or along the conception vessel to further harmonize the five-element system.

The abdominal acupoints to balance the ANS respond best to gentle needling techniques, such that the client barely feels the needle insertion. Depending on the client's size and tautness of their abdominal muscles, use a .18 to .25 gauge needle inserted between .75 and 2.0 cun. The needle angle is most often perpendicular, and in some instances, an oblique angle towards the conception vessel or the umbilicus may test best. Refrain from stimulating the needles, which can activate the sympathetic nervous system.

Five-element overlay on the abdomen

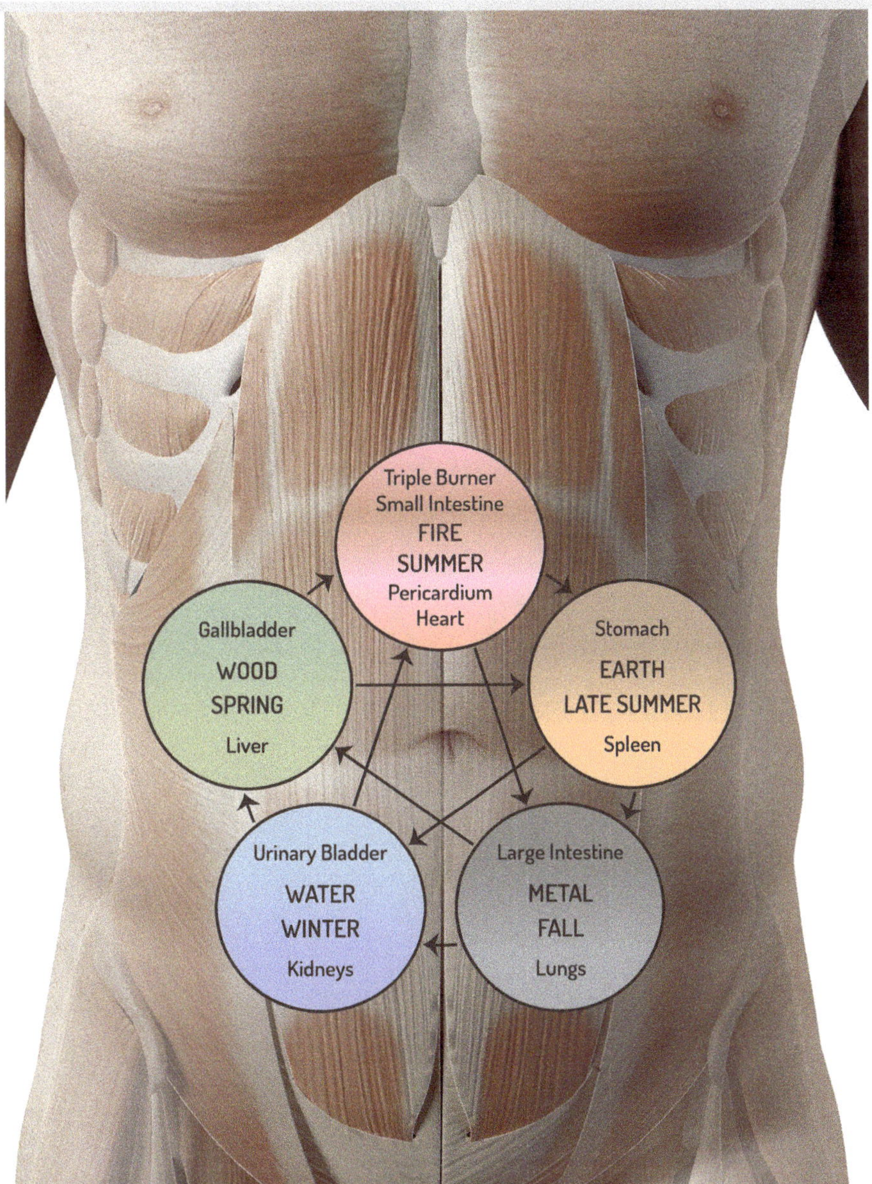

The fire element creates a vertical line above the umbilicus, and the earth, metal, water, and wood elements create diagonal lines converging at the umbilicus.

13.1.1 First Trisection Abdominal Acupoint Combinations

Harmonize metal (LU/LI) with wood (LV/GB) and fire (HT/SI)

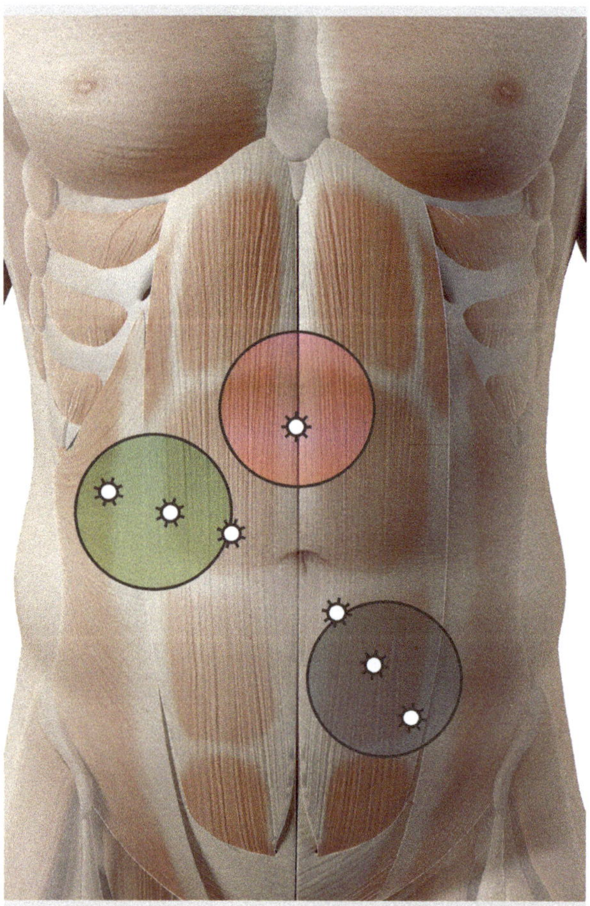

Locate and check three or four acupoints grouped together along a diagonal line in the lower left (metal) and upper right (wood) quadrants of the abdomen. Locate and check one acupoint in the upper quadrant (fire) to harmonize the metal and wood elements.

Harmonize earth (SP/ST) with water (KD/UB) and wood (LV/GB)

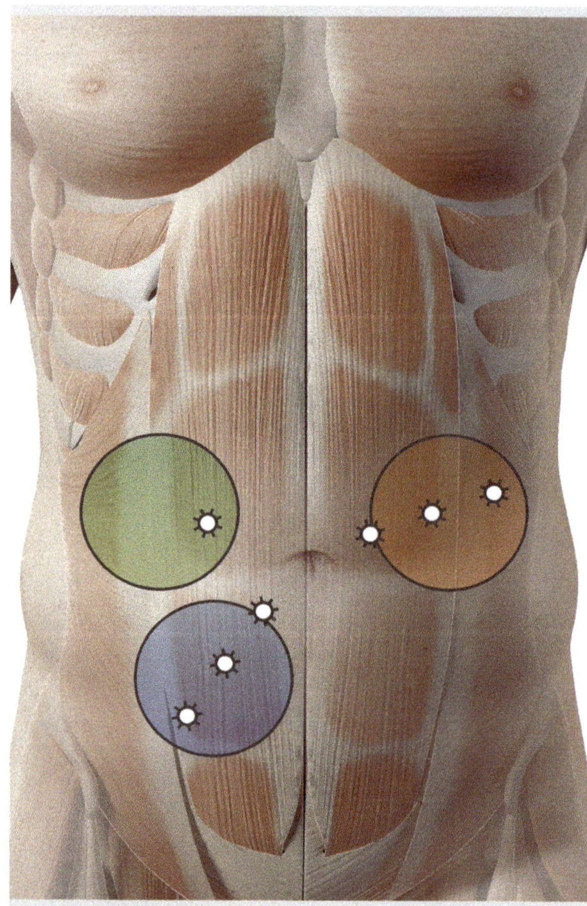

Locate and check three or four acupoints grouped together along a diagonal line in the upper left (earth) and lower right (water) quadrants of the abdomen. Locate and check one acupoint in the upper right quadrant (wood) to harmonize the earth and water elements.

13.1.2 Second Trisection Abdominal Acupoint Combinations

Harmonize imperial-fire (HT/SI) with metal (LU/LI) and water (KD/UB)

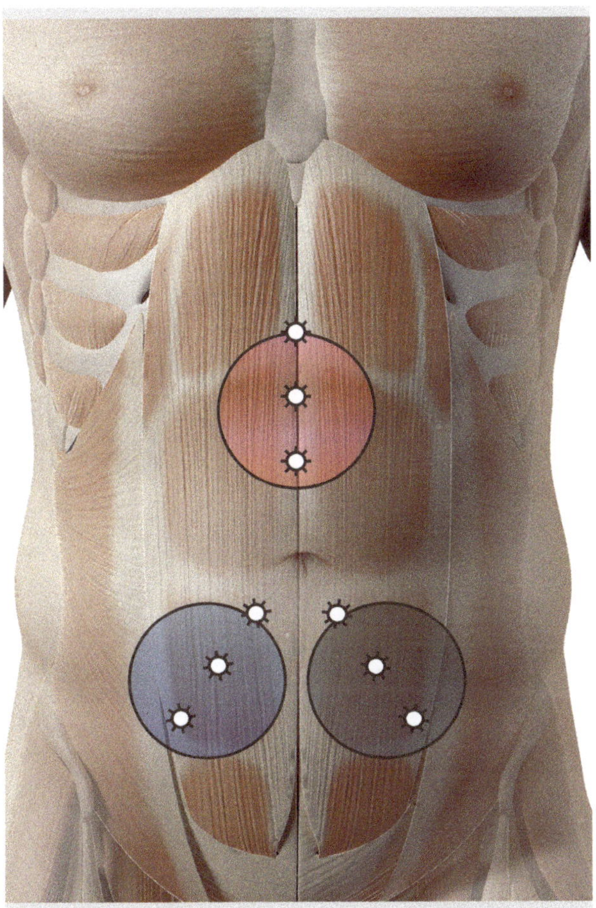

Locate and check three acupoints grouped together along the upper conception vessel (imperial-fire) between CV10 and CV14. Locate and check between one and three acupoints grouped together along a diagonal line on the lower left (metal) and lower right (water) quadrants of the abdomen.

Harmonize water (KD/UB) with earth (SP/ST) and fire (HT/SI)

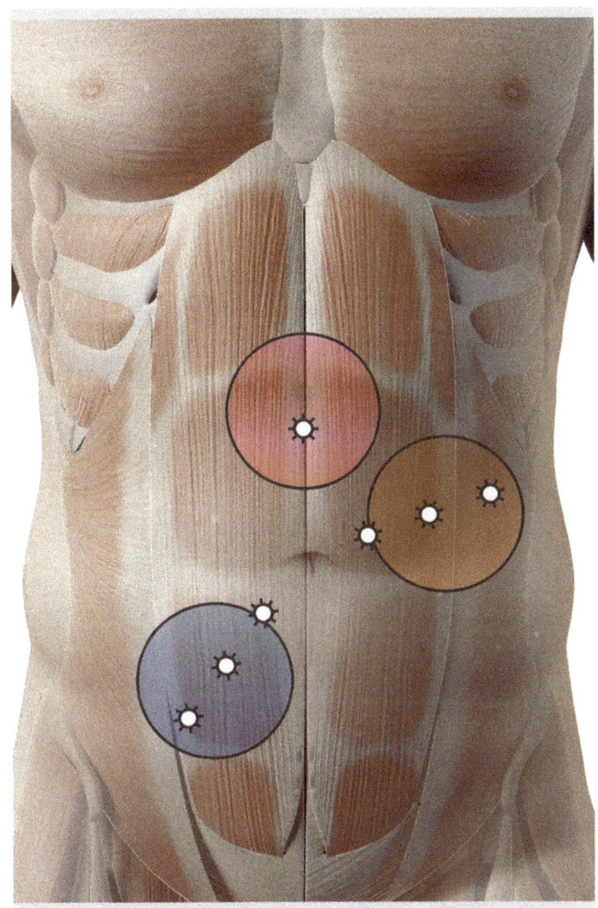

Locate and check three or four acupoints grouped together along a diagonal line on the lower right (water) and upper left (earth) quadrants of the abdomen. Locate and check one acupoint on the upper conception vessel (fire) between CV10 and CV14 to harmonize the water and earth elements.

13.1.3 Third Trisection Abdominal Acupoint Combinations

Harmonize ministerial-fire (PC/TB) with metal (LU/LI) and water (KD/UB)

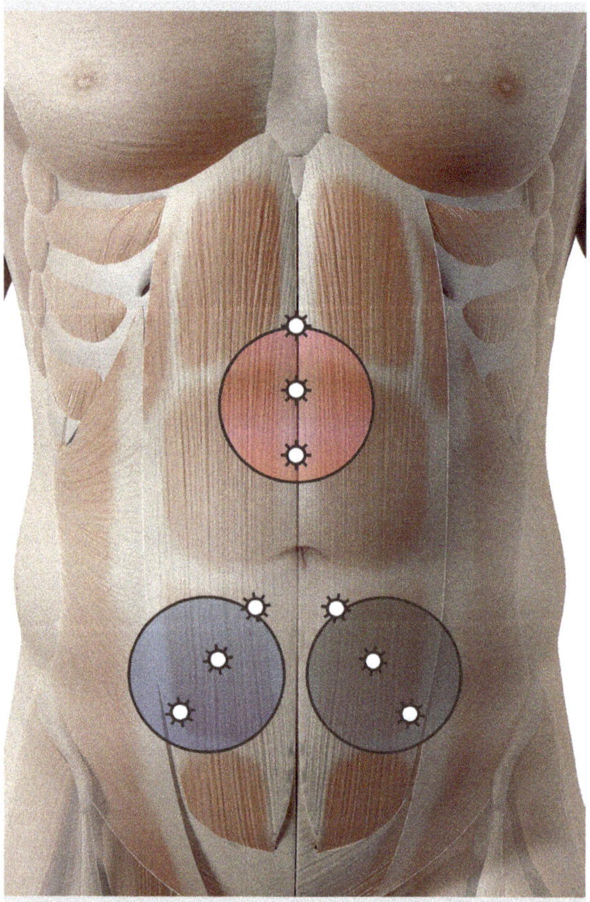

Locate and check three or four acupoints grouped together along the upper conception vessel between CV10 and CV14 (ministerial-fire). Locate between one and three acupoints grouped together along a diagonal line on the lower left (metal) and lower right (water) quadrants of the abdomen.

Harmonize wood (LV/GB) with metal (LU/LI) and earth (SP/ST)

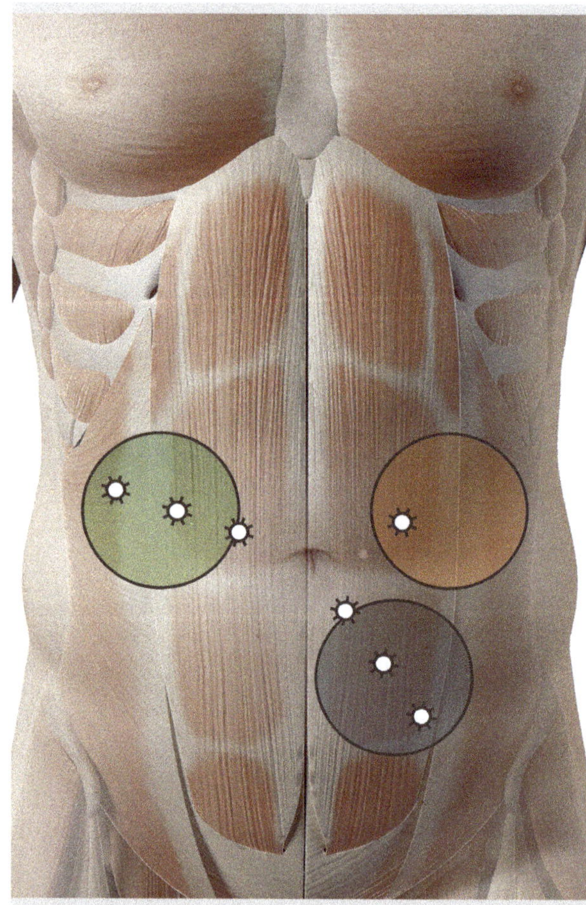

Locate and check three or four acupoints grouped together along a diagonal line in the upper right (wood) and lower left (metal) quadrants of the abdomen. Locate and check one acupoint in the upper left quadrant (earth) to harmonize the wood and metal elements.

13.1.4 Abdominal Acupoint Combinations to Harmonize Body Systems

Harmonize wood (LV/GB) and earth (SP/ST) to strengthen digestion

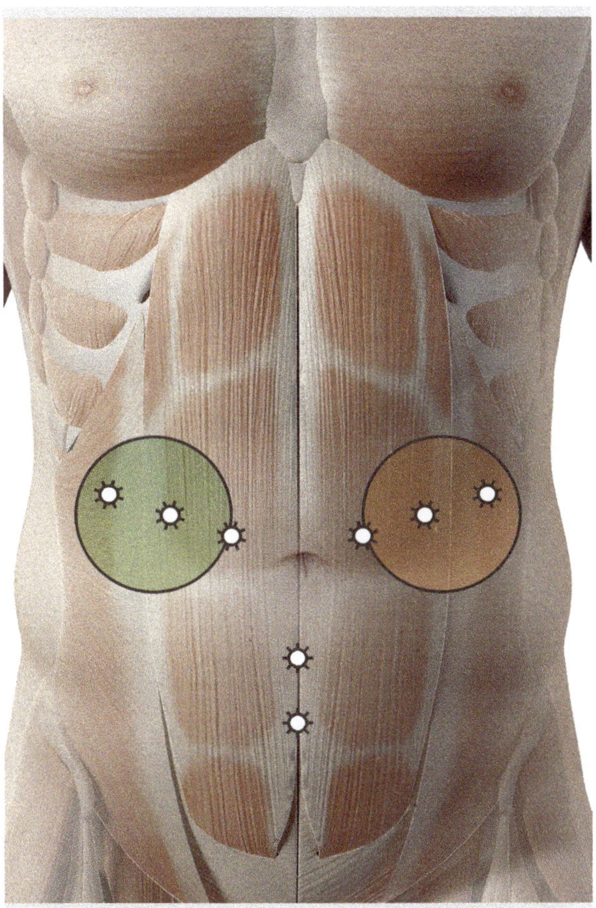

Locate and check three or four acupoints grouped together along a diagonal line in the upper right (wood) and upper left (earth) quadrants of the abdomen. Locate and check one or two acupoints grouped together between CV3 and CV6.

Harmonize metal (LU/LI) and water (KD/UB) to strengthen the immune and reproductive systems

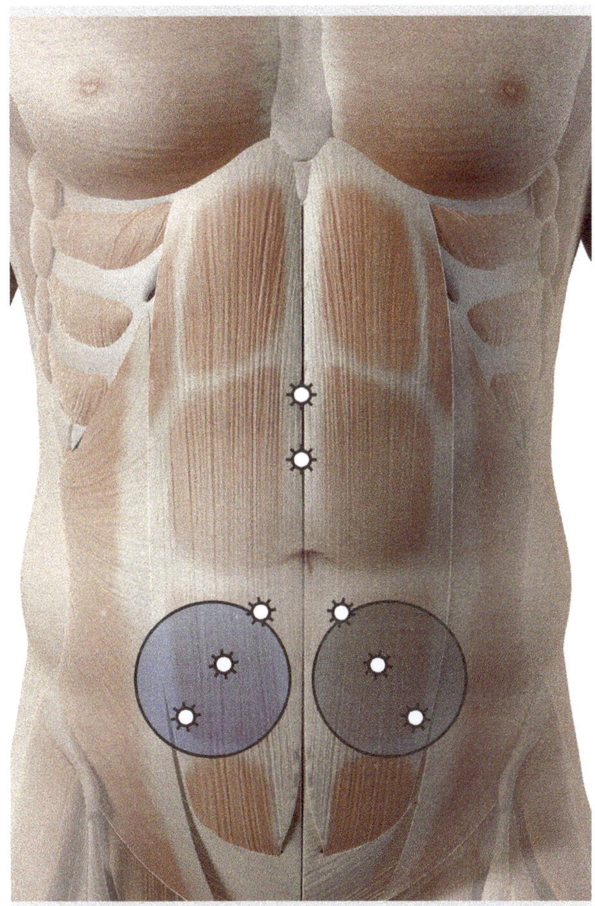

Locate and check three or four acupoints grouped together along a diagonal line in the lower left (metal) and lower right (water) quadrants of the abdomen. Locate and check one or two acupoints grouped together between CV10 and CV14.

Harmonize and strengthen the immune and digestive systems

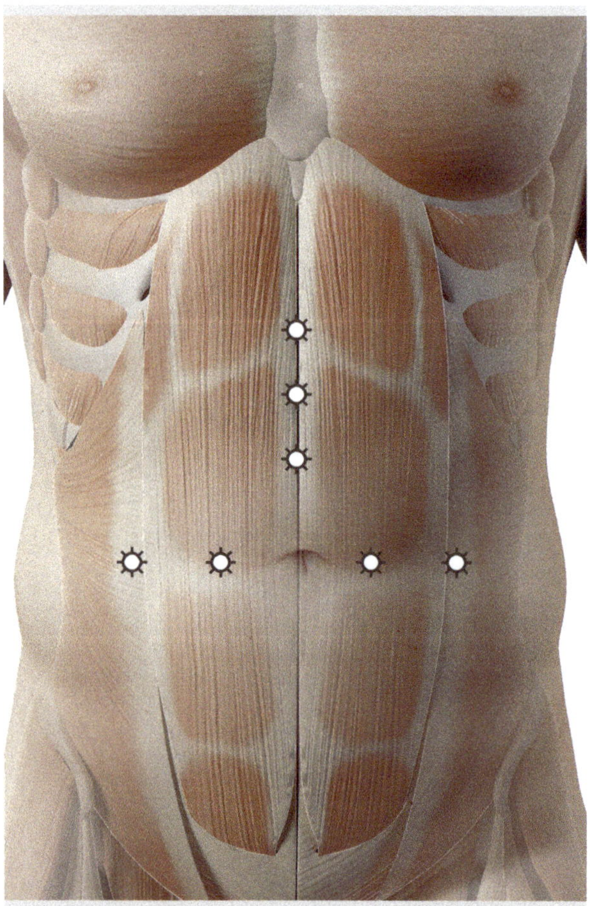

Locate and check three acupoints grouped together along the upper conception vessel between CV10 and CV14. Locate and check one or two acupoints grouped together between ST25 and SP15.

Harmonize the enteric nervous system

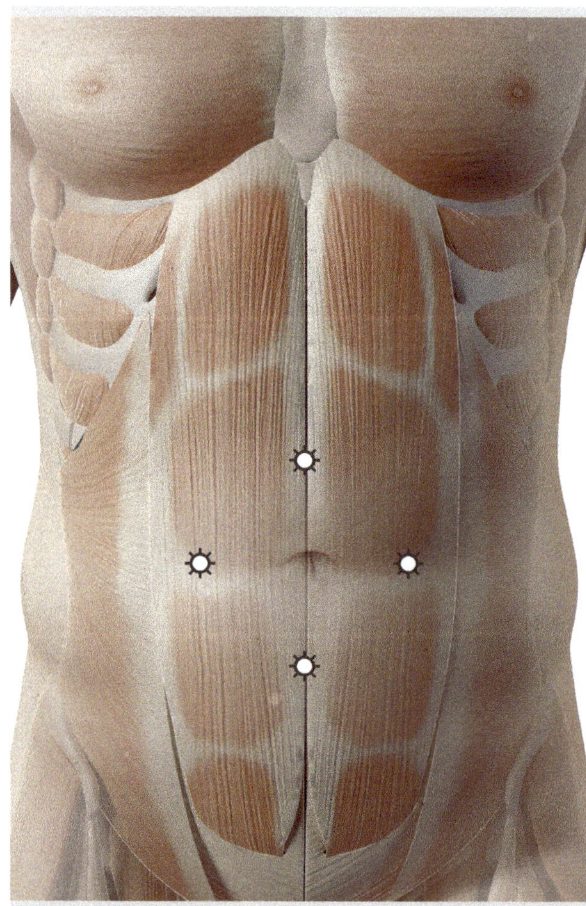

Locate and check one acupoint between CV10 and CV12, one acupoint between ST25 and SP15, and one acupoint between CV4 and CV6.

13.2 Body-Feedback Scalp and Facial Combinations

The Body-Feedback scalp and facial combinations effectively address neurological diseases, concussions, jaw misalignment, and sinus conditions, along with harmonizing the endocrine glands and different hemispheres of the brain. Mental health issues also benefit from utilizing scalp and facial acupoint combinations. Scalp ashi treatment lines (three or four acupoints per line) integrate the mind with the root treatment and strengthen brain function. Incorporate the following facial combinations for facial-rejuvenation and uneven facial features by needling different acupoint combinations for the left and right sides to improve facial symmetry. TB15 (Master Brain Alarm Point) gives rapid responses for testing acupoints located on the head and checking essential oils, herbs, and supplements that affect the brain.

The scalp acupoint combinations consist of three or four acupoints in a row that follow the trajectory of the traditional scalp and motor lines, the cranial sutures, the hairline, or the meridian pathways. Check the scalp regions for the acupoint combinations listed below and any irregularities found along the suture lines to TB15. For areas that test favorably, recheck the precise acupoint location when inserting each individual needle.

Cranial Sutures in a Newborn

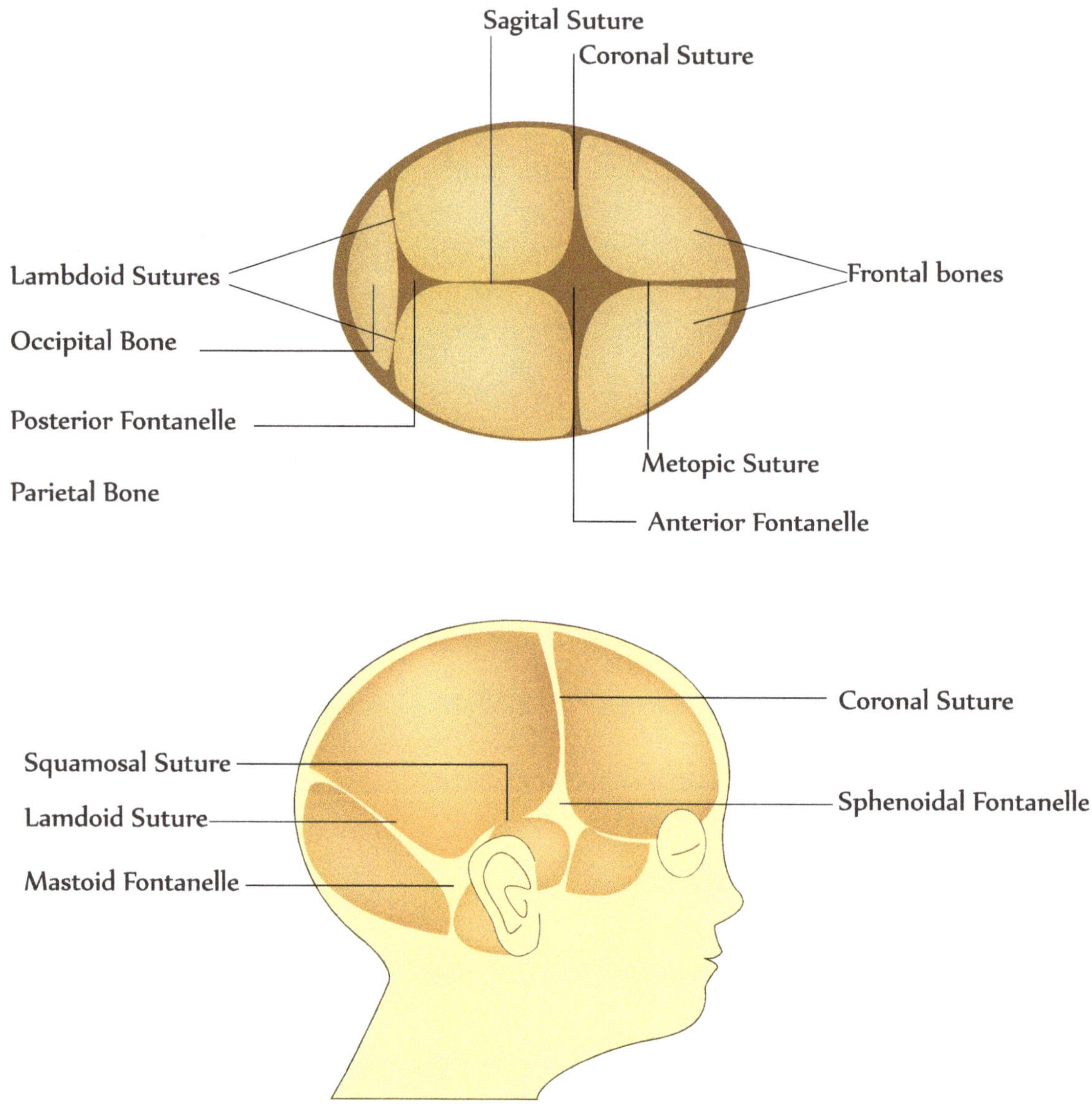

The cranial suture lines consist of dense connective tissue made from collagen. Shallow needling of the dermis layer above the cranial suture harmonizes the different regions of the brain.

Scalp Structure

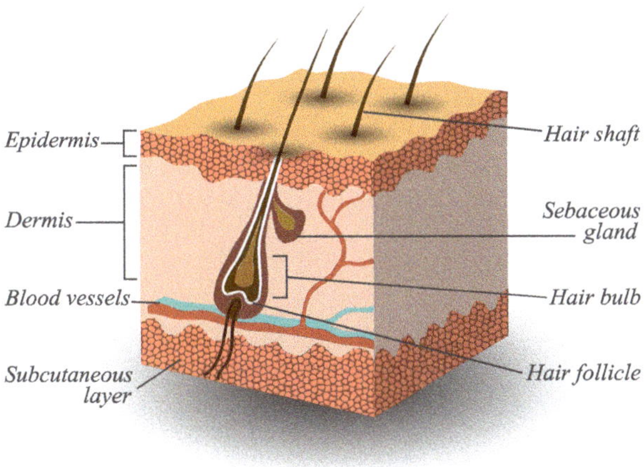

The dermis layer of the scalp is the proper needling depth. With excess conditions, the dermis layer is swollen and allows for deeper needling. With deficiency conditions, the dermis layer is compressed and requires shallower needling.

ID 91579474 © Elina Yakhontova | Dreamstime.com

Distended or swollen regions of the dermis with inflammation and stagnant fluids indicate excess conditions, which respond well to a .16- or .18-gauge needle with deeper insertion into the middle layer of the dermis. The precise acupoint aperture creates a slight palpable separation or indentation in the swollen dermis.

Compressed areas of the dermis with small divots, concavity, or rigidity indicate deficient conditions, which respond well to simply tapping a .16-gauge needle through the pipette to set the needle. The precise acupoint aperture feels like an indentation in the skull or cranial suture in the deficient regions of the scalp.

For facial acupoint combinations, use a .14- or .16-gauge needle and test the location of each acupoint. For transverse-oblique needling of the facial lines, gently pinch the skin around the point to lift it when needling to help avoid blood vessels and potential bruising on the face. Facial wrinkle lines correlate with where the body stores stress. Carefully insert the needle into the end of and underneath a wrinkle line to improve skin elasticity, release stress, and relax muscle tension. Test and compare the traditional acupoint locations to any nearby wrinkle lines. For example, test and compare Yin Tang with the two wrinkle lines commonly found lateral to it. When the wrinkle lines test better than Yin Tang, thread a .14-gauge needle downward. For horizontal wrinkles along the forehead, needle each end of a facial line inward, and again where vertical lines cross over or separations occur. For deeper and longer facial lines around the mouth, needle each end of the facial line inward and add perpendicular needles to any crevasse along the line.

BODY-FEEDBACK CLINICAL PEARLS

Systemic pathogenic heat spreads and rises upward, causing inflammation in the head and brain. When the majority of yin or yang meridians require the metal + water combination, systemic pathogenic heat is likely irritating the brain. Massage the scalp looking for swollen areas and needle three or four acupoints on each side of the head along the apex of the congested scalp tissue to release the pathogenic heat. After needling the scalp, it is easier to identify the root treatment, and fewer supporting metal + water combinations are necessary.

Chronic headaches, migraines, neurological conditions, and body weakness are common symptoms of long-term pathogenic heat with brain inflammation. Check the meridian fire alarm points before and after needling the scalp. Meridian fire alarm points that remain painful after needling the scalp can identify possible primary sources of the pathogenic heat. The meridian fire alarm points that are no longer tender after needling the scalp are meridians altered by the spreading of the heat pathogens.

Take, for example, a female client who suffers from chronic migraines and muscle weakness in the wrists and arms and has many painful meridian fire alarm points (LU10, PC8, HT8, KD2, and LV2). She has a swollen area on the scalp in the posterior region of the head and tests best to needling a total of eight acupoints in a line along the thickest area. Upon retesting the meridian fire alarm points, only LU10, KD2, and LV2 remain tender, and the pulse responds best to the liver balancing acupoint prescription. She also has discomfort on the right side of the rib cage, LV8 organ alarm point, and the sternal attachment of the pectoralis muscles (all Body-Feedback organ/meridian referral areas and muscle associations for the liver). The root liver dysfunction indicates this client has compromised detoxification, causing pathogenic heat and disrupting the immune system. Supplements and herbs to support detoxification and the liver and kidney organs are critical to restoring balance to the immune system and resolving the pathogenic heat.

13.2.1 First Trisection Scalp and Facial Acupoint Combinations

Yang-ming sinus and immune acupoint combination

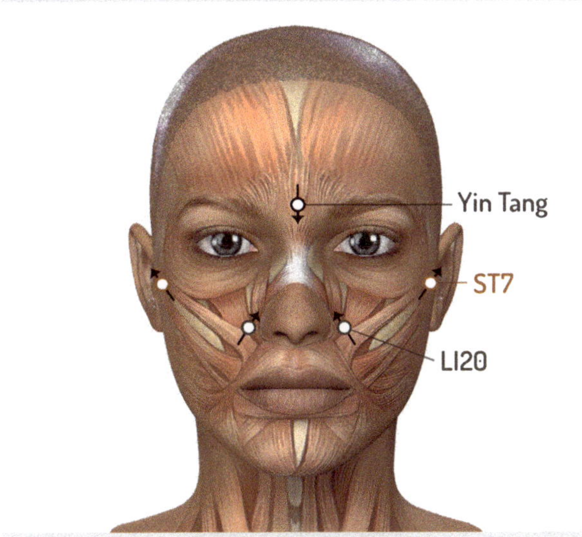

Locate and check LI20, ST7, and Yin Tang for the treatment of sinus conditions and to strengthen the immune system.

Anterior seven emotion downward with ST6

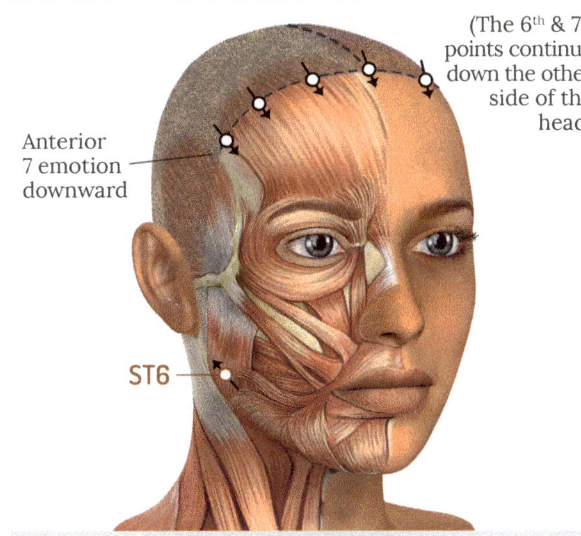

Locate and check seven acupoints at the hairline pressing downward with the middle acupoint below DU24 and three acupoints above each eyebrow. The downward direction reduces stress hormones and calms the nervous system. Locate and check ST6 to reduce jaw tension.

Anterior seven emotion upward with ST6

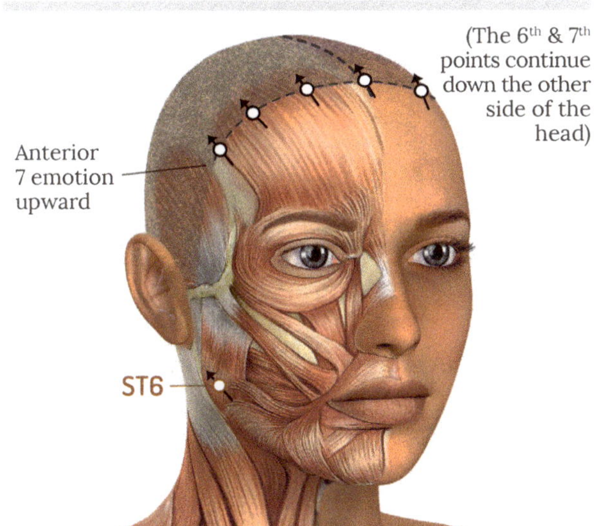

Locate and check seven acupoints at the hairline pressing upward with the middle acupoint below DU24 and three acupoints above each eyebrow. The upward direction increases energy while toning and lifting the facial muscles and skin. Locate and check ST6 to reduce jaw tension.

13.2.2 Second Trisection Scalp and Facial Acupoint Combinations

Urinary bladder meridian scalp region

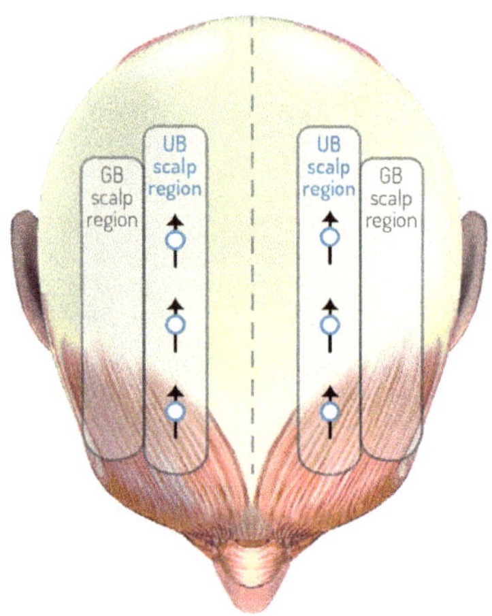

Locate and check three or four acupoints in a line along the urinary bladder meridian in the region between UB4 and UB8 to harmonize the tai-yang meridians (UB and SI) and strengthen the central nervous system.

Posterior scalp ashi region

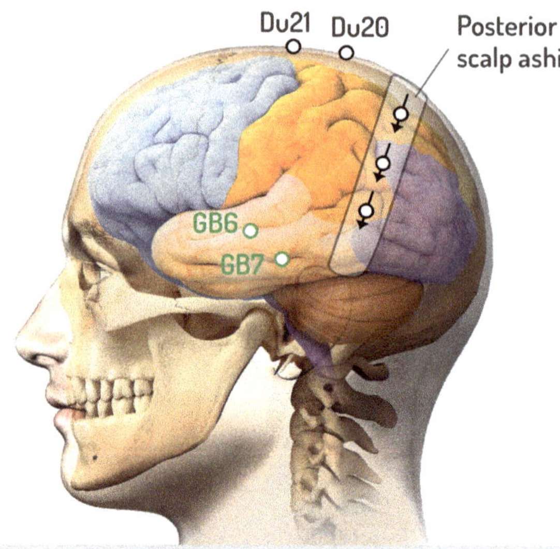

Locate and check three to four acupoints in a line downward between one and two cun behind DU20 to harmonize the imperial-fire element (HT and SI).

Harmonize the water element with UB2 + Yuyao downward and DU20

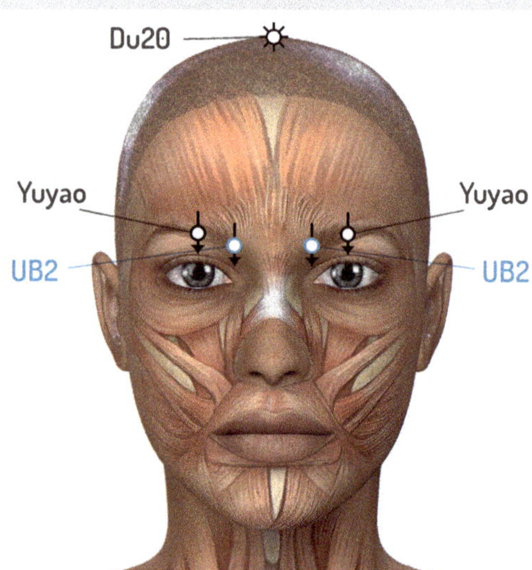

Locate and check UB2 and Yuyao pressing downward to harmonize the second trisection and calm the nervous system. Locate and check one acupoint near DU20 to harmonize the hypothalamus and pituitary axis.

Harmonize the water element with UB2 + Yuyao upward and DU20

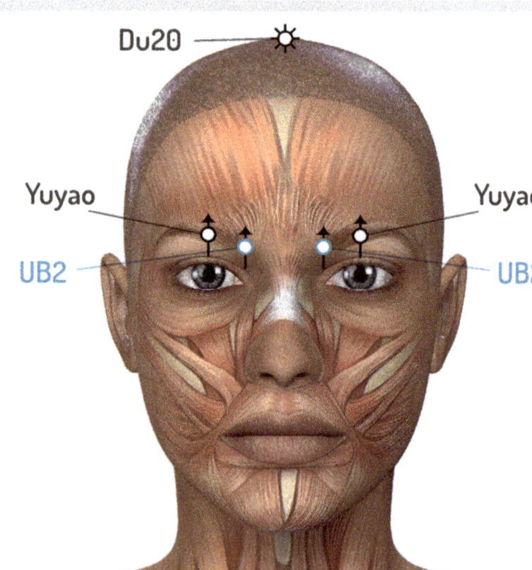

Locate and check UB2 and Yuyao pressing upward to harmonize the second trisection and lift the eyelids. Locate and check one acupoint near DU20 to harmonize the hypothalamus and pituitary axis.

13.2.3 Third Trisection Scalp and Facial Acupoint Combinations

Shao-yang sinus and headache acupoint combination

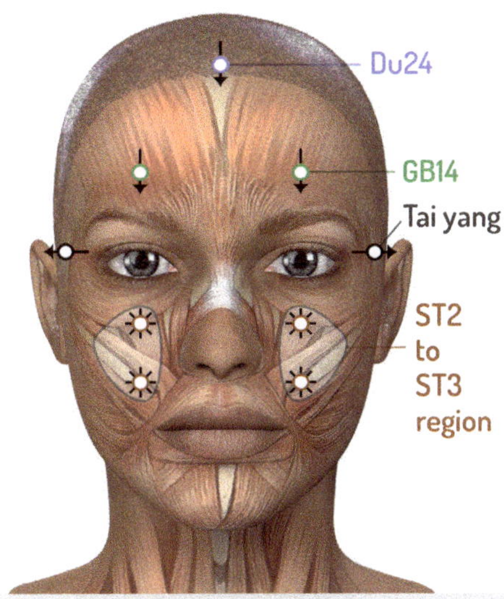

Locate and check DU24, GB14, Tai Yang, and one acupoint between ST2 and ST3 for the treatment of sinus conditions and headaches.

Gallbladder meridian scalp region

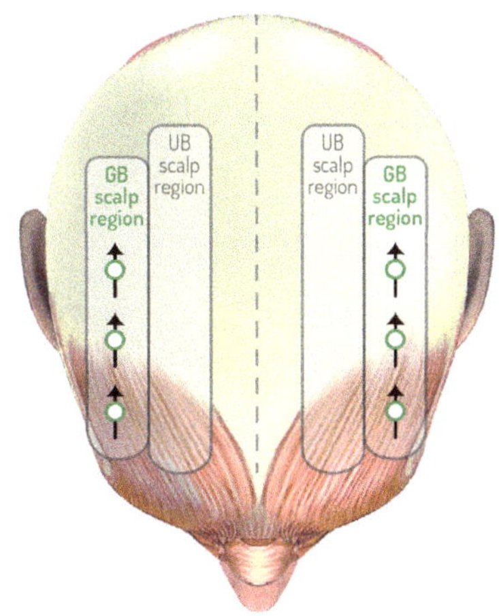

Locate and check three or four acupoints in a line along the gallbladder meridian in the region between GB15 and GB18 to harmonize the wood element.

Shao-yang scalp region

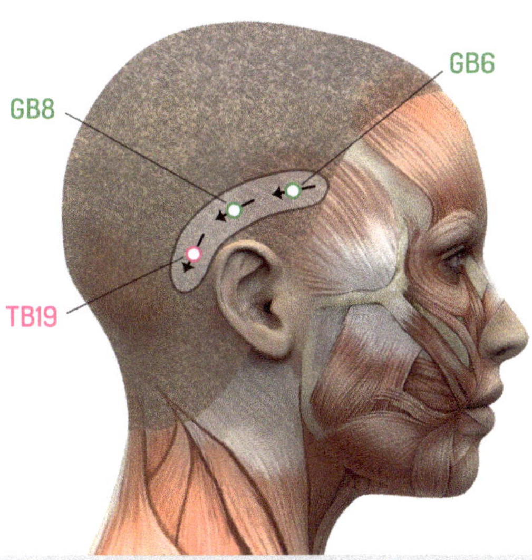

Locate and check three or four acupoints in a line on the lateral side of the head in the region between GB6, GB8, and TB19 to harmonize the shao-yang meridians (GB and TB) and strengthen the limbic system.

Posterior seven emotion

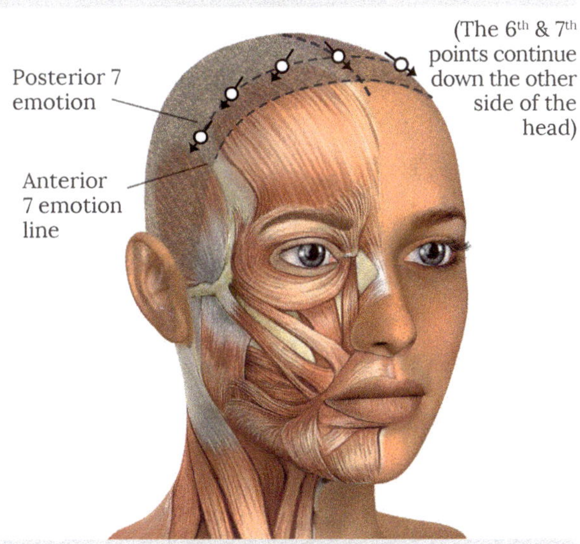

Locate and check seven acupoints approximately two to three cun posterior to the hairline with the middle acupoint near DU22 and the other three acupoints in line with each eyebrow. Needle the middle acupoint perpendicularly and the other three acupoints downward towards the ear to treat the effects of long-term stress and harmonize the wood element.

13.2.4 Scalp Acupoint Combinations to Harmonize Body Systems

ST8 to GB8 region

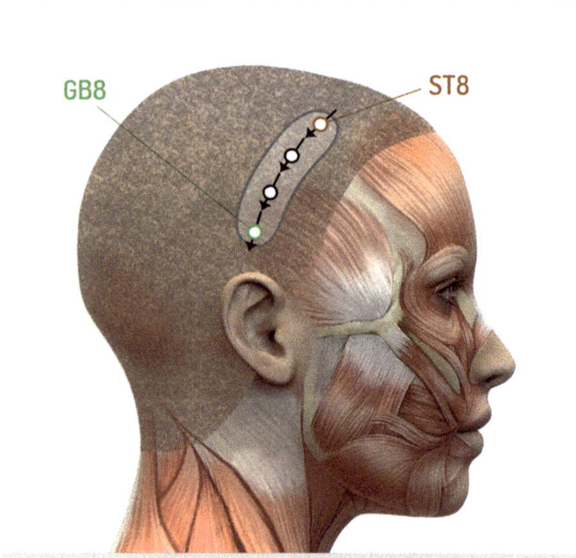

Locate and check three or four acupoints in a line on the lateral side of the head in the region between ST8 and GB8 to harmonize and strengthen the digestive and endocrine systems.

Sensory and motor scalp regions

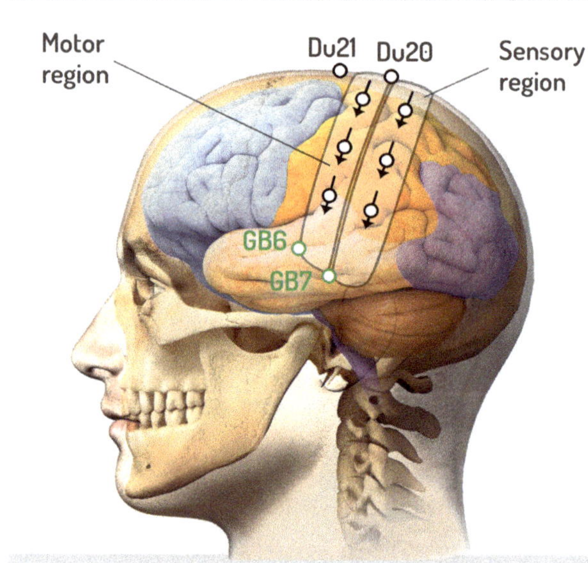

Locate and check three or four acupoints in a line approximately one cun anterior to DU20 to strengthen the motor nerves in the four extremities. Locate and check three or four acupoints in a line approximately one cun posterior to DU20 and to strengthen the sensory nerves in the four extremities.

13.3 Body-Feedback Auricular Combinations

Auricular acupoint combinations harmonize the ANS in the supine treatment position. Emotional and mental health issues, along with pain conditions, respond well to needling two or three auricular acupoints for each ear. For symmetrical treatments, test and choose the same auricular acupoints for the left and right ears. For asymmetrical treatments, check and use different acupoints for the left and right ears. Pain conditions respond best to treating the ear on the same side of the body as the region of discomfort.

Test individual auricular acupoints using the rounded tip of an acupuncture needle's handle or an ear probe to TB15. Ear acupoints can be sensitive and respond well to smaller needles (.14 x 13 mm), Vaccaria ear seeds, and 800 gauss magnetic pellets. Clients can retain the Vaccaria seeds for up to one week and the magnetic pellets for up to five days after their treatments. The magnetic pellets provide constant low-level stimulation, and clients can press the seeds, as needed, to stimulate the auricular acupoints. Remove the ear seeds and pellets immediately if irritation or itching occurs around the site.

Three Body-Feedback auricular combinations incorporate six regions of the ear to harmonize the ANS for most clients. However, on occasion, other standard auricular points may release tension and discomfort at the master alarm points better than one of these combinations. Begin by testing each region by pressing it with a thumb pad while checking TB15. Then test individual acupoints within the region that releases discomfort at the master alarm points by using the rounded tip of an acupuncture needle's handle or an ear probe to determine the precise location. If needed, test individual auricular acupoints based on the client's symptoms while checking any of the master alarm points.

- **Region 1 combination** incorporates shen men for calming the spirit and the liver to regulate the flow of qi.
- **Region 2 combination** utilizes areas of the ear to calm an overactive adrenal stress response.
- **Region 3 combination** promotes deep relaxation by regulating the flow of qi through the upper and lower areas of the body.

Balancing the ANS Ear Chart with Body-Feedback Auricular Combinations

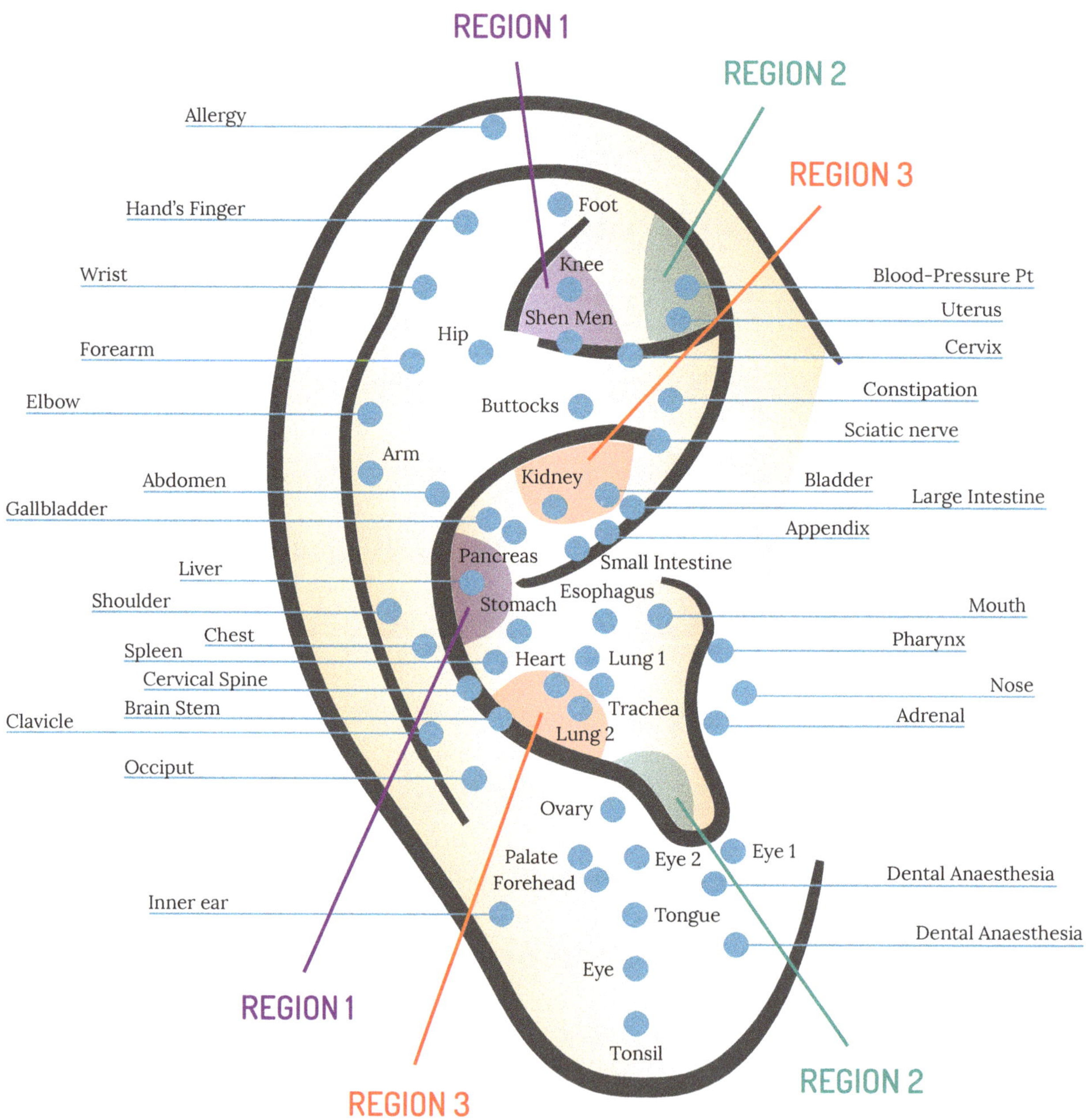

13.4 Body-Feedback Prone Treatments

The Body-Feedback prone acupoint combinations balance the ANS while focusing on the neck, shoulders, back, sacrum, and alignment of the spine. Prone combinations consist of three or four acupoints along a specific segment of the spine, sacrum, scapula, or a meridian pathway. Multiple segments work together to balance the ANS, strengthen and align the spine, and treat specific symptoms. Carefully inspect the client in the facedown position looking for differences in hip and shoulder alignment from one side to the other, along with areas that appears tighter, more excess, or that have more symptoms.

Types of Spinal Irregularities

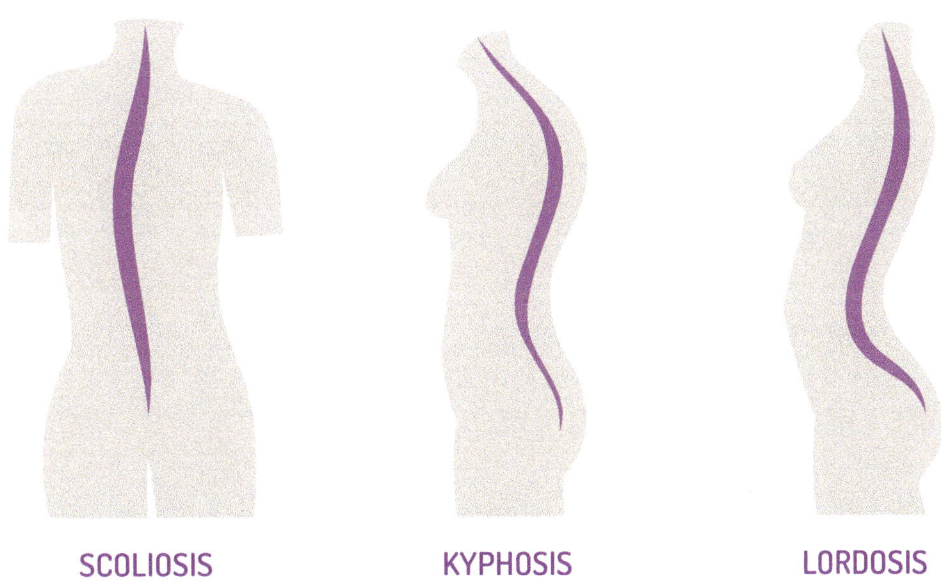

ID 80546822 © Pawel Graczyk | Dreamstime.com

Kyphosis is an exaggerated outward (convex) curve in the upper back, which over time, will cause poor posture, along with neck, shoulder, and lower back pain. Kyphosis compresses the cervical vertebrae, causes the shoulder joints to roll forward, constricts the nerves in the neck and lower lumbar region, and misaligns the sacrum.

Lordosis is an exaggerated inward (concave) curve in the lower back, which over time, will cause the head and neck to protrude forward, and the sacrum and rib cage will tilt outward from the spine, causing mid and lower back pain. Lordosis compresses the cervical and lumbar nerves and causes misalignment of the pelvis and sacroiliac joint.

Prone acupoint combinations often change at each appointment for a variety of reasons, such as changes in the nervous system, spinal alignment, recent activities, and general improvements. Prone treatments contain a significant number of acupoints, including the root sedation or tonification prescriptions, and therefore require few to no other additional supporting points. The regions to test for needling in the prone position include:

- areas of excess vertical spinal curvature, as seen in lordosis and kyphosis
- areas of excess horizontal spinal curvature, as seen in scoliosis
- around the border of phlegm nodules in the lower back
- the lower border of the sacrum
- the upper border of the PSIS originating from lumbar vertebrae five (L5 ashi)
- the lateral edge of the erector spinae muscles with excessive tightness and thickness
- the lateral edge of the spinous processes for areas of muscle weakness
- the lateral edge of the spinous processes for the cervical vertebrae
- muscle tightness along the medial border of the scapula (scapula ashi)
- muscle tightness along the upper-lateral insertions into the rotator cuff
- the lower border of the occiput from the governing vessel to the triple burner meridian

The sympathetic nervous system responds directly to needles between the thoracic vertebrae one (T1) and lumbar vertebrae two (L2). The parasympathetic nervous system responds directly to needles in the cervical vertebrae area, lumbar vertebrae three (L3) through lumbar vertebrae five (L5), and over the sacrum. Along the spine, the regions that test best usually correspond with sympathetic nerves from T1 to L2 or the parasympathetic nerves from L3 to the sacrum and in the neck. Farther away from the spine, the outer UB line and scapula points indirectly support the spinal levels that are not directly needled.

Test the prone acupoints to the same (ipsilateral) side's master alarm points due to the convenient location and quick response to any stimulation of the nervous system. The pulse, muscle memory regions (UB43-44 and UB57-58), and muscle associations for the root treatment are other options for testing the prone acupoints.

Each acupoint along the spine has the potential to affect several areas. Therefore, test and promptly needle the beneficial acupoint's aperture before proceeding to check the next one. Look for areas of overly developed muscles on the back to needle first. Check the acupoints on the governing vessel and the outer UB meridian line in the regions that appear excess due to tight muscles or spinal curvature. Then test the acupoints on the *Hua Tuo Jia Ji* line (.5 cun lateral to the spinous processes) and the inner UB meridian line for areas of muscle weakness and deficiency.

Use between four and eight needles to surround the outside the border of phlegm nodules found in the lower back and other areas of the body. Needle the phlegm nodules first to allow for longer needle retention time. If the client's symptoms affect the head, neck, shoulders, or arms, start checking and needling acupoints from the neck downward. If the client's symptoms involve the lower back, hips, pelvis, or legs, start checking and needling acupoints along the upper and lower borders of the sacrum first (L5 and sacrum ashi) and then test the spinal areas moving upward. Often with asymmetry, the right or left side tests best for the L5 ashi acupoints, while the opposite side tests best for the sacrum ashi acupoints.

For clients with scoliosis, palpate along the excess regions of the spine to find the outer border of the erector spinae or trapezius muscle that is the most pronounced for each curve. First, needle the outer edge of the curve at the apex towards the spine to release the excess tension pulling the spine outward. Then check and needle one or two acupoints above and below the peak of the curve. Check and needle all of the excess spinal curves first. For the deficient areas of the spine, either apply essential oils or gently insert two or three needles along the Hua Tuo line.

The prone acupoints to balance the ANS respond best to gentle needling techniques. The region of the body and proximity to the spine influence the preferred needle gauge, depth, and angle. In general, use a smaller gauge needle (.16 or .18) with shallow insertion (.5 cun) for root deficiency treatments, concave deficient areas on or alongside the spine, and with the acupoints on the governing vessel, inner urinary bladder line, and the Hua Tao line. For root excess treatments and acupoints along the outer urinary bladder line, sacrum, and shoulders, use a larger gauge needle (.20 to .25) with an insertion depth proportionate to the client's size (1 to 3 cun). Again, refrain from stimulating the needles, which can activate the sympathetic nervous system.

The following Body-Feedback back acupoint combinations are examples of typical treatments. Carefully inspect the back, looking for excess or deficient muscle tone or skeletal structure. Test possible treatment areas to the master alarm points to determine the regions to needle. Check individual acupoint locations by pressing the point for five seconds and monitoring the master alarm points on the same side. The prone acupoint combinations are unique to a client's needs during a session.

13.5 Body-Feedback Back Acupoint Combinations

Governing vessel example

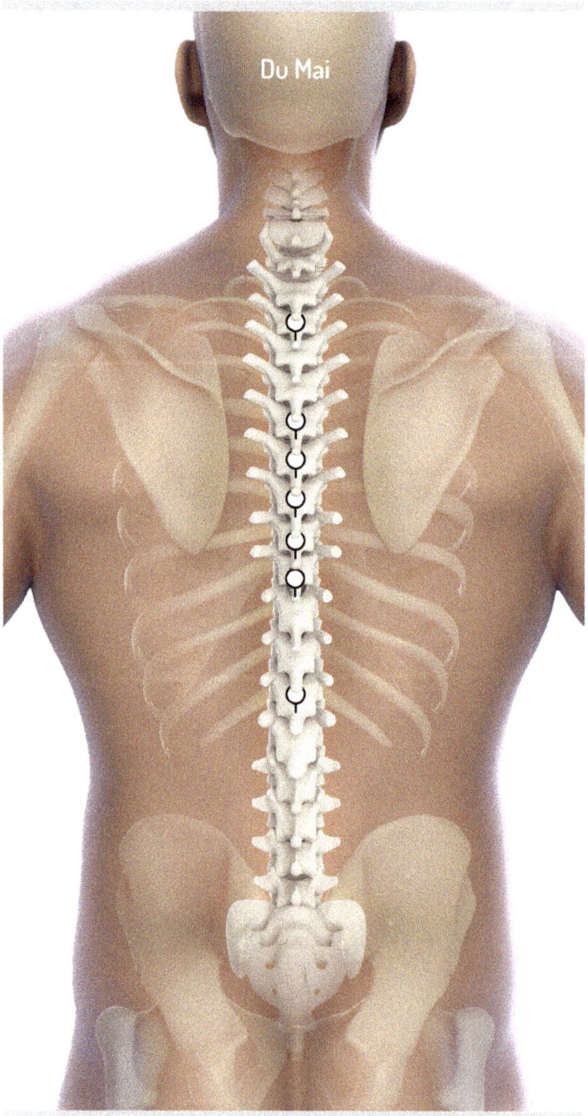

Check the acupoints along the spine in the areas of any excess convex curvature.

Hua tuo jia ji example

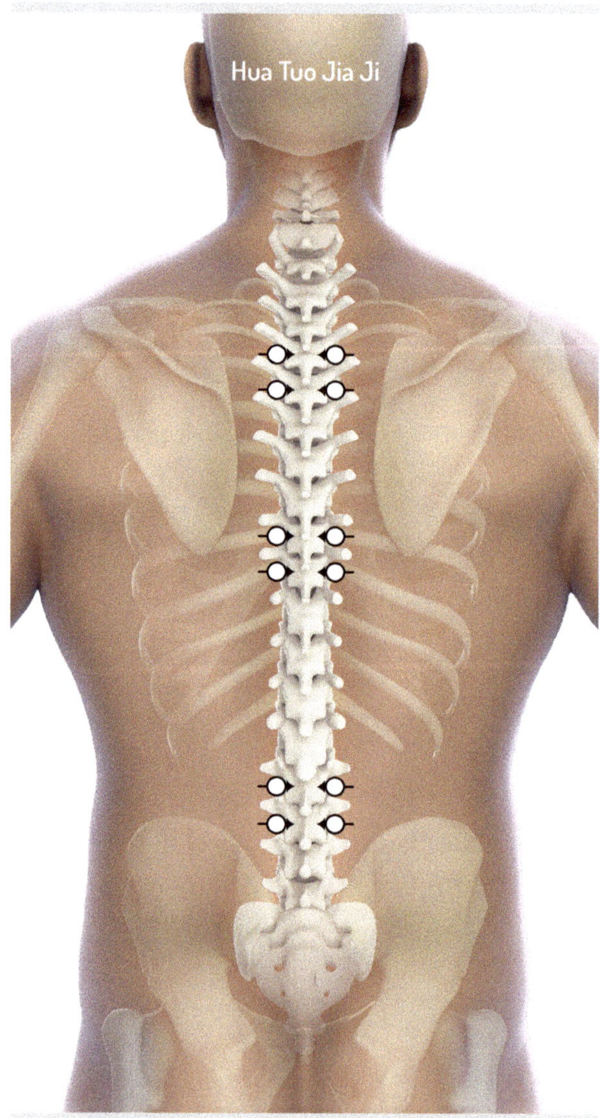

Check the acupoints .5 cun lateral to the spine in the areas of deficient concave curvature.

Outer urinary bladder line example

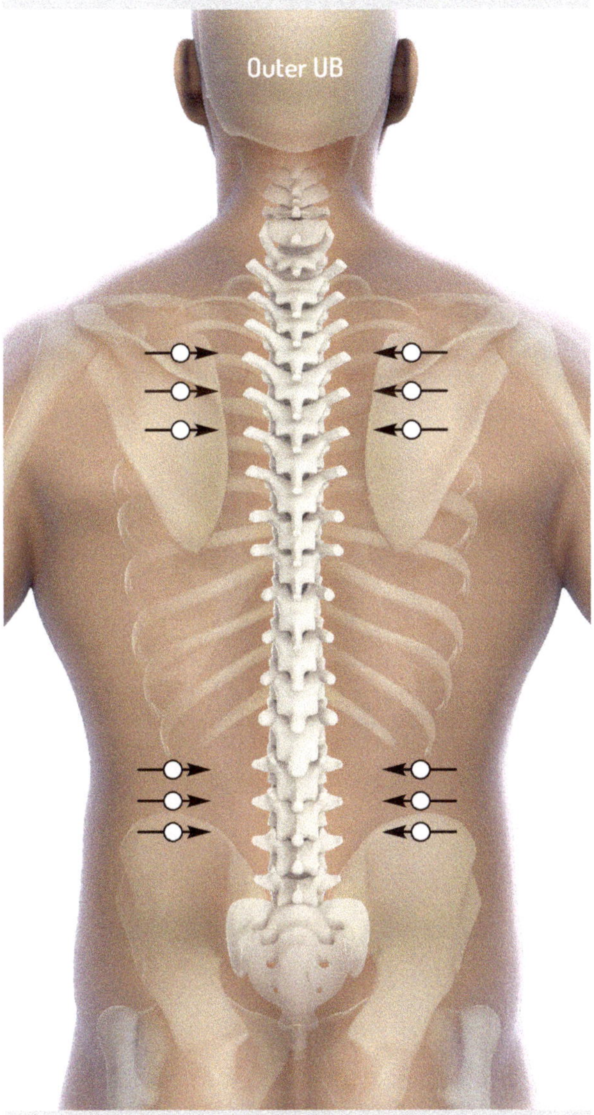

Check the acupoints 3 cun lateral to the spine in the areas of any excess convex curvature or tight erector spinae muscles.

Inner urinary bladder line example

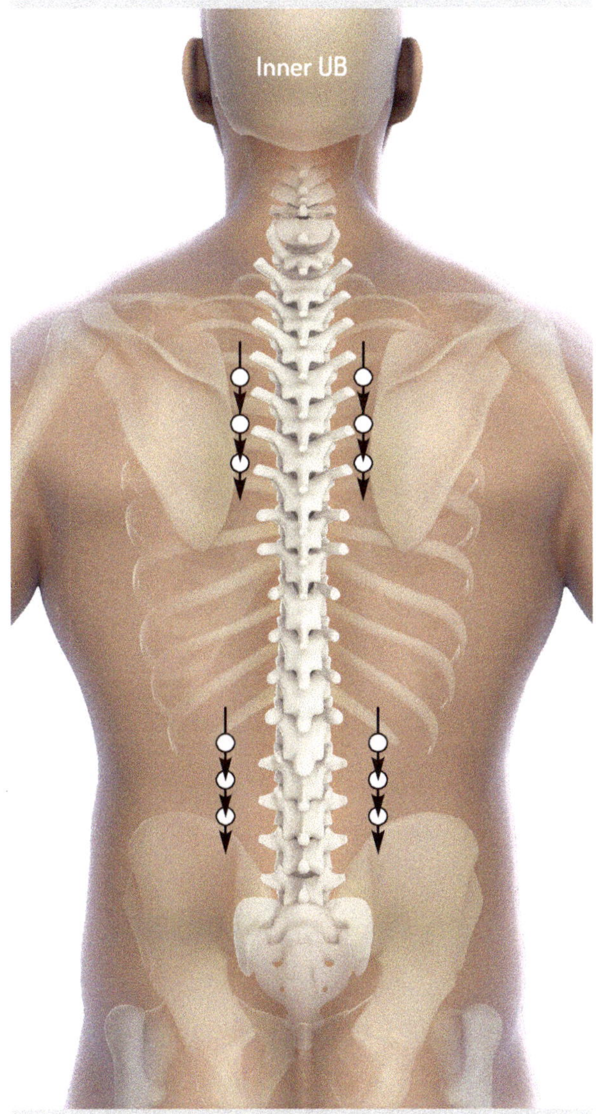

Check the acupoints 1.5 cun lateral to the spine in the areas of deficient concave curvature or weak erector spinae muscles.

Scapula ashi example

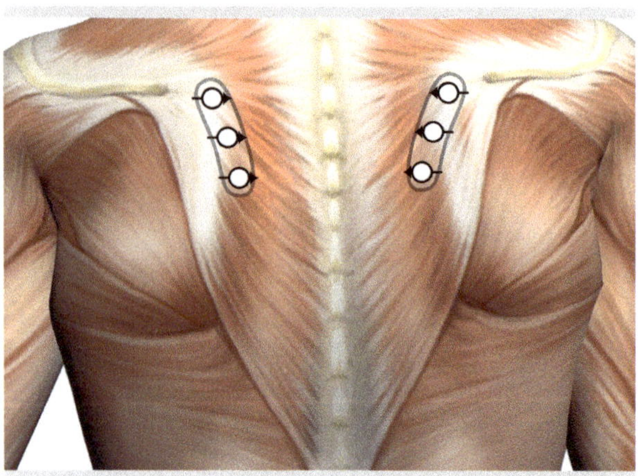

Check 3 or 4 acupoints along the lateral edge of the trapezius muscle where it meets with the medial border of the scapula in the areas of over-development or tightness.

Small intestine 9-10 example

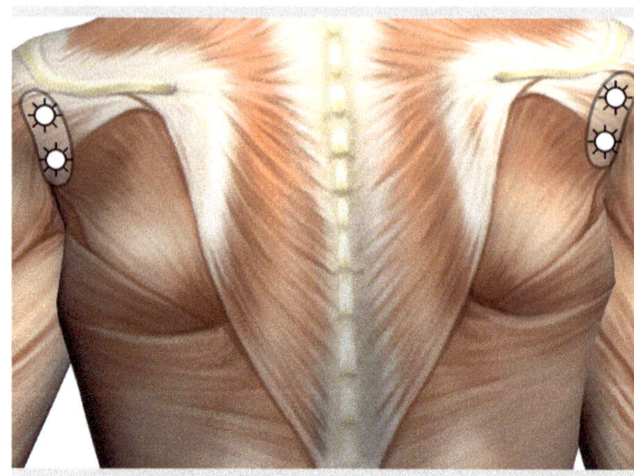

Check 2 or 3 acupoints along the posterior side or the rotator cuff in the region around SI9 to SI10 for muscle tightness.

L5 ashi example

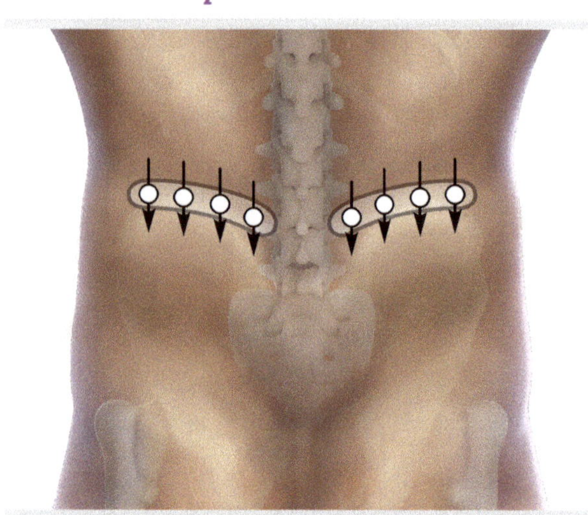

Check 3 or 4 acupoints starting at lumbar vertebrae 5 and above the border of the PSIS in areas of tightness or stored phlegm nodules.

Sacrum ashi example

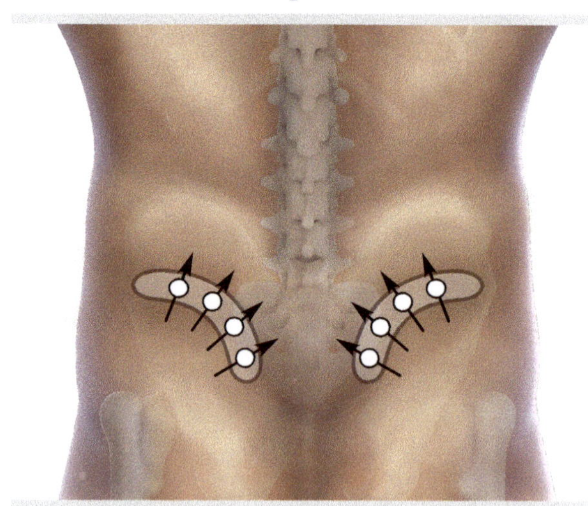

Check 3 or 4 acupoints along the medium border of the sacrum in areas of tightness.

Scoliosis treatment approach example

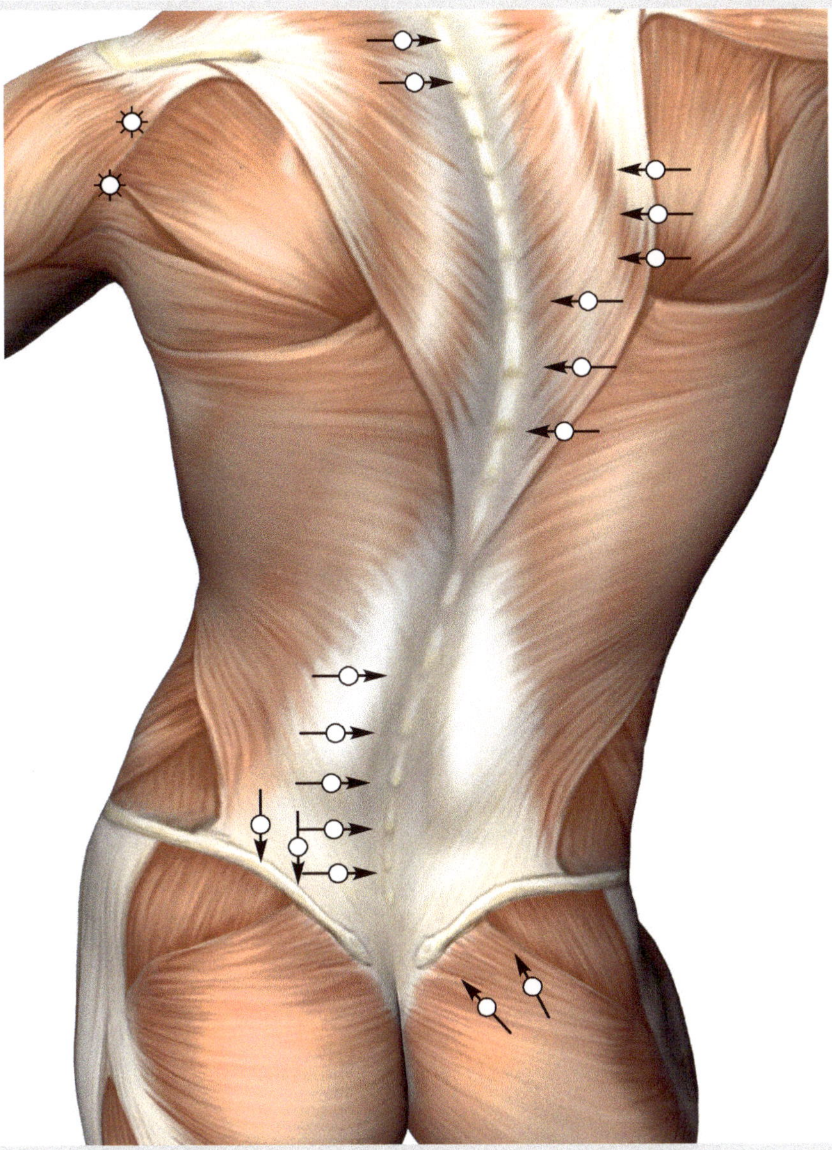

Check 2, 3, or 4 acupoints in areas of muscle tightness, starting with the sacrum and above the border of the PSIS, along with areas of excess curvature on the spine.

CHAPTER 14

The Balancing, Sedation, and Tonification Acupoints

Several options, including needles, magnets, press tacks, and moxa, are acceptable for stimulating the acupoints that comprise the Body-Feedback balancing, sedation, and tonification prescriptions. A combination of factors influences the choice of needle gauge, insertion depth, and retention time, along with the use of magnets or press tacks. These factors include the client's sensitivity to needles, age, and constitution, along with the type of treatment: sedation, tonification, one-sided, or two-sided. The Body-Feedback approach focuses on precise needle placement and angle, which allows for smaller gauge needles, shallow insertion depth, and less stimulation of the needles. This gentle treatment style utilizes an average of 20 to 40 acupoints (10 to 20 bilateral acupoints) per session.

Resolving pathogenic heat is an integral component of the Body-Feedback treatment approach, and many chronic conditions have true-heat with false-cold symptoms (see Section 3.6). *Moxa* is a technique that burns dried Chinese mugwart as a heat source to warm and energize acupoints for cold pathogens, qi stagnation, blood stasis, and deficiency conditions. Applying essential oils with warming properties, such as clove, cypress, rosemary, lemon, and orange, to the soles of the feet before inserting needles also dispels cold, moves qi stagnation, and transforms blood stasis. Incorporating the Organ Supporting and Meridian Balancing blends into treatments can eliminate the need for moxa. Moxa is optional in the Body-Feedback approach and can help treat acupoints and body regions affected by cold pathogens.

Eight-hundred gauss magnetic pellets effectively stimulate the jing-well and ying-spring acupoints for tonification treatments, sensitive clients, children, and the elderly. Leaving the magnetic pellets on the jing-well and ying-spring acupoints after an acupuncture session provides longer-term, gentle stimulation of these points. For sensitive clients new to acupuncture, use magnetic pellets on the jing-well and ying-spring acupoints for the first few sessions and transition to .14x13mm needles as needed for sedation treatments. Applying the appropriate essential oil blends to the soles of the feet can also reduce discomfort when needling sensitive acupoints.

14.1 Needling Technique to Sedate or Tonify Acupoints

The balancing shu-points can sedate excess and tonify deficient conditions by using different needle gauges, insertion depths, and retention times. Stimulate the balancing and sedation acupoints for an excess root treatment using a larger needle gauge, deeper insertion, and longer retention time. Stimulate the balancing and tonification acupoints for a deficient root treatment using a smaller needle gauge, shallow insertion, and shorter retention time.

For sedation treatments, insert and retain larger gauge needles for 25-30 minutes. Use .16x15mm for jing-well and ying-spring points, .18x15mm for shu-stream and jing-river points, and .20x30mm for he-sea points. Sensitive clients with excess conditions may respond better to smaller gauge needles with longer retention times.

For tonification treatments, insert and retain smaller gauge needles for 15-20 minutes. Sensitive clients and deficient conditions respond well to magnetic pellets applied to the jing-well points, which can remain in place until they fall off later. Use shallow needling or magnets for the jing-well points, .14x13mm for ying-spring points, .16x15mm for shu-stream and jing-river points, and .18x30mm for he-sea points. Sensitive clients or deficient conditions may respond better to fewer acupoints and shorter retention time.

Acupoints with more variation in their exact aperture location have a range indicated on the point location diagrams. Bones in the feet adjust to accommodate differences in arch height, causing the acupoint locations to shift. Knee alignment induces variations in the exact location of the he-sea points. If needed, check multiple needle placement options within a range to the pulse or master alarm points to find the precise aperture. Determine the needle size, exact location, insertion depth, and retention time while testing the sedation and tonification acupoints immediately after identifying the root balancing acupoint prescriptions.

The Body-Feedback style uses the standard angles of needle insertion: perpendicular, perpendicular-oblique, oblique, transverse-oblique, and transverse. Always insert needles in the direction a meridian flows or perpendicular to the acupoint. The five-element flow of energy does not respond favorably to inserting needles angled against the flow of a meridian. Point location diagrams throughout this text provide the recommended needle insertion direction and depth for each acupoint used in the Body-Feedback approach.

Body-Feedback testing techniques can determine the correct needle angle for each acupoint. First, press an acupoint perpendicularly and check the pulse or master alarm points, then push the skin at the acupoint in the direction the meridian flows and determine if perpendicular or oblique to transverse tests best. Recheck the needle angle if the pulse or master alarm points release more tension and discomfort during the testing process than after needle insertion. It is common to adjust the needle angle between perpendicular, oblique, and transverse while checking the pulse, neck muscles, or master alarm points.

14.2 Needling the Metal + Water Acupoint Combinations

Pathogenic heat restricts healing potential and can spread to other meridians and organs if not adequately treated. Always remember to test the metal + water substitutions for bolded points (**SP3**, **ST36**, **GB41**, and **HT8**) included in the balancing, sedation, and tonification point combinations. The cooling and nurturing effects of metal + water combinations respond best to slightly longer treatment time. Therefore, needling or applying magnets or press tacks to the metal + water combinations first allows additional treatment time for these acupoints.

Many of the Body-Feedback balancing, sedation, and tonification prescriptions include individual horary metal or water shu-points. Adding the corresponding metal or water shu-point to a horary acupoint creates the heat-clearing combination. It is most efficient to test the corresponding supporting metal or water acupoints while checking the acupoints in a root prescription (step three of the planning stage). When a meridian or organ has pathogenic heat, immediately add the supporting metal or water acupoint to the root balancing, sedation, and tonification prescriptions.

Test the following corresponding metal or water shu-points for acupoint prescriptions that include individual horary metal or water shu-points.

Acupoint prescription	Existing metal or water horary acupoint	Corresponding metal or water acupoint
LUNG SEDATION	KD10 WATER	KD7 METAL
LARGE INTESTINE SEDATION	UB66 WATER	UB67 METAL
STOMACH BALANCING	UB66 WATER	UB67 METAL
STOMACH SEDATION	LI1 METAL	LI2 WATER
HEART BALANCING	KD10 WATER	KD7 METAL
HEART BALANCING	LU8 METAL	LU5 WATER
SMALL INTESTINE BALANCING	LI1 METAL	LI2 WATER
SMALL INTESTINE BALANCING	UB66 WATER	UB67 METAL
URINARY BLADDER TONIFICATION	LI1 METAL	LI2 WATER
KIDNEY TONIFICATION	LU8 METAL	LU5 WATER
PERICARDIUM BALANCING	KD10 WATER	KD7 METAL
PERICARDIUM BALANCING	LU8 METAL	LU5 WATER
TRIPLE BURNER BALANCING	UB66 WATER	UB67 METAL
GALLBLADDER BALANCING	LI1 METAL	LI2 WATER
GALLBLADDER TONIFICATION	UB66 WATER	UB67 METAL
LIVER BALANCING	LU8 METAL	LU5 WATER
LIVER TONIFICATION	KD10 WATER	KD7 METAL

After removing the acupuncture needles, consider applying magnetic pellets or press tacks to the metal + water combinations for continued release of pathogenic heat. In cases of chronic pathogenic heat, send the clients home with extra magnetic pellets to apply to the metal + water combination when going to bed. Treating these points every night will enhance the benefits of the acupuncture sessions between appointments.

BODY-FEEDBACK CLINICAL PEARLS

On occasion, multiple organs or meridians with pathogenic heat requiring the metal + water combination can complicate the testing process. When it is difficult to determine the correct tonification or sedation prescription, needle only the metal + water combinations on the affected yin or yang meridians. For example, a client experiencing an autoimmune flareup with systemic pathogenic heat may test best for the metal + water combination on all the yin meridians. At the following appointment, this client may test for all of the metal + water combinations for the yang meridians. At follow-up appointments, the root tonification or sedation prescription with supporting metal + water combinations can be easier to identify.

14.3 Balancing, Sedation, and Tonification Point Location Diagrams

On occasion, a specific shu-point, such as UB60 and KD3, responds best to perpendicular needle insertion while the majority of the other shu-points in the same category respond best to oblique to transverse-oblique needling. These acupoints have a special image △ or ☼ indicating the preferred perpendicular insertion. Needle size or use of a press tack or magnet depends on a client's sensitivity and access to the point based on the treatment positions. The shu-points categories generally follow the preferred needle angle and gauge listed below.

Shu-point Category	Options for Sedation	Options for Tonification	Preferred Needle Angle
JING-WELL	.14, .16, or magnets	.14 or magnets	Perpendicular to oblique
YING-SPRING	.14, .16, or press tacks	.14 or magnets	Oblique to transverse-oblique
SHU-STREAM	.16 or .18	.14 or .16	Oblique to transverse-oblique
JING-RIVER	.16 or .18	.14 or .16	Oblique to transverse-oblique
HE-SEA	.18 or .20	.16 or .18	Oblique to transverse-oblique

14.3.1 Acupoint Images for the First Trisection

LUNG BALANCING ACUPOINTS:

LU10, LU11, LV1, **HT8** (compare HT4 metal + HT3 water)

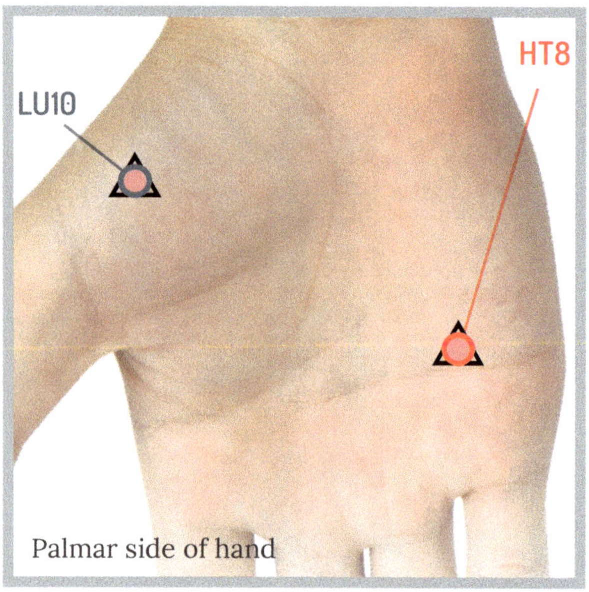

Palmar side of hand

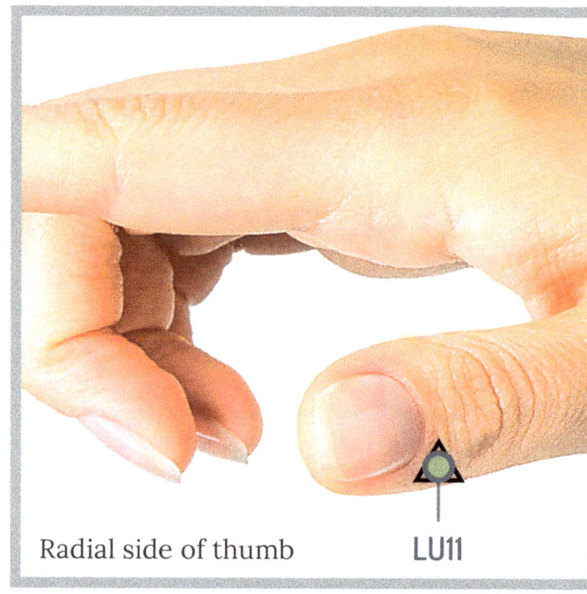

Radial side of thumb

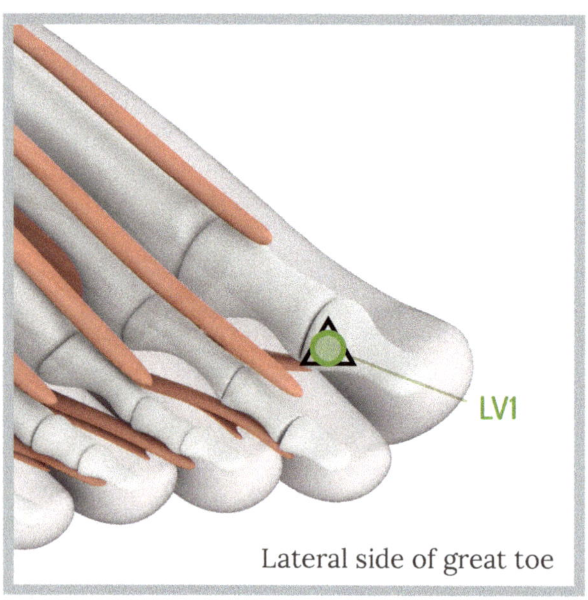

Lateral side of great toe

LUNG SEDATION ACUPOINTS:
LU5, KD10

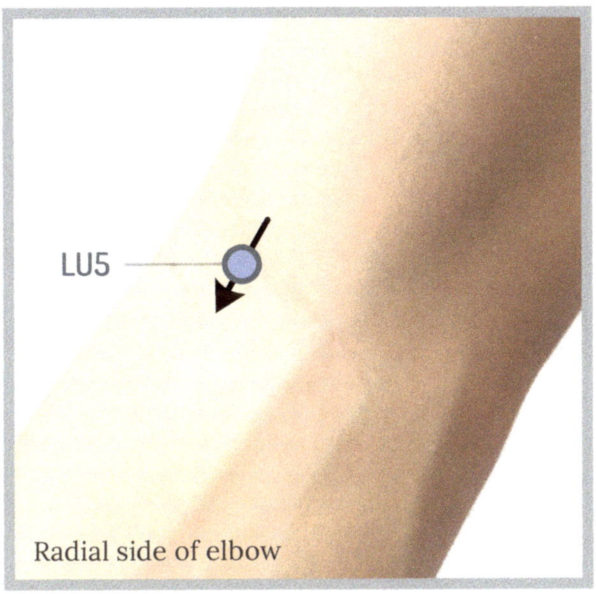

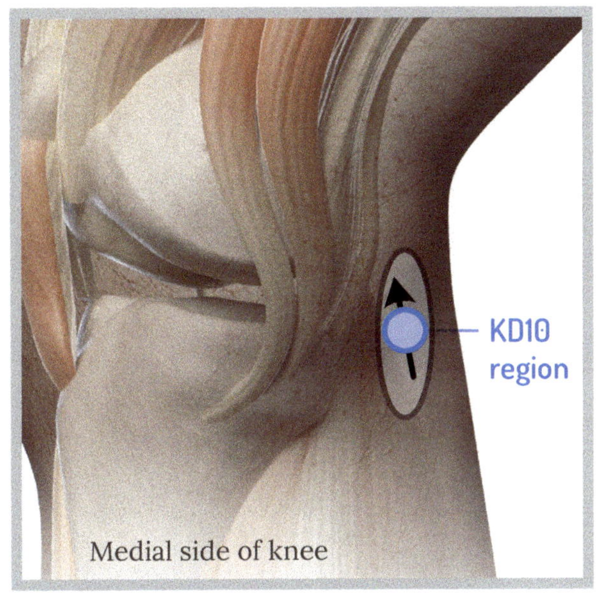

LUNG TONIFICATION ACUPOINTS:
SP3 (compare SP5 metal + SP9 water), LU9

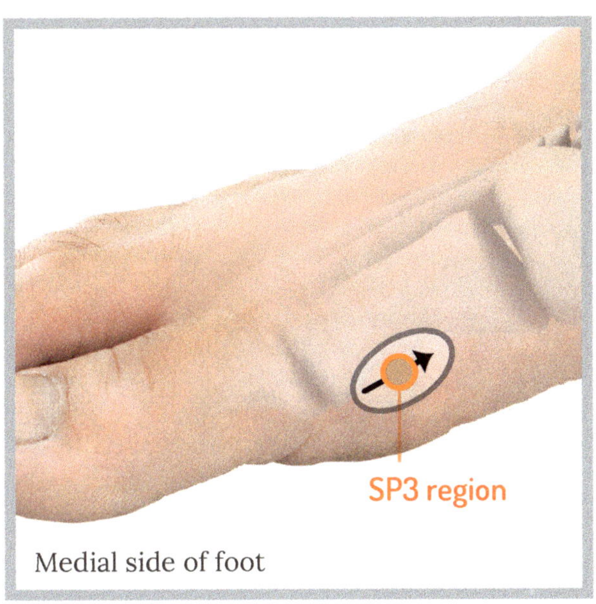

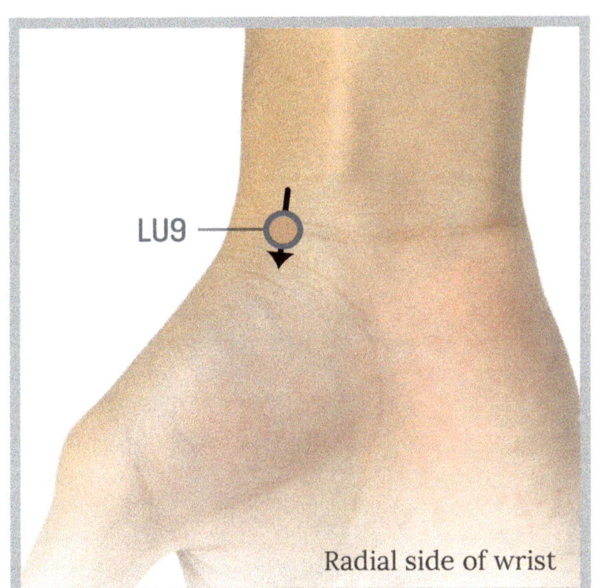

LARGE INTESTINE BALANCING ACUPOINTS:

LI5, LI3, **GB41** (compare GB44 metal + GB43 water), SI5

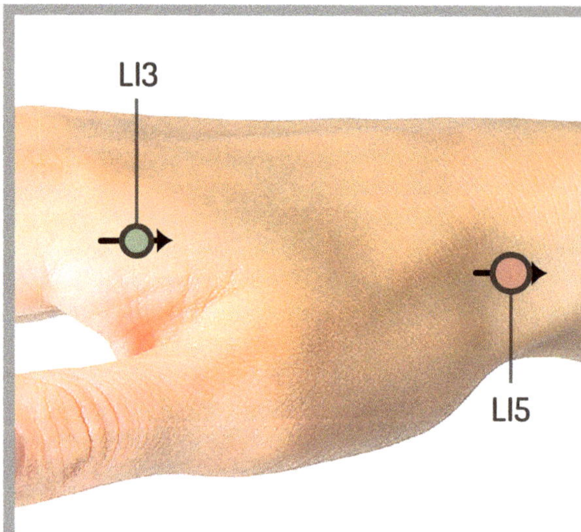

Radial side of hand

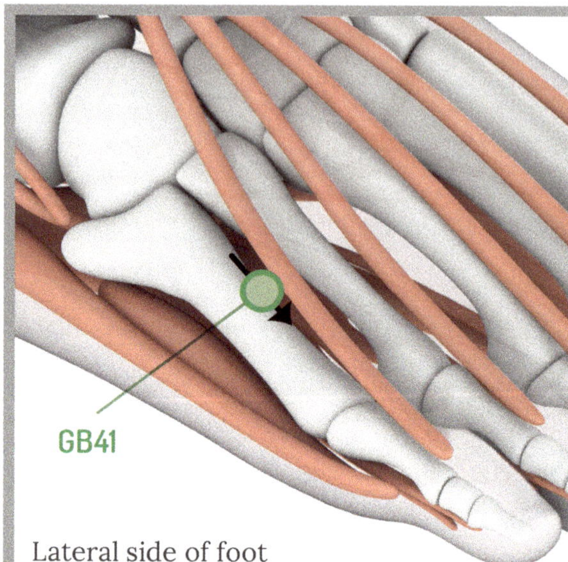

Lateral side of foot

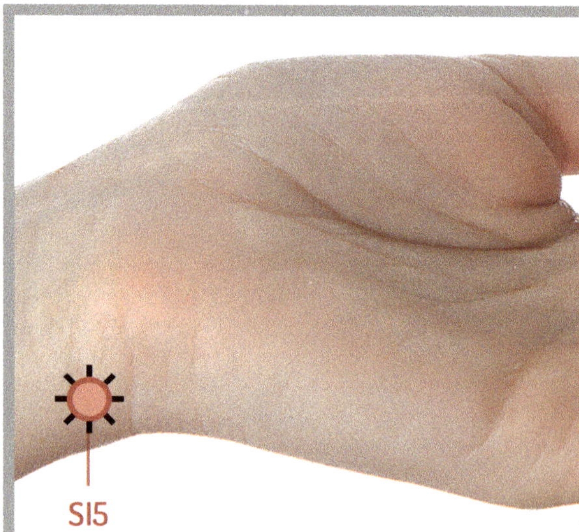

Ulnar side of wrist

LARGE INTESTINE SEDATION ACUPOINTS:
LI2, UB66

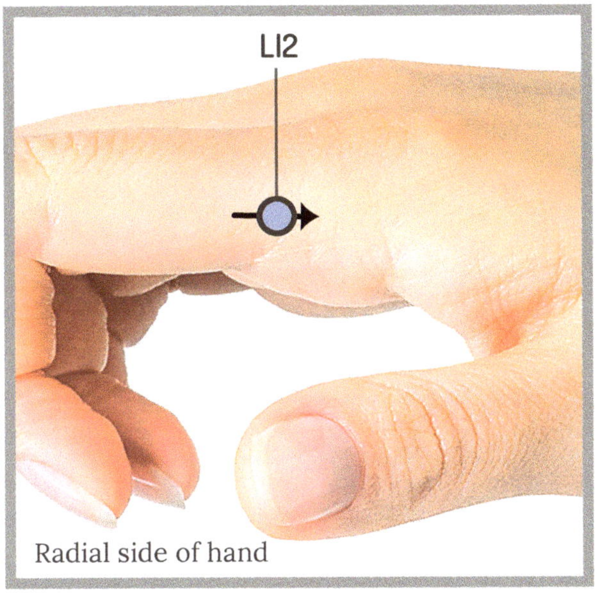

Radial side of hand

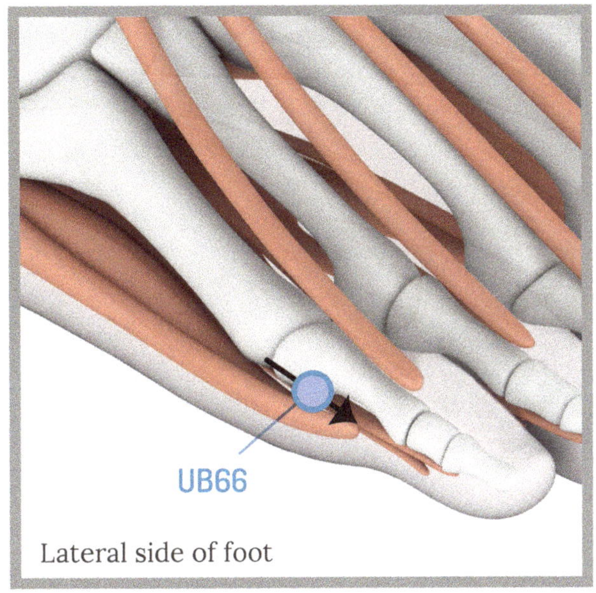

Lateral side of foot

LARGE INTESTINE TONIFICATION ACUPOINTS:
ST36 (compare ST45 metal + ST44water), LI11

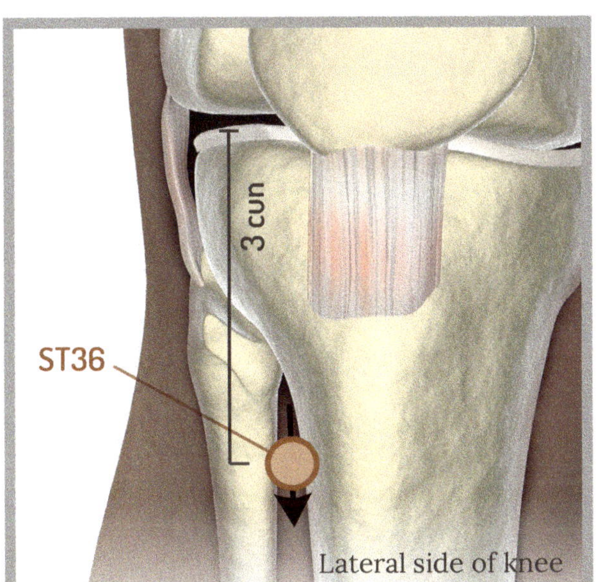

Lateral side of knee

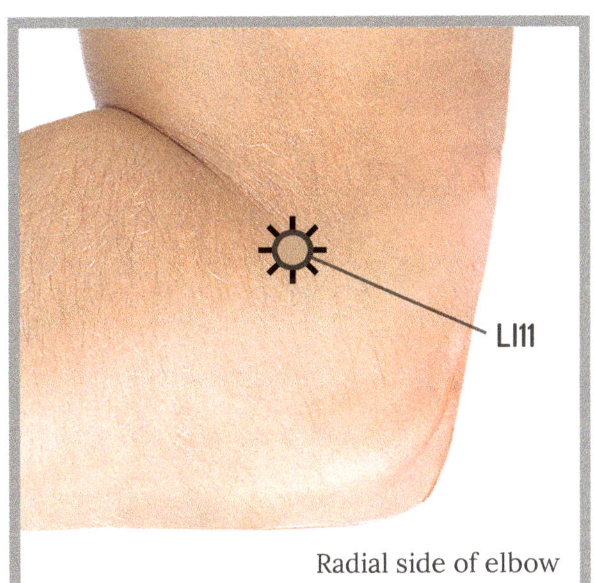

Radial side of elbow

STOMACH BALANCING ACUPOINTS:

ST43, ST44, UB66, **GB41** (compare GB44 metal + GB43 water)

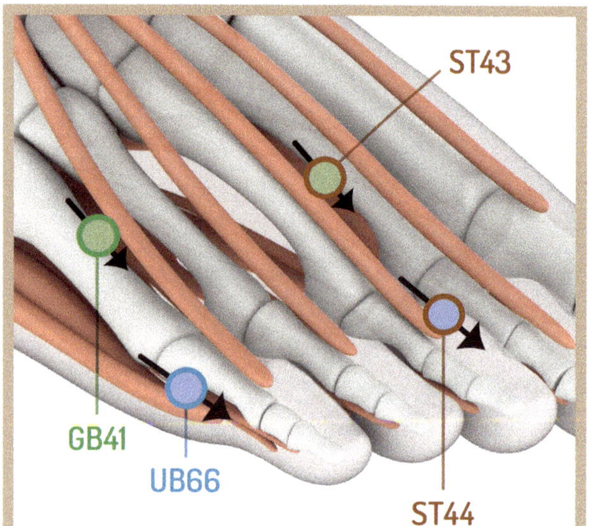

Dorsal side of foot

STOMACH SEDATION ACUPOINTS:
ST45, LI1

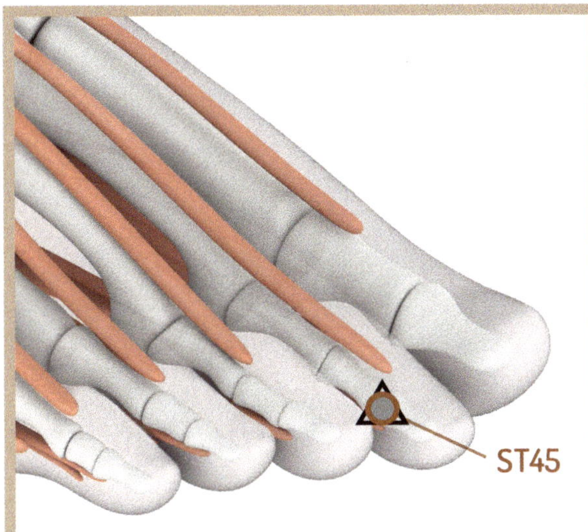

Lateral side of second toe

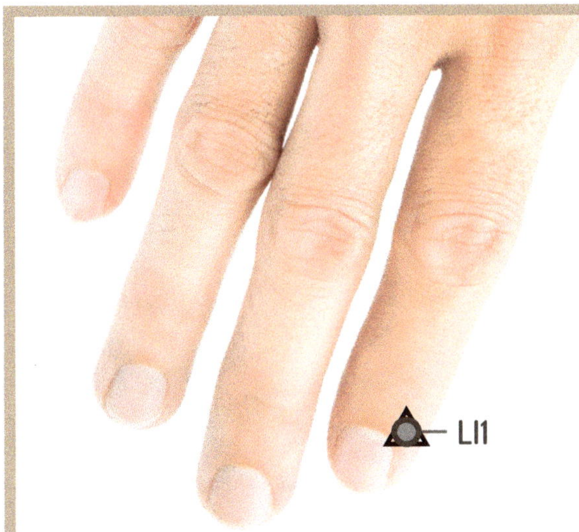

Radial side of index finger

STOMACH TONIFICATION ACUPOINTS:
SI5, ST41

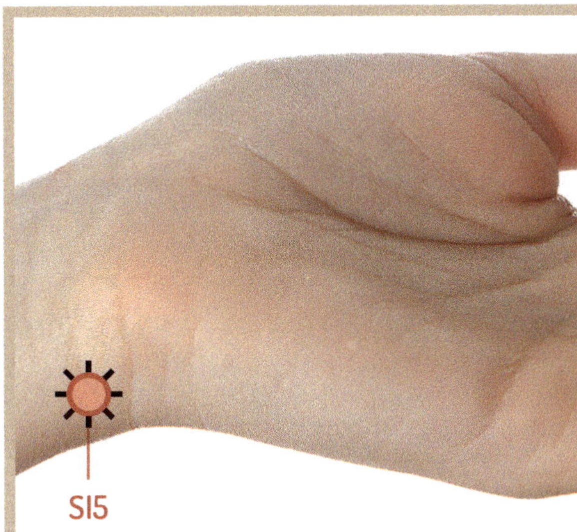

Ulnar side of wrist

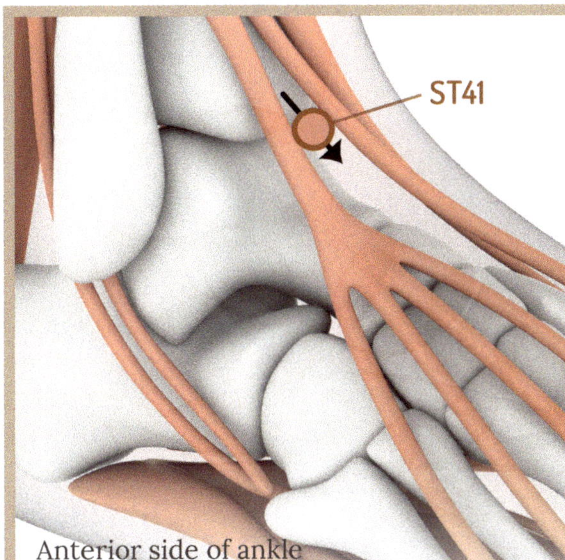

Anterior side of ankle

SPLEEN BALANCING ACUPOINTS:
SP1, SP9, LV1, KD10

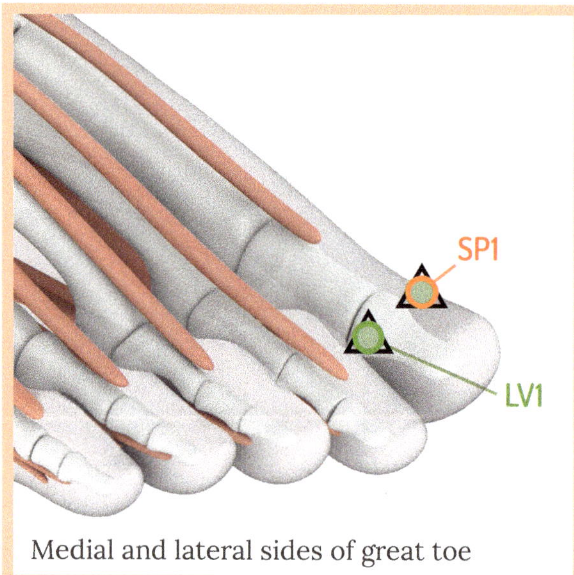

Medial and lateral sides of great toe

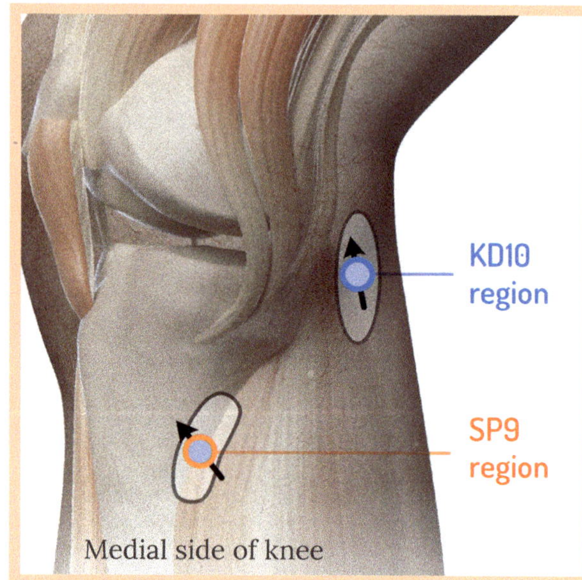

Medial side of knee

SPLEEN SEDATION ACUPOINTS:
SP5, LU8

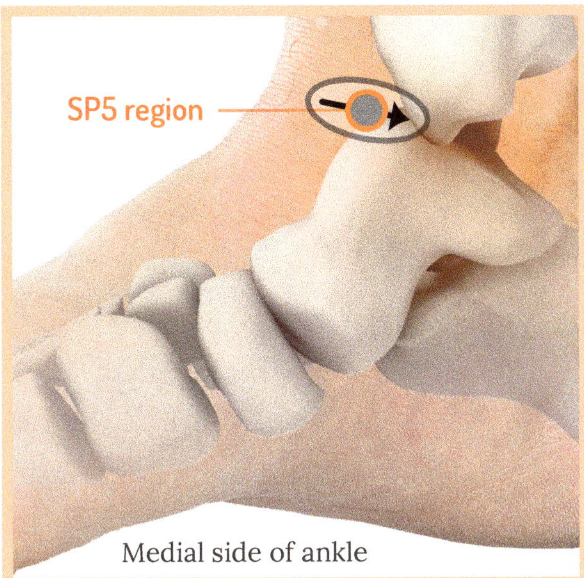

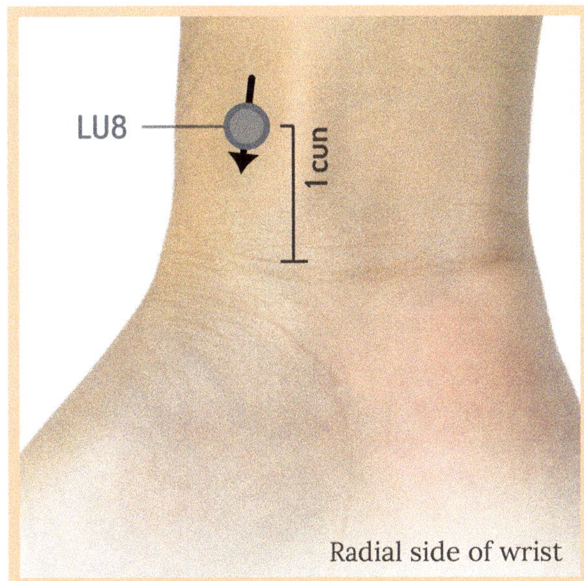

SPLEEN TONIFICATION ACUPOINTS:
HT8 (compare HT4 metal + HT3 water), SP2

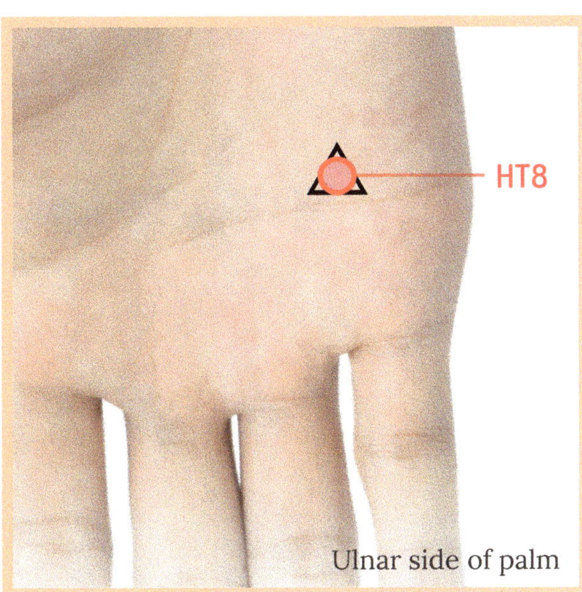

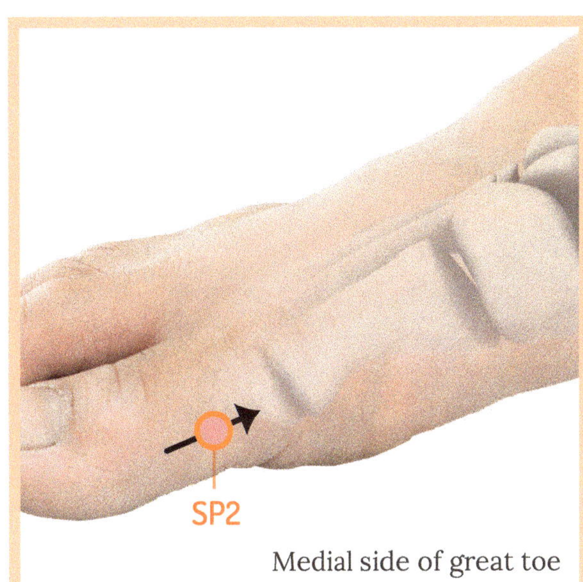

14.3.2 Acupoint Images for the Second Trisection

HEART BALANCING ACUPOINTS:
HT3, HT4, LU8, KD10

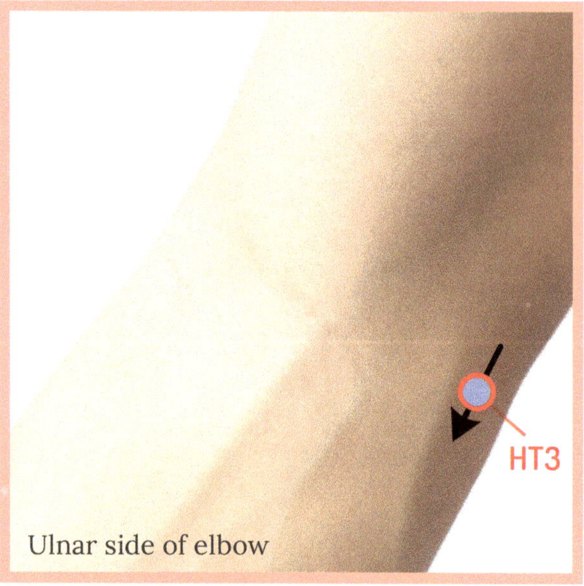

Ulnar side of elbow

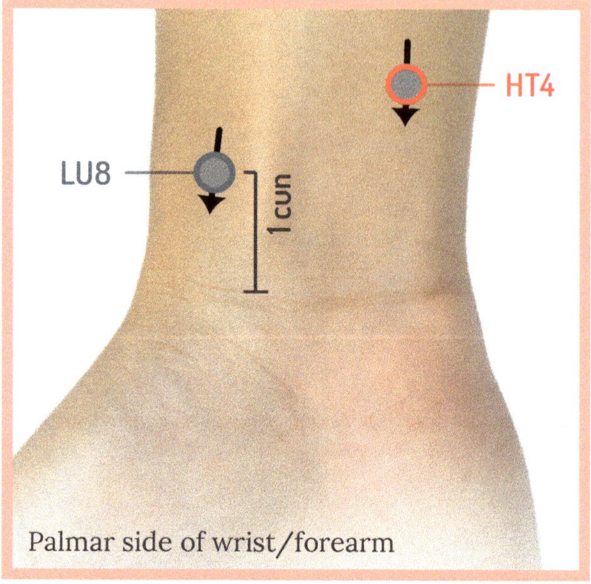

Palmar side of wrist/forearm

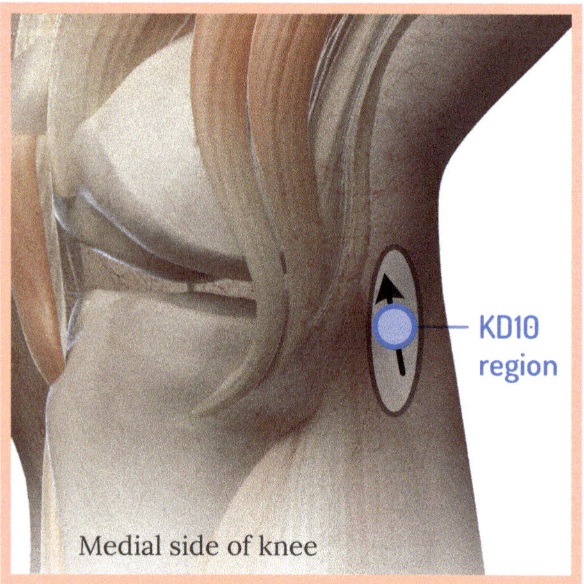

Medial side of knee

HEART SEDATION ACUPOINTS:
HT7, **SP3** (compare SP5 metal + SP9 water)

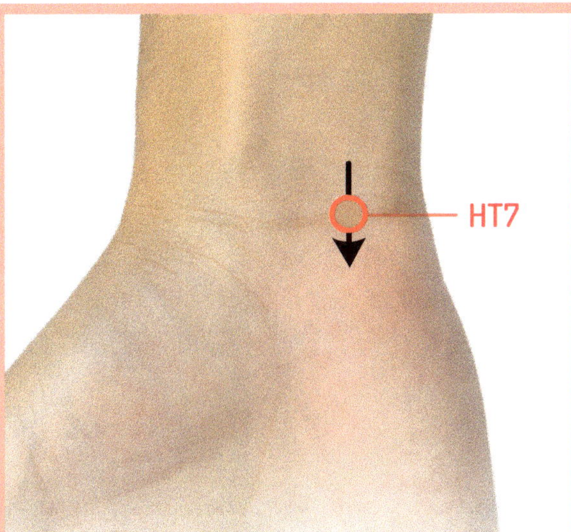

Ulnar side of wrist

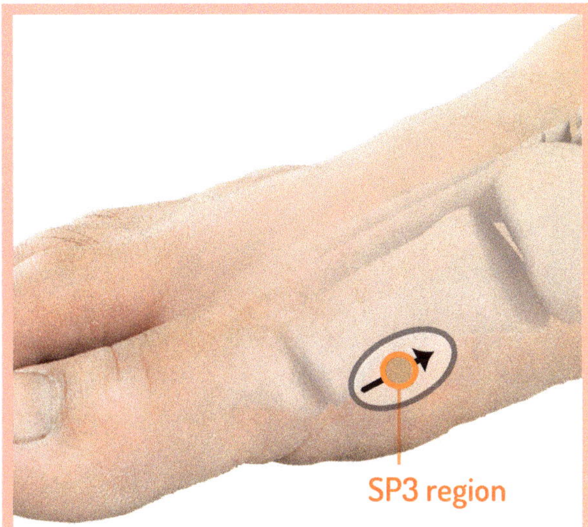

Medial side of foot

HEART TONIFICATION ACUPOINTS:
LV1, HT9

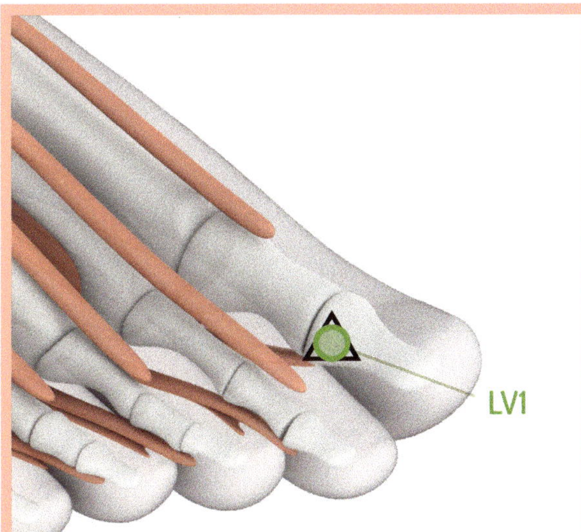

Lateral side of great toe

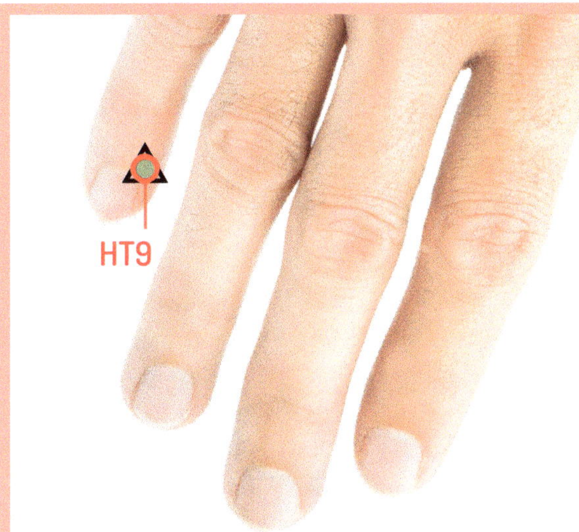

Radial side of little finger

SMALL INTESTINE BALANCING ACUPOINTS:
SI2, SI1, LI1, UB66

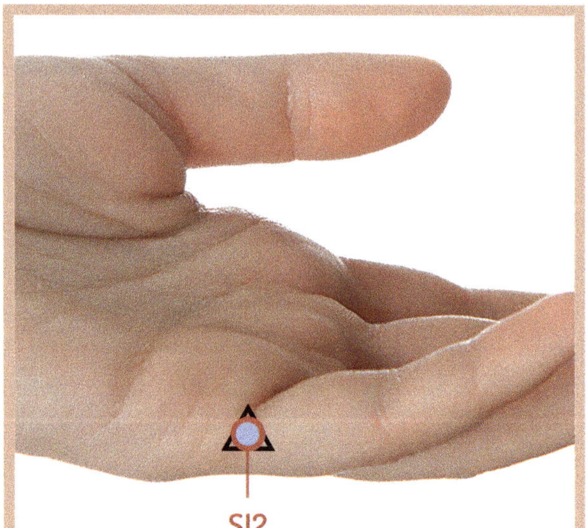

Ulnar side of hand

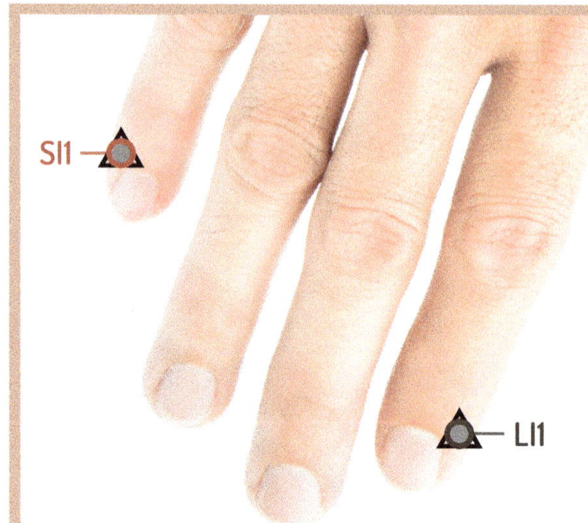

Dorsal side of fingers

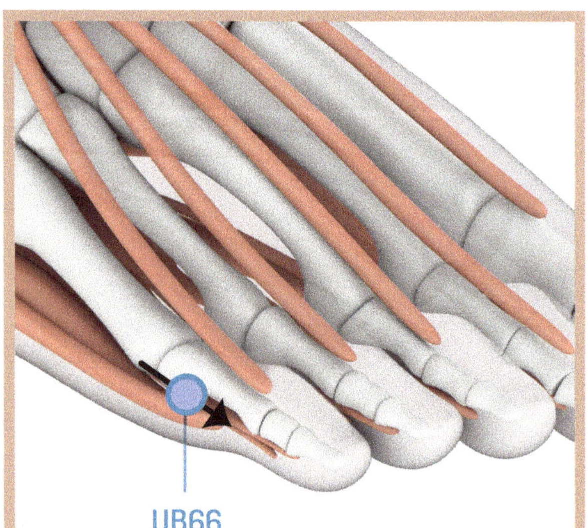

Lateral side of foot

SMALL INTESTINE SEDATION ACUPOINTS:

SI8, **ST36** (compare ST45 metal + ST44 water)

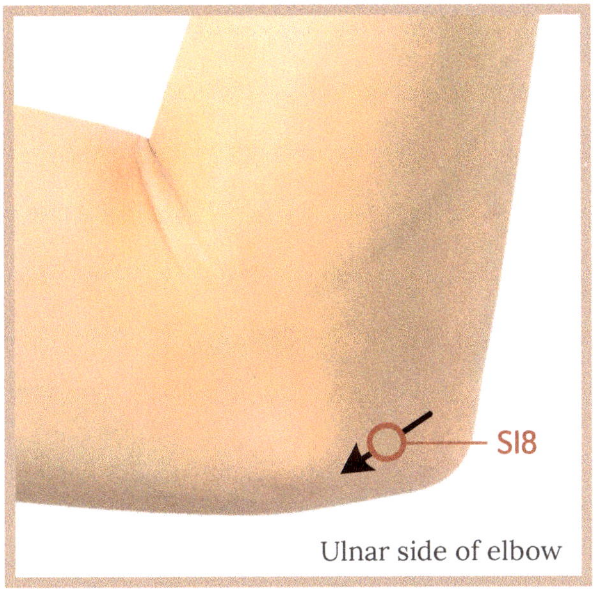

Ulnar side of elbow

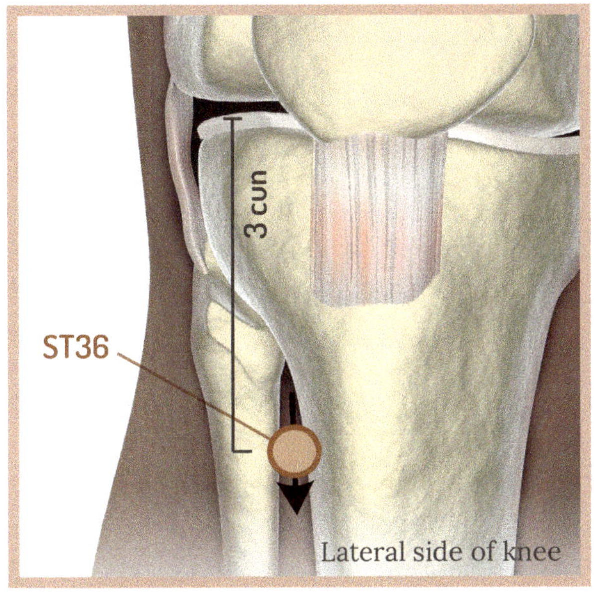

Lateral side of knee

SMALL INTESTINE TONIFICATION ACUPOINTS:

GB41 (compare GB44 metal + GB43 water), SI3

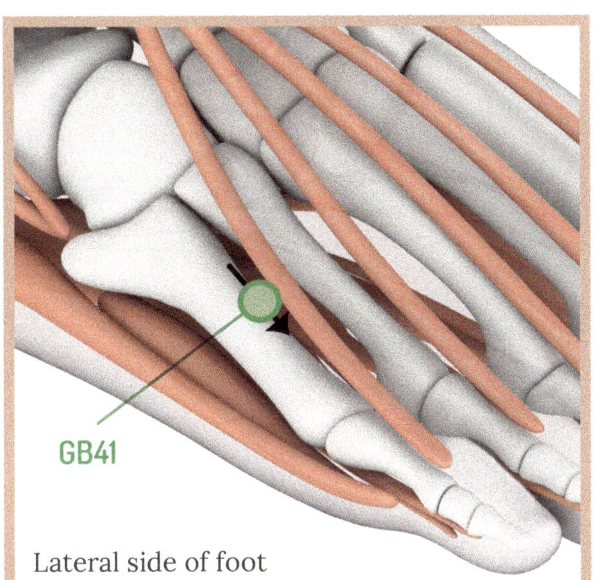

Lateral side of foot

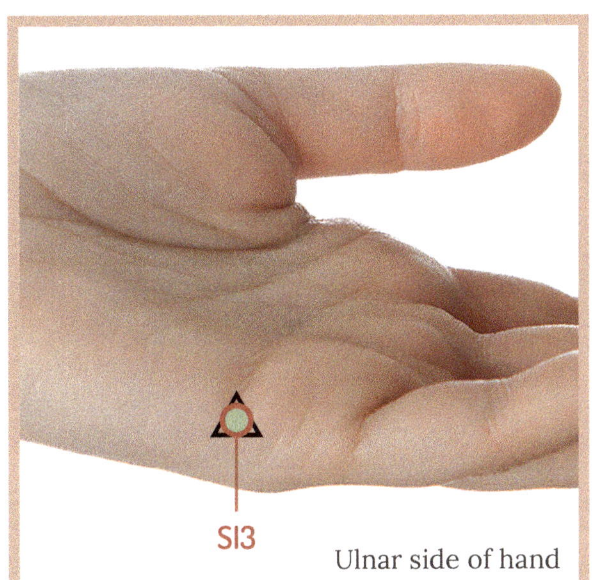

Ulnar side of hand

URINARY BLADDER BALANCING ACUPOINTS:
UB40, UB60, SI5, **ST36** (compare ST45 metal + ST44 water)

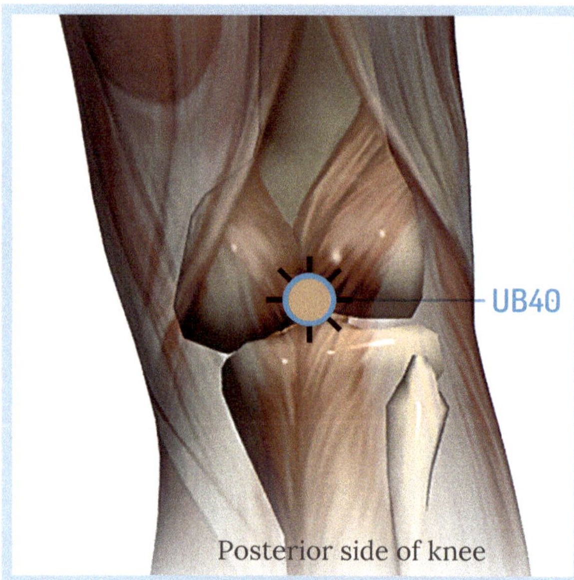

Posterior side of knee

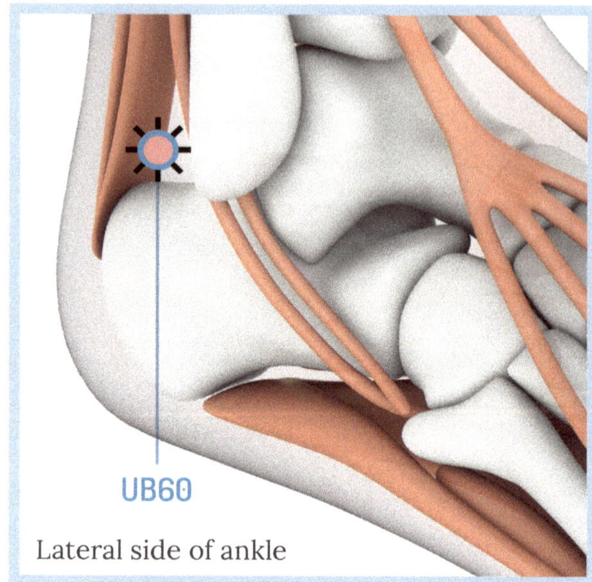

Lateral side of ankle

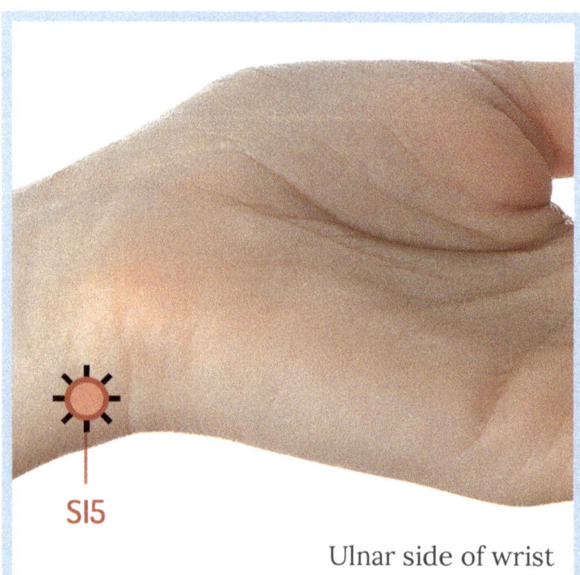

Ulnar side of wrist

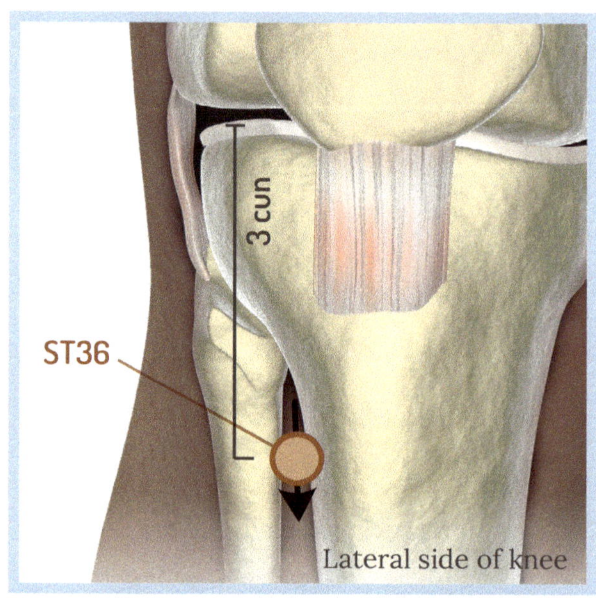

Lateral side of knee

URINARY BLADDER SEDATION ACUPOINTS:

UB65, **GB41** (compare GB44 metal + GB43 water)

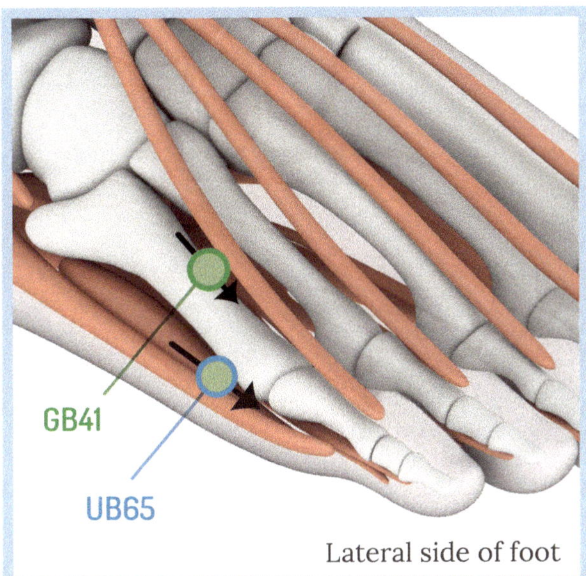

Lateral side of foot

URINARY BLADDER TONIFICATION ACUPOINTS:

LI1, UB67

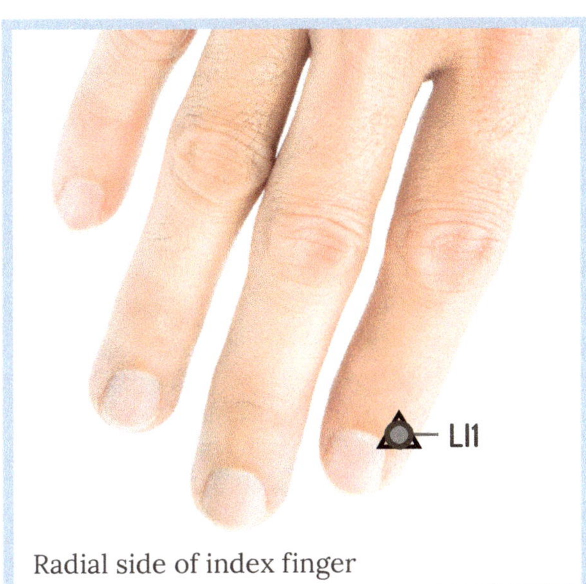

Radial side of index finger

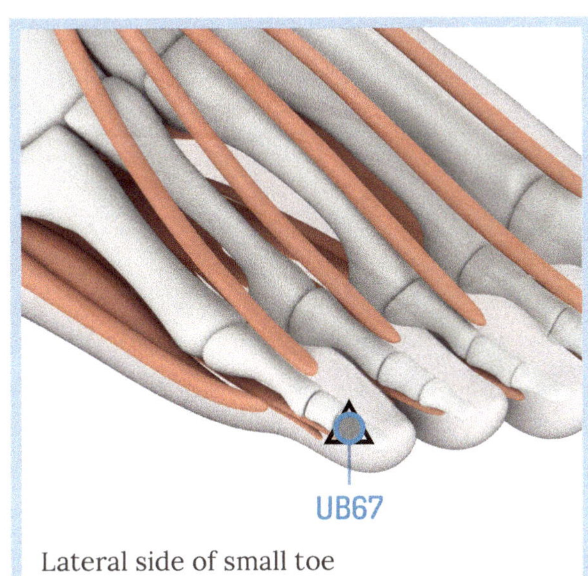

Lateral side of small toe

KIDNEY BALANCING ACUPOINTS:

KD3, KD2, **HT8** (compare HT4 metal + HT3 water),
SP3 (compare SP5 metal + SP9 water)

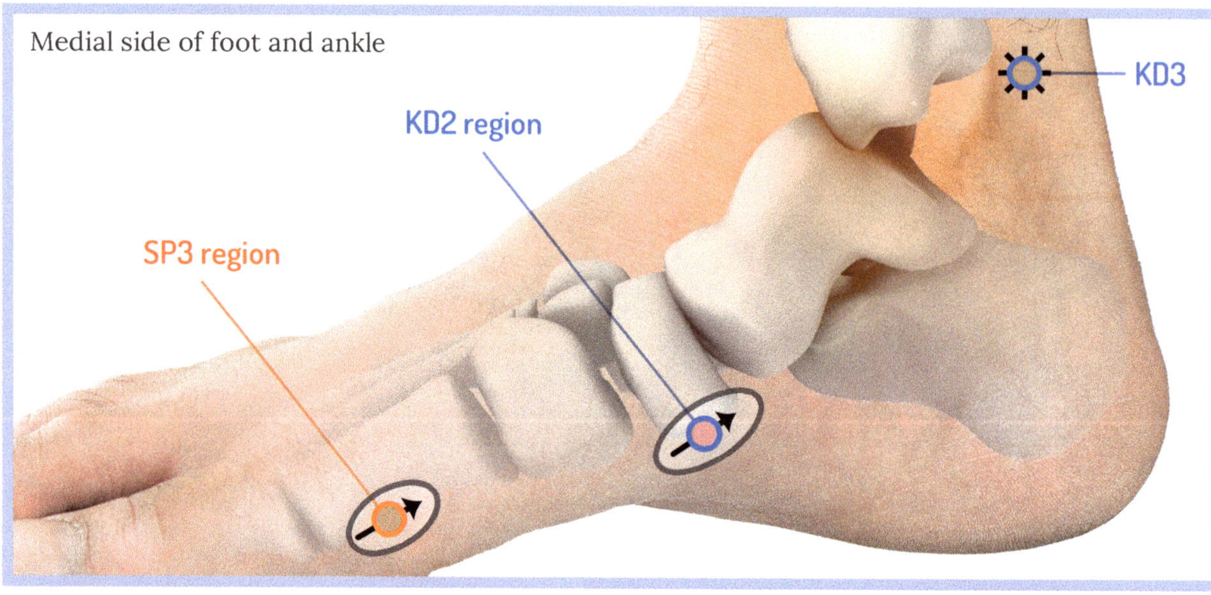

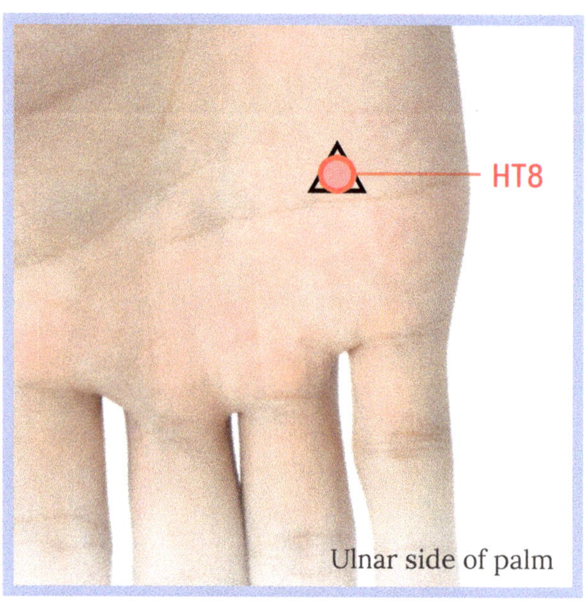

KIDNEY SEDATION ACUPOINTS:
KD1, LV1

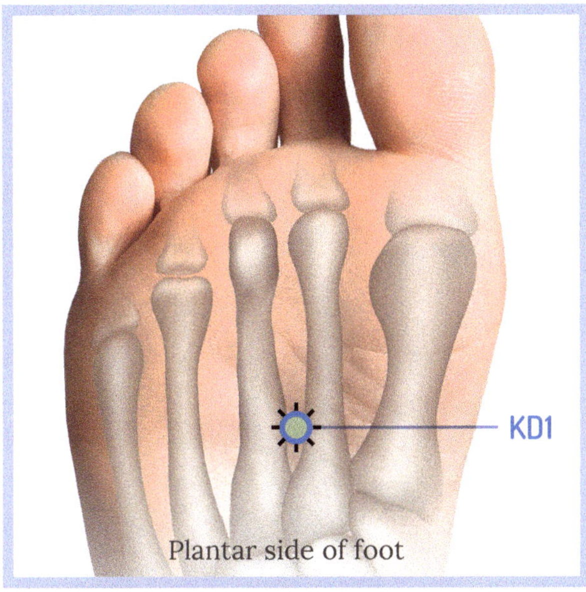

Plantar side of foot

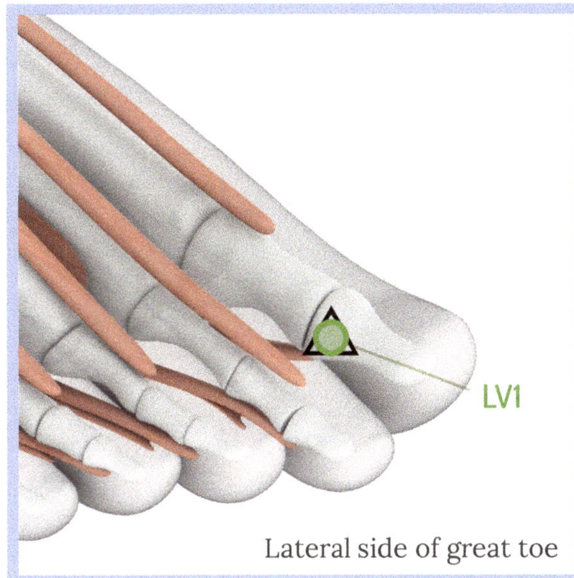

Lateral side of great toe

KIDNEY TONIFICATION ACUPOINTS:
LU8, KD7

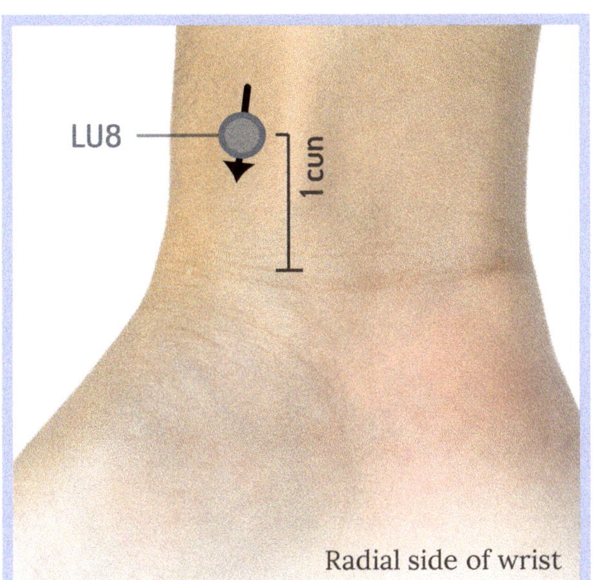

Radial side of wrist

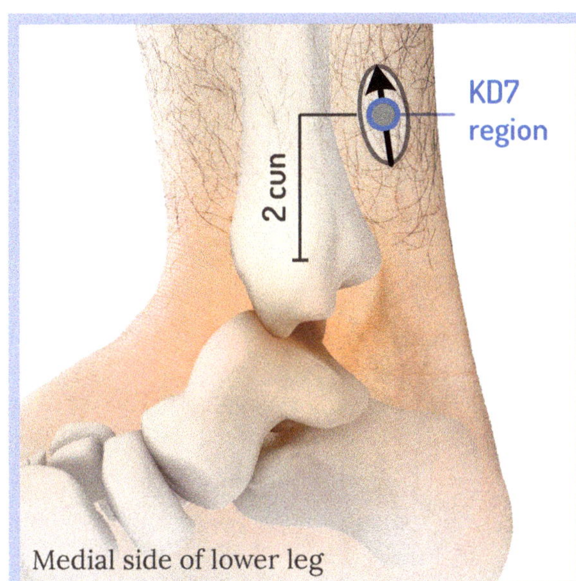

Medial side of lower leg

14.3.3 Acupoint Images for the Third Trisection

PERICARDIUM BALANCING ACUPOINTS:
PC3, PC5, LU8, KD10

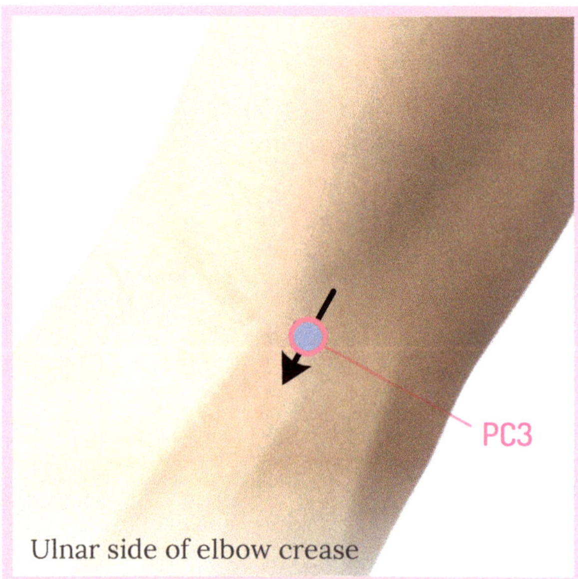

Ulnar side of elbow crease

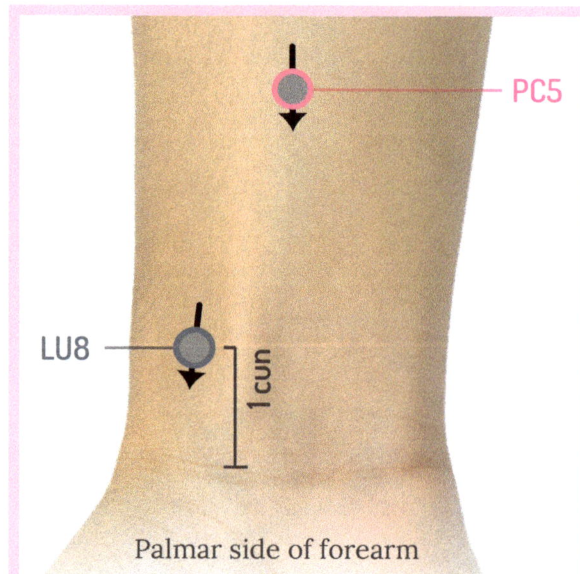

Palmar side of forearm

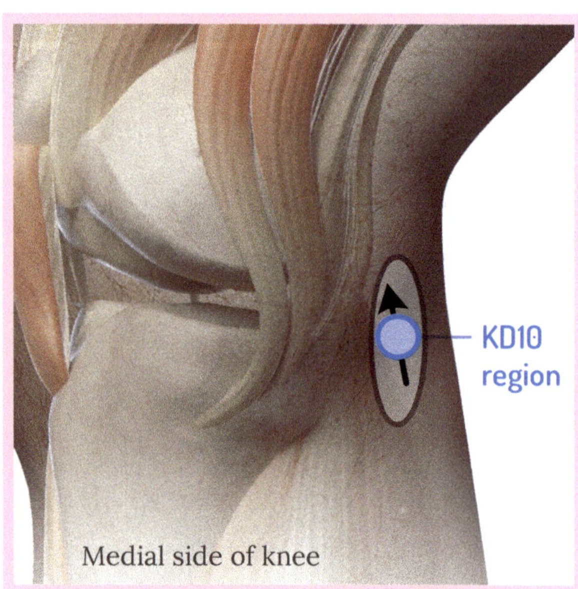

Medial side of knee

PERICARDIUM SEDATION ACUPOINTS:
PC7, **SP3** (compare SP5 metal + SP9 water)

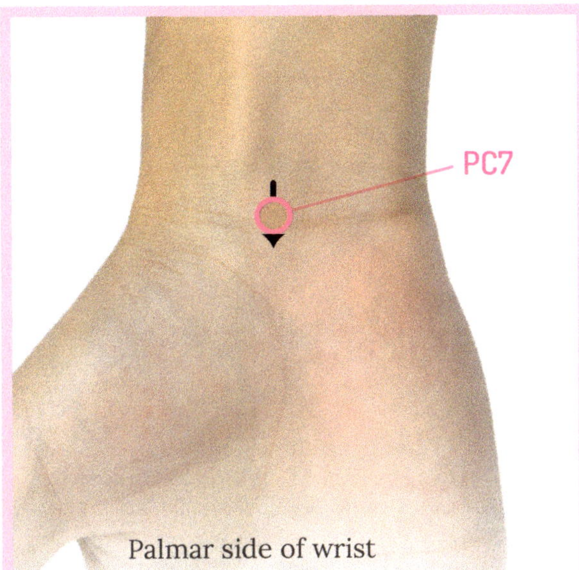

Palmar side of wrist

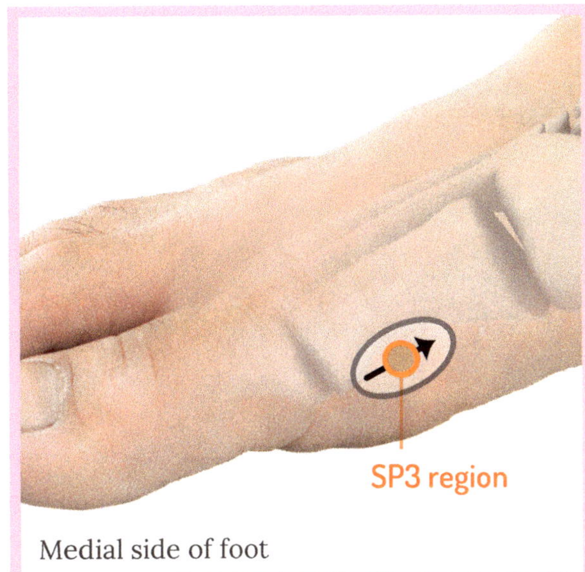

Medial side of foot

PERICARDIUM TONIFICATION ACUPOINTS:
LV1, PC9

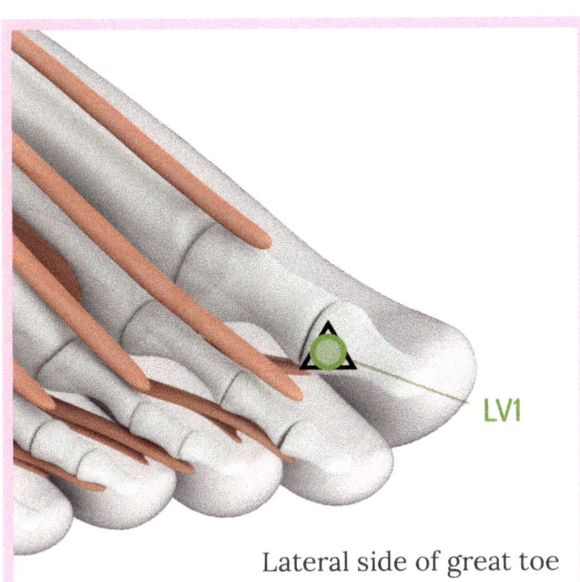

Lateral side of great toe

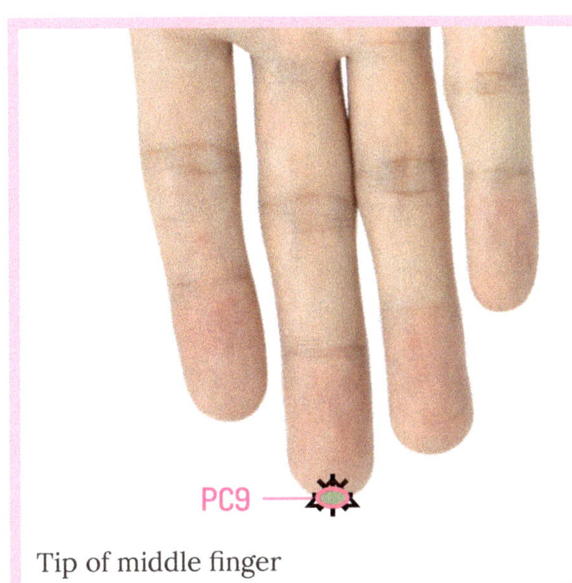

Tip of middle finger

TRIPLE BURNER BALANCING ACUPOINTS:
TB2, TB1, ST45, UB66

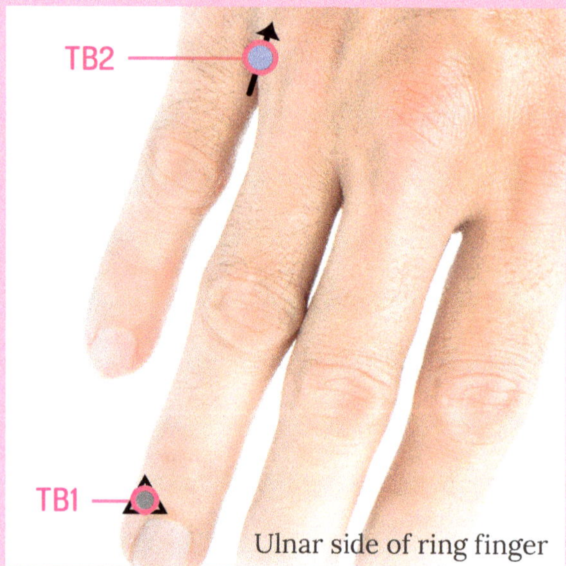

Ulnar side of ring finger

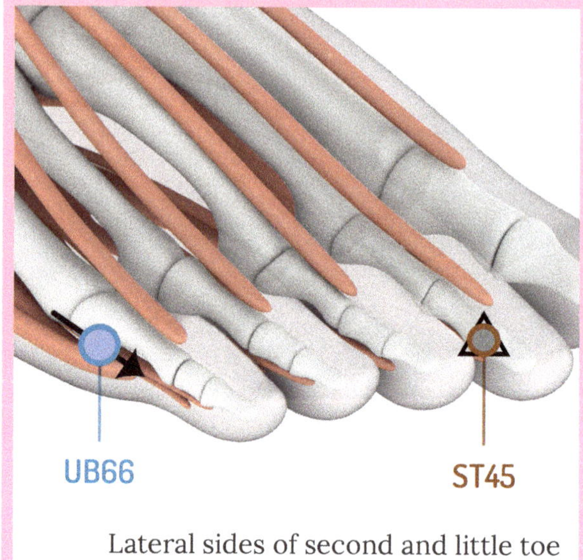

Lateral sides of second and little toe

TRIPLE BURNER SEDATION ACUPOINTS:

TB10, **ST36** (compare ST45 metal + ST44 water)

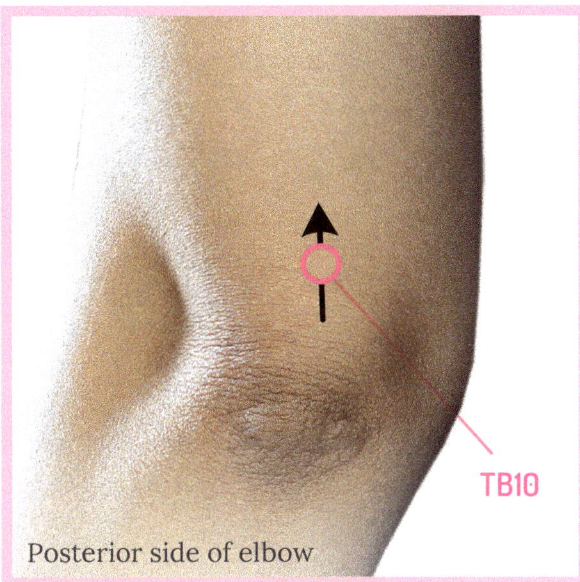

Posterior side of elbow

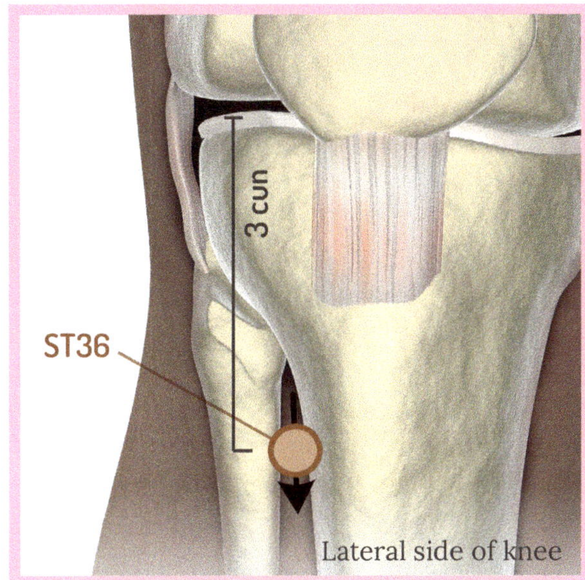

Lateral side of knee

TRIPLE BURNER TONIFICATION ACUPOINTS:

GB41 (compare GB44 metal + GB43 water), TB3

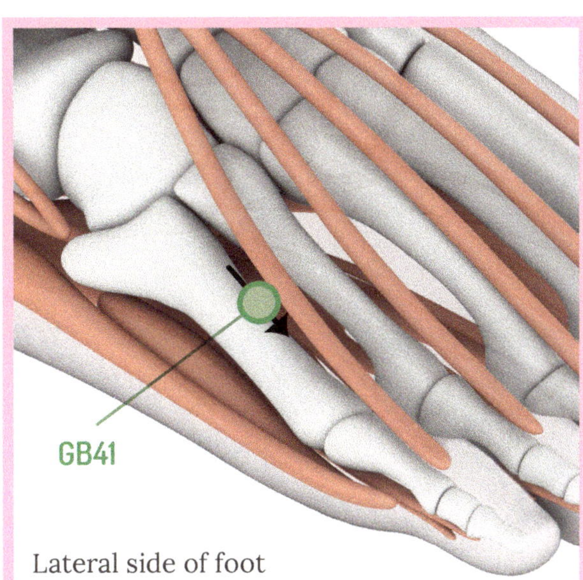

Lateral side of foot

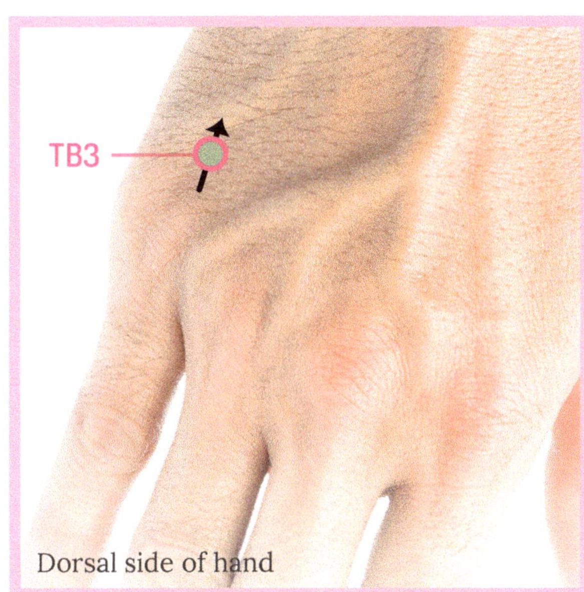

Dorsal side of hand

GALLBLADDER BALANCING ACUPOINTS:

GB44, GB34, **ST36** (compare ST45 metal + ST44 water), LI1

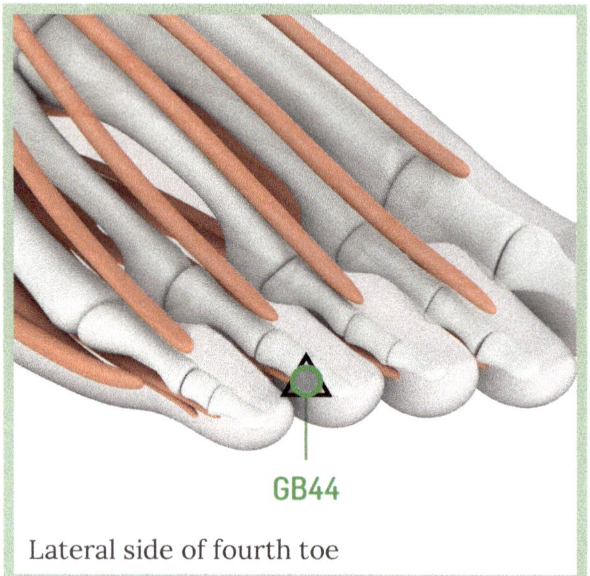

Lateral side of fourth toe

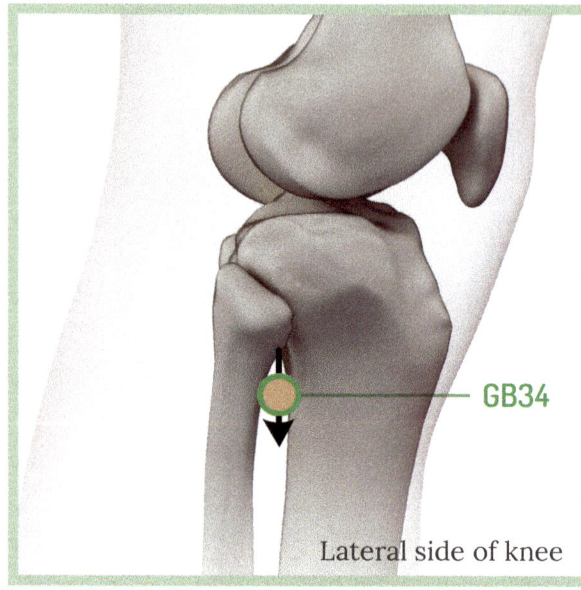

Lateral side of knee

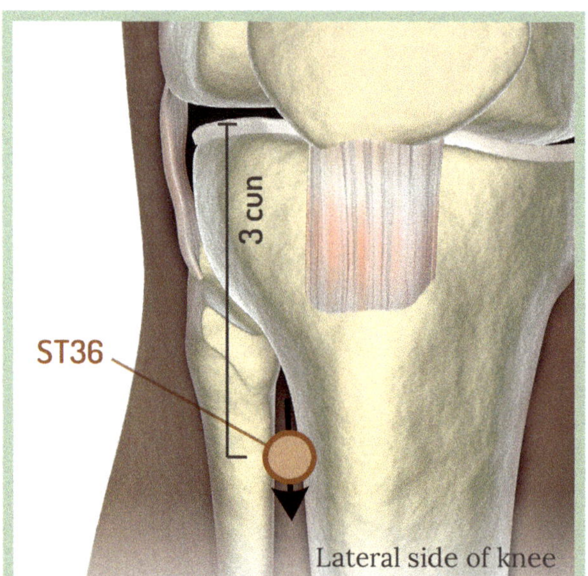

Lateral side of knee

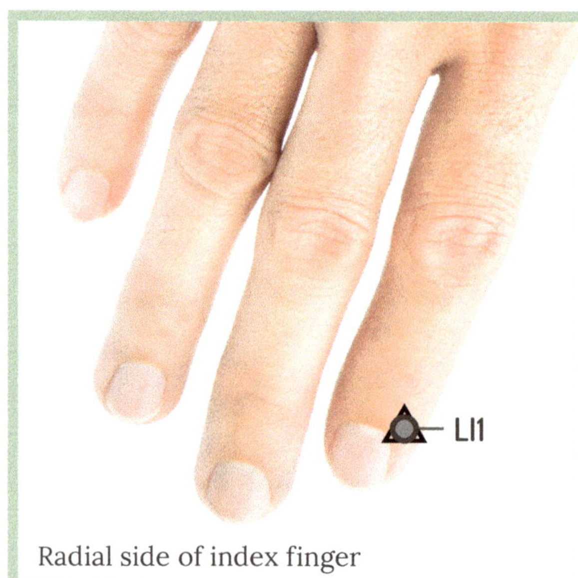

Radial side of index finger

GALLBLADDER SEDATION ACUPOINTS:
GB38, SI5

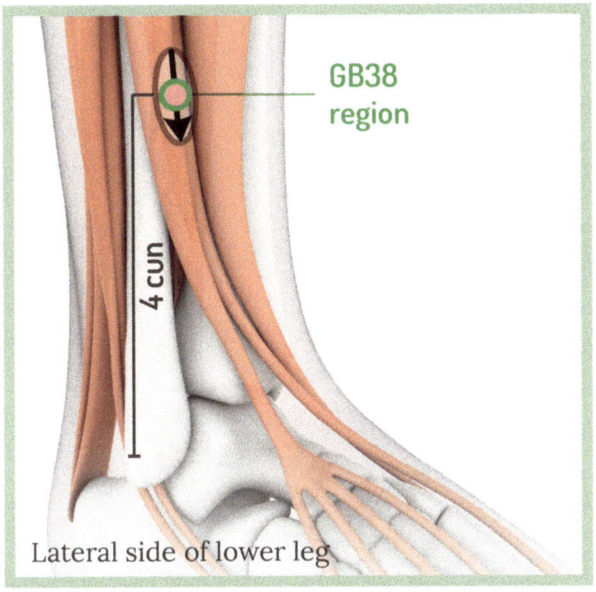

Lateral side of lower leg

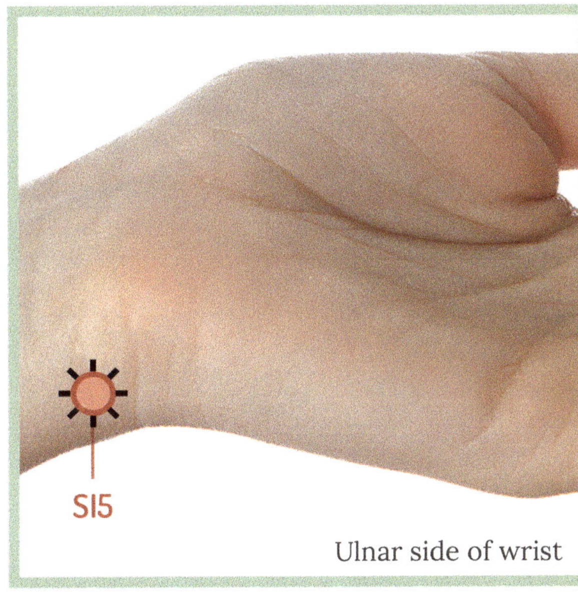

Ulnar side of wrist

GALLBLADDER TONIFICATION ACUPOINTS:
UB66, GB43

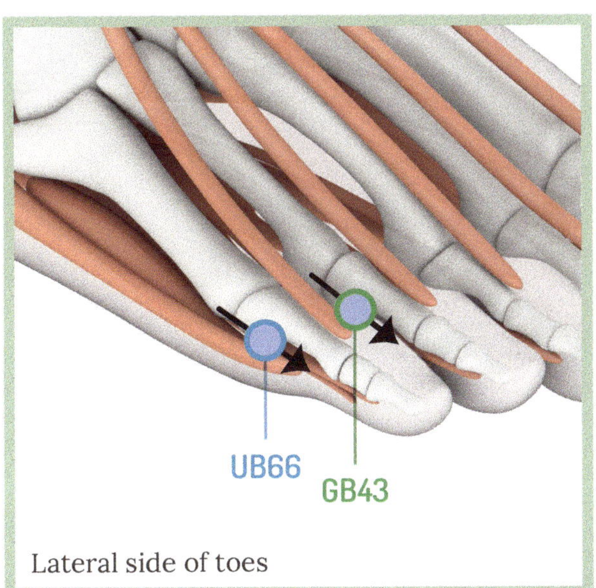

Lateral side of toes

LIVER BALANCING ACUPOINTS:
LV4, LV3, **SP3** (compare SP5 metal + SP9 water), LU8

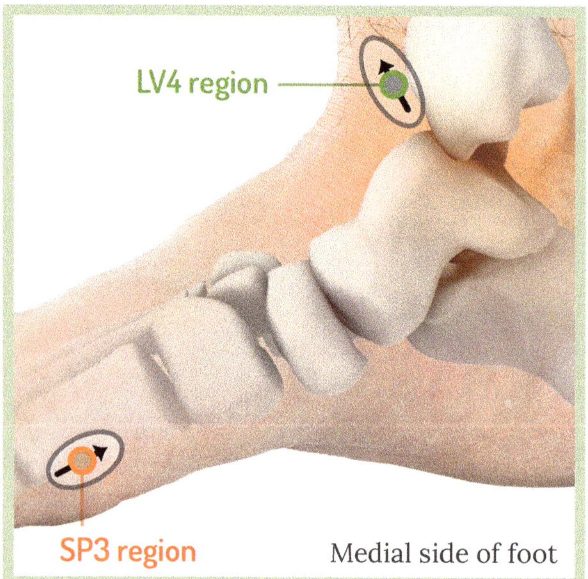

Medial side of foot

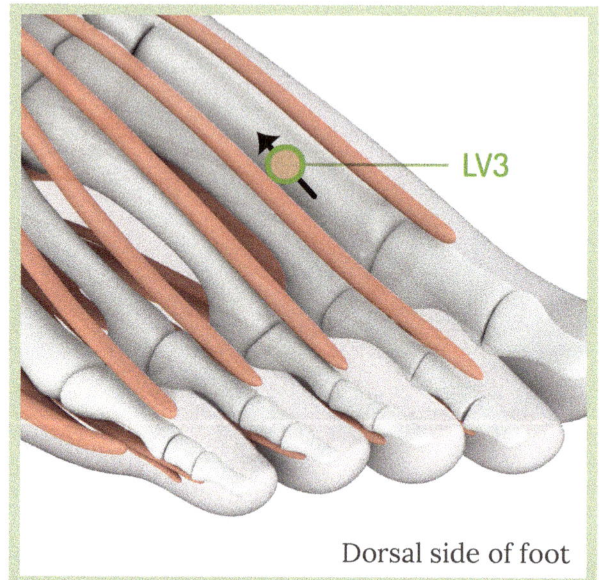

Dorsal side of foot

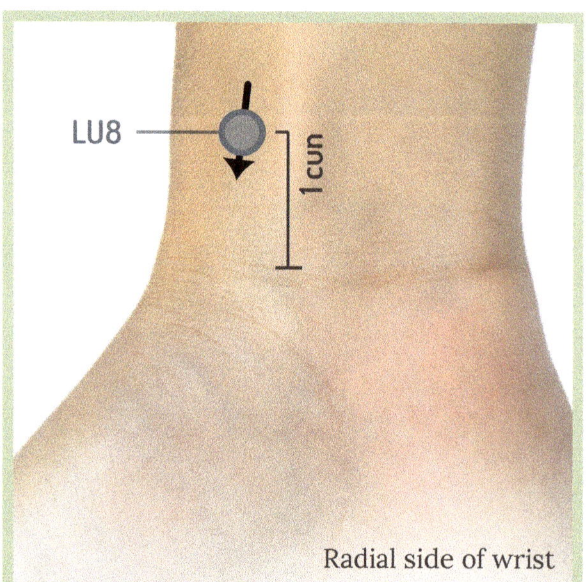

Radial side of wrist

LIVER SEDATION ACUPOINTS:
LV2, **HT8** (compare HT4 metal + HT3 water)

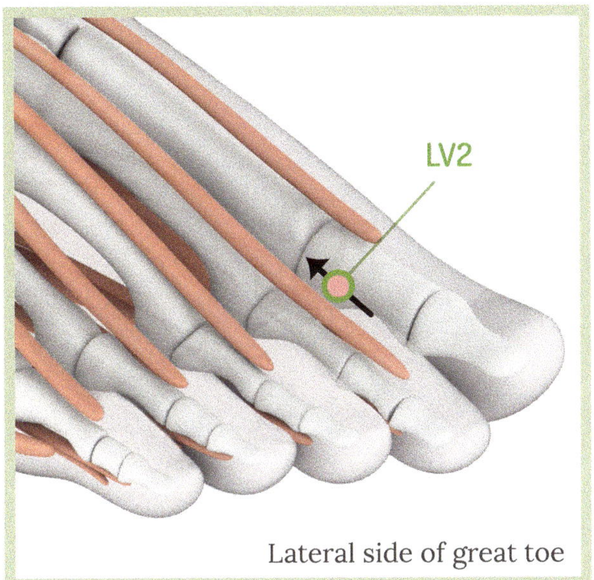

Lateral side of great toe

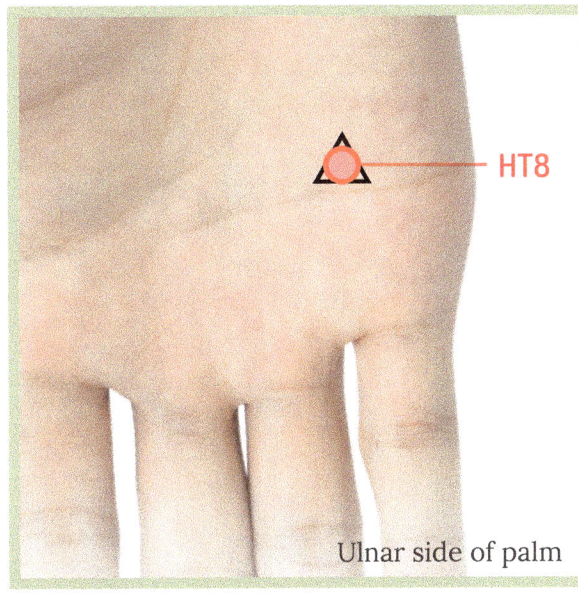

Ulnar side of palm

LIVER TONIFICATION ACUPOINTS:
KD10, LV8

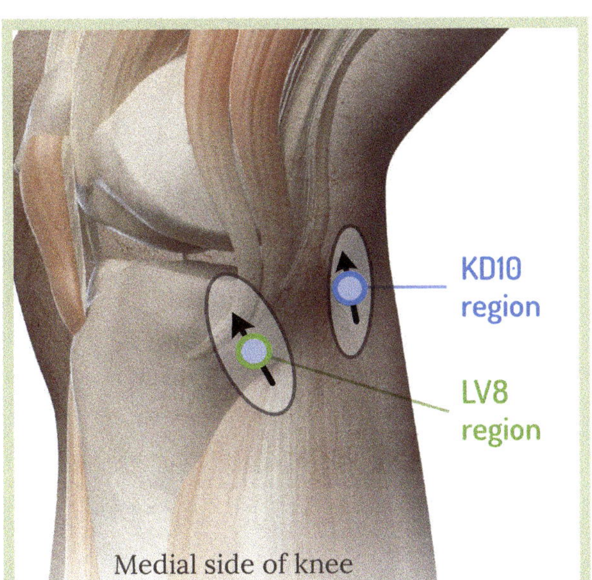

Medial side of knee

CHAPTER 15

Supporting Acupoints

Supporting acupoints enhance the Body-Feedback prescriptions, resolve pathogenic heat, integrate the extra-vessels, and address musculoskeletal symptoms. The precise combination of shu-points that create the Body-Feedback balancing, sedation, and tonification prescriptions restricts the selection of supporting acupoints to maintain the five-element root treatment approach. Always test the supporting acupoints to the pulse, master alarm points, or the root's organ/meridian referral areas and muscle associations to determine which ones are beneficial.

The supporting acupoints categories include:

- metal + water shu-points to clear pathogenic heat;
- extra-vessel controlling and linking points to support genetic and spiritual health challenges;
- xi-cleft points to treat acute trauma, pain, endocrine disorders, and the nervous system;
- luo-connecting points to harmonize the five-element pairs, unite the yin and yang meridians, and treat the extremities;
- yuan-source points on the yang meridians to strengthen qi and expel pathogens; and
- ashi points for pain, neuropathy, and musculoskeletal symptoms.

Common acceptable supporting acupoints located on the arms and legs include metal and water shu-points, along with non-shu acupoints on meridians other than those in a root acupoint prescription. On the abdomen, head, and back, supporting acupoints can come from the root treatment's meridian and its five-element pair. For instance, a root liver sedation treatment that includes LV2, LV3, LV4, SP5, SP9 (metal + water combination instead of **SP3**), **HT8**, LU8, and LU5 (additional water shu-point) avoids other acupoints on the arms and legs for the liver, spleen, heart, lung, and gallbladder meridians. The treatment may include additional supporting acupoints such as GB14, GB8, GB25, SP15, ST25, or ST3 on the head, back, and abdomen.

Test the supporting acupoints after needling the root balancing and sedation or tonification prescriptions. Any supporting acupoint that can disrupt the energy flow of the meridians included in the root Body-Feedback prescription will test negatively. Avoid the acupoints on the extremities for the root's five element pair except for the metal + water combination when pathogenic heat is present.

The metal + water combination, extra-vessel, xi-cleft, luo-connecting, and yuan-source point designations strongly support the root Body-Feedback treatments. Check these possible supporting acupoints for meridians not included in the root Body-Feedback prescription or its five-element pair. Test ashi acupoints last to address pain and musculoskeletal symptoms. For example, check SP4, SP6, and SP8 with Body-Feedback prescriptions other than a root stomach treatment and those not containing spleen shu-points.

15.1 Metal + Water Acupoints to Resolve Pathogenic Heat

The metal + water shu-point combinations are the most common supporting points added to the root Body-Feedback prescriptions. The metal + water combination resolves pathogenic heat in non-root organs and meridians, which can hinder the effectiveness of the five-element root treatment approach.

The steps for adding supporting acupoints from the metal and water shu-point categories include:

1. First, identify any unpaired water or metal shu-points already included in the balancing, sedation, or tonification prescriptions, and test the additional water or metal acupoint.
2. Second, recheck the individual radial pulse positions looking for any remaining wiry or forceful qualities. Test the metal + water combination for the meridians associated with those pulse positions.
3. Third, check the metal + water combination for any meridians traveling through areas of pain, discomfort, or musculoskeletal symptoms.
4. Finally, test the metal + water combination for the root treatment's five-element pair.

For example, a female client who has food allergies, temporal headaches, pain with her menstrual period, and Hashimoto's autoimmune thyroid disease tested favorably for a symmetrical liver sedation prescription. The root balancing treatment consisted of LV4, LV3, SP5, SP9, (metal + water combination instead of **SP3**), and LU8. The sedation prescription added LV2 and HT4 + HT3 (metal + water combination instead of **HT8**). This client tested favorably for the supporting acupoint LU5 (the water shu-point), which combined with LU8 (the metal shu-point) to release pathogenic heat from the lung organ/meridian (addressed the immune system dysfunction).

After needling the above points, rechecking the individual pulse positions found a wiry and forceful quality in the third pulse position (*chi*) on the right (ministerial-fire element). The metal + water shu-point combination for the triple burner (TB1 + TB2) tested favorably by further releasing tightness in the neck muscles.

The gallbladder metal + water combination (GB44 + GB43) further released tightness in the neck muscles and directly addressed her temporal headaches. The urinary bladder (UB67 + UB66) and stomach meridian (ST44 + ST43) metal + water combinations were checked to the neck muscles because of their proximity to the thyroid and head pain; however, these acupoints were not used in treatment because they caused tightness in the neck muscles.

LU8 METAL + LU5 WATER

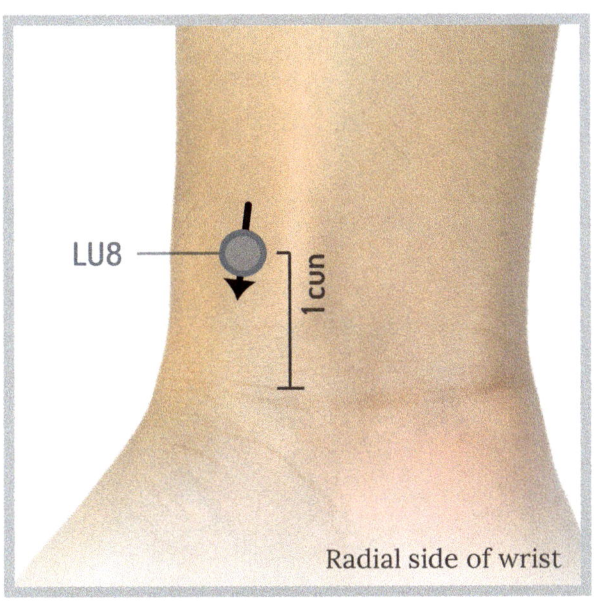

Radial side of wrist

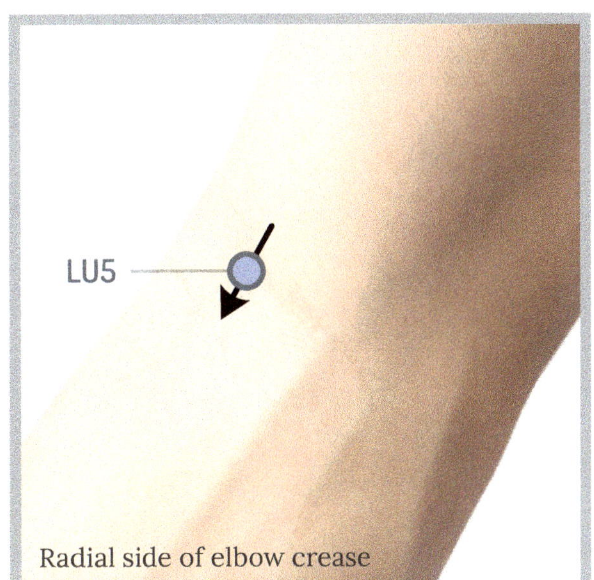

Radial side of elbow crease

LI1 METAL + LI2 WATER

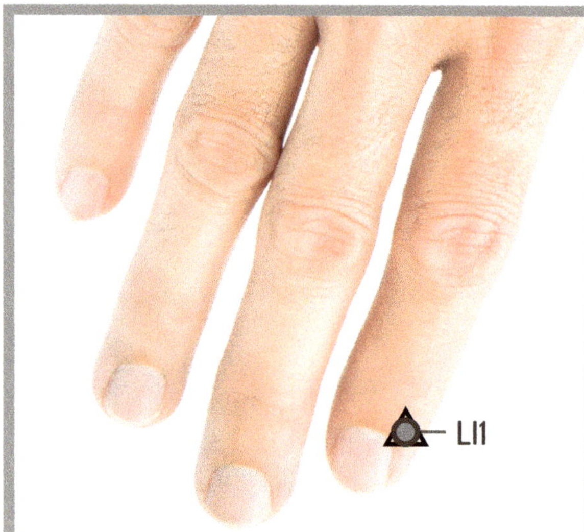

Radial side of index finger

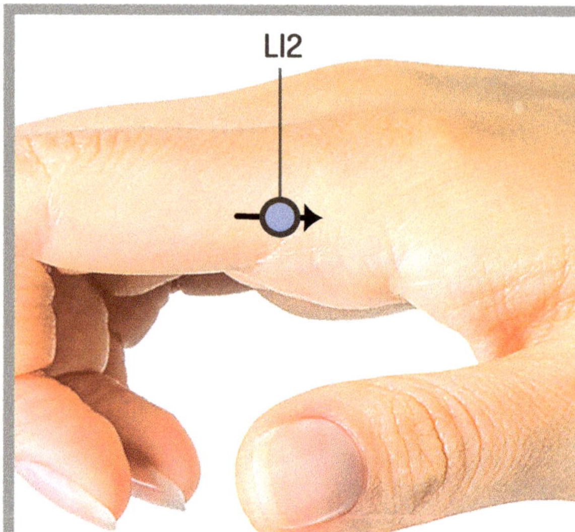

Radial side of hand

ST45 METAL + ST44 WATER

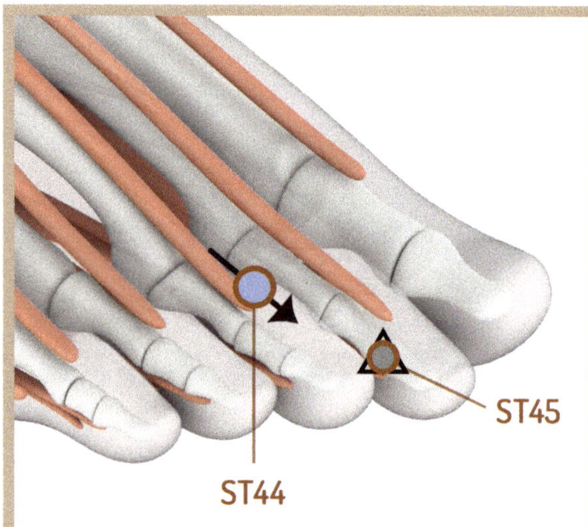

Lateral side of second toe

SP5 METAL + SP9 WATER

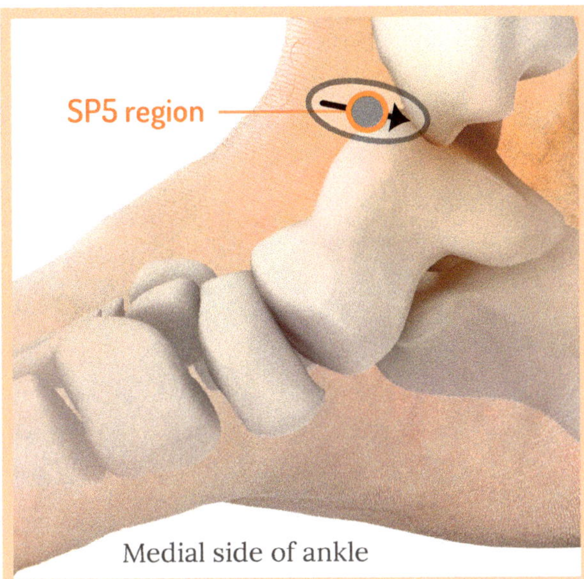

Medial side of ankle

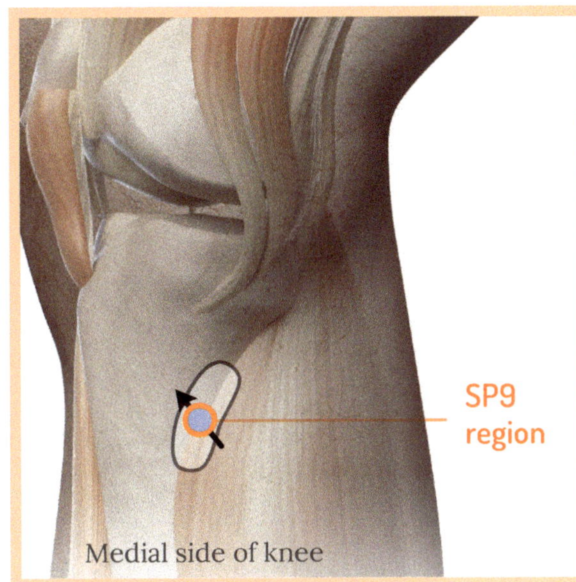

Medial side of knee

HT4 METAL + HT3 WATER

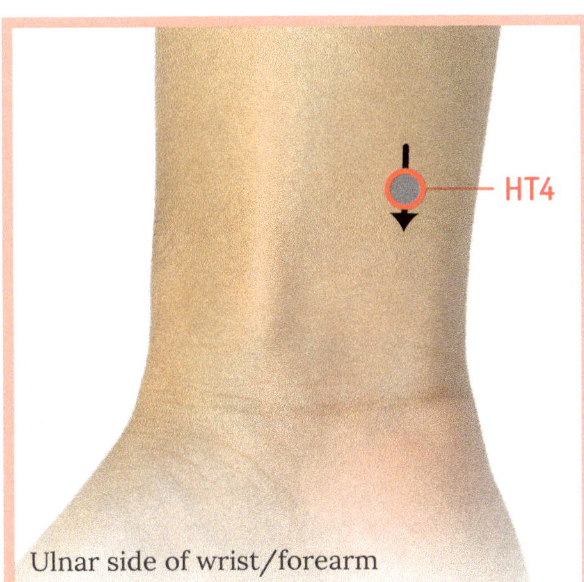

Ulnar side of wrist/forearm

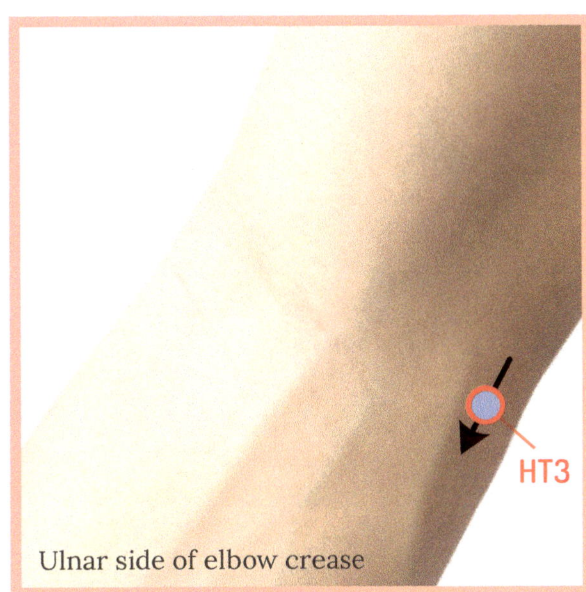

Ulnar side of elbow crease

SI1 METAL + SI2 WATER

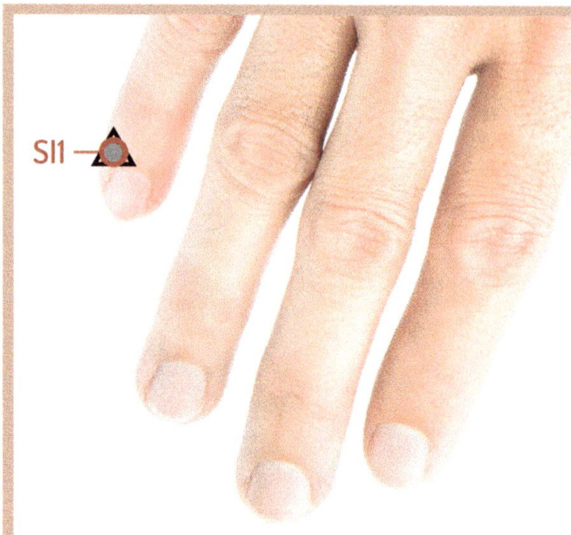

Ulnar side of little finger

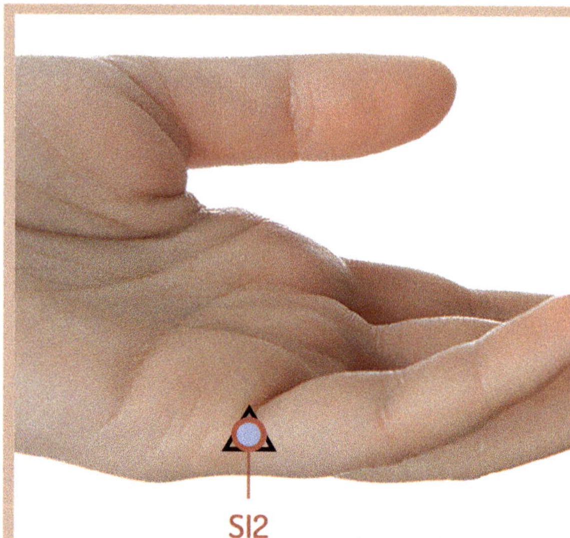

Ulnar side of hand

UB67 METAL + UB66 WATER

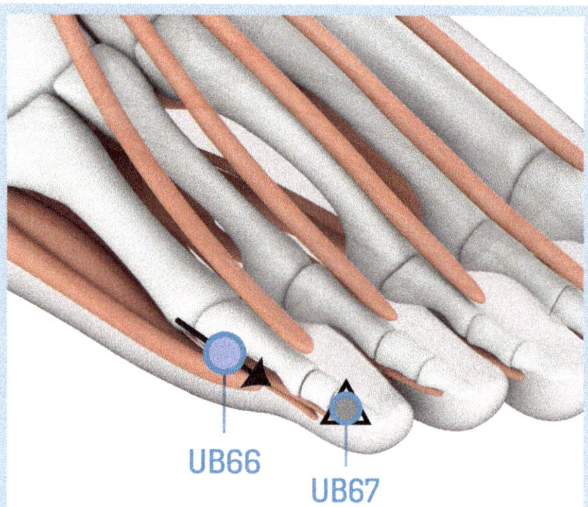

Lateral side of little toe

KD7 METAL + KD10 WATER

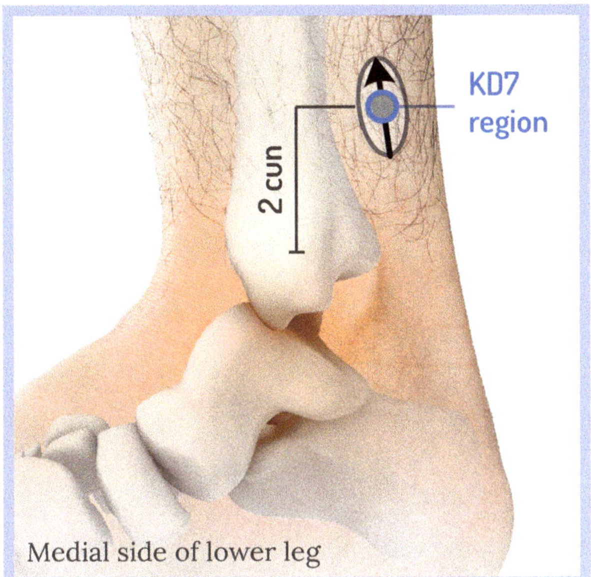

Medial side of lower leg

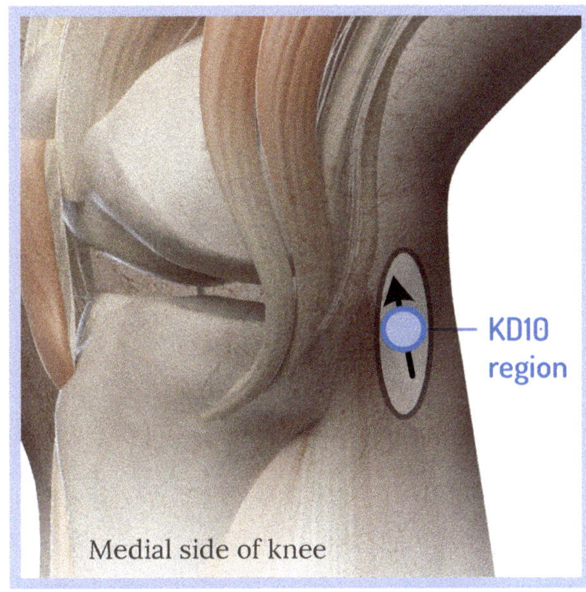

Medial side of knee

PC5 METAL + PC3 WATER

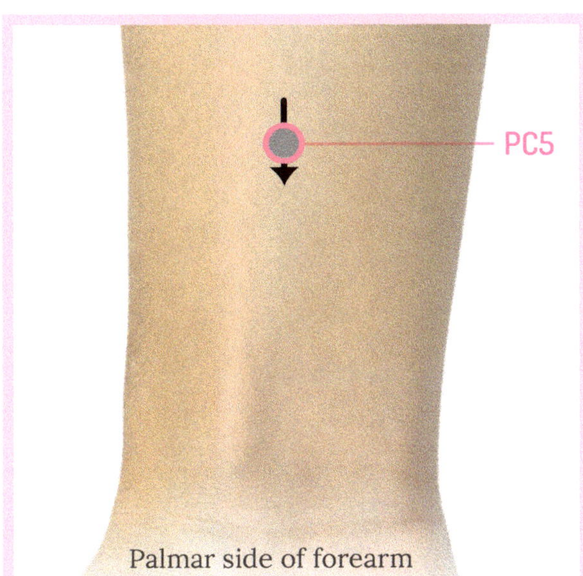

Palmar side of forearm

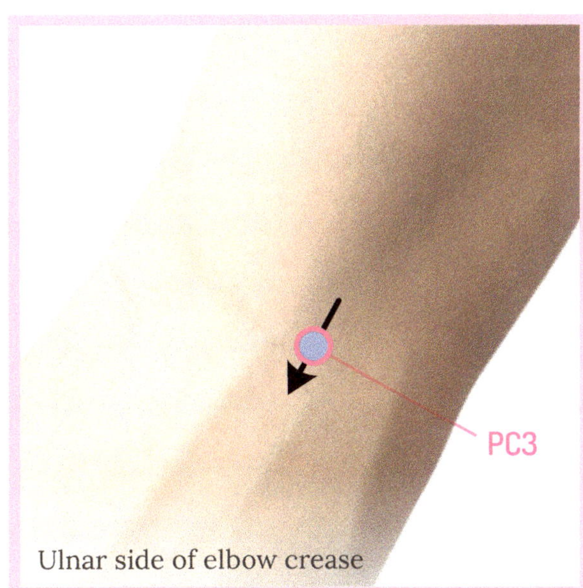

Ulnar side of elbow crease

TB1 METAL + TB2 WATER

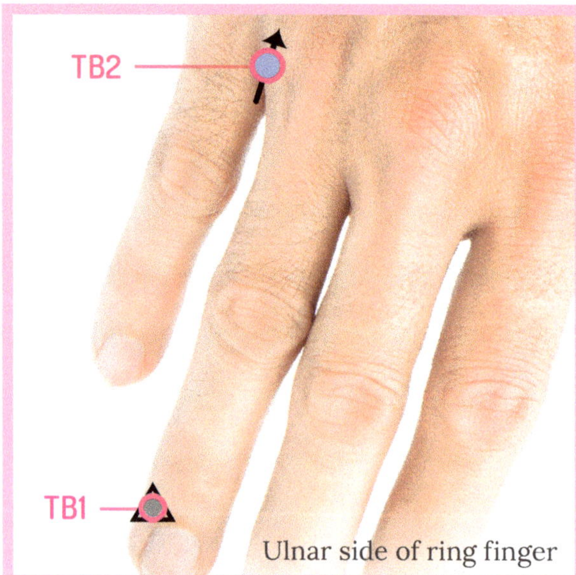

Ulnar side of ring finger

GB44 METAL + GB43 WATER

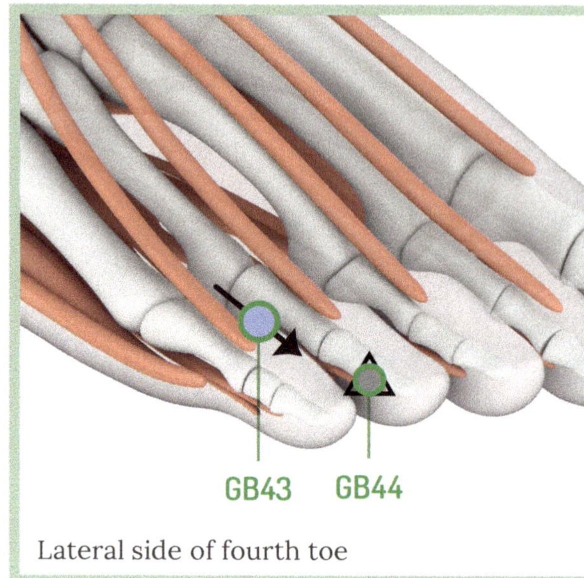

Lateral side of fourth toe

LV4 METAL + LV8 WATER

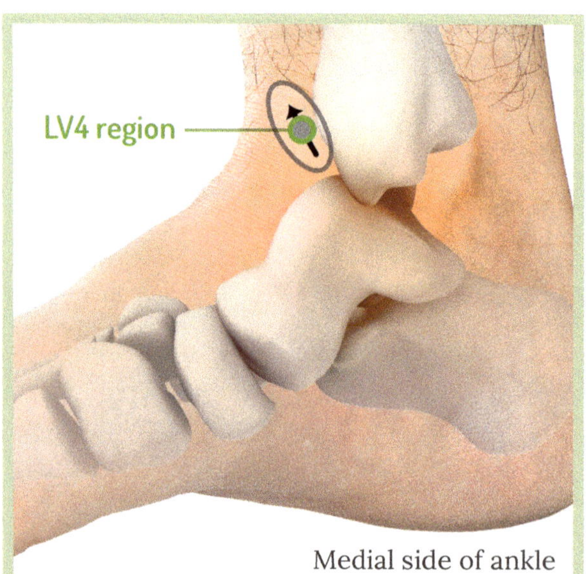

Medial side of ankle

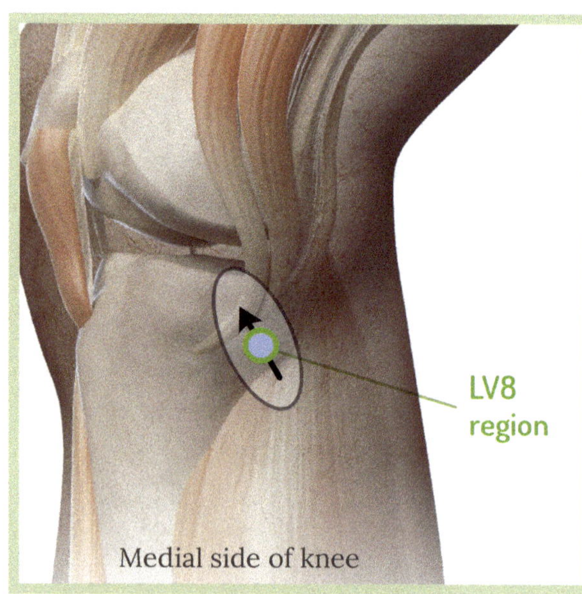

Medial side of knee

15.2 Extra-Vessel Controlling and Linking Acupoints

The eight extra-vessels form at the earliest stages of embryonic development before the twelve main meridians. The extra-vessels are active during all phases of fetal development and contain DNA programming for the entire body.

> *"The moment a sperm enters the ovum it determines a ventral and dorsal surface, which are the Directing [Conception] and Governing Vessels respectively. When the cell first divides it determines a left and a right side which are the Yin and Yang Heel Vessels. The exterior of the egg [embryo] is determined by the Yang Linking Vessel and its interior by the Yin Linking Vessel. Thus the Extraordinary Vessels, far from being 'secondary' vessels, are the primary energetic forces along which the whole body and all the other channels are formed. It is for this reason that Li Shi Zhen called them the 'Source of Creation'.*[50]
>
> *The Governing and Directing Vessels cut across the Girdle [Belt] Vessel linking it with the Heart above, the genital system below, the umbilicus in front and the Penetrating Vessel in the middle. This emphasizes why these four vessels (Governing, Directing, Penetrating, and Girdle) are interlinked for the production, circulation, discharge, and regeneration of the Essence. When these vessels are blocked, the Essence cannot be produced properly and all kinds of gynecological problems ensue.*[51]

The Body-Feedback system uses "controlling" and "joining" in place of the standard terms "master" and "couple" to describe the extra-vessel acupoints and to remove potential confusion with the Body-Feedback master alarm points, coupling five-element, and six-level pairs. These eight extra-vessels join together to create four pairs that share controlling and joining acupoints. The controlling and joining acupoints influence a myriad of body systems and personality traits programmed in DNA. These points foster the client's spiritual journey and release resistance to potential fulfillment. The controlling and joining acupoints attune the energy flow between the two pairs, strengthening the respective functions of both.

15.2.1 Governing and Yang Heel Vessels

The governing and yang heel vessels pair together. The governing vessel (*du mai*) influences the yang meridians, energy production, brain function, and warming hormones of testosterone and progesterone. The yang heel vessel (*yang qiao mai*) assists the nervous and skeletal systems. The controlling and joining acupoint SI3 is a shu-point in the small intestine tonification prescription and therefore is not viable as an extra-vessel supporting acupoint. UB62 increases motivation and drive for clients to take the next step in pursuit of their soul's highest purpose. Because of the coupling relationship, treating UB62 provides access to harmonize and support the governing vessel. The yang heel vessel's controlling acupoint (UB62) can support root treatments not containing kidney or urinary bladder shu-points.

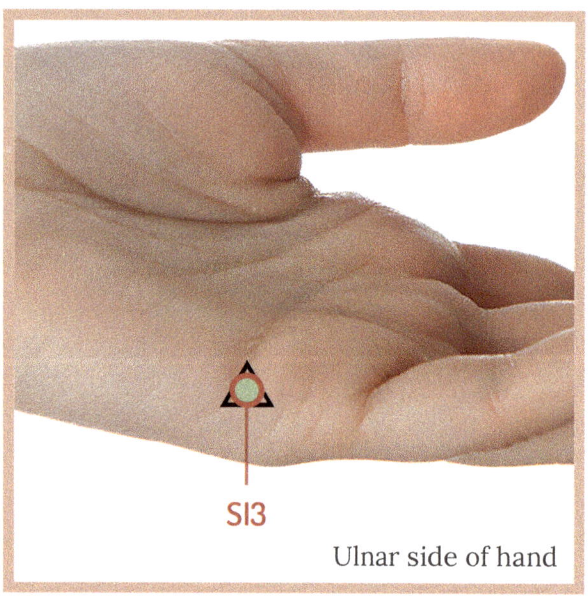

Ulnar side of hand

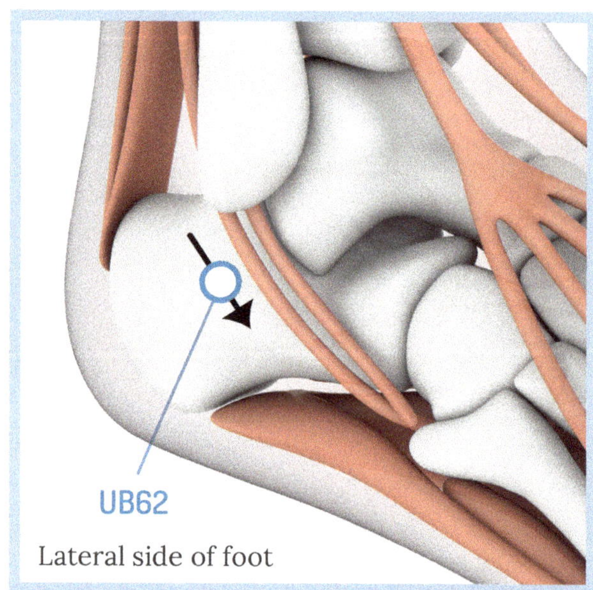

Lateral side of foot

15.2.2 Conception and Yin Heel Vessels

The conception and yin heel vessels pair together. The conception vessel (*ren mai*) influences the yin meridians, sperm production in men, egg development in women, pregnancy, rest, relaxation, and regeneration. The yin heel vessel (*yin qiao mai*), influences the muscular-skeletal, respiratory, and lymph systems. Both controlling and joining acupoints, LU7 and KD6, encourage relaxation, enhance intuition, and promote self-reflection to align with the soul's highest purpose. The yin heel vessel's controlling acupoint (KD6) can support root treatments not containing kidney or urinary bladder shu-points. The conception vessel's controlling point (LU7) can support root treatments not containing lung or large intestine shu-points.

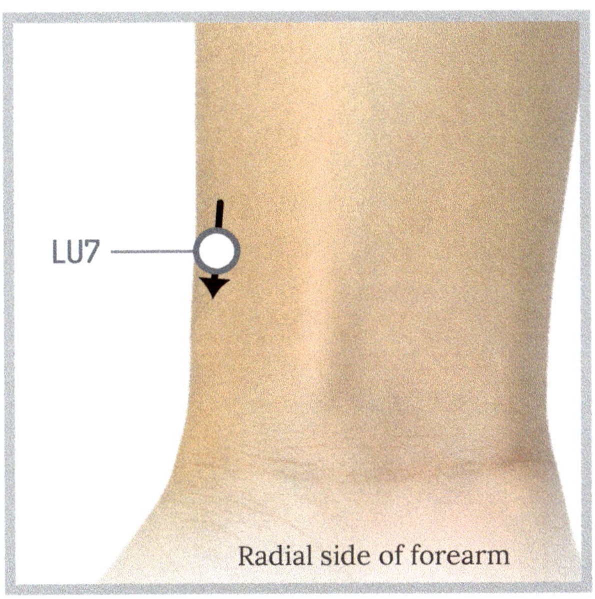

Radial side of forearm

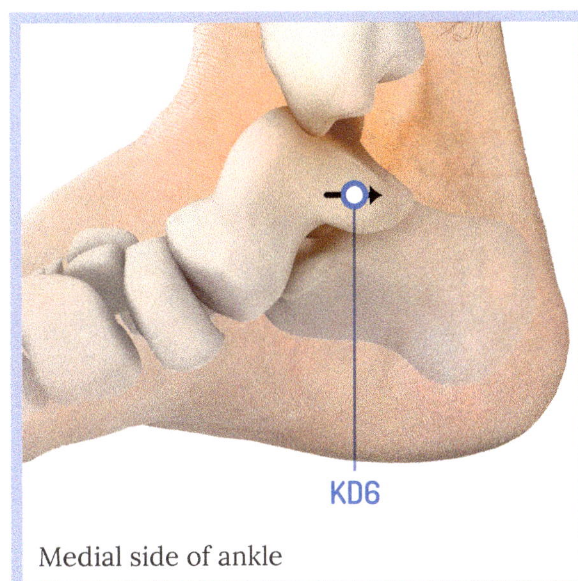

Medial side of ankle

15.2.3 Penetrating and Yin Linking Vessels

The penetrating and yin linking vessels pair together. The penetrating vessel (*chong mai*) is responsible for sending nourishment to the twelve meridians and organs through the blood vessel network. The penetrating vessel works jointly with the spleen and pericardium meridians to generate blood and hormones from the diet, and with the liver meridian to cleanse the blood and regulate its flow to the organs. The yin linking vessel (*yin wei mai*) governs the body's yin functions and unites the yin meridians. SP4 and PC6 inspire beneficial food choices, nourishing activities, and creating a lifestyle that nurtures the body, mind, and soul.

Many yang meridian root treatments utilize SP4 as a supporting acupoint, while many yin meridian root treatments include **SP3**, which is a shu-point, and therefore omits SP4 as a possible supporting acupoint. **SP3** and SP4 have differing functions; **SP3** (or metal + water combination SP5 + SP9) tonifies the qi and yang, while SP4 nourishes the blood and yin. Because the pericardium is a yin fire element, PC6 can disrupt the yin fire root balancing treatments for the heart and pericardium. In six-level theory, the pericardium meridian represents the deepest yin level of qi converting into yang, and the triple burner meridian represents the deepest yang level of qi converting into yin. Avoid PC6 with triple burner root treatments because of the shared fire-element property with the opposing flow of qi. PC6 is a common supporting acupoint for several other root treatments.

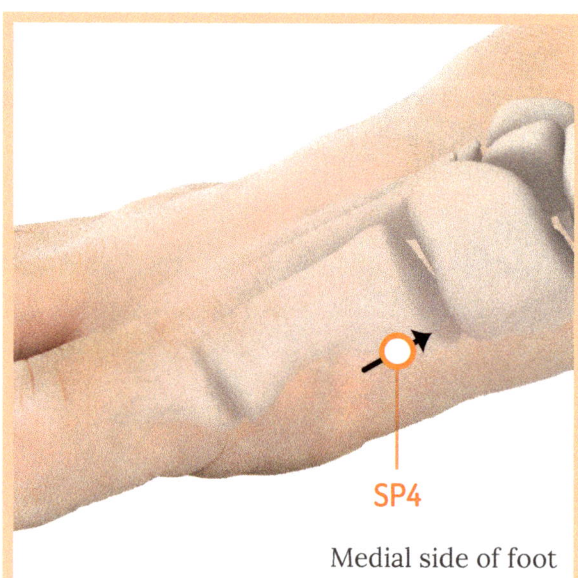

Medial side of foot

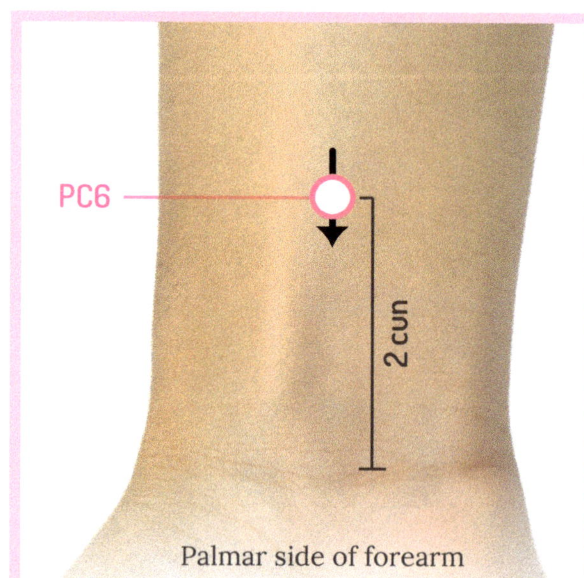

Palmar side of forearm

15.2.4 Belt and Yang Linking Vessels

The belt and yang linking vessels pair together. The belt vessel (*dai mai*), also known as the girdling vessel, is the only extra-vessel or meridian to run horizontally in the body. The belt vessel assists in securing and holding the internal organs in place, supporting pregnancy, and harmonizing the upper and lower halves of the body. The yang linking (*yang wei mai*) vessel regulates and harmonizes the yang meridians. **GB41** and TB5 encourage the outward expression of ideas, engagement in the community, and taking new insights into the world. The controlling and joining acupoint **GB41** is a shu-point on the gallbladder meridian and therefore is not viable as an extra-vessel supporting acupoint. Because only the triple burner prescriptions include triple burner shu-points, TB5 may be a supporting acupoint for all acupoint prescriptions except for the ministerial-fire element (PC and TB).

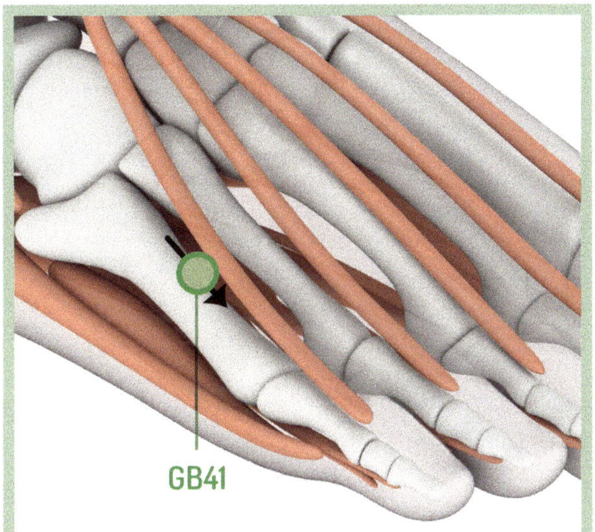

Lateral side of foot

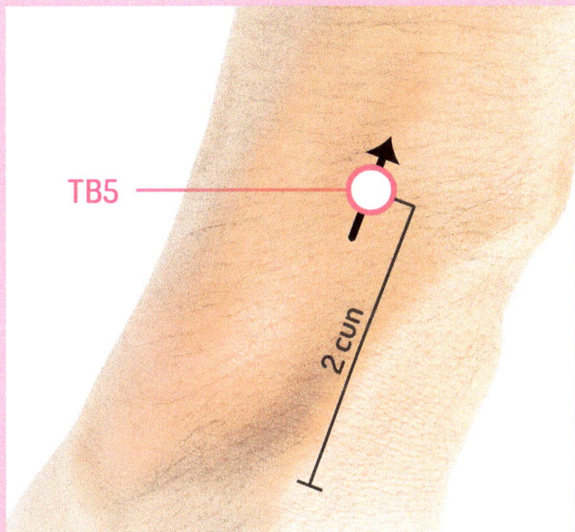

Dorsal side of forearm

15.3 Xi-Cleft Acupoints

Xi-cleft acupoints, also known as accumulation points, disperse qi stagnation and blood stasis affecting a meridian or organ. There are 16 xi-cleft acupoints, 12 on the main meridians, and 4 on the extra-vessels. The xi-cleft acupoints for the 12 main meridians energize their respective trisections and transform excess pathology to tonify the resulting deficiencies. The xi-cleft acupoints for the extra-vessels treat disorders of the endocrine and nervous systems along with genetic and constitutional weakness. All 16 xi-cleft acupoints effectively treat acute trauma and pain conditions.

Xi-cleft acupoints include:

LU6 for cough, sore throat, chest pain, or discomfort in the arm and shoulder

LI7 for headaches, sore throat, or discomfort in the arm and shoulder

ST34 for disorders of the stomach, sinuses, or discomfort in the leg and hip

SP8 for blood stasis, dysmenorrhea, or discomfort in the leg and hip

HT6 for night sweats, stress, anxiety, or discomfort in the wrist and hand

SI6 for vision, digestion, or discomfort in the wrist, arm, and shoulder

UB63 for emotions, brain function, or discomfort in the ankle, leg, back, and head

KD5 for reproductive organ dysfunction or discomfort in the lower abdomen and back

PC4 for chest pain, indigestion, stress, anxiety, or discomfort in the chest and arm

TB7 for disorders of the ear or discomfort in the wrist, arm, and shoulder

GB36 for gallbladder congestion, headaches, or discomfort in the ankle and leg

LV6 for dysmenorrhea, hormonal imbalances, or discomfort in the leg and hip

UB59 for yang heel extra-vessel, nerves, or discomfort in the head, back, and legs

KD8 for yin heel extra-vessel, reproduction, or discomfort in the lower abdomen

KD9 for yin linking extra-vessel, detoxification of used hormone metabolites, or discomfort in the lower abdomen

GB35 for yang linking extra-vessel, muscle weakness, or discomfort in the leg and hip

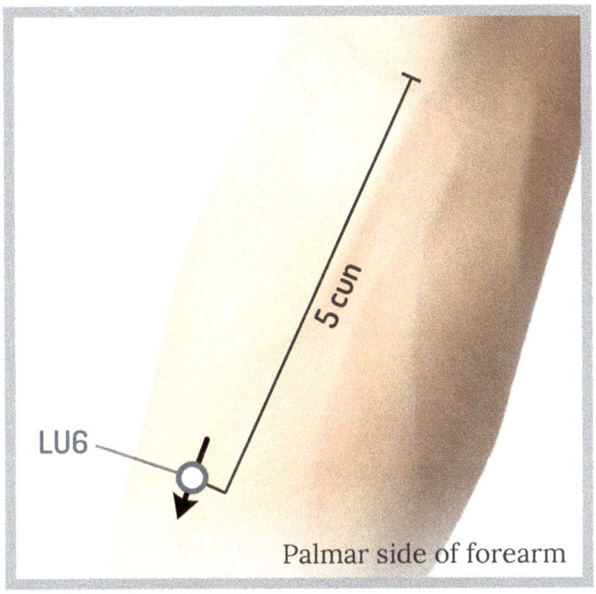

Palmar side of forearm

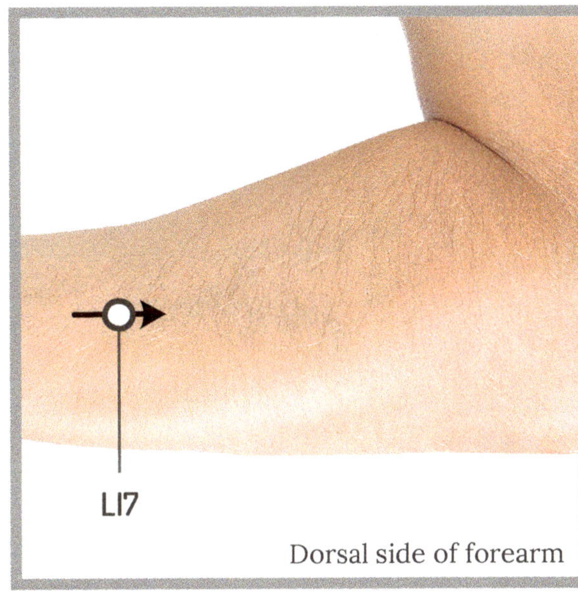

Dorsal side of forearm

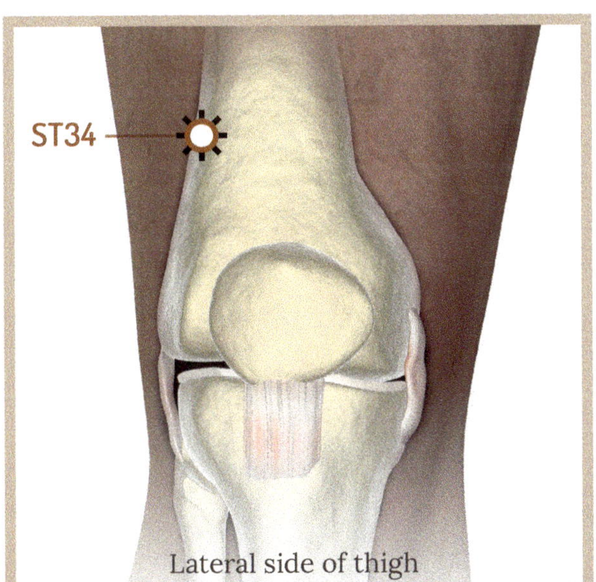

Lateral side of thigh

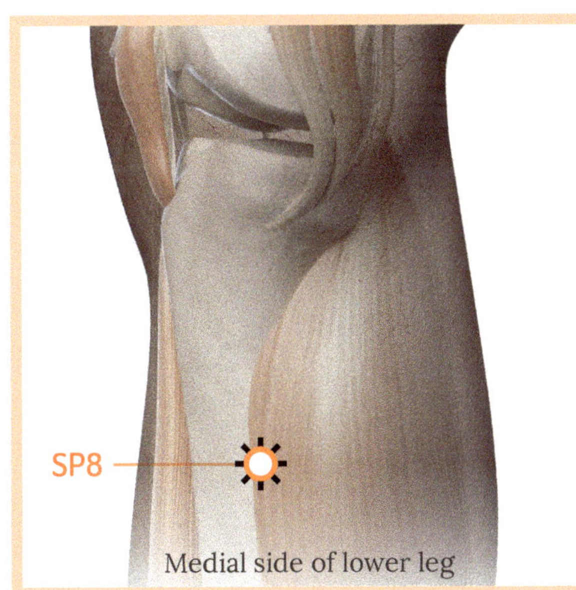

Medial side of lower leg

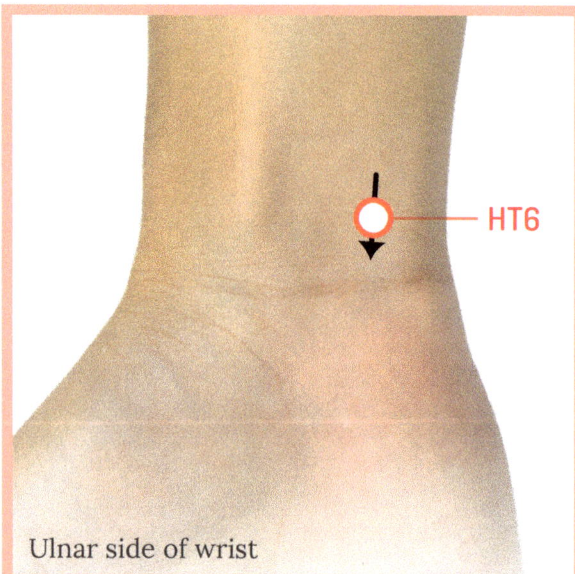

Ulnar side of wrist

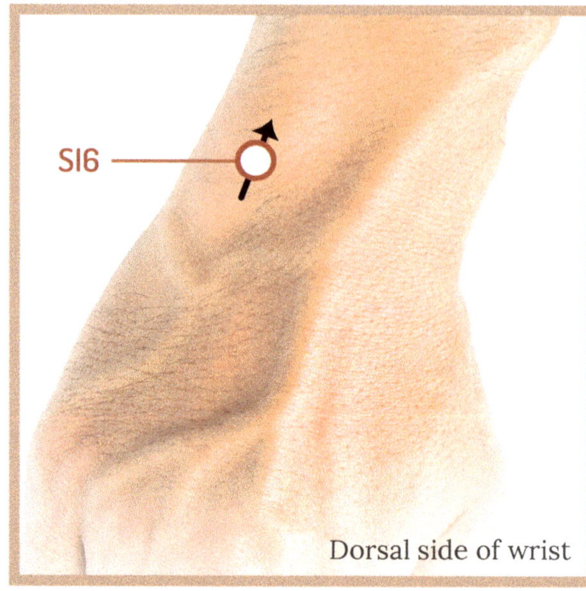

Dorsal side of wrist

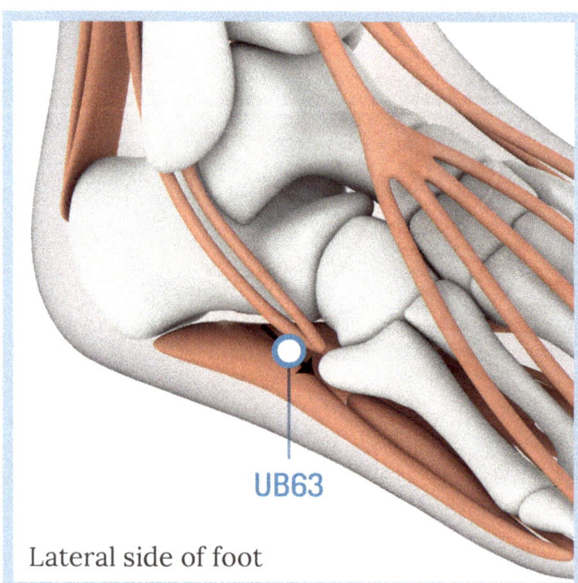

Lateral side of foot

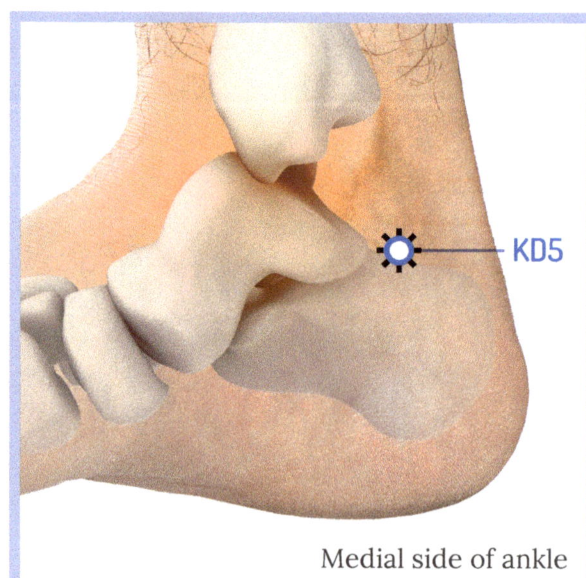

Medial side of ankle

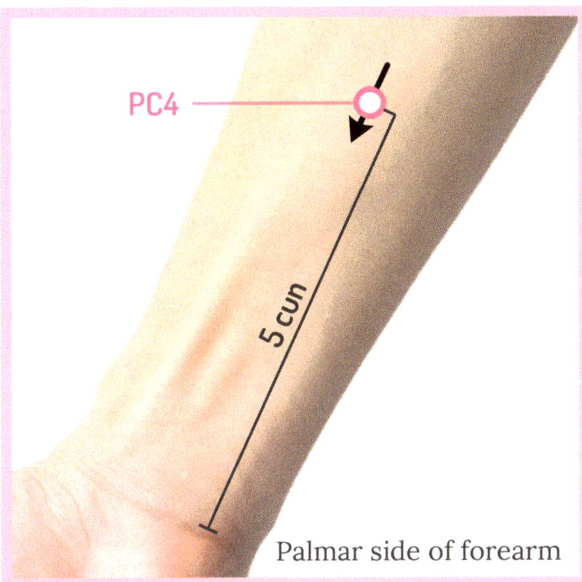

Palmar side of forearm

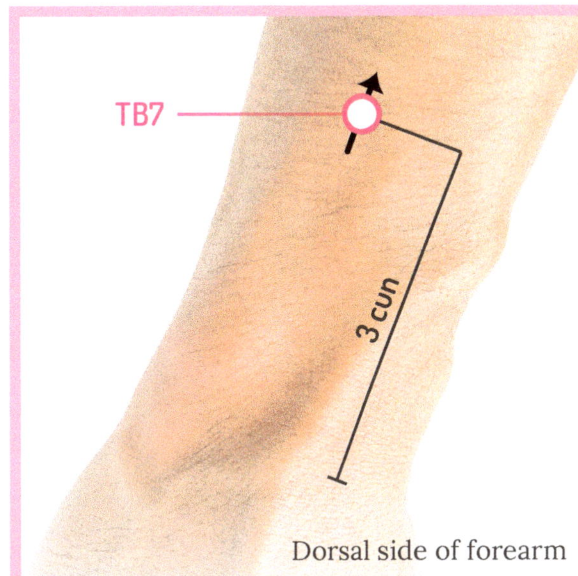

Dorsal side of forearm

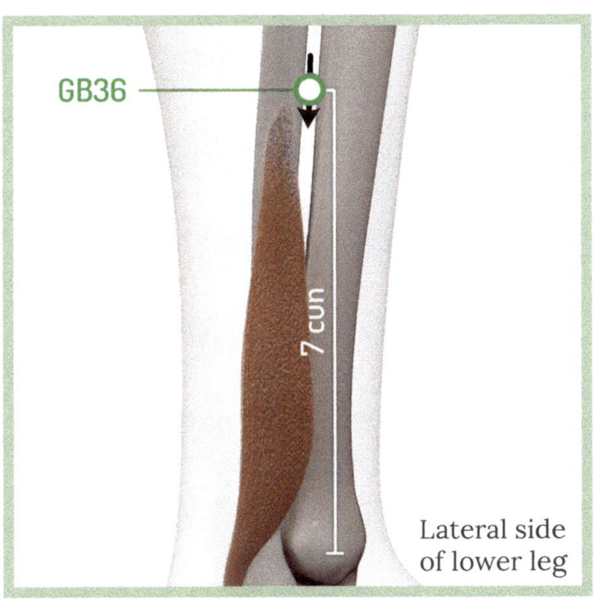

Lateral side of lower leg

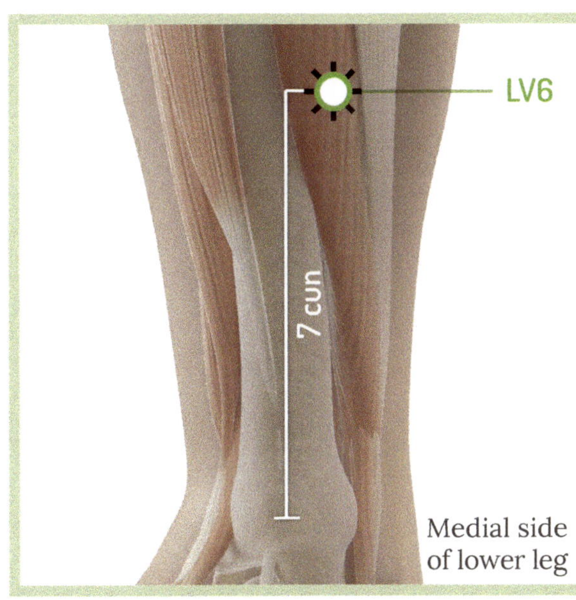

Medial side of lower leg

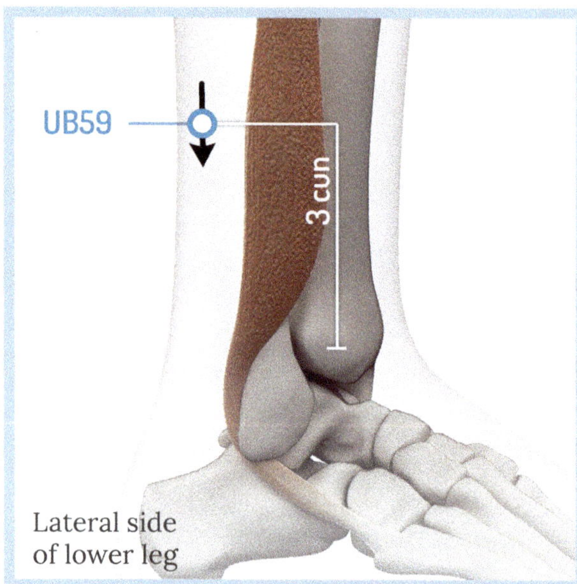
UB59
3 cun
Lateral side of lower leg

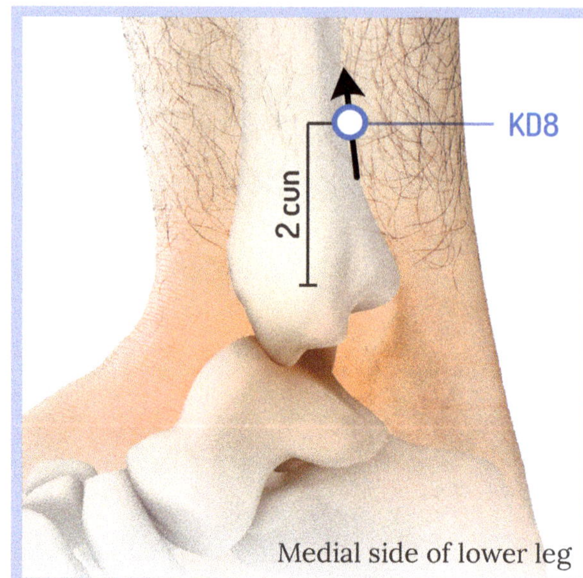
KD8
2 cun
Medial side of lower leg

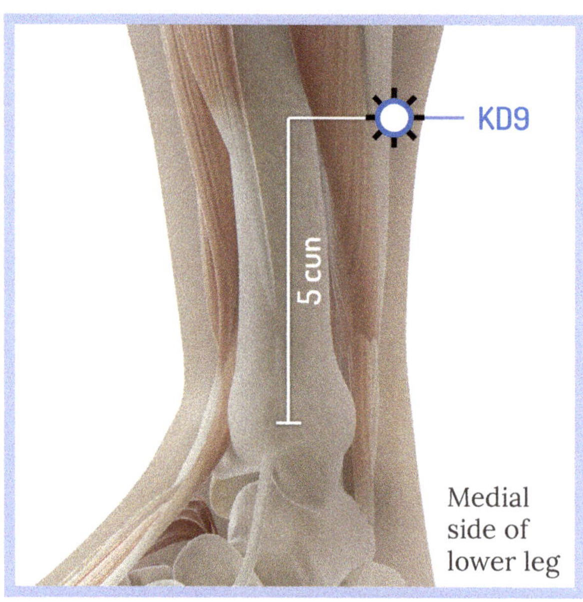
KD9
5 cun
Medial side of lower leg

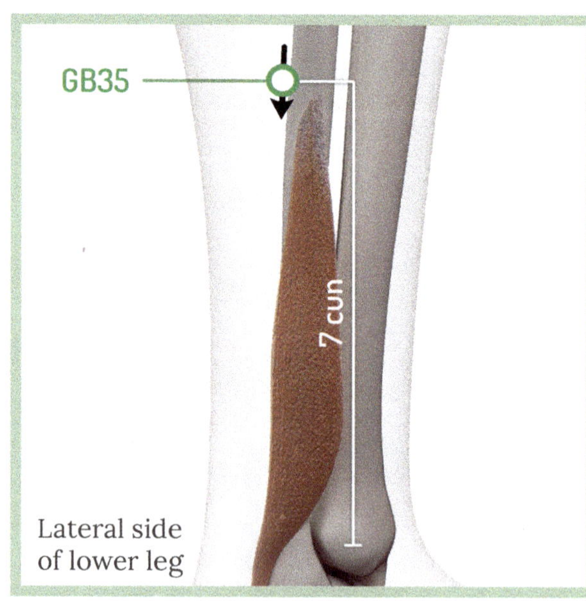
GB35
7 cun
Lateral side of lower leg

15.4 Luo-Connecting Acupoints

The luo-connecting points occur where the meridian branches off and diverges to join with its five-elemental pair. The luo-connecting points strengthen the elemental pair's organs and treat musculoskeletal conditions. Twelve luo-connecting acupoints harmonize the five elemental pairs, and the four group luo-connecting acupoints unify the yang or yin meridians for each arm or leg. Several of these points are also controlling and joining points for the extra-vessels. Because of their balancing properties, these points are especially helpful in supporting asymmetrical treatments, secondary five-element imbalances, and emotional conditions.

Luo-connecting Acupoints

LU7 and **LI6** harmonize the **metal element**.

SP4 and **ST40** harmonize the **earth element**.

HT5 and **SI7** harmonize the **imperial-fire element**.

KD4 and **UB58** harmonize the **water element**.

PC6 and **TB5** harmonize the **ministerial-fire element**.

LV5 and **GB37** harmonize the **wood element**.

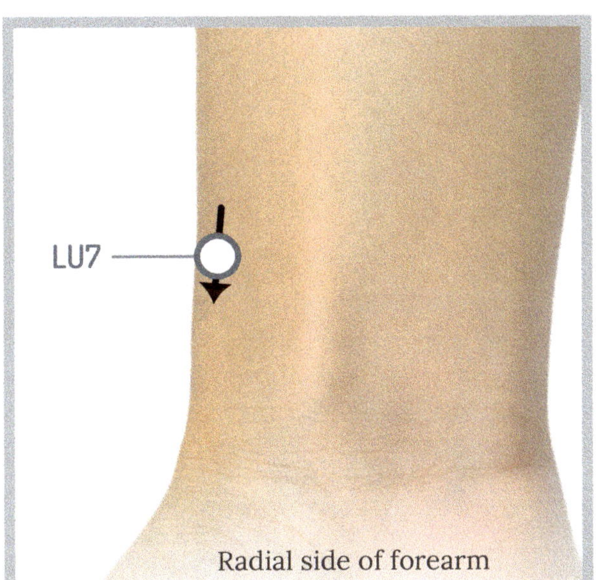

Radial side of forearm

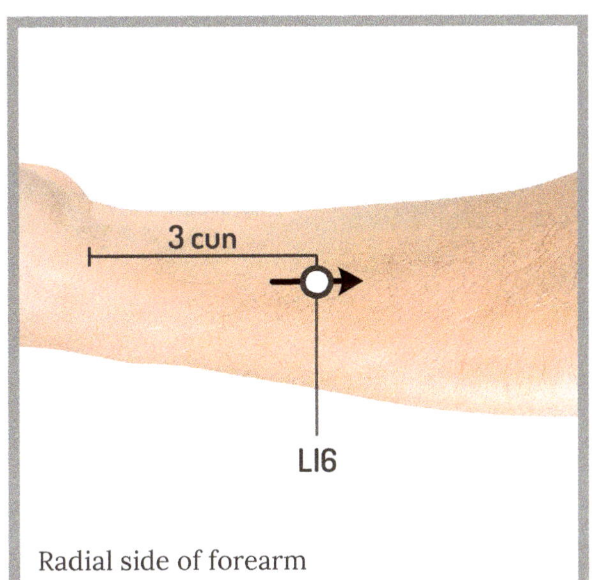

Radial side of forearm

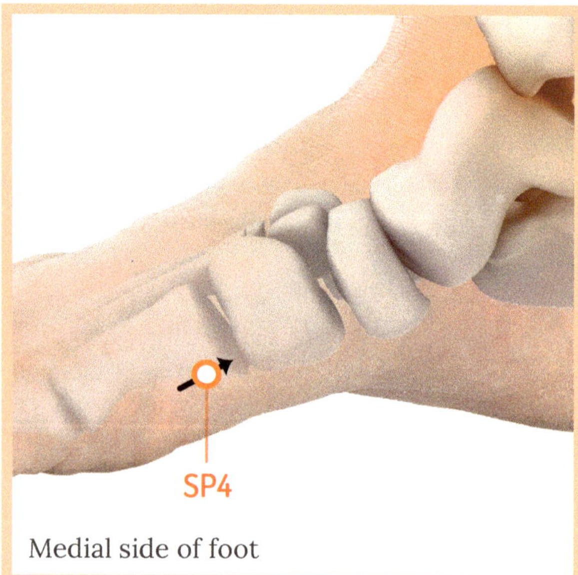

Medial side of foot

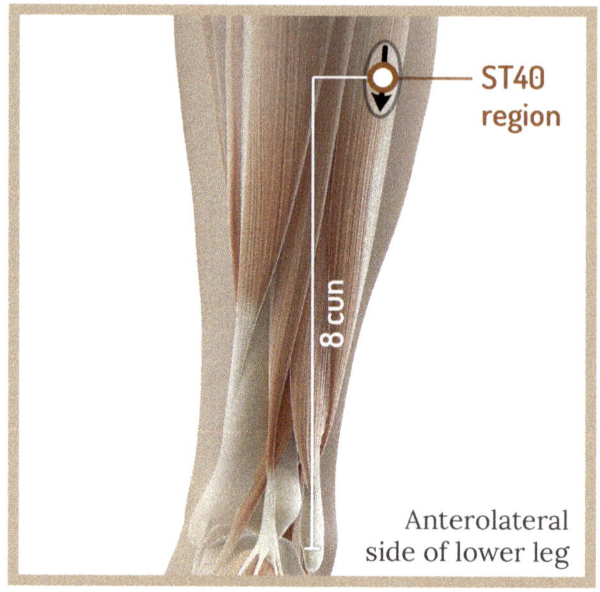

Anterolateral side of lower leg

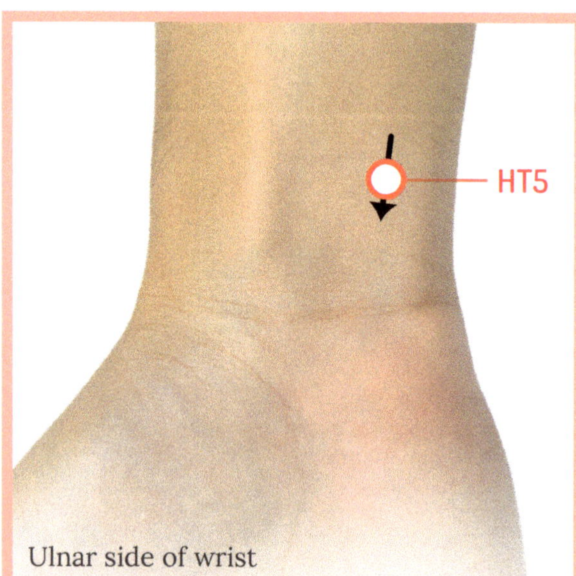

Ulnar side of wrist

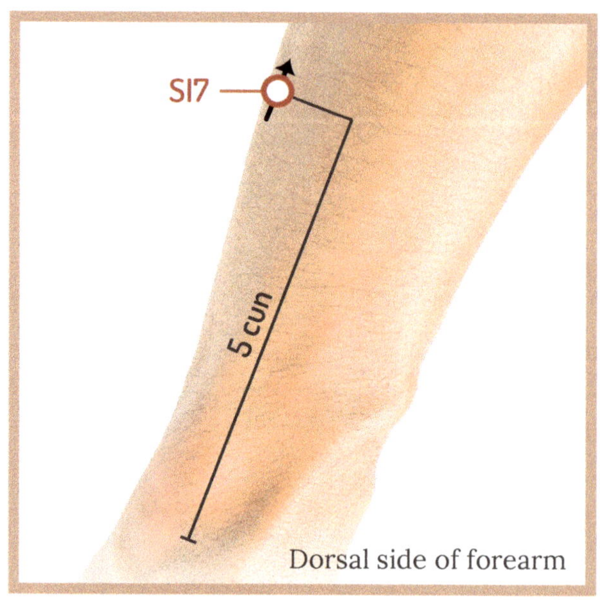

Dorsal side of forearm

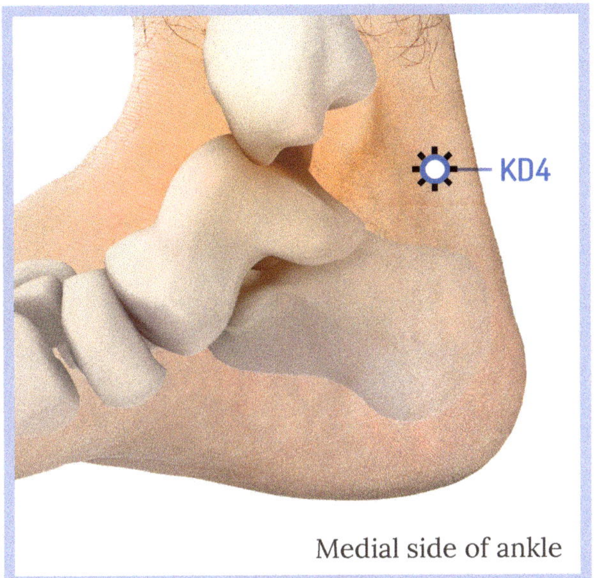

Medial side of ankle

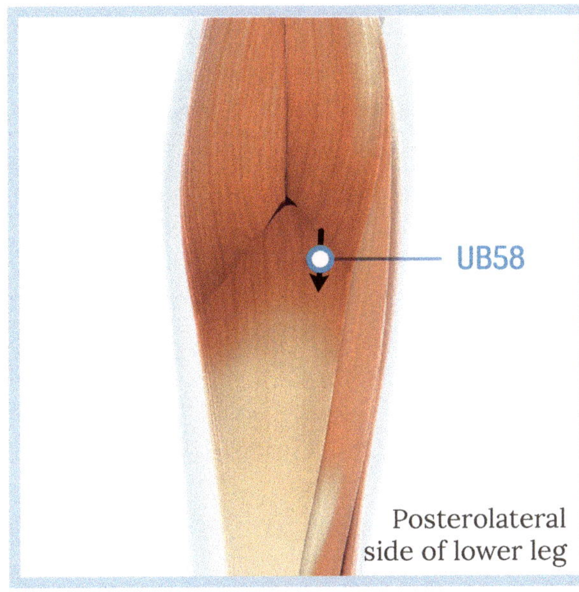

Posterolateral side of lower leg

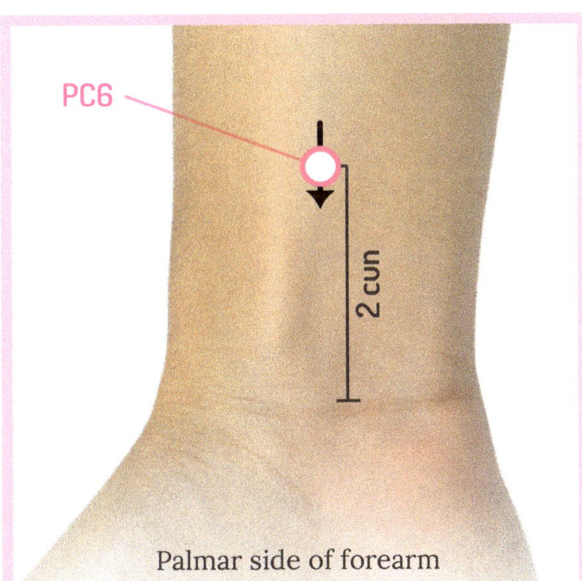

Palmar side of forearm

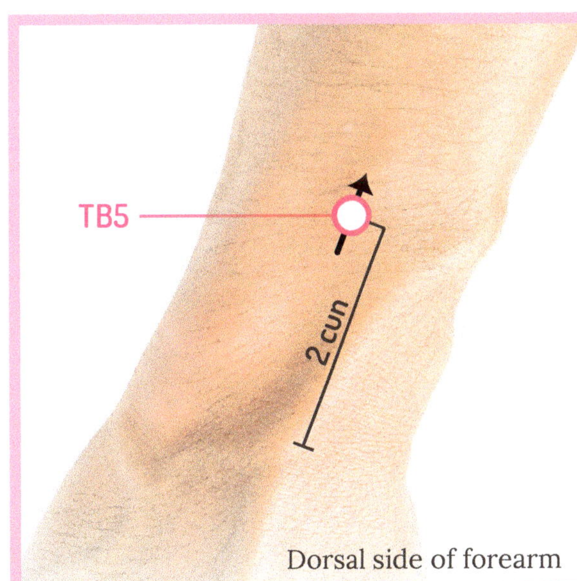

Dorsal side of forearm

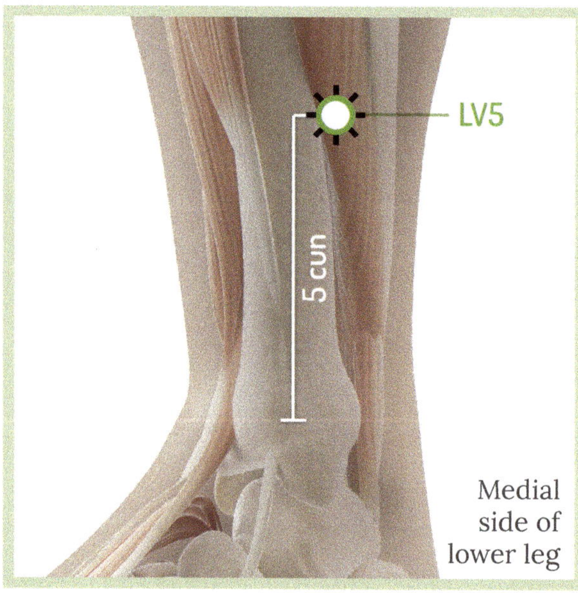

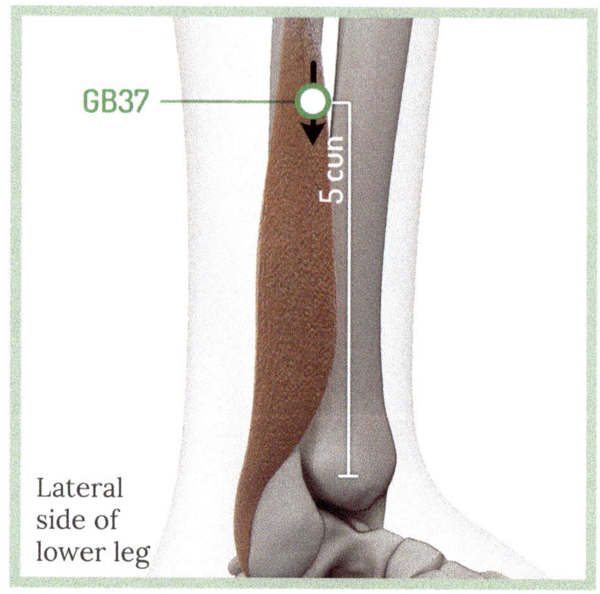

Group Luo-connecting Acupoints

TB8 harmonizes the three yang meridians of the arms (LI/SI/TB).

PC5 is used in the PC balancing acupoint prescriptions, along with the metal + water combinations, to harmonize the three yin meridians of the arms (LU/HT/PC).

GB39 harmonizes the three yang meridians of the legs (ST/UB/GB).

SP6 harmonizes the three yin meridians of the legs (SP/KD/LV).

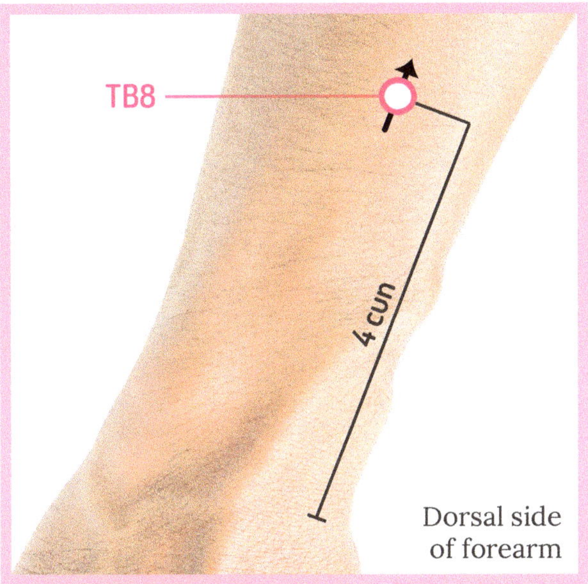
TB8
4 cun
Dorsal side of forearm

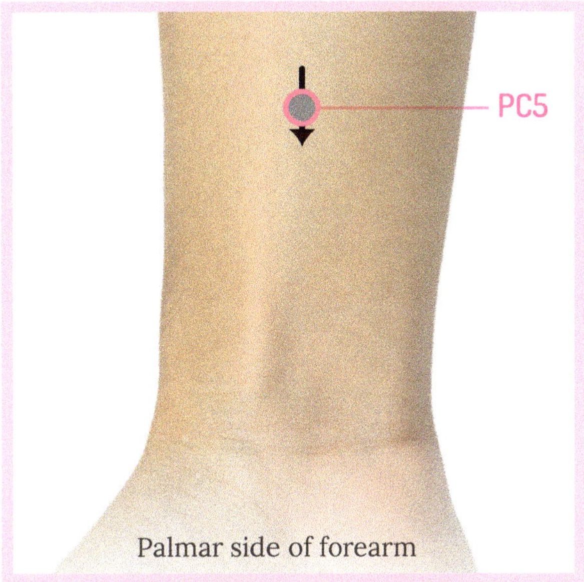
PC5
Palmar side of forearm

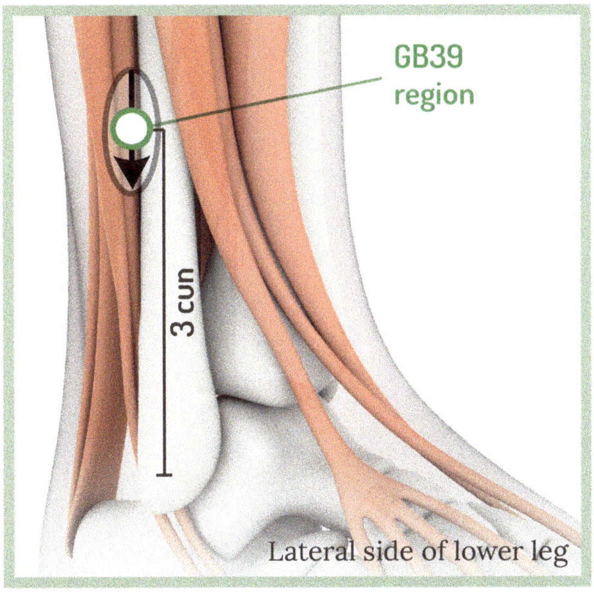
GB39 region
3 cun
Lateral side of lower leg

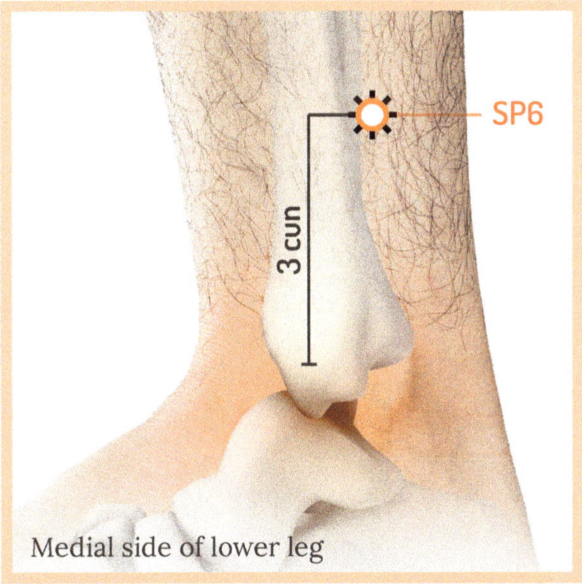
SP6
3 cun
Medial side of lower leg

15.5 Yuan-Source Acupoints for the Yang Meridians

The yuan-source acupoints boost qi in the meridians and strengthen their elements' organs. On the yin meridians, the yuan-source acupoints are the shu-stream points, which are included in the balancing, sedating, and tonifying prescriptions; therefore, they are not included as supporting acupoints. Only the yang meridian's yuan-source acupoints are options to use as support for the Body-Feedback prescriptions. The yang yuan-source acupoints expel pathogens from their corresponding six-level. For example, LI4 can release pathogens from the yang-ming level, and GB40 can release pathogens from the shao-yang level.

Yuan-source Acupoints for the Yang Meridians

LI4 to increase qi in the metal element and expel pathogens from the yang-ming level

ST42 to increase qi in the earth element and expel pathogens from the yang-ming level

SI4 to increase qi in the imperial-fire element and expel pathogens from the tai-yang level

UB64 to increase qi in the water element and expel pathogens from the tai-yang level

TB4 to increase qi in the ministerial-fire element and expel pathogens from the shao-yang level

GB40 to increase qi in the wood element and expel pathogens from the shao-yang level

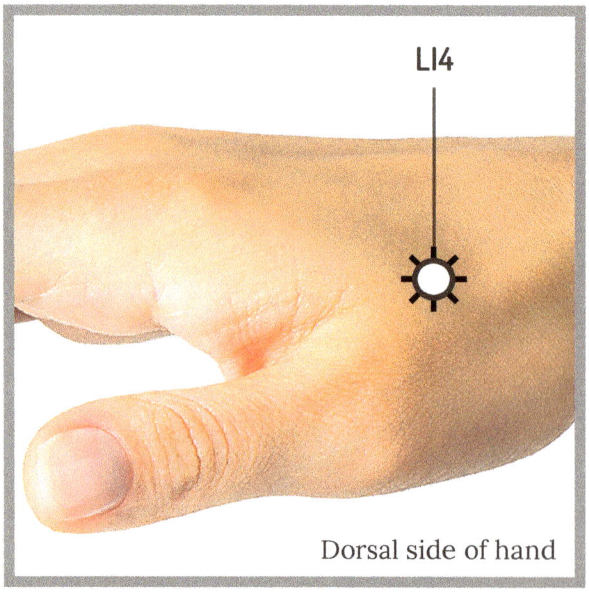

Dorsal side of hand

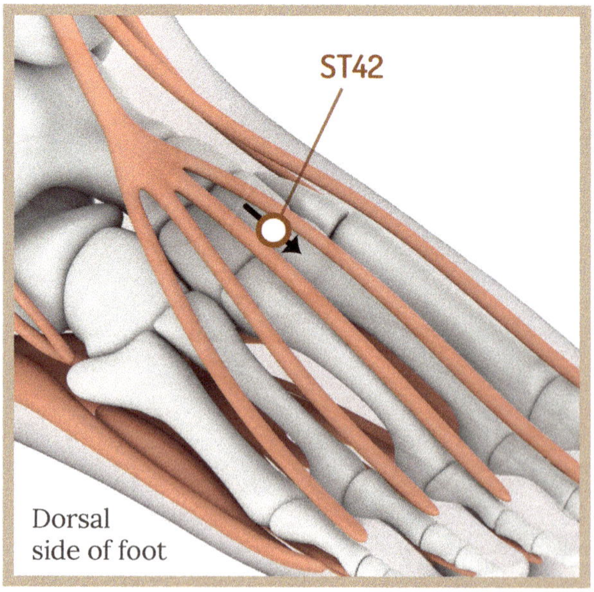

Dorsal side of foot

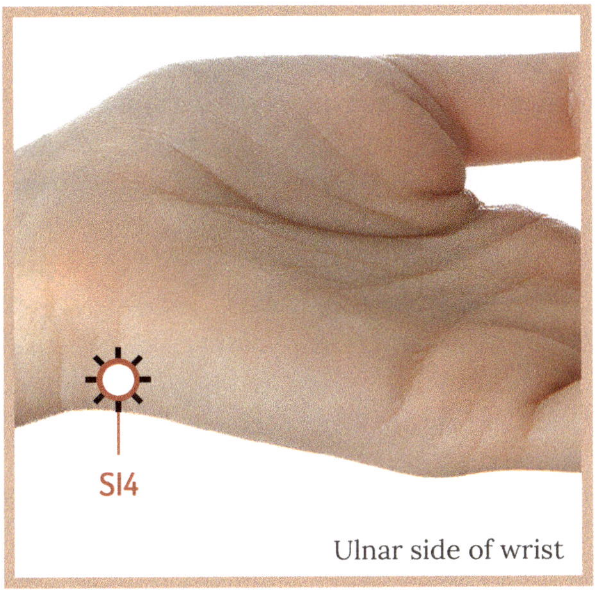

Ulnar side of wrist

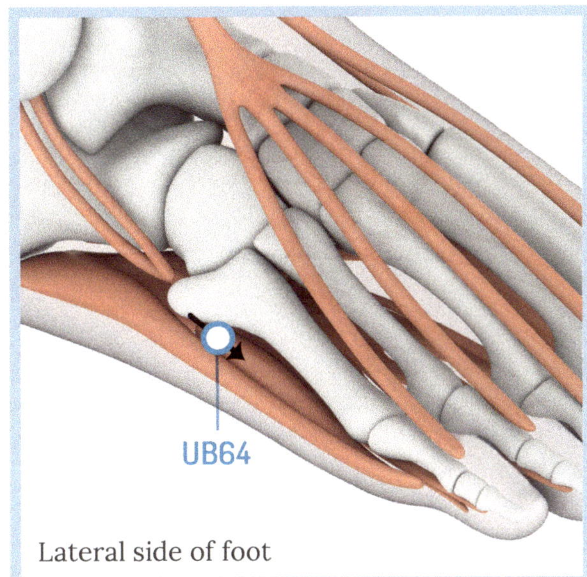

Lateral side of foot

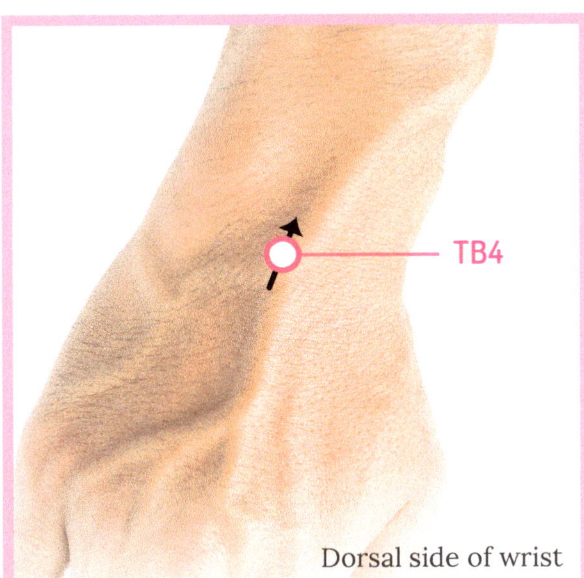

Dorsal side of wrist

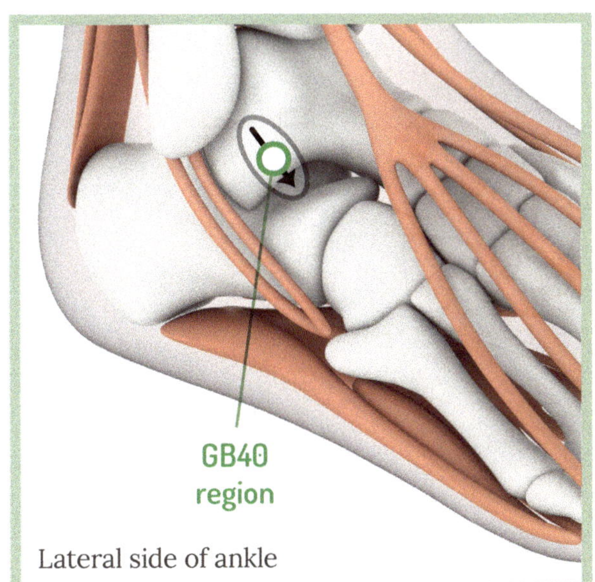

Lateral side of ankle

15.6 Ashi Acupoints for Pain, Neuropathy, and Musculoskeletal Symptoms

Ashi acupoints treat symptoms of pain, muscle tightness, weakness, and neuropathy affecting a specific musculoskeletal region or extremity. These regional ashi acupoints easily integrate with the Body-Feedback approach because they are non-shu-points. When pathogenic heat causes referred pain in a musculoskeletal region, the metal + water combination will test better as compared to the regional ashi acupoints. In this case, treat the metal + water shu-points with needles during the treatment and with magnetic pellets between acupuncture sessions to allow for local ashi needling at future appointments. When regional ashi acupoints test favorably to the pulse, master alarm points, or associated Body-Feedback areas, needle them as supporting acupoints.

For example, a new client with acute shoulder pain and tightness in the deltoid muscle tested favorably for a root spleen sedation treatment (SP1, SP9, LV1, KD10, SP5, and LU8). The supporting points included LU5 water, KD7 metal, PC5 metal, and PC3 water to create the heat-clearing combinations. At that first appointment, testing the regional shoulder ashi acupoints caused increased tightness in the master alarm points (GB21, TB15, and SI13). This client used a custom essential oil blend of marjoram, patchouli, and cedarwood on the shoulder between appointments. The shoulder ashi acupoints tested favorably for needling at subsequent appointments, as evidenced by the master alarm points releasing tension.

15.7 Practical Application of Supporting Acupoints

The supporting acupoints are the final step in the Body-Feedback treatment approach and facilitate outstanding treatment outcomes. Consider the client's symptoms and presenting complaints to determine the xi-cleft, luo-connecting, yuan-source, and ashi acupoints for testing. The steps detailed on the following page carefully guide the selection of supporting acupoints to enhance the root Body-Feedback point prescriptions.

Steps for Choosing Supporting Acupoints

1. Identify any singular water or metal shu-points already included in the root Body-Feedback acupoint prescription and test their paired water or metal acupoint.
2. Test additional metal + water combinations to the pulse or master alarm point GB21 for non-root meridians that may have pathogenic heat.
3. Check the extra-vessel-controlling and -joining acupoints on meridians not treated with a metal + water combination or included in the root prescription.
4. Test xi-cleft, luo-connecting, or yang meridian yuan-source acupoints for the root's six-level and non-paired element within the trisection.
5. Each Body-Feedback prescription includes three acupoints on the root meridian and three non-root horary shu-points. Test xi-cleft, luo-connecting, or yang meridian yuan-source acupoints for the five-element meridian pairs of the three horary shu-points included in a Body-Feedback acupoint prescription.
6. Check regional ashi acupoints for pain, neuropathy, musculoskeletal conditions, and acute symptoms.

Practical Application Example

THE BODY-FEEDBACK ACUPOINTS FOR LIVER DEFICIENCY PATHOLOGY:

STEP 1: LV4 is the restraining metal shu-point on the liver meridian.

STEP 2: LV3 is the restraining earth shu-point on the liver meridian.

STEP 3: **SP3** is the yin earth horary shu-point that engenders metal (compare SP3 to SP5 metal + SP9 water combination for pathogenic heat).

STEP 4: LU8 is the yin metal horary shu-point that restrains wood.

STEP 5: KD10 is the yin water horary shu-point that tonifies wood.

STEP 6: LV8 is the water shu-point on the liver meridian that tonifies wood.

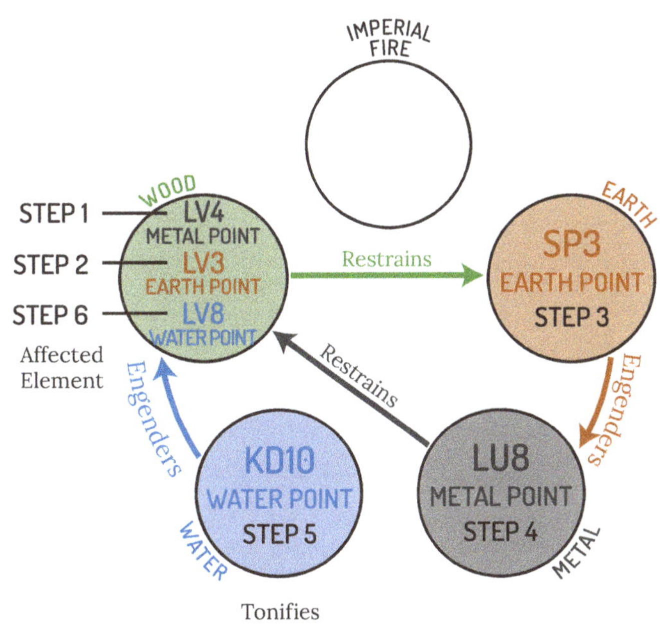

For the Practical Application Example, use the Steps for Choosing Supporting Acupoints outlined on the previous page for a liver tonification prescription (LV3,4,8, KD10, **SP3**, and LU8).

1. Identify KD10 (water shu-point) and LU8 (metal shu-point) in the root prescription and check KD7 (metal shu-point) and LU5 (water shu-point) to create the metal + water combinations when pathogenic heat is present.
2. With a wiry and forceful third (chi) pulse position on the right (ministerial-fire element), test the metal + water combinations for the pericardium (PC5 + PC3) and triple burner (TB1 + TB2).
3. Consider the extra-vessel acupoints available as support for genetic and musculoskeletal conditions (UB62, PC6, and TB5). Only check the extra-vessel acupoints when not treating the metal + water combination on that specific meridian.
4. For symptoms relating to the pericardium and triple burner meridians, check the xi-cleft (PC4 and TB7), luo-connecting (PC6, TB5, and TB8), and yang yuan-source (TB4) acupoints for the root's six-level and non-paired element within the trisection.
5. To strengthen the root prescription, check the horary shu-point's (KD10, **SP3**, LU8) five-element pair's xi-cleft (UB63, ST34, and LI7), luo-connecting (UB58, ST40, and LI6), and yang yuan-source (UB64, ST42, and LI4) acupoints for the urinary bladder, stomach, and large intestine meridians. Check the pulse to determine which meridian's acupoints to test.
6. Check regional ashi acupoints to treat pain, neuropathy, or musculoskeletal symptoms.

In practice, specific supporting acupoints commonly test best with particular root Body-Feedback prescriptions. Section 15.7.2 provides a list of these common supporting acupoints for each root Body-Feedback prescription. Resolving pathogenic heat with supporting acupoints is the first priority. After addressing pathogenic heat, consider adding a few supporting acupoints from the extra-vessel, xi-cleft, luo-connecting, or yuan-source categories. For pain and neuromuscular conditions, focus on regional ashi acupoints as support.

15.7.1 Electrostimulation of Supporting Acupoints

Electrostimulation of acupoints is an optional therapy that can be incorporated during the treatment stage using the Body-Feedback testing methods. Electrostimulation is especially helpful in treating pain and excess conditions with longstanding blood stasis and qi stagnation. It is appropriate for the xi-cleft, luo-connecting, yuan-source, and regional ashi acupoints. However, avoid electrostimulation of shu-points (including metal + water) and extra-vessel acupoints, along with any of the meridians included in the root balancing, sedation, and tonification prescriptions. For example, with a root liver tonification treatment (LV4, LV3, **SP3**, LU8, KD10, and LV8), avoid electrostimulation of acupoints on the liver, spleen, lung, and kidney meridians.

Monitor the pulse or palpate the master alarm points or neck muscles to test the electrostimulation current direction, frequency, and intensity. Choose a testing location or re-assess the pulse before adding the electrostimulation as a baseline. To apply electrostimulation, clip the electrical leads onto the chosen needles after all are inserted. Turn on the electrostimulation to the lowest frequency and intensity possible.

Test the direction of the current and choice of acupoints first. Monitor the pulse or palpate the testing locations with the current running one direction and again with the current running the opposite direction. Most electrostimulation machines provide a switch to easily change the current direction. If the acupoints with added electrostimulation and current direction are acceptable to the client's body, the pulse will feel balanced in all three positions and the testing locations will remain soft and loose when the machine is turned on the lowest setting. The current direction or the acupoints selected to be treated with electrostimulation are not beneficial when the pulse becomes wiry, forceful, or confined, and the testing locations become tight and painful. In this case, change the current direction and recheck the pulse and testing locations. If running the current both directions results in an unbalanced pulse or discomfort in the testing locations, check electrostimulation on other acupoints.

Test the frequency of the electrostimulation after the current direction and correct acupoints are confirmed. While monitoring the client's pulse or testing locations, slowly increase the frequency until the pulse becomes unbalanced or the testing locations tighten. Then slightly reduce the frequency and wait 30 seconds to recheck the pulse and testing locations. The optimal frequency will balance the pulse and loosen the testing locations.

The last step is turning up the intensity of the electrostimulation. In some instances, the ideal intensity occurs before the client feels the pulsing of the electrostimulation. Ask the client to let you know when he or she can feel the pulsing at any of the needles with the electrostimulation. Slowly increase the intensity while monitoring the pulse or palpating the testing locations until a negative response occurs in the pulse or testing locations, or the client feels the intensity is too strong. Then slightly reduce the intensity to determine the ideal setting for that treatment. In most cases, the ideal intensity will occur when the client comfortably feels the electrostimulation.

In general, clients with tonification root treatments respond best to a lower frequency and intensity. Clients with sedation root treatments respond best to a higher frequency and stronger intensity. Body-Feedback testing methods can ensure that adding electrostimulation will increase the effectiveness of the treatment. Recheck the pulse or master alarm points if increasing the intensity or frequency of the electrostimulation during the treatment. Include the electrostimulation for the entire treatment and slightly reduce the needle retention time to factor in the additional stimulation.

15.7.2 Common Supporting Acupoints for the First Trisection

LUNG BALANCING ACUPOINTS: LU10, LU11, LV1, **HT8** (compare HT4 metal + HT3 water)

LUNG SEDATION ACUPOINTS: LU5, KD10

Frequent supporting acupoints:

- KD7 metal shu to assist existing water shu in releasing heat
- SP4, TB5, or UB62 to access the extra-vessels
- ST34 xi-cleft to disperse the stomach excess
- GB40 yuan-source to strengthen the wood element

LUNG TONIFICATION ACUPOINTS: **SP3** (compare SP5 metal + SP9 water), LU9

Frequent supporting acupoints:

- KD6, UB62, or TB5 to access the extra-vessels
- KD8 or KD9 xi-clefts to release excess in the yin linking or heel extra-vessels
- TB8 group luo-connecting to harmonize the three yang arm meridians
- GB40 yuan-source to strengthen the wood element

LARGE INTESTINE BALANCING ACUPOINTS: LI5, LI3, **GB41** (compare GB44 metal + GB43 water), SI5

LARGE INTESTINE SEDATION ACUPOINTS: LI2, UB66

Frequent supporting acupoints:

- UB67 metal shu to assist existing water shu in releasing heat
- PC6, SP4, or TB5 to access the extra-vessels
- KD9 xi-cleft to disperse the yin linking extra-vessel excess
- LV5 or ST40 luo-connecting to balance the wood or earth elements

LARGE INTESTINE TONIFICATION ACUPOINTS: **ST36** (compare ST45 metal + ST44 water), LI11

Frequent supporting acupoints:

- KD6, SP4, or UB62 for the extra-vessels
- KD9 xi-cleft to disperse the yin linking extra-vessel excess
- LV5 or PC6 luo-connecting to balance the wood or ministerial-fire elements
- SP6 group luo-connecting to harmonize the three yin leg meridians

STOMACH BALANCING ACUPOINTS: ST43, ST44, UB66, **GB41** (compare GB44 metal + GB43 water)

STOMACH SEDATION ACUPOINTS: ST45, LI1

Frequent supporting acupoints:

- UB67 metal shu to assist existing water shu in releasing heat
- LI2 water shu to combine with existing metal shu
- KD6, LU7, PC6, or TB5 to access the extra-vessels
- LV5 luo-connecting to balance the wood element

STOMACH TONIFICATION ACUPOINTS: SI5, ST41

Frequent supporting acupoints:

- UB67 metal shu to assist existing water shu in releasing heat
- KD6, PC6, or TB5 to access the extra-vessels
- LV5 luo-connecting to balance the wood element
- LI4 yuan-source to strengthen the metal element

SPLEEN BALANCING ACUPOINTS: SP1, SP9, LV1, KD10

SPLEEN SEDATION ACUPOINTS: SP5, LU8

Frequent supporting acupoints:

- LU5 water shu to assist existing metal shu in releasing heat
- KD7 metal shu to assist existing water shu in releasing heat
- PC6, TB5, or UB62 to access the extra-vessels
- GB40 yuan-source to strengthen the wood element

SPLEEN TONIFICATION ACUPOINTS: **HT8** (compare HT4 metal + HT3 water), SP2

Frequent supporting acupoints:

- KD7 metal shu to assist existing water shu in releasing heat
- LU7, TB5, or UB62 to access the extra-vessels
- LI4 yuan-source to strengthen the metal element
- GB40 yuan-source to strengthen the wood element

15.7.3 Common Supporting Acupoints for the Second Trisection

HEART BALANCING ACUPOINTS: HT3, HT4, LU8, KD10

HEART SEDATION ACUPOINTS: HT7, **SP3** (compare SP5 metal + SP9 water)

Frequent supporting acupoints:

- KD7 metal shu to assist existing water shu in releasing heat
- LU5 water shu to assist existing metal shu in releasing heat
- TB5 or UB62 to access the extra-vessels
- GB40 yuan-source to strengthen the organ opposite on the 24-hour clock

HEART TONIFICATION ACUPOINTS: LV1, HT9

Frequent supporting acupoints:

- KD7 metal shu to assist existing water shu in releasing heat
- LU5 water shu to assist existing metal shu in releasing heat
- SP4, TB5, or UB62 to access the extra-vessels
- GB39 group luo-connecting to harmonize the three yin leg meridians

SMALL INTESTINE BALANCING ACUPOINTS: SI2, SI1, LI1, UB66

SMALL INTESTINE SEDATION ACUPOINTS: SI8, **ST36** (compare ST45 metal + ST44 water)

Frequent supporting acupoints:

- UB67 metal shu to assist existing water shu in releasing heat
- LI2 water shu to assist existing metal shu in releasing heat
- KD6, LU7, or SP4 to access the extra-vessels
- KD9 xi-cleft to disperse meridian excess and used hormone metabolites into the yin linking extra-vessel

SMALL INTESTINE TONIFICATION ACUPOINTS: **GB41** (compare GB44 metal + GB43 water), SI3

Frequent supporting acupoints:

- UB67 metal shu to assist existing water shu in releasing heat
- LI2 water shu to combine with existing metal shu
- KD6, LU7, or SP4 to access the extra-vessels
- KD8 xi-cleft to disperse the yin heel extra-vessel excess

URINARY BLADDER BALANCING ACUPOINTS: UB40, UB60, SI5, **ST36** (compare ST45 metal + ST44 water)

URINARY BLADDER SEDATION ACUPOINTS: UB65, **GB41** (compare GB44 metal + GB43 water)

Frequent supporting acupoints:

- LU7, PC6, or TB5 to access the extra-vessels
- LI4 yuan-source to strengthen the metal element
- LV5 or SP4 luo-connecting to balance the wood or earth elements
- SP6 group luo-connecting to harmonize the three yin leg meridians

URINARY BLADDER TONIFICATION ACUPOINTS: LI1, UB67

Frequent supporting acupoints:

- LI2 water shu to assist existing metal shu in releasing heat
- LU7, PC6, SP4, or TB5 to access the extra-vessels
- SP6 group luo-connecting to balance the three yin leg meridians
- SP8 xi-cleft to disperse the spleen excess

KIDNEY BALANCING ACUPOINTS: KD3, KD2, **HT8** (compare HT4 metal + HT3 water), **SP3** (compare SP5 metal + SP9 water)

KIDNEY SEDATION ACUPOINTS: KD1, LV1

Frequent supporting acupoints:

- LU7, TB5, or UB62 to access the extra-vessels
- SI6 xi-cleft to disperse the small intestine excess
- ST40 luo-connecting to balance the earth element
- GB35 xi-cleft to disperse the yang linking extra-vessel excess

KIDNEY TONIFICATION ACUPOINTS: LU8, KD7

Frequent supporting acupoints:

- LU5 water shu to assist existing metal shu in releasing heat
- TB5 to access the extra-vessel
- SI7 luo-connecting to balance the imperial-fire element
- GB37 luo-connecting to balance the wood element

15.7.4 Common Supporting Acupoints for the Third Trisection

PERICARDIUM BALANCING ACUPOINTS: PC3, PC5, LU8, KD10

PERICARDIUM SEDATION ACUPOINTS: PC7, **SP3** (compare SP5 metal + SP9 water)

Frequent supporting acupoints:

- KD7 metal shu to assist existing water shu in releasing heat
- LU5 water shu to assist existing metal shu in releasing heat
- UB62 to access the extra-vessel
- GB40 yuan-source to strengthen the organ opposite on the 24-hour clock

PERICARDIUM TONIFICATION ACUPOINTS: LV1, PC9

Frequent supporting acupoints:

- KD7 metal shu to assist existing water shu in releasing heat
- LU5 water shu to assist existing metal shu in releasing heat
- SP4 or UB62 to access the extra-vessels
- GB39 group luo-connecting to harmonize the three yang leg meridians

TRIPLE BURNER BALANCING ACUPOINTS: TB2, TB1, ST45, UB66

TRIPLE BURNER SEDATION ACUPOINTS: TB10, **ST36** (compare ST45 metal + ST44 water)

Frequent supporting acupoints:

- ST44 water shu to assist existing metal shu in releasing heat
- UB67 metal shu to assist existing water shu in releasing heat
- KD6, LU7, or SP4 to access the extra-vessels
- KD4 luo-connecting acupoint to balance the water element

TRIPLE BURNER TONIFICATION ACUPOINTS: **GB41** (compare GB44 metal + GB43 water), TB3

Frequent supporting acupoints:

- ST44 water shu to assist existing metal shu in releasing heat
- UB67 metal shu to assist existing water shu in releasing heat
- KD6, LU7, or SP4 to access the extra-vessels
- SP8 xi-cleft to disperse the spleen excess

GALLBLADDER BALANCING ACUPOINTS: GB44, GB34, **ST36** (compare ST45 metal + ST44 water), LI1

GALLBLADDER SEDATION ACUPOINTS: GB38, SI5

Frequent supporting acupoints:

- LI2 water shu to assist existing metal shu in releasing heat
- KD6, LU7, PC6, SP4, TB5, or UB62 to access the extra-vessels
- KD9 xi-cleft to disperse the yin heel extra-vessel excess
- SP6 group luo-connecting to harmonize the three yin leg meridians

GALLBLADDER TONIFICATION ACUPOINTS: UB66, GB43

Frequent supporting acupoints:

- UB67 metal shu to assist existing water shu in releasing heat
- LI2 water shu to assist existing metal shu in releasing heat
- KD6, LU7, PC6, SP4, or TB5 to access the extra-vessels
- SP6 group luo-connecting to harmonize the three yin leg meridians

LIVER BALANCING ACUPOINTS: LV4, LV3, **SP3** (compare SP5 metal + SP9 water), LU8

LIVER SEDATION ACUPOINTS: LV2, **HT8** (compare HT4 metal + HT3 water)

Frequent supporting acupoints:

- LU5 water shu to assist existing metal shu in releasing heat
- KD6, TB5, or UB62 to access the extra-vessels
- KD9 xi-cleft to disperse the yin linking extra-vessel excess
- LI4 yuan-source to strengthen the metal element

LIVER TONIFICATION ACUPOINTS: KD10, LV8

Frequent supporting acupoints:

- LU5 water shu to assist existing metal shu in releasing heat
- KD7 metal shu to assist existing water shu in releasing heat
- PC6, TB5, or UB62 to access the extra-vessels
- PC4 xi-cleft to disperse the pericardium excess

CHAPTER 16

The Treatment Stage Sequence

The treatment stage utilizes the information gathered during the planning stage to create a cohesive treatment strategy that relaxes the client, promotes healing, corrects the root dysfunction, and addresses specific symptoms. See Chapter 12 to review the information gathered during the pre-treatment planning stage.

Begin the treatment stage by deciding on a prone or supine position, and make any adjustments needed to regulate the autonomic nervous system if the client is in a non-optimal treatment position. Consider the location of the root prescription acupoints, the client's symptoms, and the client's ability to relax and feel comfortable when determining treatment position. In some cases, a two-sided treatment that incorporates an additional set of acupoints or cupping is best.

The treatment stage sequence is similar for the four different treatment approaches: symmetrical, asymmetrical, supine, and prone. However, there are nuances to follow for each approach detailed in the sections below. The general treatment steps are:

STEP 1 — apply essential oils

STEP 2 — regulate the autonomic nervous system

STEP 3 — treat the root

STEP 4 — support the root

16.1 The Supine Symmetrical Treatment Sequence

The symmetrical treatment indicates the hemispheres of the brain and the meridians are equalized, allowing balance between the right and left sides of the body. This approach tests well for clients with satisfactory spinal alignment or minor health challenges, along with those who are maintaining their health or seeking facial rejuvenation treatments. If the abdomen indicates the optimal treatment position is prone, but the client prefers to rest faceup, use essential oils to balance the ANS to allow for needling in the supine position. Clients may prefer the faceup position due to sinus congestion, pressure, or indentations on their forehead from resting prone in the face cradle.

16.1.1 Supine Symmetrical: Apply Essential Oils

In the supine position, several options are available for applying the essential oils that tested beneficial. The skin along the arch on the soles of the feet absorbs both undiluted and diluted essential oils quickly. It is the preferred application site for people with sensitive skin or autoimmune conditions. Another option is to apply diluted essential oils over the associated organ or Body-Feedback organ referral areas corresponding with the root treatment. For example, with a root liver treatment, apply the liver organ and meridian blends on the skin over the rib cage and liver area in the right upper quadrant of the abdomen. If the essential oils benefit the skin, apply them to the back of the neck, forehead, or hairline. Use the undiluted essential oils in areas without excessive sun exposure (mid to lower back) and the soles of the feet.

To adjust a prone optimal treatment position to supine, apply diluted essential oils along the spine and back of the neck. When using undiluted blends, spread a layer of carrier oil over the spine first and then apply the undiluted oils on top of that and to the soles of the feet. Repress the abdomen after using the essential oils and confirm the master alarm points and abdominal muscles are now relaxing, indicating the ANS is balancing.

16.1.2 Supine Symmetrical: Regulate the ANS

Locating and needling the specific abdominal, scalp, facial, or auricular acupoint apertures to regulate the ANS occurs during step two of the treatment stage. For the abdominal and scalp acupoints, lightly glide the pipette (guide tube) along the skin in the area of an acupoint to help locate the point's aperture. For facial acupoints, use transverse needle insertion underneath wrinkle lines. Confirm the precise location of each abdominal, auricular, and scalp acupoint just before inserting the needle by placing the pipette with the needle on the exact location or carefully press it with your fingertip. Recheck one of the master alarm points (GB21, TB15, or SI13) after each point's needle insertion to confirm point location accuracy.

16.1.3 Supine Symmetrical: Treat the Root

For a symmetrical treatment, the root organ/meridian dysfunction is the same on the left and right sides of the body. Needling the Body-Feedback balancing prescription along with the sedation or tonification acupoints in any order is acceptable. Remember to test and compare any horary acupoints to their metal + water substitutions for the following:

HT8 fire to HT4 metal + HT3 water

ST36 earth to ST45 metal + ST44 water

SP3 earth to SP5 metal + SP9 water

GB41 wood to GB44 metal + GB43 water

Allow additional time during the initial Body-Feedback session to determine each acupoint's precise location for that client by checking the pulse or master alarm points. At follow-up appointments, recheck the pulse or master alarm points after needling each arm or leg to verify point location accuracy of groups of points instead of individually. If the pulse became more wiry or forceful, or discomfort increased in the master alarm points, an acupoint requires re-needling. To determine if an acupoint needs re-needling, press the skin around the needle and recheck the pulse or master alarm points. If pressing on the skin around the acupoint improves the pulse or releases the discomfort in the master alarm points, remove the original needle and re-needle at the new location.

16.1.4 Supine Symmetrical: Support the Root

The supporting acupoints for each side of the body are usually the same for symmetrical treatments unless pathogenic heat affects a meridian on only the right or left side. Because pathogenic heat can jeopardize acupuncture's effectiveness, always check the metal + water shu-points on the right and left.

- Identify any unpaired water or metal shu-points already included in the root prescription and test their additional water or metal acupoint.
- Test the metal + water combination for the meridians associated with remaining wiry or forceful pulse positions.
- Check the metal + water combination for any meridians traveling through areas of pain, discomfort, or musculoskeletal symptoms.
- Test the metal + water combination for the root treatment's five-element pair.

The extra-vessel, xi-cleft, luo-connecting, and yang yuan-source supporting points are also usually the same for each side of the body unless pathogenic heat is affecting a meridian on one side. The ashi points for pain, neuropathy, musculoskeletal symptoms correspond with symptoms on the right and left sides of the body and may be symmetrical or asymmetrical.

The optimal needle retention time depends on the client's constitution, the total acupoints used, and the size of the needle. Needle retention guidelines for symmetrical treatments are 15-25 minutes for tonification root prescriptions and 20-30 minutes for sedation root prescriptions. Use shorter needle retention times when cupping or needling a second set of acupoints in the prone position.

16.2 The Supine Asymmetrical Treatment Sequence

The majority of clients experiencing an acute or chronic health crisis require the asymmetrical treatment approach. One sign of improved health is the transition from asymmetry to symmetry. With new clients experiencing complex conditions, the faceup position is more comfortable for their initial appointment to accommodate the additional time needed to test the differing acupoint prescriptions for the right and left sides.

16.2.1 Supine Asymmetrical: Apply Essential Oils

In the supine position, asymmetry uses the same application methods for beneficial essential oils as symmetry. Essential oils absorb and circulate throughout the entire body within minutes, encouraging the unification of the right and left sides of the body. Follow the recommendations in Section 16.1.1 to determine the application sites for diluted and undiluted blends.

16.2.2 Supine Asymmetrical: Regulate the ANS

The abdominal, scalp, facial, or auricular acupoints to balance the ANS for asymmetry are usually different on the right and left sides of the body. With mild asymmetry, or as the body is transitioning to symmetry, the acupoints to balance the ANS can be the same on both sides while the root prescriptions are different. After determining the acupoints on one side, check different combinations for the other side. Look for asymmetrical facial features to choose acupoints for testing. Check different combinations on the left and right sides of the body to regulate the ANS.

Phlegm nodules can form anywhere in the body and usually have an asymmetrical presentation. Surround the outer borders of a maximum of four phlegm nodules with up to six needles per nodule per treatment. Insert the needles around the nodules first to allow for additional needle retention time for this type of excess pathology.

16.2.3 Supine Asymmetrical: Treat the Root

Asymmetry requires treating two root organ/meridian dysfunctions between the left and right sides of the body. Treating the roots for asymmetry follows the same steps as in Section 16.1.3 to confirm the precise location of each acupoint. If one side is deficient and the other is excess, needle the sedation side first and the tonification side second to allow for additional needle retention time for the side requiring sedation. Remember to test and compare the metal + water combinations for **HT8**, **ST36**, **SP3**, and **GB41**. At follow-up appointments, look for signs of the body transitioning to symmetry, and consider one-sided exercises, stretches, and postural changes to encourage balance.

16.2.4 Supine Asymmetrical: Support the Root

Needling a variety of acupoints naturally occurs with asymmetrical treatments, reducing the need for additional support. Still check for pathogenic heat affecting the meridians in each side's root prescription. Identify any unpaired water or metal shu-points already included in both root prescriptions and test their additional water or metal acupoint. Test the metal + water combination for the meridians associated with remaining wiry or forceful pulse positions.

When pathogenic heat is not present, check the extra-vessel acupoints (UB62, LU7, KD6, SP4, PC6, and TB5) for each side. These extra-vessels affect genetic and structural issues, which powerfully influence the transition to symmetry. Test the right and left sides individually for ashi points for pain, neuropathy, musculoskeletal symptoms.

Needling the sedation side first accounts for the difference in needle retention time between deficiency and excess root treatments. Because the needle insertion time generally takes a little longer for asymmetry and there are a greater variety of acupoints, use the shorter time recommendations. The needle retention times for asymmetrical treatments are 15-20 minutes for tonification root prescriptions and 20-25 minutes for sedation root prescriptions. Use shorter needle retention times when cupping or needling a second set of acupoints in the prone position.

16.3 The Prone Symmetrical Treatment Sequence

The prone symmetrical treatment allows for direct treatment of the central nervous system and pain conditions affecting the neck, shoulders, and back. Positioning clients as comfortably as possible to tolerate the temporary inconvenience of lying in a face cradle allows for the increased healing offered in the prone position. Ask the client if they are comfortable before starting the treatment and use folded/rolled towels or extra pillows for comfort and support. If a client with these conditions is struggling to relax facedown, schedule additional time for a set of prone needles followed by a supine treatment.

During the pre-treatment planning stage, identify whether any of the balancing, sedation, or tonification acupoints will be resting on the treatment table or challenging to reach in the prone position. Remember to test and compare the metal + water combinations for **HT8**, **ST36**, **SP3**, and **GB41** during the pre-treatment planning stage. There are two options for applying magnetic pellets or press tacks to acupoints that are difficult to reach in the facedown position. Start the treatment faceup, apply any magnets or press tacks, and then help the client roll over to the prone position. Otherwise, before inserting needles in the prone position, ask the client to bend their knee and lift the ankle to place the magnetic pellets or press tacks on the top of their foot. Confirm that the arms are resting comfortably. The scapula is in the best position for needling when the arms are next to the torso. A rolled-up towel under the shoulders or hips can increase comfort while facedown.

16.3.1 Prone Symmetrical: Apply Essential Oils

In the prone position, apply beneficial essential oils to the soles of the feet and alongside the areas to needle. First, determine the areas to needle by comparing three or four acupoints on the governing vessel, Hua Tuo Jia Ji line, and the inner and outer urinary bladder lines. The spinal levels between T1 and L2 treat the sympathetic nerves. The cervical and sacral vertebrae, along with the spinal levels from L3 to L5, treat the parasympathetic nerves. Apply the essential oils about two cun alongside the treatment lines to needle. For areas of the skin that are frequently exposed to the sun, dilute beneficial oils first with a carrier oil or lotion and then apply the skin. Use the undiluted essential oils on the soles of the feet and in areas without excessive sun exposure (mid to lower back).

16.3.2 Prone Symmetrical: Regulate the ANS

When the root Body-Feedback prescriptions are the same on the left and right sides, the acupoints on the back are almost always symmetrical or directly over the spine. Clients with mild scoliosis, or those who have transitioned into monthly maintenance acupuncture with more severe scoliosis, may benefit from an asymmetrical back treatment with the same root treatments on the right and left sides.

Check the back acupoint combinations to balance the ANS on both the right and left sides to TB15 or the pulse to confirm precise locations before needling. Palpate the back carefully to identify possible phlegm nodules and musculoskeletal asymmetry requiring different acupoints combinations on the right and left. Needle the outer borders of the phlegm nodules and regions with excessive muscle tightness first, and acupoints to strengthen areas of weakness along the spine last.

16.3.3 Prone Symmetrical: Treat the Root

For a symmetrical treatment, the root organ/meridian dysfunction is the same on the left and right sides of the body. Needle the remaining Body-Feedback balancing prescriptions along with the sedation or tonification acupoints. Use the same techniques as in Section 16.1.3 to confirm the accuracy of the acupoints and determine if any require re-needling.

16.3.4 Prone Symmetrical: Support the Root

The back acupoints reduce the need for supporting acupoints. Always check for pathogenic heat affecting the meridians included in the acupoint prescriptions. Add back ashi points for pain, neuropathy, or musculoskeletal symptoms that may or may not be symmetrical. Additional supporting acupoints are optional.

The optimal needle retention time is shorter for treatments in the prone position because of the increase in the total acupoints and the client's ability to remain comfortable. The needle retention times for symmetrical prone treatments are 15-20 minutes for tonification root prescriptions and 20-25 minutes for sedation root prescriptions. Use shorter needle retention times when cupping or needling a second set of acupoints in the supine position.

16.4 The Prone Asymmetrical Treatment Sequence

Prone asymmetrical treatments are often complex and require additional time to treat the back accurately. With prone asymmetrical treatments, consider a two-sided treatment approach for clients experiencing an acute or chronic health crisis with nervous system involvement or musculoskeletal pain. Explain to the client how each side of the body needs a different treatment approach, and that optimal results occur with two separate sets of needles: needles for the back while facedown address the nervous system and musculoskeletal issues; needles for the front while in the faceup position address the root organ/meridian dysfunctions. A two-sided treatment approach can accelerate healing for new clients. After symptoms and the number of back acupoints reduce, consider incorporating the root treatment with the back acupoints in the facedown position.

16.4.1 Prone Asymmetrical: Apply Essential Oils

In the prone position, use the same technique for applying essential oils as the symmetrical treatment approach in Section 16.3.1. Apply the essential oils directly over the spine before needling the lateral edge of any tight erector spinae muscles causing a curve. The essential oils encourage symmetry regardless of the application site. Use the appropriate guidelines mentioned above for undiluted and diluted blends.

16.4.2 Prone Asymmetrical: Regulate the ANS

With asymmetry, the spine can have multiple curves to the right and left, or the spine can have one large curve extending the full length of the spine towards the right or left side only. Begin by testing and needling three or four acupoints in a row on the excess side of the curve. Locate these acupoints on the lateral side of the tight erector spinae muscle or the outer urinary bladder line. Then check and needle the Hua Tuo Jia Ji line towards the spine on the deficient side of the curve. If the curve runs laterally along the entire right or left side of the spine, use four or five stationary cups on the excess side and then check and gently needle between six to nine acupoints along the Hua Tuo Jia Ji or inner urinary bladder line on the deficient side. Use the same techniques for locating the asymmetrical acupoints on the back as outlined in Section 16.3.2.

16.4.3 Prone Asymmetrical: Treat the Root

A second set of needles in the faceup position to treat the root organ/meridian dysfunction can be more comfortable for new clients and those with complex symptoms. However, adding the root prescriptions in the facedown position after needling the back acupoints is perfectly acceptable. Remember to needle the sedation side first and the tonification side second, and compare the metal + water combinations for **HT8**, **ST36**, **SP3**, and **GB41** when they are included in the root acupoint prescriptions.

The initial Body-Feedback asymmetrical treatment in the prone position can take additional time to check each acupoint to TB15 or the pulse. Follow the same steps as in Section 16.1.3 to confirm the precise location of each acupoint. At follow-up appointments, look for reduced signs of asymmetry and consider one-sided exercises, stretches, and postural changes to encourage symmetry.

16.4.4 Prone Asymmetrical: Support the Root

The prone asymmetrical treatment naturally includes a wide range of acupoints, which reduces the need for additional support. Follow the same steps as in Section 16.2.4 to check for pathogenic heat and the extra-vessel acupoints. Check the ashi points for pain, neuropathy, and musculoskeletal symptoms to TB15 on the same side of the body.

Needling the sedation side first helps to account for the difference in needle retention time between deficiency and excess root treatments. The variety of acupoints for asymmetry takes longer to needle, which allows for the shorter needle retention time recommendations. Incorporate stationary cupping, as needed, during the needle retention time. The needle retention times for supine asymmetrical treatments are 15 minutes for tonification root prescriptions and 20 minutes for sedation root prescriptions.

16.5 Post Needle Removal

When removing the needles for all treatment approaches, confirm that the client was able to relax during the session. After the needles are removed, assess the pulse while the client is still lying down to evaluate improvements from the treatment before the client gets up and activates their sympathetic nervous system. The pulse should be slightly slippery and balanced in all positions. If any pulse position is wiry or forceful, check the metal + water combination for the corresponding meridians to see if pathogenic heat increased during the session.

Recheck the root treatment's Body-Feedback areas (meridian and organ alarm points, referral areas, and muscle associations). Ask if there is any remaining discomfort, and if so, what is the percentage of improvement. In general, an 80% reduction in discomfort in the Body-Feedback testing locations indicates a masterful treatment. The remaining pain should continue to reduce over the next few days. If the client's symptoms remain or pain lingers check herbs and nutritional supplements to use between appointments.

With repetition and recognizing each client's nuances, completing the four steps of the treatment stage sequence can occur in under 15 minutes. While learning the Body-Feedback treatment approach, it usually takes around 25 minutes to complete the treatment stage. Clients often recognize and appreciate this customized approach to address their healthcare needs.

SECTION

4

The Post-Treatment Stage

CHAPTER 17

Self-Care with Magnets, Press Tacks, and Seeds

Clients can extend their treatment benefits and accelerate healing by applying magnets, press tacks, and Vaccaria seeds to specific acupoints. Eight-hundred gauss magnetic pellets (sometimes called magnetic seeds) can effectively stimulate the jing-well, ying-spring, and shu-stream point categories. These small, round, 800 gauss magnetic pellets have a random pole orientation and activate acupoints without a north or south pole direction. Higher-strength magnets between 1,000 and 12,000 gauss activate the acupoints requiring deeper and stronger stimulation. These stronger flat magnets have a north or south pole direction on each side, requiring Body-Feedback testing for the correct polarity placement on the skin. Clients can reapply the stronger flat magnets indefinitely using hypoallergenic surgical tape.

Press tacks (also known as press needles) are small needles (.20-gauge by 1.0-1.5mm length) embedded in tape designed for perpendicular insertion. Due to their gauge and insertion direction, press tacks will sedate a meridian or organ when retained for more than an hour. Press tacks are useful to treat the ying-spring, shu-stream, jing-river, and he-sea points when the acupoint location is resting on the table or bolster. The client can retain the press tacks between one and 48 hours to sedate specific acupoints and drain excess conditions from the meridians and organs between appointments. If needed, use additional hypoallergenic surgical tape to secure the press tack adequately.

For additional relief of symptoms, clients can stimulate auricular acupoints as needed using Vaccaria seeds or place stronger magnets on xi-cleft or ashi acupoints daily. Unlike the small magnetic pellets that can irritate and embed in the skin after more than four days of continued use (or sooner with children whose skin regenerates quicker), Vaccaria seeds can remain in place for a week or longer without skin irritation when used with a high-quality adhesive tape, which varies by manufacturer.

17.1 Post-Treatment Self-Care Options

Determining if self-care is appropriate for a client depends on the client's interest and ability to follow through at home. Some clients appreciate and enjoy taking the time to improve their meridian system balance and organ function at home. Other clients prefer to have their practitioners manage their treatments completely. Self-care can boost the treatment results, strengthen a client's constitution, extend support for a dysfunctional organ, and provide symptom relief.

OPTION ONE:
Identify lingering pathogenic heat in the meridian system and apply magnetic pellets, press tacks, or stronger magnets to the metal + water combinations.

OPTION TWO:
Enhance the balancing treatment for a dysfunctional organ or imbalanced meridian by stimulating the root meridian's shu-points with magnetic pellets, press tacks, or stronger magnets.

OPTION THREE:
Provide symptom relief using stronger magnets with south or north pole stimulation on xi-cleft and ashi acupoints or Vaccaria seeds on specific auricular points.

17.1.1 **Option One** - Address Lingering Pathogenic Heat

The first self-care option addresses lingering pathogenic heat in an organ/meridian immediately following a treatment. Assess the three individual pulse positions on the right and left wrists after removing the acupuncture needles while the client remains resting on the treatment table. If a pulse position is wiry or forceful, check its two corresponding meridians' metal + water combinations to identify lingering pathogenic heat. For example, a client whose needles were removed after their liver sedation root treatment presented with a wiry right guan (2nd) pulse position. This indicated possible lingering pathogenic heat in the earth element's organs/meridians. The pulse was monitored while pressing ST45 and ST44 together, and then pressing SP5 followed by SP9 (due to location). The pulse improved with the ST45 + ST44 combination, and 800 gauss magnetic pellets were applied to these points and left on until they fell off at home.

In cases with excessive pathogenic heat, multiple meridians/organs can benefit from extended treatment using the metal + water combinations. Either leave the magnetic pellets or press tacks on until they fall off or explain to the client how to re-apply them at home for self-care. The healing benefits from an acupuncture treatment will last longer when there are no signs of pathogenic heat.

For some clients, pathogenic heat quickly generates due to food choices, chronic infections, autoimmune conditions, repetitive movements, low hormones, and weak digestion. Some people generate excessive inflammation with everyday activities including walking and healthy exercise because of genetically dysfunctional inflammatory cycles. These clients benefit from the metal + water combinations on the same meridians at most or all appointments. When a few meridians are chronically affected by pathogenic heat, the clients can treat their metal + water acupoints at bedtime with magnets or press tacks and remove them upon waking up. When a client has three or more meridians chronically affected by pathogenic heat, test herbs and supplements, along with dietary changes to reduce inflammation and pathogenic heat between appointments and improve the effectiveness of future treatments.

The location of a shu-point, the stimulation it needs, and the client's nervous system sensitivity determine which type of magnet, seed, or press tack to use. The yang meridians' metal + water combinations are the ying-spring and jing-well points. Magnetic pellets are appropriate for both excess and deficient conditions. Press tacks on the ying-spring points extend the heat-clearing effects and provide stronger stimulation to sedate a meridian or organ. Press tacks on the jing-well points are too painful for most clients to tolerate. Shu-points on the hands respond best to applying 800 gauss magnetic pellets at bedtime and removing them in the morning because they will fall off in the shower or with handwashing. If the feet remain mostly dry, magnetic pellets can stay on these shu-points for up to four days through showering. If the client finds that their shoes continually press on the acupoints, they may tolerate Vaccaria seeds on the jing-well or ying-spring points better than magnets.

The yin meridians' metal + water combinations are the jing-river and he-sea points. Because the ankles constantly flex and move, acupoints in this location tolerate magnetic pellets or seeds best. He-sea points respond well to stronger stimulation using press tacks or higher-strength magnets between 1,000 and 12,000 gauss to drain pathogenic heat. When using the stronger magnets for self-care, determine which pole (side of the magnet) is best for each acupoint personalized for that client. First, place the magnet flat on the he-sea point and monitor the pulse for changes or test GB21. Second, turn the magnet over on its other side and monitor the pulse for changes or test GB21. One side of the magnet, or pole, will test beneficial, while the other will test negatively.

17.1.2 **Option Two** - Enhance the Root Balancing Treatment

Enhancing the root balancing treatment has several beneficial effects. The balancing acupoints reduce the client's symptoms by stabilizing the natural fluctuation that usually occurs between excess and deficiency with organ/meridian pathology and trisection discord. The balancing acupoints focus on healing the current root organ/meridian pathology that compromises the client's ability to self-heal. For clients who are maintaining their health with acupuncture, the balancing acupoints support their constitutional or genetic weaknesses. When the same balancing prescription tests favorably for several consecutive appointments, using magnets to enhance the root treatment can extend the time the treatment remains active to invigorate health.

The root meridian's two shu-points from steps one and two of the balancing prescription dramatically enhance the acupuncture treatment. The first shu-point is the grandmother's element and the second shu-point is the grandchild's element, both on the affected meridian. For example, use LV4 and LV3 to enhance a root liver treatment. To boost the treatment, send the client home with magnetic pellets or press tacks to keep on these two acupoints until they fall off. For self-care, apply the magnetic pellets, stronger magnets, or press tacks and have the client take a picture with their phone to reference for reapplying. Magnetic pellets can remain on up to four days before they irritate the skin. Press tacks are best removed and reapplied every two days to the acupoint (clean and dry the area before reapplication). Apply stronger magnets (1,000 to 12,000 gauss) overnight or for a few hours per day. Advise clients to discontinue use if there are signs of skin irritation or a reaction to the adhesive tape.

The following list identifies a root meridian's two shu-points and the type of magnet or press tack to use for home self-care. Press tacks are sedating when used for more than five or six hours. Clients tolerate press tacks on fire and he-sea shu-points when they are comfortable. Magnetic pellets are appropriate for both excess and deficient conditions. Remember to always test the north and south pole placement for the stronger gauss magnets.

Self-Care Options for Balancing Shu-Points				
Organ/meridian	**Shu-point**	**Magnetic pellet**	**1,000+ gauss**	**Press tack**
LUNG	LU10	X	X	
LUNG	LU11	X		
LARGE INTESTINE	LI5	X		
LARGE INTESTINE	LI3	X		
STOMACH	ST43	X		
STOMACH	ST44	X		X
SPLEEN	SP1	X		
SPLEEN	SP9		X	X
HEART	HT3		X	
HEART	HT4	X		
SMALL INTESTINE	SI2	X		
SMALL INTESTINE	SI1	X		
URINARY BLADDER	UB40		X	X
URINARY BLADDER	UB60		X	X
KIDNEY	KD3		X	
KIDNEY	KD2	X		
PERICARDIUM	PC3		X	
PERICARDIUM	PC5	X		
TRIPLE BURNER	TB2	X		
TRIPLE BURNER	TB1	X		
GALLBLADDER	GB44	X		
GALLBLADDER	GB34		X	X
LIVER	LV4	X		
LIVER	LV3	X	X	

17.1.3 **Option Three** - Provide Symptom Relief

The third self-care option provides symptom relief by placing stronger magnets (1,000 to 12,000 gauss) on supporting xi-cleft or ashi acupoints and by applying Vaccaria seeds to auricular acupoints. Use 1,000 to 5,000 gauss magnets for the xi-cleft and ashi acupoints on the neck, hands, arms, feet, and ankles. Use 5,000 to 12,000 gauss magnets on the legs, back, shoulders, and abdomen. These stronger magnets are best utilized for a few hours or overnight and reapplied daily between appointments. **Avoid magnets with clients who have pacemakers.**

After removing the acupuncture needles, choose one or two supporting acupoints to test the stronger magnets. Monitor the pulse or test TB15, GB21, or SI13 after holding the magnet in place on the acupoint for 10-15 seconds. Then flip the magnet over and test its opposite pole while monitoring the pulse or checking TB15, GB21, or SI13. One magnetic pole will test favorably while the other will cause the body to respond negatively.

Self-Care Magnets for Xi-Cleft Points

Organ/meridian	Xi-Cleft Point	Magnetic Strength	Body Region Treated
LUNG	LU6	1,000 - 5,000	chest, shoulder, arm
LARGE INTESTINE	LI7	1,000 - 5,000	shoulder, arm, wrist
STOMACH	ST34	5,000 - 12,000	abdomen, hip, leg
SPLEEN	SP8	5,000 - 12,000	abdomen, hip, leg
HEART	HT6	1,000 - 5,000	chest, arm, wrist
SMALL INTESTINE	SI6	1,000 - 5,000	shoulder, arm, wrist
URINARY BLADDER	UB63	1,000 - 5,000	back, neck, leg, ankle
KIDNEY	KD5	1,000 - 5,000	pelvis, hip, leg, ankle
PERICARDIUM	PC4	1,000 - 5,000	chest, shoulder, arm
TRIPLE BURNER	TB7	1,000 - 5,000	neck, shoulder, arm
GALLBLADDER	GB36	5,000 - 12,000	back, neck, hip, leg
LIVER	LV6	5,000 - 12,000	pelvis, hip, leg
YANG HEEL	UB59	1,000 - 5,000	back, neck, leg, ankle
YIN HEEL	KD8	1,000 - 5,000	pelvis, hip, leg
YIN LINKING	KD9	5,000 - 12,000	pelvis, hip, leg
YANG LINKING	GB35	5,000 - 12,000	back, neck, hip, leg

17.2 Auricular Points

Auricular points have direct nerve connections to the entire body through the ANS, which allows them to provide immediate relief of pain or discomfort. Use the back end of a needle handle or ear probe to test corresponding regions in the ear to TB15 or while monitoring the pulse. The best testing acupoints are often painful to the client. Pain on only one side of the body usually tests favorably to auricular points on the ear of the same side. Check the corresponding regions in the ear using the following auricular chart:

Ear Reflexology Chart

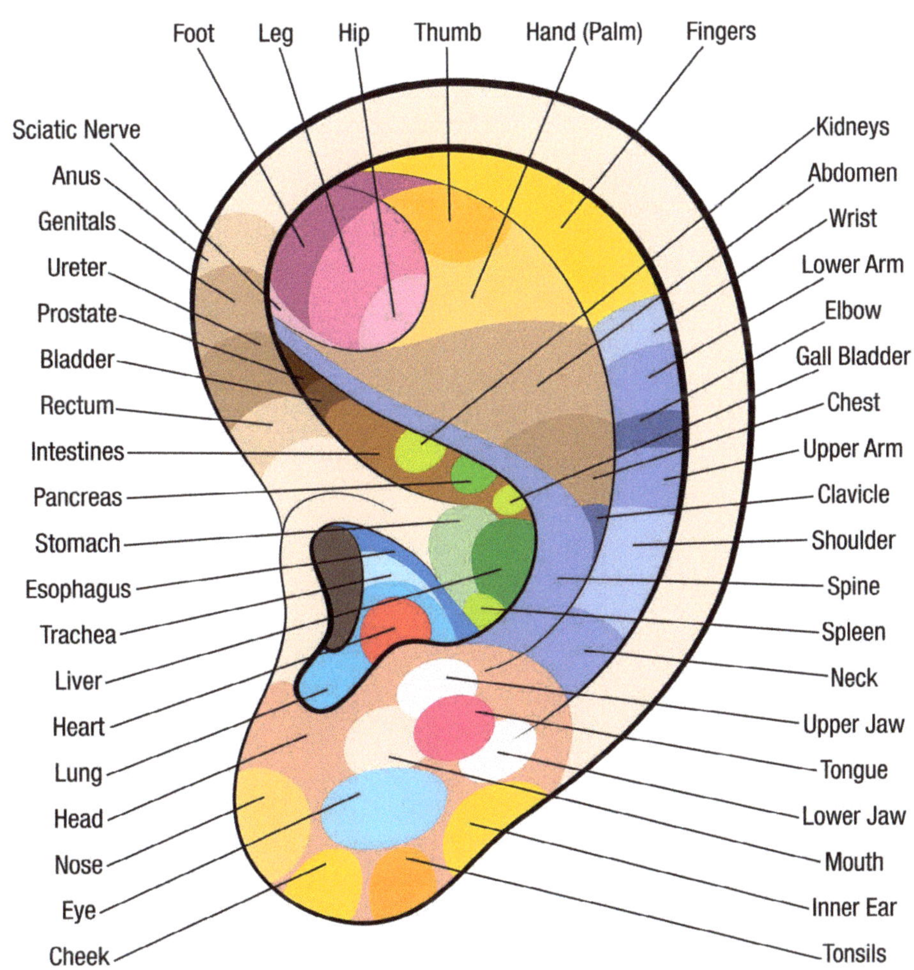

Apply a Vaccaria seed to between one and three locations on each ear. A Vaccaria seed provides low-level constant stimulation of a point, and the client can press and hold the seeds for 30-60 seconds to increase symptom relief. The seeds can remain on the ear points for a week or more as long as the skin is free of irritation and the ear's temperature is normal. Remove the ear seed early with signs of skin irritation or heat.

Some clients find self-care helpful and may need to have the ear seeds replaced or the magnets relocated before their next appointment. The body has a way of rejecting magnets and ear seeds when no longer needed. Advise clients to use the magnets and ear seeds at home daily until they fall off easily, experience an increase in symptoms, or find it more difficult to sleep. Reassess the placement of the magnets and seeds at future appointments or schedule a few minutes for the client to stop in between acupuncture sessions. As a client's health improves, they are often less interested in maintaining a self-care routine and prefer regularly scheduled maintenance acupuncture.

CHAPTER 18

Testing Herbs and Supplements

Herbology and nutrition are two of the eight foundational branches of Chinese medicine that support daily health. Body-Feedback testing methods sort through the myriad of herbs and supplements to identify the best options for each client's needs by monitoring changes in their meridians via Body-Feedback testing locations or pulse assessment. When a client is free of symptoms, maintaining good health, or managing genetic influences, the herbs and supplements that test best are stable and require minimal to no rotation. When a client is struggling with health challenges, multiple symptoms, pathogenic infections, or recent trauma, the herbs and supplements that test best can change weekly or may require frequent rotation.

Factors that influence how a client's body responds to the testing of herbs and supplements include timing (before or after an acupuncture treatment and the time of day), seasonal influences, daily intake of food and water, and pathogenic infections. For menstruating women, herbs and supplements affecting the endocrine system can test differently depending on the phase of the menstrual cycle.

Testing before an acupuncture treatment or before the application of essential oils identifies the herbs and supplements needed to manage acute health concerns and restore meridian system balance. These are short-term beneficial supplements and require frequent retesting as health progresses. Testing after optimizing the meridian system with an acupuncture treatment or application of essential oils identifies the herbs and supplements that maintain meridian system balance, support constitutional weaknesses, and manage genetic influences. Confirmation of a balanced meridian system occurs when the pulse is optimized, and the Body-Feedback locations are relatively free of discomfort. With training, clients can check their supplements at home to identify rotation needs or when to schedule a supplement recheck. It is best for the clients to check supplements at home after applying essential oils or following activities that harmonize the meridian system, such as appropriate exercise, yoga, meditation, using infrared saunas, and restful sleep.

18.1 Testing Locations for Herbs and Supplements

The neck muscles and master alarm points have an accelerated response when testing herbs and supplements after balancing the meridian system with acupuncture, magnets, or essential oils. The brain continually monitors the meridian system and responds first to a substance that negatively affects the body, causing pain and tightness in the neck muscles and master alarm points within seconds of testing. Changes in the pulse, individual organ/meridian referral areas, and muscle associations take longer to respond (a minimum of 30 seconds) because the organs and meridians instinctively attempt to manage the negative influence.

When an herb, herbal formula, or supplement tests beneficial, a release of tension or discomfort in the neck muscles and master alarm points occurs within seconds while the individual radial pulse quality can have subtle improvements after 30 seconds. During the process of testing beneficial herbs or supplements resting on the upper abdomen, the meridian system attunes to the helpful vibration of that herb or supplement. After the meridian system has acclimated to the supplement being tested, removing it causes a brief rebound of increased tightness in the client's neck muscles and master alarm points for up to 30 seconds. This rebound reflects the body's desire to continue working with the beneficial vibration of the herb or supplement.

The individual radial pulse positions that correspond with the organs or meridians affected by an herb or supplement can take up to 90 seconds to fully register changes. Detrimental items will cause the individual pulse positions to become wiry and forceful in an attempt to expel them. After helpful items optimize the pulse, removing them from the client's body causes the pulse to rebound by tightening and becoming wiry, deep, or forceful temporarily. Once herbs or supplements are determined beneficial or non-beneficial, checking them to the individual organ/meridian referral areas or muscle associations can help evaluate how they affect specific organs, meridians, or body systems.

In some instances, herbs or supplements will test beneficial at first and then negatively after 30-90 seconds, indicating the client's body is unable to fully process the changes. For instance, when the liver benefits from a release of toxins but the kidneys are unable to complete the end stages of detoxification, the herbs or supplements can test beneficial at first and then negative after about a minute. If the kidneys are unable to filter and release toxins due to genetics, illness, or type of chemical compound, the toxins then recirculate in the blood, causing headaches, nausea, and brain fog before the body stores them again in the liver or fat cells. Supporting the kidneys for several months encourages the body to detoxify stored toxins slowly. It is critical to allow a client's body sufficient time to adjust to the vibration of herbs or supplements for accurate testing.

At times, an herb or supplement can test beneficial when checking the master alarm points but test neutral when checking the root organ/meridian referral areas. This occurs when the item being tested is helpful for general health or symptom management but is not correcting the client's root dysfunction. Initially, test herbs and supplements using the master alarm points to identify the beneficial ones. Then check these herbs and supplements to the root organ/meridian referral areas or pulse to determine which ones will best address the client's root dysfunction.

The endocrine hierarchy allows for testing all hormonal herbs and supplements to the thyroid testing locations (the neck muscles or SI13 Master Hormone Alarm Point). Each level of the endocrine funnel below corresponds with specific meridians. Because the thyroid depends on optimal adrenal, hypothalamus, and pituitary function, any beneficial herb or supplement for those glands also benefits the thyroid. The adrenals, ovaries, and testes correspond with the kidney meridian for testing. The thyroid will experience dysfunction when the other glands are disrupting the kidney meridian. This explains why the thyroid can be challenging to treat due to the other glands impacting it. The third pulse position (*chi*) on the left and the second pulse position (*guan*) on the right are balanced when the entire endocrine system is optimized.

Meramour's Endocrine Funnel

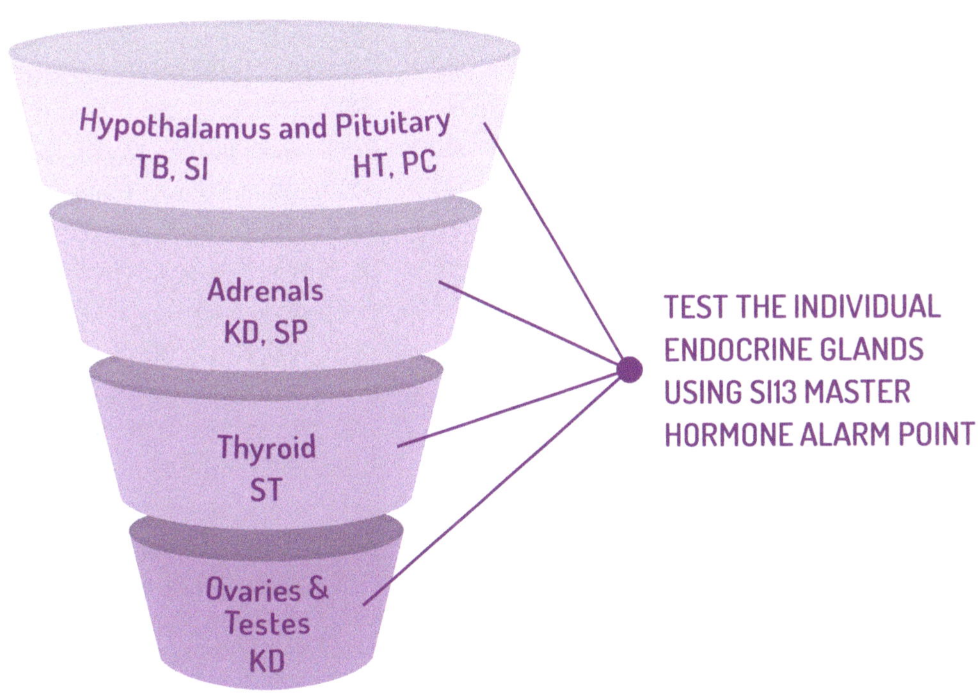

18.2 Choosing Herbs and Supplements

The Body-Feedback system integrates with herbal medicine and nutritional support in two fundamental ways. Root balancing treatments allow for identification of herbal formulas and supplements that support organ dysfunction and constitutional weaknesses. Testing methods can compare herbal formulas and supplements to confirm the correct TCM diagnosis and treatment approach. By addressing the client's root dysfunction, overall health improves quickly, the majority of symptoms resolve, and their herbal formulas require less rotation.

Compare Chinese herbal formulas that treat a client's TCM diagnosis and check them to the root balancing prescription's organ/muscle referral areas to identify the beneficial ones. For example, a twelve-year-old boy with asthma, allergies, and frequent respiratory infections received a lung balancing treatment for a lingering cough from a recent flu virus. His TCM diagnosis based on the tongue and pulse was wei qi deficiency, kidneys failing to grasp lung qi, phlegm, and dampness. The lung organ/meridian referral areas with discomfort identified during the treatment included LU10 and the deltoid muscle bilaterally. Three different Chinese herbal formulas were tested, including Yin Qiao San (for active infections), Qiang Shang Fang Feng Tang (for weak immunity with chronic low-grade infections), and Bu Fei Tang (for weak immunity without infection). Yin Qiao San tested favorably by releasing tension and discomfort at LU10 and the deltoid muscle, which indicated the presence of lingering infection. His TCM diagnosis was adjusted to include pathogenic heat in the tai-yin level.

Compare nutritional supplements that address individual symptoms or support specific body systems to identify the ones that test best. For the client above with wei qi deficiency and pathogenic heat in the tai-yin level, probiotics and immune-boosting supplements were tested. Probiotics are cultured and manufactured using three common processes: spore (or soil), dairy, and yeast. This client tested favorably for spore-cultured probiotics and a transfer factor supplement (boosts natural killer cell activity to identify intracellular pathogens and viruses). A complete release of discomfort in LU10 and the deltoid muscle occurred when the Yin Qiao San, probiotics, and transfer factor support were tested together (by placing them both on the upper abdomen at the same time).

The recommended dosages for this client began with three capsules of the Yin Qiao San twice daily with warm water on an empty stomach and one capsule of probiotics and one capsule of transfer factor support before bed for two weeks. After the initial two weeks, the recommended dose of Yin Qiao San was reduced to three capsules once a day. The one capsule of probiotics and one capsule of transfer factor support before bed remained the same for an additional two weeks. A follow-up appointment was scheduled for around five weeks to allow for one week off the above supplements before retesting. Discontinuing these supplements for one week provides time for chronic infections to register discomfort in the lung organ/meridian referral areas prior to symptoms recurring.

The following chart lists the Body-Feedback organ referral areas with corresponding TCM organ dysfunction diagnosis and common symptoms or conditions. The organ dysfunction patterns will generate tenderness, pain, muscle tightness, or muscle flaccidity at one or more of the Body-Feedback organ/meridian referral areas and muscle associations.

Organ/ Meridian Referral Area	Corresponding TCM Organ Dysfunction Diagnosis	Common Symptoms or Conditions
LUNG	Lung dysfunction with depressive heat	Allergies (environmental or food)
	Lung and kidney disharmony	Asthma
	Lung qi deficiency or lung and spleen disharmony	Immune deficiency
	Lung yin deficiency with blood heat	Autoimmune skin conditions
	Lung yin deficiency with deficient heat	Chronic cough or dry mouth
	Lung tai-yin exterior wind cold or heat with phlegm or dampness	*Shang Han Lun* six-level externally contracted diseases
LARGE INTESTINE	Large intestine depressive heat	Food allergies or pathogens
	Large intestine damp heat	Food allergies or pathogens
	Large intestine dryness	Adrenal dysfunction or dehydration
	Large intestine and stomach disharmony	Autoimmune digestive conditions or undigested food
	Large Intestine yang-ming organ pathogenic heat	*Shang Han Lun* six-level externally contracted diseases
STOMACH	Stomach depressive heat	Food intolerance or pathogens
	Stomach yin deficiency with deficient heat	Autoimmune digestive conditions or pathogens
	Stomach dysfunction	Food intolerance, acid reflux, or pathogens
	Stomach and spleen disharmony	Insufficient enzyme production or pathogens
	Stomach and gallbladder disharmony	Food intolerance or lack of bile production
	Stomach yang-ming channel pathogenic heat	*Shang Han Lun* six-level externally contracted diseases

Organ/ Meridian Referral Area	Corresponding TCM Organ Dysfunction Diagnosis	Common Symptoms or Conditions
SPLEEN/ PANCREAS	Spleen qi deficiency	Food intolerance or lack of enzymes
	Spleen qi and kidney yang deficiency	Food intolerance, pathogens, or lack of enzymes
	Spleen qi deficiency with depressive heat	Food intolerance or pathogens
	Spleen qi deficiency with damp heat	Food intolerance or pathogens
	Spleen and liver disharmony	Food intolerance or food toxins
	Spleen tai-yin exterior wind cold or heat with phlegm or dampness	*Shang Han Lun* six-level externally contracted diseases
HEART	Heart qi deficiency	Adrenal fatigue, anemia, or endocrine disorder
	Heart blood deficiency	Anemia or low hormones
	Blood heat affecting the heart	Pathogens, toxins, or autoimmune conditions
	Heart yin deficiency with deficient heat	Low hormones or autoimmune conditions
	Heart yang deficiency with dampness	Cardiovascular disease with edema
	Heart and kidney disharmony	Cardiovascular disease
	Heart shao-yin pathogenic cold (yang) or heat (yin)	*Shang Han Lun* six-level externally contracted diseases
SMALL INTESTINE	Small intestine qi deficiency	Imbalance in microbiome (dysbiosis)
	Small intestine depressive heat	Food allergies, intolerance, or pathogens
	Small intestine damp heat	Food allergies, intolerance, or pathogens
	Small and large intestine disharmony	Autoimmune digestive conditions or pathogens
	Small intestine tai-yang exterior wind cold or heat	*Shang Han Lun* six-level externally contracted diseases

Organ/ Meridian Referral Area	Corresponding TCM Organ Dysfunction Diagnosis	Common Symptoms or Conditions
URINARY BLADDER	Bladder dysfunction with depressive heat	Neurological conditions or inflammation
	Bladder dysfunction with blood heat	Autoimmune conditions or pathogens
	Bladder dysfunction with damp heat	Pathogens
	Urinary bladder tai-yang exterior wind cold or heat	*Shang Han Lun* six-level externally contracted diseases
KIDNEY/ ADRENAL	Kidney qi deficiency	Adrenal fatigue or food intolerance
	Kidney yang deficiency	Endocrine or nervous system dysfunction
	Kidney yin deficiency with deficient heat	Low hormones, endocrine or nervous system dysfunction
	Kidney essence deficiency	Genetic conditions or adrenal exhaustion
	Kidney and liver disharmony	Compromised detoxification or autoimmune conditions
	Kidney shao-yin pathogenic cold (yang) or heat (yin)	*Shang Han Lun* six-level externally contracted diseases
PERICARDIUM	Pericardium qi deficiency	Adrenal fatigue or anemia
	Pericardium blood deficiency	Endocrine dysfunction or metabolic syndrome
	Pericardium blood stasis	Endocrine dysfunction or metabolic syndrome
	Blood heat affecting the pericardium	Pathogens, toxins, or autoimmune conditions
	Pericardium jue-yin severe pathogenic cold/heat syndrome	*Shang Han Lun* six-level externally contracted diseases

Organ/ Meridian Referral Area	Corresponding TCM Organ Dysfunction Diagnosis	Common Symptoms or Conditions
TRIPLE BURNER	Dampness affecting the triple burner	Food intolerance or systemic inflammation
	Damp heat affecting the triple burner	Food intolerance, pathogens, or toxins
	Blood stasis affecting the triple burner	Pathogens, toxins, or autoimmune conditions
	Triple burner shao-yang half-interior half-exterior cold/heat pathogens	*Shang Han Lun* six-level externally contracted diseases
GALLBLADDER	Gallbladder depressive heat	Pathogens, congested bile, or gallstones
	Gallbladder damp heat	Pathogens, congested bile, or gallstones
	Gallbladder and liver disharmony	Genetic conditions or lack of bile production
	Gallbladder shao-yang half-interior half-exterior cold/heat pathogens	*Shang Han Lun* six-level externally contracted diseases
LIVER	Liver qi stagnation with depressive heat	Inflammation or excessive emotional outbursts
	Liver blood deficiency	Hormonal deficiency or anemia
	Blood heat affecting the liver	Pathogens, toxins, or hormonal imbalance
	Up-flaming of liver fire or liver yang	Food allergies, pathogens, or toxins
	Liver wind	Autoimmune or neurological conditions
	Liver jue-yin severe pathogenic cold/heat syndrome	*Shang Han Lun* six-level externally contracted diseases

18.3 Testing Daily Nutritional Supplements

Daily support with nutritional supplements can improve a client's health by providing micronutrients that are lacking in food sources, difficult to absorb, or require higher intake due to impaired genetics. Many clients notice improved energy, sleep, digestion, or mood when taking supplements chosen with Body-Feedback testing methods. If clients are taking daily supplements that increase discomfort in any of the organ/meridian referral areas or create an imbalance in the pulse, they are unable to receive the full benefits of an acupuncture treatment. Supplements that do not test beneficial can prolong a client's symptoms, organ dysfunction, and TCM diagnosis.

Multivitamin and mineral type supplements affect several different organ functions along with the corresponding organ/meridian referral areas, while individual vitamin, mineral, and amino acid supplements target fewer organs. Supplement manufacturers design standard multivitamins in proportion to meet the needs of the general public and design targeted support to include synergist vitamins and minerals to meet the needs of people with certain conditions. Some clients can test favorably for the multivitamin and mineral supplements, while others will test best for individual micronutrients or food-based supplements such as chlorella, fish oils, and turmeric. Test supplements to the organ/meridian referral areas to determine how they influence different organ functions. Certain supplements influence different organ functions more than others. Below are the five-element organ pairs and nutritional supplements commonly used to enhance their organ function.

The lung and large intestine organs are influenced by supplements that address the immune, respiratory, and digestive systems. Check probiotics, digestive enzymes, fish oils, minerals, vitamins A, C, and D, supplements with mushrooms or cultured in yeast, and herbs with anti-inflammatory or antihistamine properties using the lung and large intestine organ or meridian testing locations. People with mold allergies or chronic fungal infections will test negatively for many supplements containing mushrooms and yeast. Compare vitamin D with and without added vitamin K, as children, young adults, and people with acute pathogenic infections often test best without the vitamin K. Adults often test best for vitamin D combined with vitamin K. Iodine affects the immune system and can benefit or exacerbate immune system dysregulation depending on the client. Other factors to consider that can influence a client's reaction to iodine include consumption of iodized salt (often in processed foods) and shellfish allergies. Most clients require a blend of minerals and test best to a multimineral supplement either with or without iodine. Magnesium is a mineral some clients need alone or in addition to a multimineral supplement. Test magnesium with multimineral supplements to check for compatibility. Use the first pulse position (cun) on the right wrist for checking supplements for the lung or large intestine organs or meridians.

The spleen (pancreas) and stomach organs are influenced by supplements that address the immune, endocrine, and digestive systems. To support the initial stages of digestion by the stomach or pancreatic enzyme production, check digestive enzymes, betaine HCL, and anti-microbial herbs using the spleen or stomach organ/meridian testing locations. Check supplements that encourage healthy blood sugar levels, such as gymnema, berberine, chromium, and manganese, using the spleen organ or meridian referral areas. Check thyroid supplements, such as iodine, thyroid glandular, multivitamins, or herbal supplements, using the stomach meridian (which connects with the thyroid) muscle referral testing locations. Use the second pulse position (guan) on the right wrist for checking supplements for the pancreas, thyroid, spleen, or stomach organs or meridians.

The heart and small intestine organs are influenced by supplements that address the cardiovascular, endocrine, nervous, and digestive systems. Check supplements to support the cardiovascular system, such as fish oil, antioxidants, CoQ10 (as ubiquinol or ubiquinone), magnesium, heart glandular, multivitamins, B-vitamins, probiotics, or herbs using the heart organ or meridian testing locations. To enhance the absorption of nutrients, correct dysbiosis, address pathogens, or affect the enteric nervous system, check digestive enzymes, betaine HCL, probiotics, antimicrobial, and other digestive supplements using the small intestine organ testing locations. Check pituitary, hypothalamus, and adrenal supplements using the heart or small intestine meridian testing locations or SI13 due to the endocrine and nervous system interactions. Use the first pulse position (cun) on the left wrist for checking supplements for the pituitary, hypothalamus, and heart and small intestine organs or meridians.

The kidney and urinary bladder organs are influenced by supplements that address the endocrine, detoxification, and nervous systems. Check supplements to support detoxification and the kidney organs, such as alpha-lipoic acid, antioxidants, n-acetyl cysteine, resveratrol, chlorella, minerals, and kidney glandular, using the kidney organ or meridian testing locations. Check cranberry extract, uva ursi, corn silk, and horsetail supplements to the urinary bladder organ testing locations. To enhance the endocrine and nervous systems, test fish oil (compare different ratios of EPA and DHA), pregnenolone, DHEA, melatonin (test in the evening), and minerals using the urinary bladder meridian testing locations. Check pituitary, hypothalamus, and adrenal supplements using the kidney or urinary meridian testing locations or SI13 due to the endocrine and nervous system interactions. Use the third pulse position (chi) on the left wrist for checking supplements for the adrenals, ovaries, testes, and kidney and urinary bladder organs or meridians.

The pericardium and triple burner (lymph nodes) organs are influenced by supplements that address the endocrine, immune, lymph, detoxification, nervous, and digestive systems. Check antimicrobial supplements, probiotics (compare different types of sources), vitamin D (with and without K), antioxidants, chlorella, activated charcoal, and minerals using the pericardium or triple burner organ testing locations. Check nerve, pituitary, hypothalamus, and brain support supplements, such as fish oil, resveratrol, phosphatidylserine, and phosphatidylcholine, using the pericardium or triple burner meridian testing locations, SI13 or TB15. Use the third pulse position (chi) on the right wrist for checking supplements for the hypothalamus, pituitary, lymph nodes, lymph channels, and pericardium and triple burner organs or meridians.

The liver and gallbladder organs are influenced by supplements that address the detoxification, digestive, endocrine, and nervous systems. Check all supplements using the liver or gallbladder organ/meridian testing locations due to the interconnectedness of these two organs. To support general liver function, enzyme production, and digestion of fats, check digestive enzymes that target fats, choline, B-vitamins (including folate and SamE), antioxidants, turmeric, berberine, reishi mushroom, and liver glandular supplements. To assist with detoxing heavy metals and environmental toxins, check chlorella, activated charcoal, topical magnesium, bath salts, milk thistle, and mineral supplements. To assist with detoxing used hormone metabolites and xenoestrogens (environmental toxins that bind to estrogen receptor sites), check cruciferous vegetable supplements, probiotics, and quercetin. Use the second pulse position (guan) on the left wrist for checking supplements for the liver and gallbladder organs or meridians.

18.4 Practical Application for Testing Herbs and Supplements

Testing herbs and supplements can add between 5-15 minutes to the post-treatment stage, depending on the treatment position and number of items to assess. With the client in the prone treatment position, remove the needles and allow the client to turn over and get comfortable in the supine position for testing. With the client in the supine treatment position, remove the needles to begin testing. Sedation treatments respond best to longer needle retention time. Therefore, if the root treatment is sedating, another option for testing herbs and supplements can occur after removing only the abdominal acupoints leaving the other ones in for additional treatment time. In general, three to five herbs or supplements are manageable to test as part of an acupuncture appointment. For complex cases while testing more than six items, schedule 15 minutes after an acupuncture session for testing.

Limiting the time for testing herbs and supplements to 15 minutes maintains the integrity of the acupuncture treatment or application of essential oils to optimize the meridian system. Ask every new client to bring all supplements and medications they are currently taking to their initial acupuncture session. If a new client has been taking supplements that are not testing favorably, ask them to refrain from taking them to allow the acupuncture treatment to hold and to return to retest the supplements within a few days to a week. If the client requires a medication, herb, or supplement that is not testing favorably, check essential oil blends with the necessary item to identify the compatible combinations that change their body's response to neutral or beneficial. Instruct the client to apply the essential oils to the soles of the feet just before taking these medications, herbs, or supplements.

When a client is experiencing a significant health challenge, the root organ dysfunction requires the majority of support. Herbs or supplements that support other non-root organs can test negatively because they are supporting a different organ, which further distresses the root organ. As a client's constitution strengthens and their general health improves, a wider variety of herbs and supplements will test beneficial. Retest herbs and supplements before refilling them to identify when rotation is necessary or when new items can be added.

Several factors can cause a supplement or herb not to test beneficial, including the raw materials used, manufacturing process, the time of day the supplement is taken, and whether the supplement is taken with or without food. Testing supplements with hormonal influence may require coordination with a woman's menstrual cycle. If an herb or supplement causes an adverse effect after testing favorably, change the recommended time of day or take with food. With pathogenic infections, a client may respond best to slowly titrating the dose for a few weeks until reaching the desired dose. Leaky gut syndrome is a condition that allows food, herbs, and supplements to seep through the intestinal wall and trigger an unwanted immune response. If a client has leaky gut syndrome, they will have an intolerance to regularly ingested foods or food allergies and will respond best to fewer supplements with a four-day rotation schedule.

The quality of herbal formulas and nutritional supplements can vary significantly by manufacturer. Herbal manufacturers use different binding agents to create tablets and tea pills, and some use anticaking agents to prevent herbal granules from clumping and hardening. Where the herbs are grown, how they are harvested, and the manufacturing process impacts the quality of a supplement. Supplement manufacturers use different raw materials that can vary significantly and affect the testing results. For instance, magnesium supplements can contain any one or combination of the following types of raw materials: citrate, oxide, chloride, lactate, malate, taurate, glycinate, orotate, and L-threonate. The type of or blend of magnesium that tests favorably depends on magnesium's functions and a client's symptoms.

As health improves, a client will eventually only require support for constitutional or genetic weaknesses. The journey to wellness can occur within a few months for some and take years for others. The herbs or supplements to support constitutional or genetic deficiencies will test beneficial after a client's symptoms have resolved.

CHAPTER 19

Testing Foods and Personal Care Products

Foods, beverages, and personal care products applied topically to the skin significantly impact any type of medical treatment's potential healing benefits. The skin absorbs topically applied products (lotion, bug spray, makeup, perfume, and deodorant), along with clothing materials (polyester contains estrogen-mimicking particles), laundry detergent, and fabric softener. Women with estrogen dominance or going through menopause can have increased sensitivity to environmental toxins containing xenoestrogens.

Body-Feedback testing can identify beneficial foods, beverages, and personal care products that diminish tenderness in the organ/meridian testing locations. When foods or personal care products increase organ dysfunction or disrupt energy flow through the meridian system, discomfort in the testing locations increases, the pulse becomes imbalanced, and the benefits from acupuncture, essential oils, herbs, or supplements decrease.

An individual's genetics and constitution influence how well their body can tolerate certain food groups, along with chemicals found in personal care products and non-organic or processed foods and beverages. Clients with a more robust constitution can tolerate more frequent exposure to chemicals and non-organic foods. However, chemicals, fertilizers, genetically modified foods, and herbicides will still burden their digestive, immune, and detoxification systems, thereby reducing the effectiveness of their acupuncture treatments. Some clients require natural personal care products and organic fresh foods to support their health. Current farming practices of genetically modified wheat and gluten products cause adverse testing responses for many clients, while organic wheat products test fine for some.

Body-Feedback testing can help each client understand their individual needs and develop a healthier lifestyle. Training clients to check their testing locations or pulse before and after eating, and before purchasing personal care products, allows them to make educated choices and learn how their body responds to certain foods and products. To support health and longevity, continual monitoring of the testing locations allows clients to gather information and adjust their diet and personal care products as needed.

19.1 Testing Foods and Beverages

Some people tolerate certain foods groups (grains, dairy, legumes, or fats) better than others based on their genetics and constitution. The Body-Feedback testing methods can identify challenging food groups to avoid or consume with digestive enzymes. Testing of foods and beverages can occur both before and after an acupuncture session, but the results may differ. Before an acupuncture treatment, a client will generally have more foods that test negatively due to organ dysfunction within the wood element or first trisection. A client can tolerate more foods and beverages after acupuncture or using supplements and digestive enzymes. Testing foods or beverages with and without the digestive enzymes can indicate how helpful the supplement will be for digestion of those items. In general, it is best to test foods and beverages to TB15 or the neck muscles during the post-treatment stage.

Three common conditions that challenge the digestive and immune systems include an excessive histamine response to foods, excessive inflammation production with digestion, and the inability to digest fats properly. Excessive histamine and inflammation can damage the small intestine, causing leaky gut syndrome and irritate the large intestine and nervous system. Excessive histamine always causes additional inflammation, while inflammation by itself does not create a histamine response. Use the master pathogenic heat alarm point (GB21) and the meridian fire alarm points to test foods and beverages that may cause excess inflammation alone. Use the lung and large intestine testing locations to check for excessive histamine response to foods.

Most allopathic food allergy testing identifies foods that trigger a severe IgE anaphylactic response, such as peanut and other nut allergies. These extreme IgE allergies differ from the more common IgG and IgA immune response that challenges digestion. The IgG response is a delayed immune reaction that can create antibodies that disrupt the immune functions for over 30 days after consuming the food allergen. The IgG response can trigger an autoimmune response affecting any organ, endocrine gland, or musculoskeletal tissue in the body. Currently, while there are tests to identify which foods are causing the abnormal IgG response, there is no way to determine which part of the body is affected by the autoimmune response. Because of the delayed immune response of IgG, people are often unaware of a particular food causing an unwanted immune response. The IgA response is an immediate immune response that creates antibodies that cause organ dysfunction of the small or large intestines. Often, people associate IgA response with a recent meal that causes digestive pain, constipation, or diarrhea. The IgE and IgG responses cause discomfort in the lung and stomach testing locations. The IgA response causes discomfort in the small and large intestine testing locations.

Healthy fats are a source of fuel for the brain and the body, and they become cholesterol that converts into hormones. The proper digestion of healthy fats is required to complete the healing cycle caused by excessive histamine or inflammation. The final stages of cellular repair depend on a combination of hormones and omega-three fatty acids. Sources of omega-three fatty acids include fish oil, olives, olive oil, avocados, avocado oil, coconut, coconut oil, palm oil, walnuts, walnut oil, grass-fed dairy products, and grass-fed meats. Omega-six fatty acids found in other nuts, seeds, and the oils are challenging to digest. If the ratio of omega-three fats is too low compared to omega-six fats, additional inflammation occurs.

The immune system is responsible for a healthy inflammatory response that initiates and completes the tissue regeneration process. Properly digested healthy fats and hormones provide the raw materials needed for tissue regeneration. The adrenals produce cortisone that signals the end of an inflammatory cycle. If a client consumes excessive amounts of inflammatory foods, has compromised digestion, or has low hormone levels, he or she will remain in an unproductive inflammatory cycle that damages the body and compromises health.

Clients who produce excessive histamine and remain in an unproductive inflammatory cycle or who have difficulty digesting fats from their diet can benefit significantly from digestive enzymes. Most supplement manufacturers provide a variety of enzyme-based products to address different aspects of digestive support. Some enzymes help reduce an excessive histamine response from certain food groups, reduce the inflammatory response to certain food types, or assist with the digestion of fats. Check between three to six different digestive enzyme supplements to the master alarm points, neck muscles, or second pulse positions on both wrists.

After optimizing the meridian system with acupuncture or essential oils, test organic foods from the common disruptive food groups along with healthy fats and fish oil supplements. If organic foods or fish oil supplements cause discomfort in the testing locations, digestive enzymes are going to be beneficial. Check two or three items from the common inflammatory and allergen food groups, including gluten, dairy, sugar, legumes, soy, nuts, and corn.

Common Food Allergen and Intolerance Groups

Gluten: compare organic to conventional bread products, pasta, and flour products.

Dairy: compare organic to conventional yogurts, milk, butter, and cheeses.

Sugar: compare organic to conventional cane sugar, honey, and maple syrup.

Legumes: compare organic to conventional and canned to dried beans and lentils.

Soy: compare organic to conventional tofu, soy sauce, and other soy-based products.

Nuts: compare organic to conventional and raw to roasted cashews, almonds, and walnuts.

Corn: compare organic to conventional corn chips, popcorn, and cornmeal.

Oils: compare omega 3 (fish, avocado, coconut, olive, and walnut) to omega 6 (sunflower, safflower, sesame, and canola).

Many people experience increased discomfort in the testing locations from coffee, because a volatile oil in the coffee bean causes an adrenal stress response and high levels of acid result from the roasting process. When coffee causes increased discomfort in the testing locations, the client might find that the caffeine in tea may be easier to tolerate. Check coffee, tea, and other regularly consumed beverages to the master alarm points, neck muscles, or second pulse positions on both wrists.

Recheck foods that initially tested negatively, along with beneficial enzyme products placed together on the upper abdomen. Foods or beverages a client can tolerate with the digestive enzymes will test neutral or favorably. A client should continue to avoid foods and beverages that test unfavorably with the digestive enzymes. Recommend clients follow a four-day rotation for foods tolerated with digestive enzymes.

The digestive and immune systems reset at night after several hours of inactivity. Intermittent fasting promotes healing by allowing the digestive system to rest, the immune system to remove damaged cells, the liver to focus on detoxification, and the nervous system to regenerate. Waiting 12-15 hours between dinner and breakfast is ideal. Tea, coffee, and other clear beverages under 50 calories are acceptable during the fasting period. Ingesting a collagen powder (which includes protein) in water instead of an early breakfast stabilizes blood sugar, reduces hunger, and helps with tissue repair. Recommend eating dinner by 6 p.m., drinking tea or water before bed and upon waking, taking collagen protein powder early in the morning, and eating a healthy breakfast or snack between 9 a.m. and 10 a.m. Intermittent fasting with collagen powder early in the morning may help stabilize the immune and digestive systems for chronic and autoimmune conditions. Remember to check the collagen powder to the master alarm points, neck muscles, or to the first trisection organ or meridian testing locations.

19.2 Testing Personal Care Products

Personal care products absorb through the skin and then circulate into the lymph system and bloodstream. Items beneficial for health will assist with detoxification and immune functions while bypassing the digestive system. Unfavorable personal care items disrupt self-healing by congesting the liver, gallbladder, and lymph system, burdening detoxification pathways, and creating undesirable immune responses. Clients who have chronic detoxification or immune system dysfunction can make choices in the use of personal care products to improve their health. By choosing organic lotions, body wash, soaps, and laundry detergents that test beneficial, the acupuncture, essential oils, herbs, or supplements can achieve their full potential.

Third trisection organs detoxify the blood and lymph system, manage the absorption and utilization of fats, and create cholesterol for conversion into hormones. Clients who are struggling with excessive weight and cellulite have dysfunctional third trisection organs. Adding a few drops of essential oil to an organic lotion and applying a few times a week to areas where fat is stored will enable the oil to bind with toxins and improve detoxification. Essential oils that are beneficial for the skin and aid with detoxification include geranium, cypress, and lavender. Essential oils that are beneficial for the lymph system and weight reduction include spearmint, grapefruit, and lime. Note that citrus oils increase skin sensitivity and photosensitivity. Dilute citrus essential oils with an organic lotion or carrier oil and only use on skin not currently exposed to or previously damaged by the sun.

Test any products containing essential oils, including natural body wash, deodorant, lotion, laundry soap, and dryer products to ensure they are supporting a client's health. Check personal care products using the master alarm points, neck muscles, individual liver testing locations, or pulse either before or after the acupuncture session. The quality of the essential oils, the ingredients in the personal care products, and the organs they support influence how these items test using Body-Feedback techniques. Clients with skin sensitivities, autoimmune conditions, or hives usually test best for products that are fragrance-free and contain no essential oils.

19.3 Assessing Foods, Beverages, and Personal Care Products

Check foods, beverages, and personal care products using the master alarm points, individual Body-Feedback testing locations, and wrist pulses. Testing these items before and after balancing the meridian system causes a response in the same manner as testing herbs and supplements.

- Testing before balancing the meridian system with acupuncture or essential oils more easily identifies foods, beverages, and personal care products that improve organ function.
- Testing after balancing the meridian system with acupuncture or essential oils more easily identifies acceptable foods, beverages, and personal care products to use long-term, and those to avoid.
- After balancing the meridian system, the neck muscle and master alarm points respond first because the brain continually monitors for any disturbance from a substance that negatively affects the body.
- After balancing the meridian system, changes in the pulse, individual organ/meridian referral areas, and muscle associations have a delayed response (a minimum of 30 seconds) because the organs and meridians instinctively attempt to manage negative influences.
- While testing a beneficial item, the meridian system attunes to the helpful vibration of the food or product, and removing it causes a temporary rebound of increased tightness in the client's neck muscles and master alarm points lasting up to 30 seconds. This rebound effect is the body's desire to continue working with the beneficial vibration of the food or product.
- Limit the time for testing foods, beverages, and personal care products to a maximum of 15 minutes to maintain the integrity of the acupuncture treatment.

The individual Body-Feedback testing locations provide clarity for possible causes of dysfunction and provide options for checking the body's response to foods, beverages, and personal care products. The amount of time spent on testing these items depends on each client's lifestyle and individual needs. Some clients will commit to making lifestyle changes and schedule acupuncture less often (from four to eight weeks). Others prefer to make fewer lifestyle changes and will schedule acupuncture more regularly (every one to three weeks). Clients often find making gradual changes toward a healthier lifestyle is easier to maintain long-term than changing too many things at once.

Focusing on changes in diet and personal care products to support the root organ dysfunction brings noticeable changes that provide positive reinforcement for continuing to follow recommendations. Gradually introduce more recommendations at an agreeable rate. Some clients like ideas for improving their lifestyle at every appointment, while others seem more open to changes in conjunction with New Year's resolutions, spring detox, or preparing for cold and flu season. The chart below provides suggestions for foods, beverages, and personal care products to test in combination with a client's root organ dysfunction.

Organ/Meridian	Possible Causes of Dysfunction
LUNG	Environmental toxins, excessive histamine response, chronic inflammation
LARGE INTESTINE	Histamine response to carbohydrates, yeast, sugar, leaky gut syndrome, excessive inflammation
STOMACH	Environmental toxins, food allergies, low enzyme production
SPLEEN	Inflammation response to carbohydrates, yeast, sugar, low enzyme production
HEART	Immune dysfunction affecting autonomic nervous system, endocrine disrupting skin care products
SMALL INTESTINE	Immune dysfunction affecting enteric nervous system, immune response due to low enzyme production
URINARY BLADDER	Immune dysfunction affecting central nervous system, endocrine disrupting skin care products
KIDNEY	Compromised detoxification, environmental toxins, inflammation from oxalates, insulin resistance
PERICARDIUM	Environmental toxins, food allergies, endocrine disrupting skin care products
TRIPLE BURNER	Environmental toxins, chronic inflammation, excessive histamine response
GALLBLADDER	Compromised detoxification of used hormones, lack of digestive bile for fats
LIVER	Environmental toxins, leaky gut syndrome, lack of digestive enzymes for fats

For example, a new client with autoimmune thyroid dysfunction had pain and muscle tension in all three of the master alarm points (GB21, TB15, and SI13), neck muscles, liver organ referral areas, and lung, liver, and gallbladder meridian alarm points. The root treatment at the initial appointment was a liver sedation treatment. A fish oil supplement only tested favorably after combining it with a digestive enzyme supplement to aid with the digestion of fats. Organic yogurt and cheese tested positively, while conventional cheese and milk tested negatively. This client was willing to change to organic food and dairy products.

Weekly acupuncture sessions showed improvements with reduced pain and discomfort in the original testing locations. After four weekly acupuncture treatments, the liver organ referral areas, along with the lung and liver meridian alarm points, remained tender. The client agreed to check personal care products and scheduled an additional 15-minute testing session after the next acupuncture session. This testing identified makeup foundation, lipstick, body lotion, and eye cream that caused increased discomfort in the master alarm points and neck muscles. Instructions on how to self-test LU10 and the liver organ referral area allowed her to test new products while shopping.

There are several ways to train clients to self-test using Body-Feedback methods. They usually gravitate to checking the wrist pulse, an organ referral area, or the neck muscles. Clients need guidance to identify the testing method that is easiest for them and supervision to gain confidence. One option is to schedule an additional 15-minute testing session after an acupuncture appointment. Seasonal or regularly scheduled 90-minute workshops for clients to practice self-testing provide an opportunity to improve health and lifestyle choices continually. For instance, offer self-testing workshops for immune-boosting supplements and essential oils before cold and flu season, detoxification support in the spring, and testing foods for the new year.

CHAPTER 20

The Post-Treatment Testing Stage

The positive effects of acupuncture on organ function and the meridian system are strongest immediately following a Body-Feedback session. An acupuncture treatment (using needles or magnets) or the application of essential oils removes the trisection discord resulting from the root dysfunction to accelerate the healing of multiple body-systems. Immediately following treatment, the vibration of qi traveling through each meridian attunes to cellular regeneration and allows for clear testing of items by way of the Body-Feedback locations. Testing items following an acupuncture treatment produces predictable and duplicatable results by enabling unencumbered communication between the practitioner and the client's body in a state of regeneration.

During the post-treatment testing stage:

- Use magnets, seeds, or press tacks as continuing self-care.
- Test herbs and supplements to support for the root dysfunction and constitutional health.
- Check foods and personal care products to enhance a healthy lifestyle.
- Determine a treatment schedule for future appointments.
- Monitor the natural progression of healing.

Healthy lifestyle choices and self-care with magnets immediately after an acupuncture treatment can continue to aid a client's root dysfunction after removing the needles. Accelerated healing resulting from a Body-Feedback style treatment can last up to one month with a healthy lifestyle and beneficial herbs, supplements, or essential oils. Continued cellular regeneration occurs when a client can maintain a balanced and slightly slippery pulse between appointments, representing robust organ and meridian activity.

After treatment, the meridian system responds clearly to testing for up to 15 minutes with palpable changes in muscle tension and pulse quality. During this time, a client can easily feel the changes in discomfort at master alarm points and tension in neck muscles. Use pulse assessment to identify any remaining discord in the individual organ/meridian testing locations and to confirm the compatibility of herbs or supplements. In some instances, checking items to the testing locations is straightforward, while at other times the pulse can be more obvious. Pregnant women and children under the age of twelve are highly sensitive to changes. For these clients, monitoring the pulse reflects this heightened awareness and checking items using pulse assessment can be easier.

20.1 Practical Application of the Post-Treatment Testing Stage

The complexity of each client's needs, in combination with the recommended 15-minute post-treatment testing time, limits the number of items to check during each session. With all new clients, allow for 15 minutes of post-treatment testing immediately following their initial treatment. At this appointment, create a treatment plan that provides for one or two additional 15-minute post-treatment testing sessions to have the client bring in foods and personal care products for testing. Allow for five-minutes of post-treatment testing with regular follow-up acupuncture sessions. Schedule a future 15-minute session for clients with routine follow-up appointments who need additional post-testing time. Use magnets or essential oils to quickly balance the meridian system before testing when not immediately following an acupuncture session.

Self-care with magnets, press tacks, and seeds provides options to enhance the acupuncture's effectiveness and fine-tune the Body-Feedback root treatments. Step one options fine-tune the Body-Feedback root acupoint prescriptions. While removing needles, determine if the client was able to sleep or experience deep relaxation during the acupuncture treatment, which indicates a state of accelerated healing. After removing the needles, recheck the pulse (on one or both wrists) and confirm that it is slightly slippery and balanced. In most instances, if one side's radial pulse is balanced, the other will also be. If the practitioner and the client are satisfied with the improvements in health between appointments, and deep relaxation along with the pulse indicates a successful treatment, self-care options with magnets, press tacks, and seeds may not be needed. If the pulse indicates lingering pathogenic heat or the client desires more substantial treatment results, use time during the post-treatment stage to focus on the step one options below.

Options for self-care with magnets, press tacks, and seeds include:

- Identify lingering pathogenic heat in the meridian system and apply magnetic pellets, press tacks, or stronger magnets to the metal + water combinations.
- Enhance the balancing treatment for a dysfunctional organ or imbalanced meridian by stimulating the root meridian's shu-points with magnetic pellets, press tacks, or stronger magnets.
- Provide symptom relief using stronger magnets with south or north pole stimulation on xi-cleft and ashi acupoints or Vaccaria seeds on specific auricular points.

The amount of time to spend checking herbs and supplements during the post-treatment stage depends on a client's needs. There are two options for testing herbs and supplements when implementing Body-Feedback treatments with existing clients. For complex clients on multiple herbs or supplements, schedule an extra 15-minute testing session following their acupuncture to recheck what they are currently taking. For clients who are on fewer herbs and supplements, recheck their current recommendations before refilling them. Clients appreciate the time taken to ensure they are taking beneficial supplements as they can also feel the changes during testing.

Options for choosing herbs and supplements to support the root dysfunction and provide relief of symptoms include:

- Check all vitamins, supplements, and herbs a client takes daily. Consider phasing in or rotating herbs and supplements over multiple appointments to allow a client's body time to adjust.
- Test all herbs or supplements the client takes to ensure the current routine is supporting their needs. Recheck before refilling herbs and supplements to identify when rotation is needed.
- Test essential oils and other topical treatments for symptom relief while between appointments.
- Identify herbs or supplements that support detoxification and digestion first.
- If needed, check additional herbs and supplements to support the immune system.
- If a client's constitutional weakness occurs in the second trisection, choose additional herbs or supplements to support the endocrine and nervous systems.

Testing foods and personal care products can help identify hindrances to healing. Schedule additional 15-minute sessions following acupuncture to test up to ten items. With complex cases, it can be helpful to start with food allergy or intolerance testing. Test for food allergies when discomfort remains in the lung or large intestine testing locations. Test for food intolerances when discomfort remains in the spleen or stomach testing locations. Test the water a client drinks at home and work, including any bottled water regularly consumed. Reverse osmosis water can have severe health consequences when consumed without additional mineral supplementation for extended periods.

Soaps, lotions, cosmetics, detergents, and fabric softeners absorb through the skin and enter into the lymph system. Test these personal care products when a client has discomfort in the liver, lung, or triple burner testing locations at consecutive appointments. Training clients to self-test foods and personal care products reduces the need for additional sessions.

Options for testing foods and personal care products to create a healthy lifestyle include:

- Place digestive enzymes on the upper abdomen when testing foods if a client is or will be taking enzymes with their meals.
- Have a client bring with them two or three items from the common inflammatory and allergen food groups, including gluten, dairy, sugar, legumes, soy, nuts, and corn.
- Have a client bring with them foods that they notice cause digestive or immune symptoms.
- Have a client bring with them beverages they drink daily, including coffee, tea, juice, and soda. Test water in small glass jar containers and have high-quality spring water for comparison on hand.
- Have a client bring their personal care products or train them how to check these items at home.

Advise clients that a supportive lifestyle influences cellular aging and the ability to heal. Daily habits can limit or enhance the potential effectiveness of acupuncture treatments, herbs, and supplements. In some instances, relief of symptoms occurs only after making changes to foods, water, or personal care products. A client's root treatments can provide insights for further investigation into items for testing. Some clients require more time for post-treatment testing than others, depending on their current lifestyle.

CHAPTER 21

The Natural Progression of Healing

The two-hour segments of peak organ activity correspond with yin and yang's daily rhythms to harmonize with nature. The natural progression of healing follows these peak organ times in the twelve earthly branches order, beginning with the third trisection's wood element during the night. The first trisection organs correspond with the rising of the sun and increased activity in that geographical region. The heart's peak organ time occurs mid-day when the sun is the fullest, representing extreme yang transitioning into yin. As the sun withdraws, yin governs the second trisection's organs and glands, influencing the nervous and endocrine systems. The natural progression of healing ends with the ministerial-fire organs, the eleventh and twelfth earthly branches, developing stem cells in the lymph system and bloodstream for cellular regeneration.

Through restorative sleep, each day provides new opportunities for healing. Reducing excess conditions, such as qi stagnation, blood stasis, dampness, or external pathogens, allows for supplementing qi, blood, yin, and yang, along with regeneration. Optimal organ function throughout the day is key to enhancing quality-of-life and renewing cells.

> According to the *Yellow Emperor's Classic of Medicine*, the cycle of the twelve earthly branches corresponds with the five elemental phases, six atmospheric influences, and the three yin and yang steps [six-level pairs]. These twelve earthly branches begin with the first branch, known as *Zi*, that corresponds with the hours between eleven p.m. and one a.m. [the time of peak gallbladder organ activity]. The second branch, known as *Chou*, relates to the hours between one a.m. and three a.m. [the time of peak liver organ activity].[52]

21.1 Healing Depends on the Wood Element

According to the *Energy Almanac*, the natural healing process begins with the first earthly branch, the gallbladder, followed by the second earthly branch, the liver. All other organs depend on the wood element to function optimally. Supporting gallbladder and liver functions increase the concentration of qi available that transfers forward throughout the day. The liver and gallbladder organs produce bile and enzymes required for digestion and the processing of fats, which store and release toxins, create and dispose of hormones, provide raw materials to complete a healthy inflammatory cycle, and remove cellular byproducts from everyday activities. The liver meridian regulates qi flow throughout each organ to release stagnation and promote regeneration during its corresponding two-hour period of peak activity.

Quality sleep during peak gallbladder and liver organ times (11 p.m. to 3 a.m.) is necessary for cleansing blood, releasing toxins, and managing qi flow. Improving sleep enables acupuncture treatments, essential oils, herbs, and supplements to promote healing. Liver or gallbladder organ dysfunction or meridian imbalance can disrupt sleep during the respective peak organ time. Dual spleen and liver dysfunction can cause people to wake up every two hours during the organ transition times of 11 p.m., 1 a.m., and 3 a.m. Supporting detoxification and blood sugar regulation using herbs, essential oils, and nutritional supplements to encourage sleep promotes accelerated healing from acupuncture treatments.

The body replenishes its energy reserves and resets the daily flow of peak organ activity during the night for the following day. When a client works third shift or regularly remains awake between 11 p.m. and 3 a.m., support their sleep cycle with calming and relaxing herbs, supplements, or essential oils before bed and qi-boosting or energizing ones upon waking. Augmenting irregular or abnormal sleep cycles using herbs or supplements before going to bed and upon waking rectifies disrupted gallbladder and liver functions that occur between 11 p.m. and 3 a.m.

BODY-FEEDBACK CLINICAL PEARLS

A menstruating woman's cycle represents the significance of releasing the old to allow for the new. Day one of a monthly menstrual cycle begins with the first day of full flow that releases the last cycle's uterine lining. If a menstrual period fails to release used hormones and older blood, the following menstrual cycle is compromised. Leftover hormones delay egg maturation during the first half of a new cycle (the follicular phase) and compromise egg quality. Environmental synthetic estrogens clog hormone receptor sites and linger, causing estrogen-dominance. If estrogen-dominance continues, conditions such as endometriosis, fibroids, and infertility may eventually occur.

Mid-cycle ovulation depends on healthy estrogen levels and egg maturation activity during the follicular phase. Delayed ovulation, pain during ovulation, or lack of fertile cervical mucus indicates that follicular phase dysfunction has compromised the ovulation phase. Progesterone significantly increases during post-ovulation to balance estrogens and promote pregnancy if conception has occurred. Progesterone production depends on healthy liver and gallbladder organ function, along with a balanced endocrine system. The first step in improving reproductive health is to achieve a full release of old hormones, which comprise the uterine lining, so the new cycle can begin in an optimal state.

The Natural Progression of Healing Through the Twelve Earthly Branches

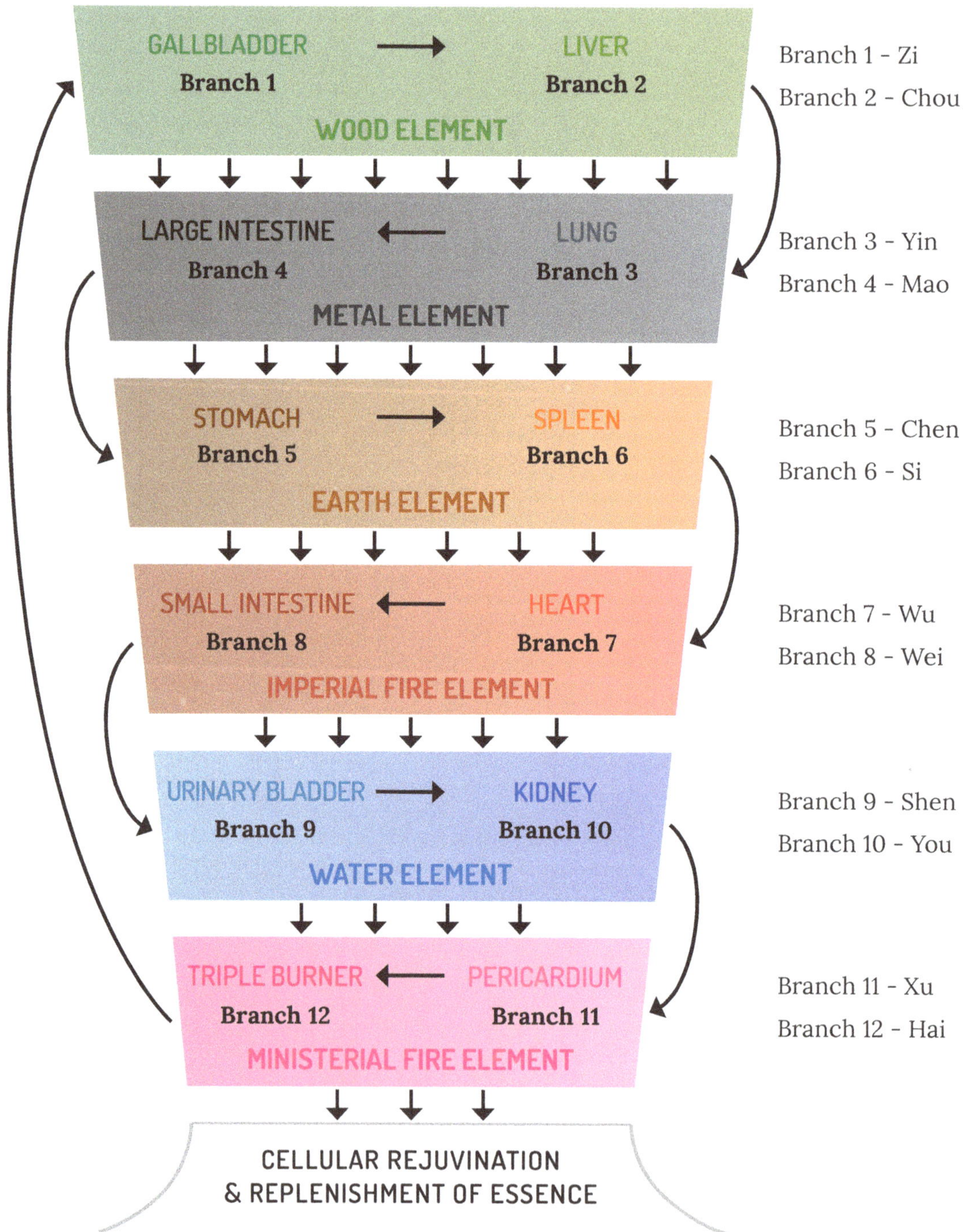

21.2 Healing Through the Twelve Earthly Branches

The client's earthly branch requiring attention determines the Body-Feedback root treatment at each appointment. For clients with a robust constitution, acupuncture accelerates healing of the root dysfunction for up to three weeks and optimizes the entire meridian system. For clients with multiple dysfunctional organs or chronic illness, acupuncture strengthens the weakest root organ, adds benefits to the other organ dysfunctions, and accelerates healing for about one week.

Weekly treatments for new clients and for those with a chronic illness will often address different root organs that follow the order of the twelve earthly branches. For instance, a new client's first root treatment was liver. The second appointment was a root gallbladder treatment. The third appointment was a lung root treatment. She then settled into spleen root treatments to support her constitution. As health improves for clients with chronic disease, the root Body-Feedback treatments will repeat cycling through specific twelve earthly branches, such as gallbladder, liver, large intestine, gallbladder, liver, large intestine, and so on.

Environmental toxins, poor water quality, and synthetic estrogens burden the gallbladder and liver organs. The most common root treatments are liver and gallbladder to support digestion and detoxification pathways. Negative emotions can result from or be the origin of a meridian imbalance in the wood element that contributes to organ dysfunction. Liver congestion can cause or result from irritability and frustration. Gallbladder dysfunction can cause or result from a lack of willpower. Optimizing liver and gallbladder function is critical for accessing the natural healing rhythms and allows the body to focus on the metal element's immune functions next.

The metal element organs (lungs and large intestine) generate the majority of immune system cells, such as IgG, IgE, IgA, white blood cells, neutrophils, lymphocytes, basophils, eosinophils, mast cells, and histamine. The lungs and large intestine construct the body's permeable borders to absorb qi by making contact with air and food. These barriers can make it challenging for the immune system to differentiate self from non-self, as in autoimmune conditions. Stress, sadness, and grief suppress immune function and can lead to or exacerbate autoimmune diseases. With immune system dysfunction, the lungs or large intestine might be the client's constitutional root treatment. Clients may need the occasional metal element root treatment when exposed to bacteria or viruses. Optimizing the wood and metal elements allows the body to focus on the earth element next.

The stomach and spleen influence metabolic rates, the thyroid, and muscle tone. The spleen also includes pancreatic functions. The early stages of digestion depend on healthy stomach acid, pancreatic enzyme production, and blood sugar regulation. Excessive sugar consumption, history or family history of diabetes, food allergies, and autoimmune endocrine diseases compromise the earth element organs. Stomach qi maintains the downward movement of energy throughout the digestive system. Feeling emotionally stuck or failing to put ideas into action can arise from or lead to stomach meridian imbalance. Spleen qi maintains the upward movement of energy to hold the organs in place. Spleen meridian imbalance can cause a client to feel unsupported or to lack pleasure in everyday life.

After optimizing the wood element and the first trisection, access to the second trisection organs and endocrine glands becomes available. The shao-yin level translates to deepest yin and corresponds with genetics, cellular regeneration, aging, cognition, and mental health. The tai-yang level translates to greatest yang and represents the most superficial aspects of the body's borders and how the nervous system is perceiving the environment. This trisection's five-element pairs internalize the external world on a cellular level, causing people to feel emotions like joy, fear, hope, frustration, or satisfaction generated through the nervous and endocrine systems. Emotions result from certain neurotransmitters and hormones combining, and they can change when a client changes how he or she perceives the world. This trisection includes the autonomic nervous system, hypothalamus, pituitary, and adrenals. Root treatments in this trisection can reduce the effects of stress on the body and change how clients perceive stress.

The imperial-fire element includes the heart and small intestine organs and meridians. TCM associates the heart with emotional and mental health (shen), which relates to the hypothalamus-pituitary axis and enteric nervous system. The heart represents the pituitary, and the small intestine represents the enteric nervous system and a portion of the hypothalamus. A heart deficiency root treatment often corresponds with organ weakness. A heart excess root treatment calms the response to stress in the hypothalamus and pituitary through optimizing hormones and neurotransmitters of the brain.

The small intestine organ generates neurotransmitters for the enteric nervous system and the meridian generates neurotransmitters in the brain for the hypothalamus. Root treatments for the small intestine organ and meridian impact mental health and organ function simultaneously. Food sensitivities, childhood abuse, and long-term stress can cause an imperial-fire constitutional weakness.

The water element includes the urinary bladder and kidney organs and meridians. TCM associates the kidneys with life-force, which corresponds with the adrenals, ovaries, and testes. Chronic stress and fear can cause water element discord that disrupts the hypothalamus-pituitary-adrenal axis, and overtime can lead to adrenal dysfunction. The urinary bladder meridian relates to the central nervous system's interaction with the hypothalamus. In the early stages of adrenal dysfunction, urinary bladder root treatments (either sedation or tonification) modulate the response to and perception of chronic stress. During later stages of adrenal dysfunction, root kidney tonification treatments revitalize exhausted adrenal glands. The water element influences the cellular aging and replication process.

Kidney sedation treatments help disperse kidney stones or infections. Kidney tonification treatments support organ and adrenal function and enhance cortisol production, sperm development, and egg maturation. Urinary bladder sedation and tonification treatments address organ function and optimize the hypothalamus and central nervous system. Optimizing the water element can address adrenal dysfunction, neurological diseases, infertility due to egg or sperm quality, accelerated aging, and cognitive decline.

The ministerial-fire element represents the last two branches in the natural progression of healing and corresponds with the body's ability to regenerate through adult stem cells, hormones, and new blood. The pericardium correlates with the pituitary's production of progesterone and testosterone from cholesterol and the creation of blood from digestion. Healthy nerve conduction conveyed through its myelin sheath depends on nutrient-rich blood and these hormones. The triple burner meridian encompasses the lymph vessels and aspects of the hypothalamus, and the organ includes lymph nodes and lymphocytes. The ministerial-fire element influences aspects of the HP axis and the endocrine system.

The ministerial-fire element protects a person's shen, the heart organ, and the body's deeper yin levels. Heat pathogens often cause excess conditions in this element and require sedation treatments. Outbursts and overreactions to stress cause excess pathology in the pericardium, and emotional rigidity affects the triple burner. Hematopoietic cells are adult stem cells that become monocytes, macrophages, neutrophils, basophils, eosinophils, erythrocytes, T cells, B cells, natural killer cells, and innate lymphoid cells, which protect the body and correspond with this element. Optimizing organ function for the previous ten earthly branches allows the body to focus on regeneration through the ministerial-fire element.

21.3 The Healing Journey

The natural progression of healing, often called the healing journey, is unique for each client and depends on multiple factors. Body-Feedback treatments identify the earthly branch's root organ dysfunction, which disrupts a client's healing progression. A client's genetic or constitutional weaknesses will become apparent when their root treatments are predominantly within the same element. A client with two or more dominant root dysfunctions will require asymmetrical treatments.

Many clients new to holistic medicine and organic lifestyles require liver and gallbladder support. If liver or gallbladder root treatments occur in the first few sessions, focus on detoxification of environmental toxins, xenoestrogens (plastics that mimic estrogen and clog the receptor sites), heavy metals, and excessive hormone metabolites (used hormones). The next priority is to promote healthy sleep patterns. From here, the client's body will identify where assistance is needed to complete the natural progression of healing and enhance peak organ activity. Clients with genetic liver or gallbladder root dysfunctions require continual detoxification and digestive support to improve all types of health challenges.

On occasion, an atypical root treatment will test best for a client who is under unusual stress, fighting a cold or flu, eating excessive sugar during the holidays, or recovering from a recent trauma. The point prescriptions will normally rotate between sedation and tonification when treatments target a constitutional or genetic weakness. This rotation of draining and supplementing acupoint prescriptions depends on diet, sleep, stress, exercise, time of year, and phase of the menstrual cycle for menstruating women.

Maximizing the daily healing cycle supports cellular renewal and longevity, which occurs when the pulse remains balanced, and minimal discomfort in the root treatment's testing locations occurs at multiple appointments. Some minor pain and tension in the master alarm points and neck muscles is normal and results from everyday activities. As health improves, root treatments strengthen the constitution so a client can overcome future health challenges. A client usually senses a root treatment is no longer active by a decline in energy, stamina, or emotional health. Use this guideline to determine the ideal length of time between appointments when creating a schedule for maintenance acupuncture.

How long the healing journey takes depends on age, lifestyle, constitutional health, and genetics. Recovery time is proportional to the duration of organ dysfunction and the severity of symptoms. For genetic or constitutional weaknesses, a healthy lifestyle with maintenance treatments enhances cellular regeneration, longevity, and quality of life. Caring for clients with compassion and appreciation for the opportunity to help them along their healing journey fosters life-long healthy relationships.

SECTION

5

Case Studies

The Integration of Body-Feedback and TCM Diagnosis

The Body-Feedback treatment approach integrates with and substantiates TCM differential pattern diagnosis. The inherent advantages of TCM, which ensure its continual existence, arise from its abilities to integrate with allopathic medicine, embrace advances in technology, and treat modern forms of chronic illness. TCM uses five-element and six-level theories in combination with the eight principles of pattern identification (interior or exterior, yin or yang, hot or cold, and excess or deficiency) to analyze new information and understand its effects on a client's health. New information can be assimilated into classical patterns and treatment principles using traditional differential diagnosis.

A client's constitutional weakness is the root of the TCM diagnosis and the earthly branch that disrupts the natural progression of healing. The TCM diagnosis for a new client with complex symptoms includes multiple pathologies representing several dysfunctional organs. At the time of treatment, the dysfunctional organ or meridian contributing the most symptoms to the TCM diagnosis is the root of the trisection discord that corresponds with the Body-Feedback balancing point prescription.

As a client's health improves, and their consequential symptoms resolve, the number of pathologies identified in their TCM diagnosis reduces until only constitutional weaknesses remain. Body-Feedback root treatments will rotate as a client overcomes superficial pathologies. When Body-Feedback root treatments repeat at multiple sessions, the constitutional weakness matches a client's TCM diagnosis.

The Body-Feedback system relies on the identification of discord in the trisection, along with standard TCM tongue and pulse assessment, to formulate a client's diagnosis. The number of pathologies reflects the extent of a trisection discord. In general, symmetrical treatments have fewer pathologies than asymmetrical treatments. The most significant difference in formulating a client's diagnosis between TCM and the Body-Feedback approach is the stage of treatment in which it occurs. Standard TCM establishes a diagnosis first, which controls the formulation of an acupoint prescription. Body-Feedback uses a treatment's acupoint prescription to identify trisection discord and then formulates a TCM diagnosis.

The following case studies outline the Body-Feedback approach using the pre-treatment, treatment, and post-treatment stages. Information gathered during the treatment process, along with tongue and pulse assessment, formulates the TCM diagnosis.

CHAPTER 22

Case Study One: Symmetrical Supine

Appointment #1 New Client Assessment

Case Study One (CS1) was a female, age 37 at the first appointment, with a two-year-old child that she conceived naturally. CS1 had gained 40 pounds during pregnancy and lost most of the weight during maternity leave. She has slowly gained 60 pounds over the last two years. Over the previous six months, her menstrual cycles increased from 28 to 38 days, and her periods had become very light. She experienced severe premenstrual syndrome (PMS) symptoms the day prior to her periods that included headache, anger, and lower back pain. She described her headaches as severe pain in the temples and forehead that started in the back of the head and moved forward. She also reported having experienced severe headaches during the first trimester of her pregnancy. CS1 indicated she would like to have a second baby, but she felt too unhealthy to try and conceive at this time.

CS1's health history had six symptoms indicated in the wood element section and three symptoms in the ministerial-fire element section. The form suggested a third trisection discord with a likely root wood element imbalance and branch ministerial-fire element imbalance. The treatments focused on testing acupoint prescriptions, herbs, and supplements to support liver and gallbladder organ function.

SUBJECTIVE INFORMATION

CS1 scheduled acupuncture to address tailbone pain, bilateral hip pain, and hyper-joint mobility that began after the labor and delivery of her first child. Over the previous few months, she had very tight calf muscles and woke up most days with bilateral foot pain and occasional muscle cramps in her lower legs. CS1 went to physical therapy, as recommended by her medical doctor, but experienced no improvement in her symptoms.

CS1 regularly skipped breakfast because of nausea upon waking and would overeat carbohydrates during the evening. She had urgent and loose bowel movements after eating that became more frequent during her menstrual periods. Since her pregnancy, CS1 had been taking a prenatal vitamin, D3, and fish oil she purchased at a retail store. She said that her vitamin D level had always registered below normal on bloodwork since her doctors started monitoring it.

BODY-FEEDBACK for Health, LLC
Confidential Health History

Name *Case Study 1*

Please Check All That Apply

METAL ELEMENT

- ○ Frequent colds, rhinitis, or sinusitis
- ○ Allergies, asthma, or autoimmune conditions
- ● Frequent cough, post-nasal drip, or congestion
- ○ Dry skin or sensitive skin
- ○ Hives, eczema, or rashes
- ● Constipation, loose stools, irregular bowels
- ○ Colon polyps or history of any type of cancer
- ○ Low back or hip pain worse in the morning
- ○ Shortness of breath or exercise induced asthma
- ○ Cold sores or herpes or other viral infections
- ○ Easily disappointed or offended
- ○ Sadness, low self-esteem, or excessive grief

EARTH ELEMENT

- ● Muscle weakness or lack of strength
- ○ All over puffiness or water retention
- ● Bruises easily, varicose, or spider veins
- ○ Low energy or fatigue after eating
- ○ Hypo or hyper thyroid function
- ○ Indigestion, bloating, or gas
- ○ Craves sugar, sweets, or carbohydrates
- ○ Neck pain or left sided pain in body
- ○ Diabetes, pre-diabetes, or hypoglycemia
- ○ Pain that worsens with cold or damp weather
- ○ Headaches or migraines triggered by weather
- ○ Easily worried or upset with changes or obsessive

WATER ELEMENT

- ○ Frequent, urgent, or difficult urination
- ○ Swollen or puffy ankles or feet
- ○ Low energy or needs more than 8 hours sleep
- ○ Low libido, sex drive, or reduced sexual function
- ○ Kidney stones, disease, or dysfunction
- ○ Forgetful or poor short term memory
- ○ Low back pain worse at end of day
- ● Headaches or migraines triggered by fatigue or hormone changes
- ○ Adrenal or thyroid dysfunction (hyper or hypo)
- ● Scoliosis, osteoarthritis, osteoporosis, (osteopenia)
- ○ Hormonal imbalances or endocrine dysfunction
- ○ Fearful, depression, or lack of motivation

FIRE ELEMENT

- ○ Insomnia, difficulty sleeping, or waking early
- ○ Excessive dreaming or nightmares
- ○ Dry skin and increased desire for fluids
- ○ Heart palpitations or irregular heartbeat
- ● Easy flushing, red type acne, dislike heat
- ○ Hot flashes or night sweats
- ○ Heart disease or family history of
- ○ Anxiety, restlessness, panic attack, or mind racing with physical exhaustion
- ○ High blood pressure or Low blood pressure
- ● Pain in sacrum, SI joint, or tailbone
- ○ Mouth sores, bleeding gums, or burning tongue
- ○ Headaches triggered by heat or excessive sun

WOOD ELEMENT

- ● Muscle tension, cramps, tightness
- ○ Sensitive to noise, strong odors, and tastes
- ○ Dry, red, or weak eyes
- ○ Coarse or brittle hair or nails or premature gray hair
- ● Tendon, ligament, or meniscus weakness or pain
- ● Fibromyalgia or all over joint pain
- ○ Numbness and tingling with sleep or inactivity
- ○ Seizures, tremors, or Parkinson's
- ● Pain or tightness in right shoulder or side of neck
- ● Bloating, diarrhea, or stomach pains after eating
- ○ Headaches or migraines triggered by stress
- ● Anger, irritability, or easily frustrated

MINISTERIAL-FIRE ELEMENT

- ○ High-pitched ringing or congestion in the ears
- ○ Headaches or migraines that move around in head
- ○ Swollen lymph nodes or chronic infections
- ○ Chronic sinus or ear congestion
- ● Stiff movements or general tightness
- ○ Belching, burping, or heartburn
- ● Difficulty losing weight or obesity in family
- ○ Polycystic ovarian syndrome or ovarian cysts
- ○ Cystic acne, boils, or cysts
- ● Sciatic pain or (tailbone pain)
- ○ Overly optimistic or unrealistic
- ○ Feeling oppressed or unable to make changes

www.Body-Feedback.com 608-535-9144 2014 Yahara Place, Madison WI 53704

OBJECTIVE INFORMATION

Pulse - overall choppy and tight, and forceful in the PC/TB and HT/SI positions
Tongue - medium white coating with a full, light purple body

ASSESSMENT

TCM: liver blood deficiency with uprising of liver yang, phlegm, blood stasis, and damp heat
Body-Feedback: third trisection discord with hypothalamus-pituitary dysfunction

PLAN

Treatment principle: nourish liver blood, anchor liver yang, transform phlegm and blood stasis, drain damp heat, harmonize the third trisection, and support the hypothalamus-pituitary axis.

Appointment #1 Pre-Treatment Planning Stage

PLANNING STEP ONE: ASSESS FOR ASYMMETRY

Visual assessment of the hips, feet, and shoulders indicated symmetry. TB15, SI13, and GB21 were painful upon palpation, tighter on the right, and increased discomfort upon palpation on the right. The neck muscles were symmetrical in size but tighter on the right.

PLANNING STEP TWO: REGULATE THE AUTONOMIC NERVOUS SYSTEM

Checking the abdomen decreased the tightness at TB15, SI13, and GB21, and indicated supine as the optimal treatment position. The wood and earth regions on the abdomen regulated the ANS at this appointment.

PLANNING STEPS THREE AND FOUR: DETERMINE THE BALANCING AND SEDATION OR TONIFICATION PRESCRIPTIONS

Based on the health history form and the most excessive pulse positions, the following exclusive shu-points were tested to the pulse bilaterally to determine this treatment's root prescription: LV3, GB34, PC3, HT3, TB2, and SI2. The pulse improved and became slightly choppy to balanced when pressing GB34, the gallbladder balancing prescription, and the sedation prescription bilaterally. Testing the same acupoints for both sides of the body confirmed a symmetrical supine treatment position. As part of the balancing prescription, **ST36** was checked and compared to ST45 metal + ST44 water; **ST36** tested favorably, as evidenced in the pulse.

PLANNING STEP FIVE: ASSESS THE CORRESPONDING TESTING LOCATIONS

CS1's symptoms indicated she'd had a wood element organ/meridian dysfunction for several years. Therefore, both the gallbladder and liver testing locations were checked for pain, discomfort, and muscle tightness. The testing locations with corresponding signs of organ/meridian dysfunction included:

- right rib cage shared regions with liver- and gallbladder-referred pain
- bilateral liver-referred discomfort at sternal attachment of pectoralis major muscle
- bilateral gallbladder-referred tightness and pain in anterior head of deltoid muscle
- bilateral LV2 and GB38 fire alarm points tender
- bilateral LV8 and GB34 organ alarm points tender

PLANNING STEP SIX: TEST ESSENTIAL OILS

The Liver and Gallbladder Organ Supporting and Meridian Balancing blends were tested individually, and only the Gallbladder Organ Supporting Blend released tightness in the master alarm points. Then the Triple Burner and Pericardium Organ Supporting and Meridian Balancing blends were tested individually, and only the Pericardium Organ Supporting Blend released tightness in the master alarm points. Finally, the Gallbladder and Pericardium blends were tested together and released the tightness and reduced the pain better than when tested individually.

PLANNING STEP SEVEN: CHECK FOR PHLEGM NODULES

There were no palpable phlegm nodules in the lower back along PSIS. This area was only checked during this first appointment.

Third Trisection Discord Root Gallbladder Excess

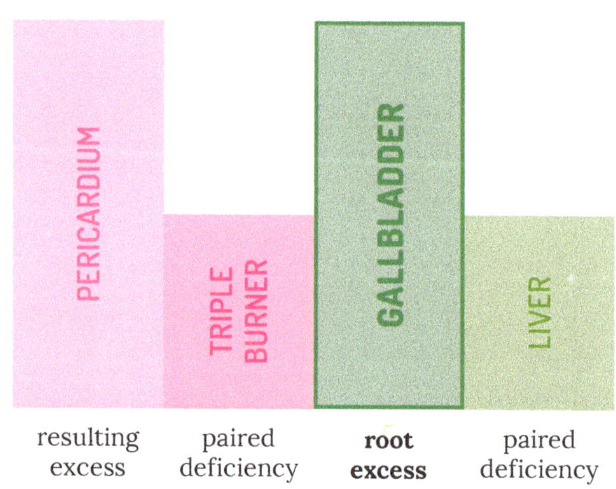

Appointment #1: Treatment Stage

TREATMENT STEP ONE: APPLY ESSENTIAL OILS

Applied 3 drops each of the Gallbladder and Pericardium Organ blends to the soles of the feet.

TREATMENT STEP TWO: REGULATE THE AUTONOMIC NERVOUS SYSTEM

Needled 4 acupoints along a horizontal line to harmonize wood and earth, along with CV6 to regulate the ANS at this appointment.

TREATMENT STEP THREE: TREAT THE ROOT

Needled the gallbladder balancing and sedation prescriptions including GB44, GB34, **ST36**, LI1, GB38, and SI5.

TREATMENT STEP FOUR: SUPPORT THE ROOT

Needled the supporting acupoints, including LI2 (additional individual water point), ST37 (large intestine lower he-sea), ST39 (small intestine lower he-sea), Yin Tang + Si Shen Cong (supports the hypothalamus-pituitary axis), and UB62 (yang-heel extra-vessel controlling point).

Root Gallbladder Sedation Prescription

STEP 1: GB44 is the restraining metal shu-point on the gallbladder meridian.

STEP 2: GB34 is the restraining earth shu-point on the gallbladder meridian.

STEP 3: **ST36** is the yang earth horary shu-point that engenders metal (compare **ST36** to ST45 metal + ST44 water combination for pathogenic heat).

STEP 4: LI1 is the yang metal horary shu-point that restrains the wood element.

STEP 5: GB38 is the fire shu-point on the gallbladder meridian that sedates wood.

STEP 6: SI5 is the yang imperial-fire horary shu-point that sedates wood.

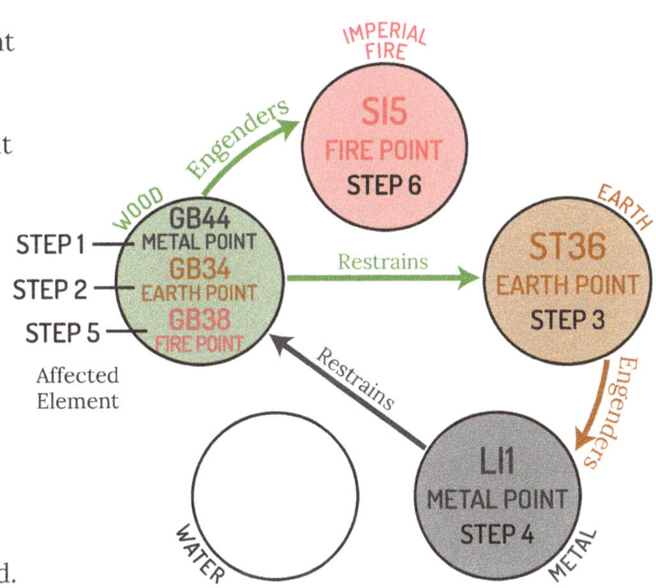

Appointment #1 Post-Treatment Stage

TEST SUPPLEMENTS AND HERBS

CS1 was taking a prenatal vitamin and fish oil that increased the pain and tightness in the neck muscles and master alarm points upon testing. She experienced reduced pain and tightness in neck muscles, master alarm points, and gallbladder testing locations with the herbal formula Wen Dan Tang. The vitamin D supplement tested neutral and didn't affect the neck muscles or master alarm points.

TEST ESSENTIAL OILS TO USE BETWEEN APPOINTMENTS

Marjoram essential oil released tightness in the calf muscles, anterior head of the deltoid (gallbladder muscle referral), and neck muscles. Orange essential oil released remaining pain in the right side of the rib cage (liver/gallbladder referral area).

We discussed dietary changes that focused on detoxification with support for the liver and gallbladder. CS1 had followed the Whole 30 diet in the past and had experienced improvements in general health; she agreed to follow it again.

Recommended 1 teaspoon Wen Dan Tang (for gallbladder support) with 3 drops of orange essential oil (for liver support) twice daily as a tea.

Recommended to temporarily stop the current vitamins and retest the vitamins at the next appointment.

Recommended applying 3-6 drops of marjoram essential oil to the soles of her feet before bed (for gallbladder support and to relax muscles).

Recommended follow-up appointments every 2-3 weeks for next three months and to follow the Whole 30 diet for a minimum of two months.

Appointment #2 Follow-up

SUBJECTIVE INFORMATION

CS1 returned for a follow-up appointment three weeks after the initial session. She reported increased energy and feeling happier since the last treatment. Her calves felt better for about ten days, hips felt better for about five days, and the tailbone pain resolved. The previous menstrual cycle was 30 days, and her period had increased clots in the menstrual blood. She experienced an all-day headache that occurred two days before her period with less anger and frustration. A week before this appointment, CS1 noticed swelling in her left foot and ankle, and her peroneus tendon had been painful. She had used ice on the left foot and ankle nightly for the week prior to this appointment. CS1 had followed recommendations for Wen Dan Tang tea and essential oils, but she hadn't changed her diet and was planning to start Whole 30 the next week.

OBJECTIVE INFORMATION

Pulse - overall slightly choppy to wiry, and forceful in the LV/GB and SP/ST positions
Tongue - medium white coating with a full, purple body

ASSESSMENT

The assessment remained the same as at the first appointment.
TCM: liver blood deficiency with uprising of liver yang, phlegm, blood stasis, and damp heat
Body-Feedback: third trisection discord with hypothalamus-pituitary dysfunction

PLAN

The plan remained the same as at the first appointment.
Treatment principle: nourish liver blood, anchor liver yang, transform phlegm and blood stasis, drain damp heat, harmonize the third trisection, and support the hypothalamus-pituitary axis.

Appointment #2 Pre-Treatment Planning Stage

PLANNING STEP ONE: ASSESS FOR ASYMMETRY

Visual assessment of the hips, feet, and shoulders indicated symmetry. TB15, SI13, and GB21 were still painful upon palpation and tighter on the right. The neck muscles were symmetrical in size.

PLANNING STEP TWO: REGULATE THE AUTONOMIC NERVOUS SYSTEM

Checking the abdomen decreased the tightness at TB15, SI13, and GB21 and indicated supine as the optimal treatment position. The wood and earth regions on the abdomen regulated the ANS at this appointment.

PLANNING STEPS THREE AND FOUR: DETERMINE THE BALANCING AND SEDATION OR TONIFICATION PRESCRIPTIONS

Based on the last appointment and this appointment's most excessive pulse positions, the following exclusive shu-points were tested to the pulse bilaterally to determine this treatment's root prescription: LV3, GB34, ST43, and SP1. The pulse improved and became slightly choppy to balanced when pressing GB34, the gallbladder balancing prescription, and the sedation prescription bilaterally. Testing the same acupoints for both sides of the body confirmed a symmetrical supine treatment position. As part of the balancing prescription, **ST36** was checked and compared to ST45 metal + ST44 water; the metal + water combination tested favorably, as evidenced in the pulse, and indicated pathogenic heat.

PLANNING STEP FIVE: ASSESS THE CORRESPONDING TESTING LOCATIONS

The same gallbladder and liver testing locations were checked as at the first appointment. There was a reduction in pain, discomfort, and muscle tightness from the first appointment. The testing locations with corresponding signs of organ/meridian dysfunction included:

- right rib cage shared regions with liver- and gallbladder-referred pain
- bilateral liver-referred discomfort at sternal attachment of pectoralis major muscle
- bilateral gallbladder-referred tightness and pain in anterior head of deltoid muscle
- bilateral LV2 and GB38 fire alarm points tender
- bilateral LV8 and GB34 organ alarm points tender

PLANNING STEP SIX: TEST ESSENTIAL OILS

The Gallbladder and Pericardium Organ Supporting blends were rechecked together, as they tested the best at the last appointment. The tension in the neck muscles released, along with reduced tightness and pain in the master alarm points, when both bottles were placed on the upper abdomen.

Appointment #2 Treatment Stage

TREATMENT STEP ONE: APPLY ESSENTIAL OILS

Applied 3 drops each of the Gallbladder and Pericardium Organ blends to the soles of the feet.

TREATMENT STEP TWO: REGULATE THE AUTONOMIC NERVOUS SYSTEM

Needled 4 acupoints along a horizontal line to harmonize wood and earth, along with CV6 to regulate the ANS.

TREATMENT STEP THREE: TREAT THE ROOT

Needled the gallbladder balancing and sedation prescriptions GB44, GB34, ST44 + ST45, LI1, GB38, and SI5.

TREATMENT STEP FOUR: SUPPORT THE ROOT

Needled the supporting acupoints, including LV4 + LV8 and KD7 + KD10 (additional metal + water shu-points for pathogenic heat affecting the liver and kidney meridians), Yin Tang (supports the hypothalamus-pituitary axis), and UB62 (yang-heel extra-vessel controlling point).

Appointment #2 Post-Treatment Stage

TEST SUPPLEMENTS AND HERBS

CS1 again experienced reduced pain and tightness in neck muscles, master alarm points, and gallbladder testing locations with the herbal formula Wen Dan Tang. The prenatal vitamin and fish oil increased pain in the right side of the rib cage and increased tension in the neck muscles. The vitamin D supplement tested neutral again and didn't affect the neck muscles or master alarm points.

TEST ESSENTIAL OILS TO USE BETWEEN APPOINTMENTS

Marjoram essential oil again released tightness in the calf muscles, anterior head of the deltoid (gallbladder muscle referral), and neck muscles. Orange and spearmint essential oils released remaining pain in the right side of the rib cage (liver and gallbladder organ testing location).

We discussed the implications of the increased pathogenic heat in her liver and kidney meridians that indicated detoxification support was needed. I recommended she begin following the Whole 30 diet starting immediately. I explained that changing her diet to support detoxification functions was necessary to lose weight and to help her body heal.

Recommended 1 teaspoon Wen Dan Tang (for gallbladder support) with 3 drops of orange and 1 drop of spearmint essential oils (for liver support) twice daily as a tea and to retest vitamins at next appointment.

Recommended applying 3-6 drops of marjoram essential oil to the soles of the feet before bed (for gallbladder support and to relax muscles).

Recommended to temporarily stop the current vitamins and test for new vitamins at the next appointment after following the Whole 30 diet.

Appointment #3 Follow-up

SUBJECTIVE INFORMATION

CS1 returned for another follow-up appointment three weeks later. She started the Whole 30 diet and reported feeling much better. Her pain was significantly reduced in the feet and legs, with mild pain remaining in the right foot. She noticed improved sleep and digestion with formed stools. The previous menstrual cycle was 31 days, had fewer clots, with fatigue just before the menstrual flow, and no premenstrual headache. CS1 reported a slight reduction in her weight, but her abdominal bloating and fluid retention in legs improved significantly. The appointment occurred on day 11 of her current cycle. She requested to test for new vitamin supplements to assist with detoxification.

OBJECTIVE INFORMATION

Pulse - overall slightly wiry, and forceful in the KD/UB and PC/TB positions (likely due to endocrine system dysfunction and preparing to ovulate)
Tongue - thin white coating with a medium pink body

ASSESSMENT

The assessment was changed from the last appointment. The uprising of liver yang and damp heat were removed because of the improvements in digestion and no premenstrual headache.
TCM: liver blood deficiency with phlegm and blood stasis
Body-Feedback: third trisection discord with hypothalamus-pituitary dysfunction

PLAN

The plan was adjusted to remove the anchor liver yang and drain damp heat from the last appointment.
Treatment principle: nourish liver blood, transform phlegm and blood stasis, harmonize the third trisection, and support the hypothalamus-pituitary axis.

Appointment #3 Pre-Treatment Planning Stage

PLANNING STEP ONE: ASSESS FOR ASYMMETRY

CS1's master alarm points and neck muscles had reduced discomfort and mild tightness bilaterally.

PLANNING STEP TWO: REGULATE THE AUTONOMIC NERVOUS SYSTEM

Checking the abdomen decreased the tightness at TB15, SI13, and GB21 and indicated supine as the optimal treatment position. Harmonizing and strengthening the immune and digestive systems' point combination on the abdomen regulated the ANS at this appointment.

PLANNING STEPS THREE AND FOUR: DETERMINE THE BALANCING AND SEDATION OR TONIFICATION PRESCRIPTIONS

Based on the last appointment and this appointment's most excessive pulse positions, the following exclusive shu-points were tested to the pulse bilaterally to determine this treatment's root prescription: LV3, GB34, KD3, UB60, PC3, and TB2. The pulse became slightly slippery to balanced when pressing LV3, the liver balancing prescription, and the tonification prescription bilaterally. As part of the balancing prescription, **SP3** was checked and compared to SP5 metal + SP9 water; **SP3** tested favorably, as evidenced in the pulse.

PLANNING STEP FIVE: ASSESS THE CORRESPONDING TESTING LOCATIONS

The same gallbladder and liver testing locations were checked as at the first appointment. There was a significant reduction in pain, discomfort, and muscle tightness compared to the last appointment. The testing locations with corresponding signs of organ/meridian dysfunction included:

- right rib cage shared region with liver- and gallbladder-referred pain
- bilateral liver-referred discomfort at sternal attachment of pectoralis major muscle
- bilateral gallbladder-referred tightness and pain in anterior head of deltoid muscle
- bilateral LV8 organ alarm point tender

PLANNING STEP SIX: TEST ESSENTIAL OILS

The Gallbladder and Pericardium Organ Supporting blends were retested (together and individually) but caused increased tightness in neck muscles and master alarm points. Then the following blends were tested individually: Liver Organ Supporting, Liver Meridian Balancing, Stomach Organ Supporting, and Stomach Meridian Balancing. The stomach blends were tested due to pathogenic heat identified in the meridian at this and the previous appointment. The Liver Organ Supporting and Stomach Meridian Balancing blends both released tightness in the neck muscles and master alarm points and the muscles relaxed the most when both of these blends were checked simultaneously.

Third Trisection Discord Root Liver Deficiency

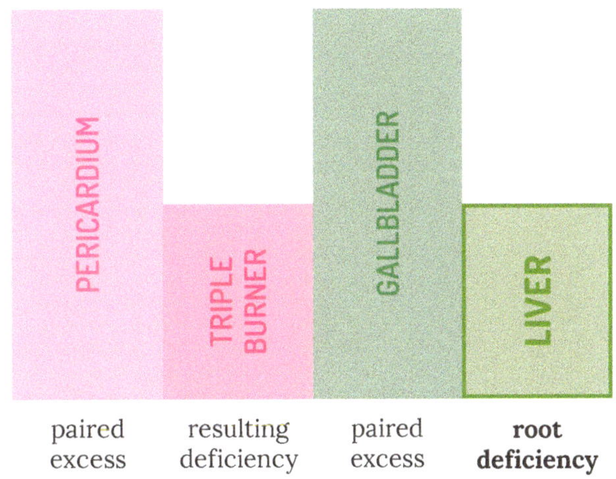

Appointment #3 Treatment Stage

TREATMENT STEP ONE: APPLY ESSENTIAL OILS

Applied 3 drops each of the Liver Organ and Stomach Meridian blends to the soles of the feet.

TREATMENT STEP TWO: REGULATE THE AUTONOMIC NERVOUS SYSTEM

Needled 3 acupoints along a vertical line between CV10 and CV14 and 2 acupoints bilaterally along a horizontal line between ST25 and SP15 to harmonize and strengthen immune and digestive systems and to regulate the ANS.

TREATMENT STEP THREE: TREAT THE ROOT

Needled the liver balancing and tonification prescriptions LV4, LV3, **SP3**, LU8, KD10, and LV8.

TREATMENT STEP FOUR: SUPPORT THE ROOT

Needled the supporting acupoints KD7 (additional metal shu-point), SP10 (nourishes and cools blood), ST45 metal + ST44 water combination, PC6 (yin linking extra-vessel controlling point), and 7 emotion downward along the hairline on the forehead (calms stress hormones).

Root Liver Tonification Prescription

STEP 1: LV4 is the restraining metal shu-point on the liver meridian.

STEP 2: LV3 is the restraining earth shu-point on the liver meridian.

STEP 3: **SP3** is the yin earth horary shu-point that engenders metal (compare **SP3** to SP5 metal + SP9 water combination for pathogenic heat).

STEP 4: LU8 is the yin metal horary shu-point that restrains wood.

STEP 5: KD10 is the yin water horary shu-point that tonifies wood.

STEP 6: LV8 is the water shu-point on the liver meridian that tonifies wood.

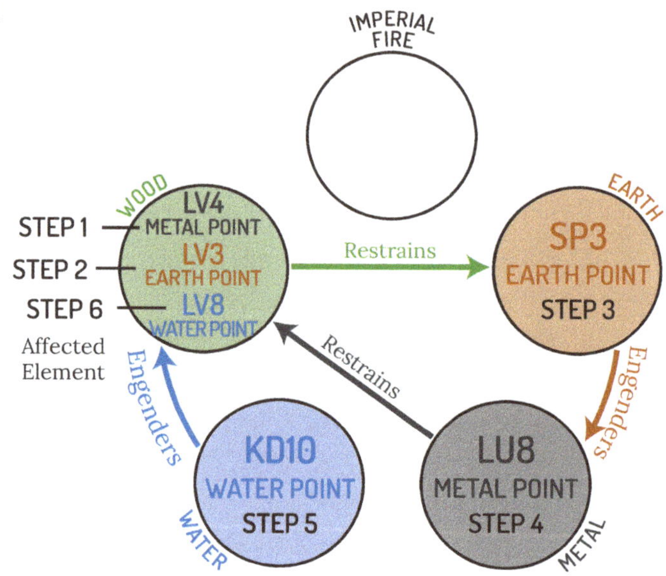

Appointment #3 Post-Treatment Stage

TEST SUPPLEMENT AND HERBS

The same types of supplements using different raw materials were tested to identify the ones that further released tension in the neck muscles and master alarm points. CS1 tested favorably for new supplements that included a non-methylated B-complex (compared to methylated B-complex), a mineral complex with iodine (compared to without iodine), vitamin D drops without K (compared to vitamin D with K), and choline tables (for gallbladder support). The Wen Dan Tang continued to test favorably. All supplements also reduced pain in the liver and gallbladder testing locations.

TEST ESSENTIAL OILS TO USE BETWEEN APPOINTMENTS

The marjoram, orange, and spearmint essential oils continued to test favorably.

We discussed CS1's progress and improved digestion, noticed since following the Whole 30 diet, to encourage continued beneficial food choices. The improvements seen at this appointment included transitioning to a liver root treatment in the progression of natural healing, alternating from draining sedation points to supportive tonification points, and a reduced number of metal + water combinations that indicated less pathogenic heat.

Recommended reducing the 1 teaspoon Wen Dan Tang (for gallbladder support) with 3 drops of orange and 1 drop of spearmint essential oils (for liver support) to once daily as a tea.

Recommended 2 B-complex tablets, 3 multi-mineral capsules, and 2 drops of vitamin D with breakfast, and 1 tablet of choline with breakfast and dinner.

Recommended applying 3-6 drops of marjoram essential oil to the soles of the feet before bed (for gallbladder support and to relax muscles).

Appointment #4 Follow-up

SUBJECTIVE INFORMATION

CS1 returned for another follow-up appointment four weeks later. She had tried to incorporate foods back into her diet during the previous week. After eating black beans, she experienced a 12-hour headache, increased stomach pain, bloating that night, and diarrhea the next day. CS1 decided to remain in the first phase of the Whole 30 diet that is more restrictive. She noticed mild spring allergies started last week. CS1 reduced her weight by 25 pounds over the previous six weeks. CS1 reported her legs were feeling better with only a little tightness on the bottom of the heel. She had experienced mild seasonal allergies over the previous week. Her last menstrual cycle was longer, and ovulation occurred around day 25 or 26. The post-ovulation luteal phase was ten days with no PMS symptoms, and menstrual flow was lighter and lasted three full days.

OBJECTIVE INFORMATION

Pulse - overall slightly wiry, and forceful in the KD/UB and PC/TB positions (likely due to hypothalamus and pituitary dysfunction)
Tongue - thin white coating with a thin pink body

ASSESSMENT

The assessment remained the same as at the third appointment.
TCM: liver blood deficiency with phlegm and blood stasis
Body-Feedback: third trisection discord with hypothalamus-pituitary dysfunction

PLAN

The plan remained the same as at the third appointment.
Treatment principle: nourish liver blood, transform phlegm and blood stasis, harmonize the third trisection, and support the hypothalamus-pituitary axis.

Appointment #4 Pre-Treatment Planning Stage

PLANNING STEP ONE: ASSESS FOR ASYMMETRY

CS1's master alarm points and neck muscles had minimal discomfort and tightness bilaterally.

PLANNING STEP TWO: REGULATE THE AUTONOMIC NERVOUS SYSTEM

Checking the abdomen decreased the tightness at TB15, SI13, and GB21 and indicated supine as the optimal treatment position. Harmonizing and strengthening the immune and digestive systems' point combination on the abdomen regulated the ANS at this appointment.

PLANNING STEPS THREE AND FOUR: DETERMINE THE BALANCING AND SEDATION OR TONIFICATION PRESCRIPTIONS

Based on the last appointment and this appointment's most excessive pulse positions, the following exclusive shu-points were tested to the pulse bilaterally to determine this treatment's root prescription: LV3, GB34, KD3, UB60, PC3, and TB2. The pulse became slightly slippery to balanced when pressing LV3, the liver balancing prescription, and the tonification prescription bilaterally. As part of the balancing prescription, **SP3** was checked and compared to SP5 metal + SP9 water; the metal + water combination tested favorably, as evidenced in the pulse, and indicated pathogenic heat.

PLANNING STEP FIVE: ASSESS THE CORRESPONDING TESTING LOCATIONS

The same gallbladder and liver testing locations were checked as at the first appointment. There was a continued reduction in pain, discomfort, and muscle tightness compared to the last appointment. The testing locations with corresponding signs of organ/meridian dysfunction included:

- right rib cage shared liver- and gallbladder-referred pain reduced
- bilateral liver-referred discomfort at sternal attachment of pectoralis major muscle
- bilateral LV8 organ alarm point tender

PLANNING STEP SIX: TEST ESSENTIAL OILS

The Liver Organ Supporting and Stomach Meridian Balancing blends from the last session were tested individually and caused increased tightness in the neck muscles and master alarm points. The Liver Meridian Balancing Blend was tested because it corresponded with the root treatment, and it released tension in the neck muscles and master alarm points. Spleen Organ Supporting and Meridian Balancing blends were tested individually due to pathogenic heat identified at this appointment. The Liver and Spleen Meridian Balancing blends both released tightness in the neck muscles and master alarm points and the muscles relaxed the most when both of these blends were checked simultaneously.

Appointment #4 Treatment Stage

TREATMENT STEP ONE: APPLY ESSENTIAL OILS

Applied 3 drops each of the Liver and Spleen Meridian blends to the soles of the feet.

TREATMENT STEP TWO: REGULATE THE AUTONOMIC NERVOUS SYSTEM

Needled 3 acupoints along a vertical line between CV10 and CV14 and 2 acupoints bilaterally on a horizontal line between ST25 and SP15 to harmonize and strengthen immune and digestive systems and regulate the ANS.

TREATMENT STEP THREE: TREAT THE ROOT

Needled the liver balancing and tonification prescriptions LV4, LV3, SP5 + SP9, LU8, KD10, and LV8.

TREATMENT STEP FOUR: SUPPORT THE ROOT

Needled the supporting acupoints, including KD7 (additional metal shu-point), PC6 (yin linking extra-vessel controlling point), Yin Tang, LI20, and ST7 (for seasonal allergies).

Appointment #4 Post-Treatment Stage

TEST SUPPLEMENTS AND HERBS

The multi-minerals and Wen Dan Tang were tested and refilled. CS1 tested favorably for a chaste tree supplement to support the hypothalamus-pituitary axis and improve the menstrual cycle.

TEST ESSENTIAL OILS TO USE BETWEEN APPOINTMENTS

The marjoram, orange, and spearmint essential oils continued to test favorably.

Recommended continuing 1 teaspoon Wen Dan Tang (for gallbladder support) with 3 drops of orange and 1 drop of spearmint essential oils (for liver support) once daily as a tea.

Recommended applying 3-6 drops of marjoram essential oil to the soles of the feet (for gallbladder support and to relax muscles).

Recommended continuing 2 B-complex tablets, 3 multimineral capsules, and 2 drops of vitamin D with breakfast, and 1 tablet of choline with breakfast and dinner.

Recommended adding 2 chaste tree tablets with dinner daily.

Appointment #5 Follow-up

SUBJECTIVE INFORMATION

CS1 returned for another follow-up appointment four weeks later. She had tried to eat a hamburger bun and experienced an immediate and excessive histamine response with itchy dry eyes, sneezing, chapped lips, stuffy nose, and itchy skin all over the next day. She started to feel better after three days. CS1 was subsequently able to incorporate a small amount of yogurt and cheese back into her diet and seemed fine. CS1 and her husband had decided that they would like to start trying to conceive a second child now that she felt better and understood how food choices were impacting her health. The previous menstrual cycle was 36 days, and the luteal phase was two days longer for a total of 12 days. Treatment this day was on day 17 of the current menstrual cycle, and she had been getting high fertility readings for five days. She reported having a frontal headache that didn't respond to Tylenol for the first two days after starting the chaste tree supplement.

OBJECTIVE INFORMATION

Pulse - overall slightly slippery, and forceful in PC/TB position (likely due to hypothalamus and pituitary dysfunction)
Tongue - thin white coating with a thin pink body

ASSESSMENT

The assessment changed from appointment #4 to remove the blood stasis (due to no clots with menstrual period) and add spleen qi deficiency (the cause of the blood stasis, shorter luteal phase, and lighter menstrual periods), and represents her constitutional weakness.
TCM: liver blood and spleen qi deficiency with phlegm
Body-Feedback: third trisection discord with hypothalamus-pituitary dysfunction

PLAN

The plan from appointment #4 was adjusted to remove transform blood stasis and add tonify spleen qi.
Treatment principle: nourish liver blood, tonify spleen qi, transform phlegm, harmonize the third trisection, and support the hypothalamus-pituitary axis.

Appointment #5 Pre-Treatment Planning Stage

PLANNING STEP ONE: ASSESS FOR ASYMMETRY

CS1's master alarm points and neck muscles had minimal discomfort and tightness bilaterally.

PLANNING STEP TWO: REGULATE THE AUTONOMIC NERVOUS SYSTEM

Checking the abdomen decreased the tightness at TB15, SI13, and GB21, and indicated supine as the optimal treatment position. The ministerial-fire, metal, and water regions on the abdomen regulated the ANS at this appointment.

PLANNING STEPS THREE AND FOUR: DETERMINE THE BALANCING AND SEDATION OR TONIFICATION PRESCRIPTIONS

Based on the last appointment and this appointment's most excessive pulse positions, the following exclusive shu-points were tested to the pulse bilaterally to determine this treatment's root prescription: LV3, GB34, PC3, and TB2. The pulse became slightly slippery to balanced when pressing PC3, the pericardium balancing prescription, and the sedation prescription bilaterally. CS1's root dysfunction transitioned from the wood element to the ministerial-fire element at this appointment. As part of the sedation prescription, **SP3** was checked and compared to SP5 metal + SP9 water; **SP3** tested favorably, as evidenced in the pulse.

PLANNING STEP FIVE: ASSESS THE CORRESPONDING TESTING LOCATIONS

The root treatment transitioned to the ministerial-fire element; therefore, the pericardium and triple burner testing locations were checked at this appointment for pain, discomfort, and muscle tightness. The testing locations with corresponding signs of organ/meridian dysfunction included:

- bilateral rib cage pericardium-referred pain and discomfort
- bilateral pericardium-referred discomfort in piriformis and gluteus medius muscles
- bilateral PC8 fire meridian alarm point tender
- bilateral triple burner-referred discomfort in teres minor muscle
- bilateral lymph-system-referred pain along sagittal plane in mid torso affecting a larger region on the right side (which overlaps with liver, gallbladder, and pericardium organ testing locations)

PLANNING STEP SIX: TEST ESSENTIAL OILS

The Liver and Pericardium Organ Supporting and Meridian Balancing blends were tested individually at this appointment. The Liver and Pericardium Organ Supporting blends caused increased tightness in neck muscles and master alarm points. The Liver and Pericardium Meridian Balancing blends released tension in the neck muscles and master alarm points. The pericardium meridian corresponds more closely with the hypothalamus-pituitary axis, which is related to CS1's endocrine and metabolic dysfunctions. The Liver and Pericardium Meridian Balancing blends were rechecked together, and the neck muscles and master alarm points relaxed the most when both of these blends were checked simultaneously.

Third Trisection Discord Root Pericardium Excess

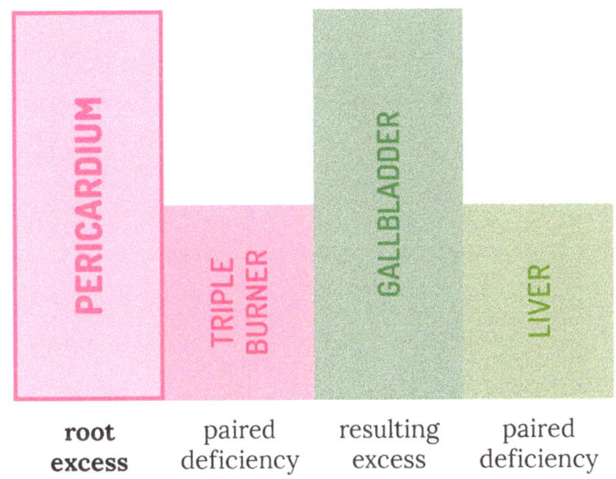

Appointment #5 Treatment Stage

TREATMENT STEP ONE: APPLY ESSENTIAL OILS

Applied 3 drops each of the Liver and Pericardium Meridian blends to the soles of the feet and 3 drops of each over right side of the upper abdomen.

TREATMENT STEP TWO: REGULATE THE AUTONOMIC NERVOUS SYSTEM

Needled 3 acupoints along a vertical line between CV10 and CV14, and 2 acupoints bilaterally along a diagonal line in the lower left and the lower right quadrants to harmonize ministerial-fire with metal and water.

TREATMENT STEP THREE: TREAT THE ROOT

Needled the pericardium balancing and sedation prescriptions PC3, PC5, LU8, KD10, **SP3** and PC7.

TREATMENT STEP FOUR: SUPPORT THE ROOT

Needled supporting acupoints, including KD7 (additional individual metal shu-point), ST34 (xi-cleft point), and GB40 (yuan-source point).

Root Pericardium Sedation Prescription

STEP 1: PC3 is the restraining water shu-point on the pericardium meridian.

STEP 2: PC5 is the restraining metal shu-point on the pericardium meridian.

STEP 3: LU8 is the yin metal horary shu-point that engenders water.

STEP 4: KD10 is the yin water horary shu-point that restrains ministerial-fire.

STEP 5: PC7 is the earth shu-point on the pericardium meridian that sedates ministerial-fire.

STEP 6: **SP3** is the yin earth horary shu-point that sedates ministerial-fire (compare **SP3** to SP5 metal + SP9 water combination for pathogenic heat).

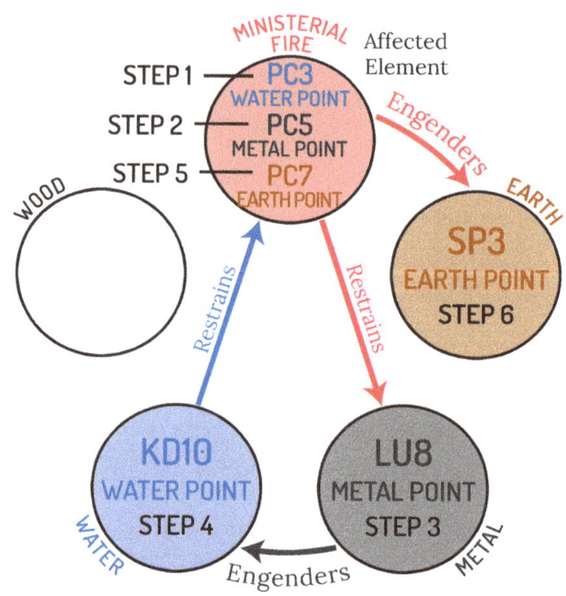

Appointment #5 Post-Treatment Stage

The treatment goals and recommendations were changed at this appointment to reflect the desire for a healthy pregnancy. The treatment focus optimized the endocrine system to encourage a healthy pregnancy.

TEST SUPPLEMENTS AND HERBS

The B-complex, vitamin D, and chaste tree were tested and refilled. Two different high-quality prenatal vitamins were tested; increased tightness in the neck muscles and master alarm points indicated individual supplements were needed. Tested additional non-methylated folate, vitamin A, vitamin C, and fish oil to create a custom prenatal supplement routine.

TEST ESSENTIAL OILS TO USE BETWEEN APPOINTMENTS

Recommended continuing 1 teaspoon Wen Dan Tang (for gallbladder support with damp heat) with 3 drops of orange and 1 drop of spearmint essential oils (for liver support) once daily as a tea.

Recommended applying 3-6 drops of marjoram essential oil to the soles of the feet (for gallbladder support and to relax muscles) starting with the menstrual period and discontinuing at ovulation. Recommended applying 3-4 drops of the Liver Meridian blend over the lower abdomen during and after ovulation.

Recommended a new supplement routine to use as a custom prenatal: With breakfast, take 1 B-complex tablet, 1 non-methylated folate capsule, 2 multimineral capsules, 2 drops of vitamin D, 1 vitamin C capsule, 1 vitamin A gel capsule, and 1 choline tablet. With dinner, take 1 B-complex tablet, 1 vitamin C capsule, 1 multimineral capsule, and 1 choline tablet.

Recommended increasing chaste tree to 2 tablets with breakfast and dinner (total of 4 tablets daily) and discontinuing with a positive pregnancy test.

CS1 Conclusion Summary

CS1's constitutional weakness was the third trisection and became apparent after she changed her diet and followed the detoxification Whole 30 meal plan. Her root treatments addressed third trisection organ/meridian dysfunction at all appointments. There are likely food allergies and compromised digestion due to genetics causing the final TCM pattern diagnosis of liver blood and spleen qi deficiency with phlegm. The spleen component created branch symptoms and affected her penetrating (*chong mai*) and yin linking (*yin wei mai*) extra-vessels. CS1 had the typical body type of someone with Polycystic Ovarian Syndrome (PCOS), which included being overweight, a barrel chest with overdeveloped breasts, excessive facial hair, thin waist, and deep voice. However, she did not have a PCOS diagnosis and, therefore, likely has metabolic syndrome disrupting the endocrine system and causing the irregular and prolonged menstrual cycles.

CS1's natural progression of healing followed the twelve earthly branches. By releasing the gallbladder first (appointments one and two), the liver was able to be strengthened (appointments three and four). The pericardium dysfunction affecting the hormones became apparent (appointment five) once she had the correct supplements and food choices to support the liver. The luteal phase defect, evidenced by the headaches, PMS, and reduced number of days after ovulation, matched the TCM pattern of spleen qi deficiency. However, CS1's root of endocrine dysfunction was the pericardium's influence on the hypothalamus-pituitary axis, which was continuously challenged by its six-level pair, the liver. Her genetic and constitutional weakness occurred in the third trisection and alternated between the wood element and jue-yin pairs.

During the reintroduction phase of the Whole 30 diet, CS1's health continuously improved as long as she remained on a gluten-free and legume-free diet of healthy, unprocessed foods. She embraced this lifestyle and discontinued her acupuncture when she achieved her treatment goals. She also understood the importance of having vitamins that supported her liver function and continued to use food-based, non-methylated B-vitamins for daily support.

CHAPTER 23

Case Study Two: Asymmetrical Supine

Appointment #1 New Client Assessment

Case Study Two (CS2) was a female, age 86 at her first appointment. She was in good health and had an active lifestyle that included downhill skiing. She has had three surgeries: a torn meniscus on the right knee, a hysterectomy, and a varicose vein stripped. Her significant traumas included a broken right leg at age 38 and a broken back at age 71, both from downhill skiing and neither requiring surgery.

CS2's health history form indicated only one symptom in each of the earth and fire elements. The lack of symptoms in the form represented her robust constitution, even with her age. The treatment focused on addressing her acute symptoms, and after these resolved, she discontinued the acupuncture treatments.

SUBJECTIVE INFORMATION

CS2 scheduled acupuncture to address sharp, burning nerve pain on the right side of her head that resulted from an outbreak of shingles 14 months prior. Her acute shingles rash was mild with minimal sores; however, nerve pain continued on the right temporal and occipital areas of the head after the rash resolved. Her pain was most intense and concentrated around the outer right ear along the gallbladder meridian. CS2 noticed her nerve pain was worse after drinking wine, and it increased with stress and at other times for unknown reasons. The time of day did not change her level of pain.

On a pain scale of zero to ten, with zero representing no pain and ten representing extreme pain, her nerve pain was a five at the first appointment. The nerve pain dropped as low as three and could increase to an eight when touched. She experienced a sharp, bruised sensation on the right side of her head when pressing the area. She took Gabapentin, as prescribed by her doctor, for three months and then stopped because she only experienced a minimal pain reduction, and her memory was negatively affected. CS2 had a mild loss of hearing that gradually worsened over the years and was not affected by the shingles.

BODY-FEEDBACK for Health, LLC

Confidential Health History

Name Case Study #2

Please Check All That Apply

METAL ELEMENT

○ Frequent colds, rhinitis, or sinusitis
○ Allergies, asthma, or autoimmune conditions
○ Frequent cough, post-nasal drip, or congestion
○ Dry skin or sensitive skin
○ Hives, eczema, or rashes
○ Constipation, loose stools, irregular bowels
○ Colon polyps or history of any type of cancer
○ Low back or hip pain worse in the morning
○ Shortness of breath or exercise induced asthma
○ Cold sores or herpes or other viral infections
○ Easily disappointed or offended
○ Sadness, low self-esteem, or excessive grief

WATER ELEMENT

○ Frequent, urgent, or difficult urination
○ Swollen or puffy ankles or feet
○ Low energy or needs more than 8 hours sleep
○ Low libido, sex drive, or reduced sexual function
○ Kidney stones, disease, or dysfunction
○ Forgetful or poor short term memory
○ Low back pain worse at end of day
○ Headaches or migraines triggered by fatigue or hormone changes
○ Adrenal or thyroid dysfunction (hyper or hypo)
○ Scoliosis, osteoarthritis, osteoporosis, osteopenia
○ Hormonal imbalances or endocrine dysfunction
○ Fearful, depression, or lack of motivation

WOOD ELEMENT

○ Muscle tension, cramps, tightness
○ Sensitive to noise, strong odors, and tastes
○ Dry, red, or weak eyes
○ Coarse or brittle hair or nails or premature gray hair
○ Tendon, ligament, or meniscus weakness or pain
○ Fibromyalgia or all over joint pain
○ Numbness and tingling with sleep or inactivity
○ Seizures, tremors, or Parkinson's
○ Pain or tightness in right shoulder or side of neck
○ Bloating, diarrhea, or stomach pains after eating
○ Headaches or migraines triggered by stress
○ Anger, irritability, or easily frustrated

EARTH ELEMENT

○ Muscle weakness or lack of strength
○ All over puffiness or water retention
○ Bruises easily, varicose, or spider veins
○ Low energy or fatigue after eating
○ Hypo or hyper thyroid function
● Indigestion, bloating, or gas
○ Craves sugar, sweets, or carbohydrates
○ Neck pain or left sided pain in body
○ Diabetes, pre-diabetes, or hypoglycemia
○ Pain that worsens with cold or damp weather
○ Headaches or migraines triggered by weather
○ Easily worried or upset with changes or obsessive

FIRE ELEMENT

● Insomnia, difficulty sleeping, or waking early
○ Excessive dreaming or nightmares
○ Dry skin and increased desire for fluids
○ Heart palpitations or irregular heartbeat
○ Easy flushing, red type acne, dislike heat
○ Hot flashes or night sweats
○ Heart disease or family history of
○ Anxiety, restlessness, panic attack, or mind racing with physical exhaustion
○ High blood pressure or Low blood pressure
○ Pain in sacrum, SI joint, or tailbone
○ Mouth sores, bleeding gums, or burning tongue
○ Headaches triggered by heat or excessive sun

MINISTERIAL-FIRE ELEMENT

○ High-pitched ringing or congestion in the ears
○ Headaches or migraines that move around in head
○ Swollen lymph nodes or chronic infections
○ Chronic sinus or ear congestion
○ Stiff movements or general tightness
○ Belching, burping, or heartburn
○ Difficulty losing weight or obesity in family
○ Polycystic ovarian syndrome or ovarian cysts
○ Cystic acne, boils, or cysts
○ Sciatic pain or tailbone pain
○ Overly optimistic or unrealistic
○ Feeling oppressed or unable to make changes

www.Body-Feedback.com 608-535-9144 2014 Yahara Place, Madison WI 53704

OBJECTIVE INFORMATION

Examination of the right leg identified a two-inch scar with muscle tension in the area between acupoints KD9 and LV7, resulting from a varicose vein removal over 40 years ago. The muscles in the right calf felt rigid and tight, and CS2 said they were painful upon palpation.
Pulse - slightly wiry overall, and wiry and forceful in the UB/KD and LU/LI positions
Tongue - medium white coat with pink full body and deep vertical center crack

ASSESSMENT

TCM: blood stasis, blood deficiency, dampness, and qi stagnation with depressive heat
Body-Feedback: third trisection discord with wood element dysfunction

PLAN

Treatment principle: transform blood stasis, nourish blood, drain dampness, rectify qi to resolve depressive heat, harmonize the third trisection, and optimize the wood element.

Appointment #1 Pre-Treatment Planning Stage

PLANNING STEP ONE: ASSESS FOR ASYMMETRY

Visual assessment of the hips, feet, and shoulders indicated asymmetry. The right hip, knee, and ankle were rotated externally with the right foot lying closer to the table. The anterior superior iliac spine crest (ASIS) on the right was forward and lower when compared to the left side. The master alarm points (GB21, TB15, and SI13) were significantly more painful on the right side. Her neck muscles felt broader, thicker, and tighter on the right lateral side, and smaller and weaker on the left lateral side.

PLANNING STEP TWO: REGULATE THE AUTONOMIC NERVOUS SYSTEM

Checking the abdomen decreased the tightness at TB15, SI13, and GB21 on the right and indicated supine as the optimal treatment position. The scalp acupoint combinations to regulate the ANS caused additional tightness in the master alarm points on the right when checked. The wood and metal regions on the abdomen regulated the ANS at this appointment.

PLANNING STEPS THREE AND FOUR: DETERMINE THE BALANCING AND SEDATION OR TONIFICATION PRESCRIPTIONS

Based on the nerve pain trajectory (wood element) and the most excessive pulse positions, the following exclusive shu-points were tested to the pulse bilaterally to determine this treatment's root prescriptions: GB34, LV3, UB60, KD3, LU10, and LI5. The right wrist's pulse positions became slightly slippery to balanced when pressing GB34, the gallbladder balancing prescription, and the tonification prescription on the right side, along with LV3, the liver balancing prescription, and the tonification prescription on the left. The tension and pain in her master alarm points on the right side also diminished when pressing on these acupoints. The different root prescriptions within the wood element confirmed an asymmetrical supine treatment position.

On the right side, as part of the balancing and tonification prescriptions, **ST36** was checked and compared to ST45 metal + ST44 water; **ST36** tested favorably, as evidenced in the pulse. UB67 metal (to combine with UB66 water) was checked and tested favorably, as evidenced in the pulse. LI2 water (to combine with LI1 metal) was checked and tested favorably, as evidenced in the pulse.

On the left side as part of the balancing and tonification prescriptions, **SP3** was checked and compared to SP5 metal + SP9 water; the metal + water combination tested favorably, as evidenced in the pulse. LU5 water (to combine with LU8 metal) was checked and tested favorably, as evidenced in the pulse. KD7 metal (to combine with KD10 water) was checked and tested favorably, as evidenced in the pulse.

The number of metal + water acupoint combinations in this treatment indicated an excessive amount of pathogenic heat and inflammation, hindering CS2's capacity to heal. The gallbladder and liver tonification prescriptions also included the metal + water combination on their root meridians. The root prescription's individual metal or water points all tested favorably to adding the other point to create the heat-clearing combination. Pathogenic heat affected both metal and water element meridian pairs, causing the two corresponding pulse positions to feel wiry and forceful.

PLANNING STEP FIVE: ASSESS THE CORRESPONDING TESTING LOCATIONS

CS2's symptoms and prescriptions to correct her asymmetry related to the wood element. Therefore, both the gallbladder and liver testing locations were checked for pain, discomfort, and muscle tightness. The testing locations with corresponding signs of organ/meridian dysfunction included:

- right rib cage and scapula shared gallbladder- and liver-referred pain
- bilateral gallbladder-referred tightness and pain in anterior head of deltoid muscle
- bilateral liver-referred discomfort at sternal attachment of pectoralis major muscle
- right GB34 organ and GB38 fire alarm points painful
- bilateral LV8 organ and LV2 fire alarm points painful
- right UB43-UB44 upper body muscle memory region tight and painful
- right UB57-UB58 lower body muscle memory region tight and painful

PLANNING STEP SIX: TEST ESSENTIAL OILS

Manufactured products containing essential oils were tested and used to provide pain relief and bioidentical hormone precursors for nerve repair. The lotion for pain relief contains the active ingredients of menthol, methyl salicylate, green tea extract, and organic aloe leaf juice, along with the essential oils of peppermint, wintergreen, oregano, niaouli, lavender, blue cypress, elemi, vetiver, caraway, dorado azul, and matricaria. The hormonal lotion for regeneration contains pregnenolone, MSM, the extracts of wild yam, aloe vera, kelp, black cohosh, blue cohosh, eleuthero root, and green tea, along with the essential oils of wintergreen, lycium, calendula, Roman chamomile, rose, peppermint, Douglas fir, oregano, and other ingredients.

The above two lotions reduced the muscle tightness and pain in the master alarm points on the right side when tested individually. Together, these products eliminated muscle tightness and pain at the master alarm points and reduced her sharp bruised sensation when pressing the outside of the right ear.

PLANNING STEP SEVEN: CHECK FOR PHLEGM NODULES

There were no palpable phlegm nodules in the lower back along PSIS. This area was only checked during this first appointment.

Asymmetrical Third Trisection Discord

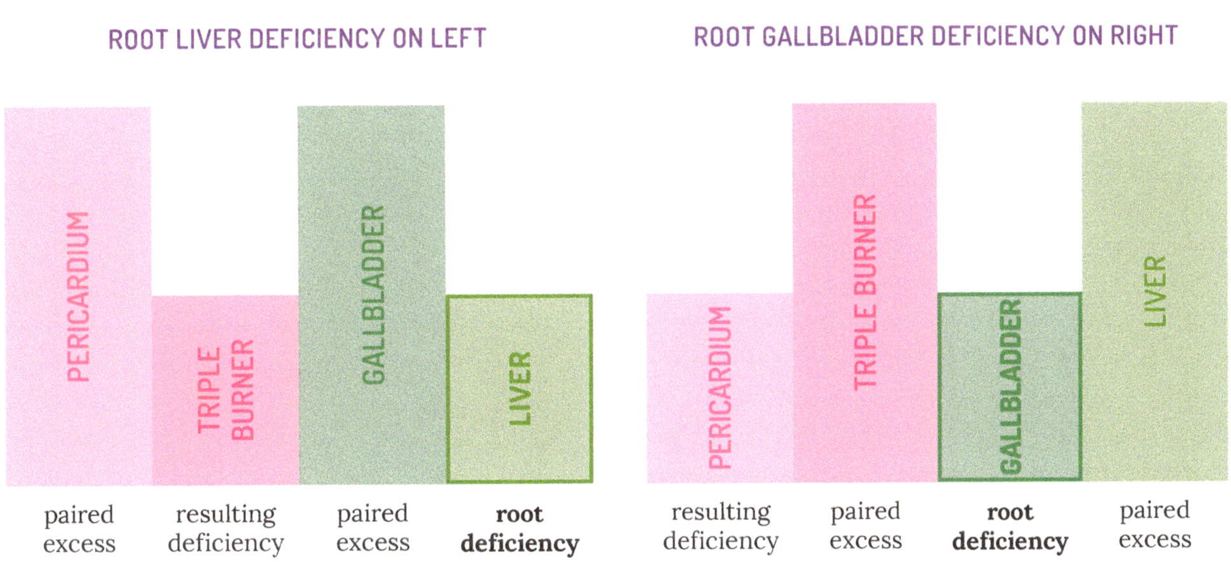

Appointment #1 Treatment Stage

TREATMENT STEP ONE: APPLY ESSENTIAL OILS

A thin layer of hormonal lotion was applied first along CS2's spine in the upper back and neck region, the occipital area below the hairline, around the outside of the right ear, and over the scar on the right calf. A thin layer of the pain-relief lotion was applied atop the hormonal lotion.

TREATMENT STEP TWO: REGULATE THE AUTONOMIC NERVOUS SYSTEM

The ANS was regulated by needling 3 acupoints along a diagonal line in both the upper right (wood) and lower left (metal) quadrants of the abdomen for a total of 6 acupoints.

TREATMENT STEP THREE: TREAT THE TWO ROOTS

On the right side, needled the gallbladder balancing and tonification prescriptions GB44, GB34, **ST36**, LI1, UB66, and GB43.

On the left side, needled the liver balancing and tonification prescriptions LV4, LV3, SP5 + SP9, LU8, KD10, and LV8.

TREATMENT STEP FOUR: SUPPORT THE ROOT

Scalp acupoints were tested around the right ear and caused increased tightness in the master alarm points, which indicated the need to avoid direct needling of this area at this appointment. The supporting acupoints released pathogenic heat from the meridians affecting the right side of the head and tightness in the right calf. The supporting acupoints on the right included LI2 (additional individual water point), UB67 (additional individual metal point), TB1 metal + TB2 water combination, and 4 ashi points around the scar area on the right calf. The supporting acupoints on the left included KD7 (additional individual metal point), LU5 (additional individual water point), and 2 ashi points between UB61 and UB62 to release the remaining tightness in the muscle memory testing regions.

Root Liver Tonification Prescription on left

STEP 1: LV4 is the restraining metal shu-point on the liver meridian.

STEP 2: LV3 is the restraining earth shu-point on the liver meridian.

STEP 3: **SP3** is the yin earth horary shu-point that engenders metal (compare **SP3** to SP5 metal + SP9 water combination for pathogenic heat).

STEP 4: LU8 is the yin metal horary shu-point that restrains wood.

STEP 5: KD10 is the yin water horary shu-point that tonifies wood.

STEP 6: LV8 is the water shu-point on the liver meridian that tonifies wood.

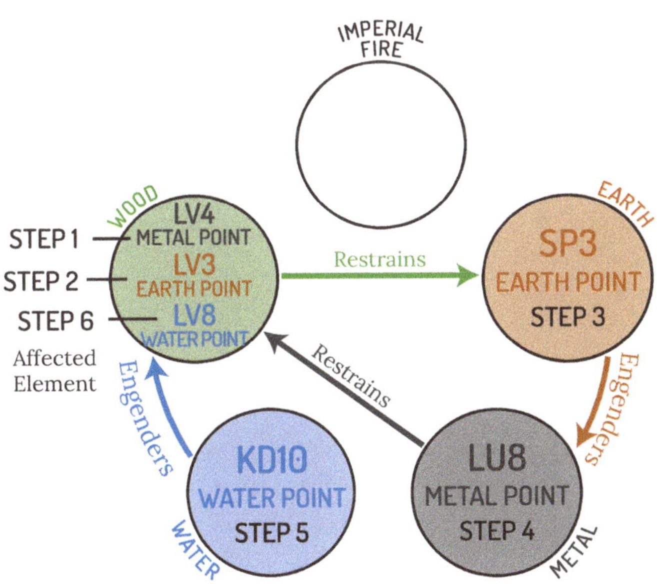

Root Gallbladder Tonification Prescription on right

STEP 1: GB44 is the restraining metal shu-point on the gallbladder meridian.

STEP 2: GB34 is the restraining earth shu-point on the gallbladder meridian.

STEP 3: **ST36** is the yang earth horary shu-point that engenders metal (compare **ST36** to ST45 metal + ST44 water combination for pathogenic heat).

STEP 4: LI1 is the yang metal horary shu-point that restrains the wood element.

STEP 5: UB66 is the yang water horary shu-point that tonifies wood.

STEP 6: GB43 is the water shu-point on the gallbladder meridian that tonifies wood.

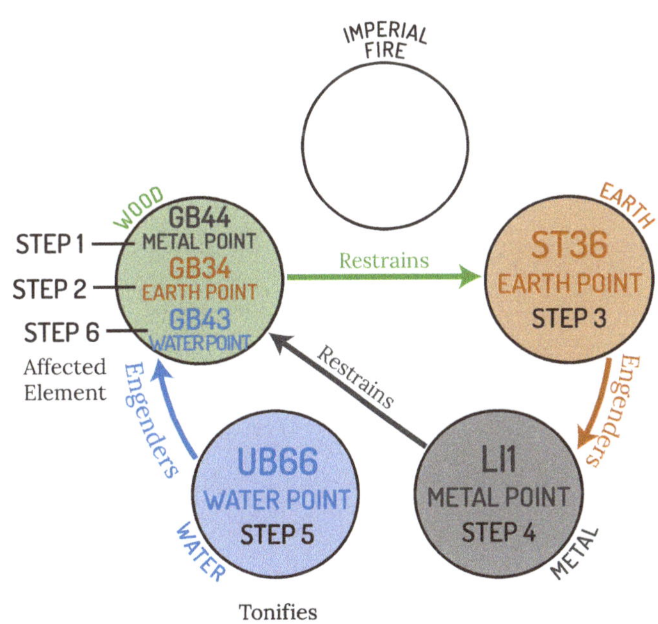

Appointment #1 Post-Treatment Stage

TEST SUPPLEMENTS AND HERBS

CS2 typically ate a very healthy diet of home-grown or local organic produce and meats. She preferred to use only the topical essential oil lotions, so no supplements or herbs were tested.

TEST ESSENTIAL OILS TO USE BETWEEN APPOINTMENTS

CS2 felt immediate benefits from the pain-relief and hormonal essential oil lotions and agreed to purchase them.

Recommended applying a thin layer of the hormonal lotion followed by the pain relief lotion to the base of the head under the hairline, the right side of the neck, and the outside of the right ear twice daily.

Recommended follow-up appointments weekly for the next two weeks and then every three weeks until the nerve pain resolved.

Appointment #2 Follow-up

SUBJECTIVE INFORMATION

CS2 returned for a follow-up appointment one week later. She reported the sharp, burning nerve pain reduced after her treatment for a few days and now feels about the same as at the initial appointment. She noticed that the area around the right eye looked darker, like a bruise, and was swollen for one day after the acupuncture treatment. She was surprised by the changes around her eye, as there was no direct treatment on the face and scalp. At this appointment, the nerve pain was about a three on a scale of one to ten. In the previous week (after her initial appointment), CS2 experienced one day with a pain level of six. The bruised sensation around the outside of the right ear had continued after the last appointment.

OBJECTIVE INFORMATION

Pulse - slightly choppy overall, and choppy and forceful in the LV/GB position
Tongue - medium white coat with pink full body and deep vertical center crack

ASSESSMENT

The assessment remained the same as at the first appointment.
TCM: blood stasis, blood deficiency, dampness, and qi stagnation with depressive heat
Body-Feedback: third trisection discord with wood element dysfunction

PLAN

The plan remained the same as at the first appointment.
Treatment principle: transform blood stasis, nourish blood, drain dampness, rectify qi to resolve depressive heat, harmonize the third trisection, and optimize the wood element.

Appointment #2 Pre-Treatment Planning Stage

PLANNING STEP ONE: ASSESS FOR ASYMMETRY

Visual assessment of the hips, feet, and shoulders indicated the same asymmetry as at the first appointment. The right hip, knee, and ankle were rotated externally with the right foot lying closer to the table. The anterior superior iliac spine crest (ASIS) on the right was forward and lower when compared to the left side. The master alarm points were significantly more painful on the right side. Her neck muscles felt broader, thicker, and tighter on the right lateral side, while the left lateral side felt smaller and weaker.

PLANNING STEP TWO: REGULATE THE AUTONOMIC NERVOUS SYSTEM

Checking the abdomen decreased the tightness at TB15, SI13, and GB21 on the right and indicated supine as the optimal treatment position. The scalp acupoint combinations to regulate the ANS caused additional tightness in the master alarm points on the right when checked. The wood and metal regions on the abdomen regulated the ANS at this appointment.

PLANNING STEPS THREE AND FOUR: DETERMINE THE BALANCING AND SEDATION OR TONIFICATION PRESCRIPTIONS

Based on the last appointment and the most excessive pulse position, the only exclusive shu-points tested to the pulse bilaterally were GB34 and LV3, which determined this treatment's root prescriptions. The right wrist's pulse positions became slightly slippery to balanced when pressing GB34, the gallbladder balancing, and the tonification acupoints on the right side, along with LV3, the liver balancing, and tonification acupoints on the left. The tension and pain in her master alarm points on the right side also diminished when pressing on these acupoints. The different root prescriptions within the wood element confirmed an asymmetrical supine treatment position.

On the right side, as part of the balancing and tonification prescriptions, **ST36** was checked and compared to ST45 metal + ST44 water; the metal + water combination tested favorably, as evidenced in the pulse. UB67 metal (to combine with UB66 water) was checked and tested favorably, as evidenced in the pulse. LI2 water (to combine with LI1 metal) was checked and tested unfavorably, as evidenced in the pulse.

On the left side as part of the balancing and tonification prescriptions, **SP3** was checked and compared to SP5 metal + SP9 water; the metal + water combination tested favorably, as evidenced in the pulse. LU5 water (to combine with LU8 metal) was checked and tested favorably, as evidenced in the pulse. KD7 metal (to combine with KD10 water) was checked and tested favorably, as evidenced in the pulse.

The number of metal + water combinations that tested favorably indicated that CS2 continued to have excessive amounts of pathogenic heat and inflammation.

PLANNING STEP FIVE: ASSESS THE CORRESPONDING TESTING LOCATIONS

CS2's symptoms and root acupoint prescriptions to correct her asymmetry were the same as at the last appointment. Therefore, the gallbladder and liver testing locations were checked again, and the level of pain, discomfort, and muscle tightness were the same as the last appointment. The testing locations with corresponding signs of organ/meridian dysfunction included:

- right rib cage and scapula shared gallbladder- and liver-referred pain
- bilateral gallbladder-referred tightness and pain at anterior head of deltoid muscle
- bilateral liver-referred discomfort at sternal attachment of pectoralis major muscle
- right GB34 organ and GB38 fire alarm points painful
- bilateral LV8 organ and LV2 fire alarm points painful
- right UB43-UB44 upper body muscle memory region tight and painful
- right UB57-UB58 lower body muscle memory region tight and painful

PLANNING STEP SIX: TEST ESSENTIAL OILS

The same two lotions containing essential oils were tested and used again to provide pain relief and bioidentical hormones to repair the nerves. Nerve regeneration requires healthy fats, along with testosterone for both men and women, and additional progesterone for women.[53,54,55,56] The two products were tested together and eliminated the muscle tightness and pain in the master alarm points and reduced the sensation of a bruise when pressing around the outside of the right ear.

Appointment #2 Treatment Stage

TREATMENT STEP ONE: APPLY ESSENTIAL OILS

The essential oil lotions were applied the same as at the first appointment: a thin layer of hormonal lotion applied along spine in upper back and neck region, occipital area below hairline, around outside of right ear, and over scar on right calf, and a thin layer of pain-relief lotion applied atop hormonal lotion.

TREATMENT STEP TWO: REGULATE THE AUTONOMIC NERVOUS SYSTEM

The same acupoints regulated the ANS as at the first appointment: 3 acupoints were needled along a diagonal line in both the upper right (wood) and lower left (metal) quadrants of the abdomen for a total of 6 acupoints.

TREATMENT STEP THREE: TREAT THE TWO ROOTS

On the right side, needled the gallbladder balancing and tonification prescriptions GB44, GB34, ST45 + ST44, LI1, UB66, and GB43.

On the left side, needled the liver tonification prescriptions LV4, LV3, SP5 + SP9, LU8, KD10, and LV8.

TREATMENT STEP FOUR: SUPPORT THE ROOT

Scalp acupoints were tested around the right ear and caused increased tightness in the master alarm points, indicating the need to avoid direct needling of this area at this appointment. The supporting acupoints needled cleared pathogenic heat and released tightness in the right calf. The supporting acupoints on the right included UB67 (additional individual metal point), TB1 metal + TB2 water combination, and 3 ashi points around the scar area on the right calf. The supporting acupoints on the left included KD7 (additional individual metal point), LU5 (additional individual water point), and 2 ashi points between UB61 and UB62 to release the remaining tightness in the muscle memory testing regions.

Appointment #2 Post-Treatment Stage

TEST SUPPLEMENTS AND HERBS

No supplements or herbs were tested.

TEST ESSENTIAL OILS TO USE BETWEEN APPOINTMENTS

CS2 continued to apply the essential oil lotions twice daily, as recommended in the first session.

Appointment #3 Follow-up

SUBJECTIVE INFORMATION

CS2 returned for another follow-up appointment one week later. She reported her nerve pain reduced again after the treatment for a few days, along with a few hours with no pain. She still has the same bruised sensation on the scalp around her right ear, and the ear itself felt as if it was asleep. At this appointment, the nerve pain was a three on a scale of one to ten, and she experienced a pain level of five during one day between sessions. Her chronic muscle tightness in the right leg was noticeably better since the last session and she felt improved circulation in both legs.

OBJECTIVE INFORMATION

Pulse - slightly choppy overall, and choppy and forceful in the LV/GB position
Tongue - thin white coat with pink full body and reduced vertical center crack

ASSESSMENT

The assessment remained the same as at the first and second appointments.
TCM: blood stasis, blood deficiency, dampness, and qi stagnation with depressive heat
Body-Feedback: third trisection discord with wood element dysfunction

PLAN

The plan remained the same as at the first and second appointments.
Treatment principle: transform blood stasis, nourish blood, drain dampness, rectify qi to resolve depressive heat, harmonize the third trisection, and optimize the wood element.

Appointment #3 Pre-Treatment Planning Stage

PLANNING STEP ONE: ASSESS FOR ASYMMETRY

Visual assessment of the hips, feet, and shoulders indicated asymmetry. The right knee and ankle rotated a little less laterally, and the right foot was more aligned with the left foot's resting position. The pain when pressing the master alarm points was slightly reduced, although more intense on the right side. The difference in her neck muscles was becoming less noticeable.

PLANNING STEP TWO: REGULATE THE AUTONOMIC NERVOUS SYSTEM

Checking the abdomen decreased the tightness at TB15, SI13, and GB21 on the right and indicated supine as the optimal treatment position. The wood and metal regions on the abdomen regulated the ANS at this appointment.

PLANNING STEPS THREE AND FOUR: DETERMINE THE BALANCING AND SEDATION OR TONIFICATION PRESCRIPTIONS

Based on the last appointment and the most excessive pulse position, the only exclusive shu-points tested to the pulse bilaterally were GB34 and LV3, which determined this treatment's root prescriptions. The right wrist's pulse positions became slightly slippery to balanced when pressing GB34, the gallbladder balancing, and the tonification acupoints on the right side, along with LV3, the liver balancing, and the sedation acupoints on the left. The tension and pain in her master alarm points on the right side also diminished when pressing on these acupoints. The different root prescriptions within the wood element confirmed an asymmetrical supine treatment position. At this appointment, the root liver treatment transitioned from tonification to sedation.

On the right side as part of the balancing and tonification prescriptions, **ST36** was checked and compared to ST45 metal + ST44 water; the metal + water combination tested favorably, as evidenced in the pulse. UB67 metal (to combine with UB66 water) was checked and tested favorably, as evidenced in the pulse. LI2 water (to combine with LI1 metal) was checked and tested favorably, as evidenced in the pulse.

On the left side as part of the balancing and sedation prescriptions, **SP3** was checked and compared to SP5 metal + SP9 water; the metal + water combination tested favorably, as evidenced in the pulse. **HT8** was checked and compared to HT4 metal + HT3 water; the metal + water combination tested favorably, as evidenced in the pulse. LU5 water (to combine with LU8 metal) was checked and tested favorably, as evidenced in the pulse.

CS2 had continued to have an excessive amount of pathogenic heat and inflammation indicated by the number of metal + water combinations and the liver fire shu-point at this appointment. In the root prescriptions, the gallbladder, spleen, and heart included the metal + water combination and the liver sedation included LV2.

PLANNING STEP FIVE: ASSESS THE CORRESPONDING TESTING LOCATIONS

CS2's symptoms and root acupoint prescriptions to correct her asymmetry were the same as at the last appointment. Therefore, the gallbladder and liver testing locations were checked again, and the level of pain, discomfort, and muscle tightness diminished slightly compared to the first appointment. The testing locations with corresponding signs of organ/meridian dysfunction included:

- right rib cage and scapula shared gallbladder- and liver-referred pain
- bilateral gallbladder-referred tightness and pain in anterior head of deltoid muscle
- bilateral liver-referred discomfort at sternal attachment of pectoralis major muscle
- right GB34 organ and GB38 fire alarm points painful
- bilateral LV8 organ and LV2 fire alarm points painful
- right UB43-UB44 upper body muscle memory region tight and painful
- right UB57-UB58 lower body muscle memory region tight and painful

PLANNING STEP SIX: TEST ESSENTIAL OILS

The same two lotions containing essential oils were tested and used again to provide pain relief and bioidentical hormones to repair the nerves. The two products tested together eliminated the muscle tightness and pain in the master alarm points and reduced the sensation of a bruise when pressing around the outside of the right ear.

Asymmetrical Third Trisection Discord

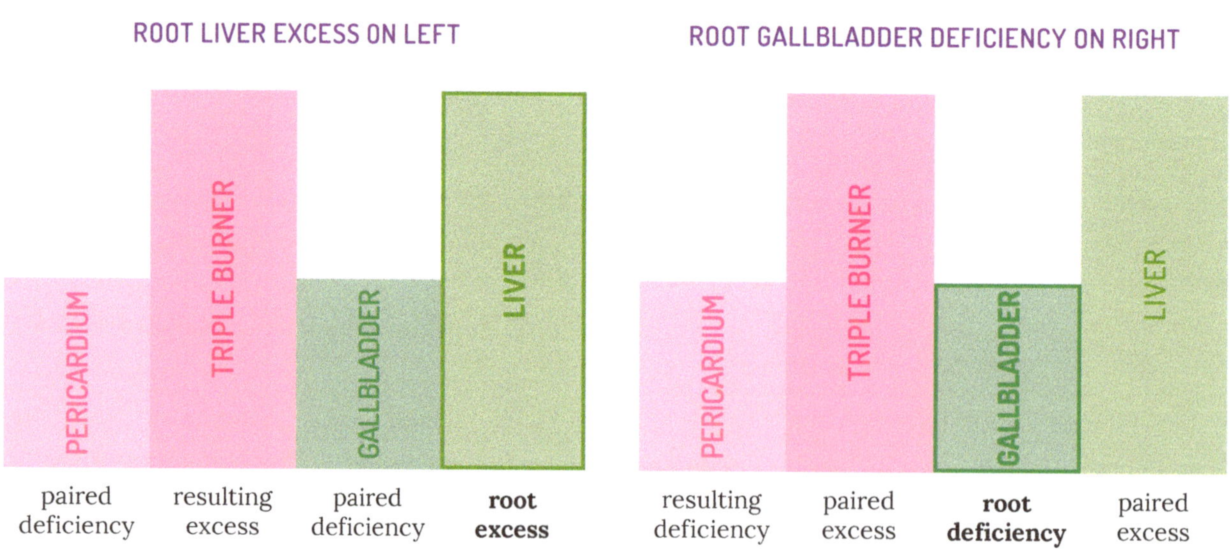

Appointment #3 Treatment Stage

TREATMENT STEP ONE: APPLY ESSENTIAL OILS

The essential oil lotions were applied the same as at the first and second appointments: a thin layer of hormonal lotion applied along spine in upper back and neck region, occipital area below hairline, around outside of right ear, and over scar on right calf; a thin layer of pain-relief lotion applied atop hormonal lotion.

TREATMENT STEP TWO: REGULATE THE AUTONOMIC NERVOUS SYSTEM

The same acupoints regulated the ANS as at the first two appointments: 3 acupoints were needled along a diagonal line in both the upper right (wood) and lower left (metal) quadrants of the abdomen for a total of 6 acupoints.

TREATMENT STEP THREE: TREAT THE TWO ROOTS

On the left side first, needled the liver balancing and sedation prescriptions LV4, LV3, LU8, SP5 + SP9, LV2, and HT4 + HT3.

Then on the right side, needled the gallbladder balancing and tonification prescriptions GB44, GB34, ST45 + ST44, LI1, UB66, and GB43.

TREATMENT STEP FOUR: SUPPORT THE ROOT

The first indication of reduced inflammation and pathogenic heat on the right side of the head was verified when the scalp acupoints finally tested beneficial by releasing tightness in the master alarm points on the right side. The supporting acupoints needled cleared pathogenic heat and provided local treatment around the right ear. The supporting acupoints on the left included KD9 (xi-cleft for the yin linking extra-vessel) and LU5 (additional individual water point). The supporting acupoints on the right included UB67 (additional individual metal point), LI2 (additional individual water point), TB8 (group luo-connecting for the arm yang meridians), and 3 ashi scalp acupoints from the GB7 to GB9 region.

Root Liver Sedation Prescription on left

STEP 1: LV4 is the restraining metal shu-point on the liver meridian.

STEP 2: LV3 is the restraining earth shu-point on the liver meridian.

STEP 3: **SP3** is the yin earth horary shu-point that engenders metal (compare **SP3** to SP5 metal + SP9 water combination for pathogenic heat).

STEP 4: LU8 is the yin metal horary shu-point that restrains wood.

STEP 5: LV2 is the fire shu-point on the liver meridian that sedates wood.

STEP 6: **HT8** is the yin imperial-fire horary shu-point that sedates wood (compare **HT8** to HT4 metal + HT3 water combination).

Root Gallbladder Tonification Prescription on right

STEP 1: GB44 is the restraining metal shu-point on the gallbladder meridian.

STEP 2: GB34 is the restraining earth shu-point on the gallbladder meridian.

STEP 3: **ST36** is the yang earth horary shu-point that engenders metal (compare **ST36** to ST45 metal + ST44 water combination for pathogenic heat).

STEP 4: LI1 is the yang metal horary shu-point that restrains the wood element.

STEP 5: UB66 is the yang water horary shu-point that tonifies wood.

STEP 6: GB43 is the water shu-point on the gallbladder meridian that tonifies wood.

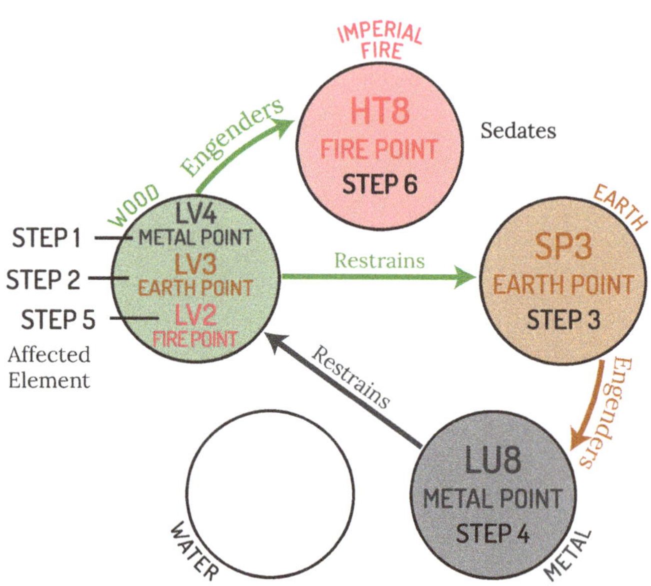

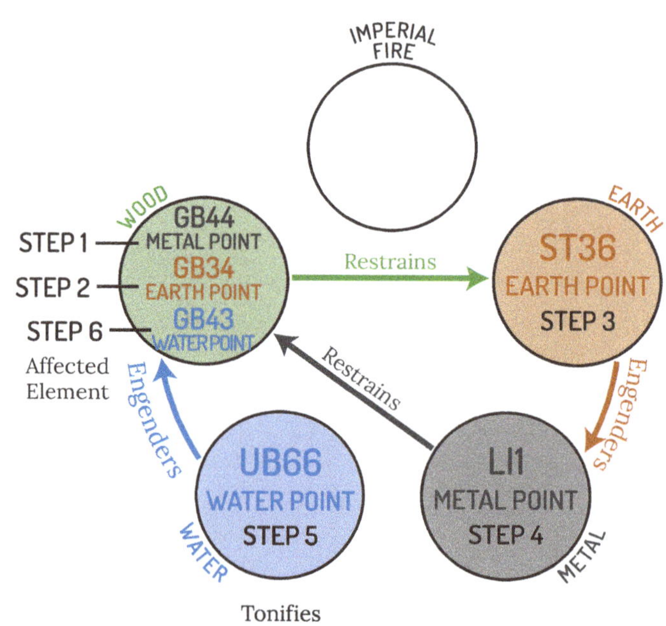

Appointment #3 Post-Treatment Stage

TEST SUPPLEMENTS AND HERBS

No supplements or herbs were tested.

TEST ESSENTIAL OILS TO USE BETWEEN APPOINTMENTS

CS2 continued to apply the essential oil lotions twice daily, as recommended in the first session.

Appointment #4 Follow-up

CS2 returned for another follow-up appointment after three weeks. She reported no nerve pain for four days after the last treatment, and then the pain returned with less burning intensity and no sharpness. The ear felt better and had no nerve sensations. At this appointment, the nerve pain was between one and two on a scale of one to ten. She had little to no muscle tightness in the right leg and noticeably better circulation in both legs.

CS2's pulse was slightly choppy and balanced, which indicated her body was healing at an accelerated rate and she was maintaining balanced qi flow in the meridian system. This appointment was identical to the previous session and included the exact same acupoints to regulate the ANA, treat the gallbladder and liver asymmetrical roots, and support the roots.

Appointment #5 Follow-up

SUBJECTIVE INFORMATION

CS2 returned for another follow-up appointment three weeks later. She said the nerve pain was a different type of dull sensation for one week after the last treatment, and then the pain disappeared and hasn't returned. She reported everything else is fine and feeling back to normal.

OBJECTIVE INFORMATION

Pulse - slightly choppy and balanced
Tongue - medium white coat with pink full body and reduced vertical center crack

ASSESSMENT

The assessment remained the same as at the first and all subsequent appointments.
TCM: blood stasis, blood deficiency, dampness, and qi stagnation with depressive heat
Body-Feedback: third trisection discord with wood element dysfunction

PLAN

The plan remained the same as at the first and all subsequent appointments.
Treatment principle: transform blood stasis, nourish blood, drain dampness, rectify qi to resolve depressive heat, harmonize the third trisection, and optimize the wood element.

Appointment #5 Pre-Treatment Planning Stage

PLANNING STEP ONE: ASSESS FOR ASYMMETRY

Visual assessment of the hips, feet, and shoulders indicated symmetry at this appointment. The right knee and ankle were aligned with the left foot's resting position. The pain when pressing the master alarm points was reduced, and slightly more intense on the right side. The tension in her neck muscles was the same side to side; however, the neck muscles on the right side felt broader and thicker.

PLANNING STEP TWO: REGULATE THE AUTONOMIC NERVOUS SYSTEM

Checking the abdomen decreased the tightness at TB15, SI13, and GB21 on the right and indicated supine as the optimal treatment position. The acupoints along the conception vessel regulated the ANS at this appointment.

PLANNING STEPS THREE AND FOUR: DETERMINE THE BALANCING AND SEDATION OR TONIFICATION PRESCRIPTIONS

Based on the last appointment and the balanced pulse, the only exclusive shu-points tested to the pulse bilaterally were GB34 and LV3, which determined this treatment's newly symmetrical root prescription. The right wrist's pulse positions became slightly slippery to balanced when pressing LV3, the liver balancing, and the tonification acupoints on the right and left sides. The same root prescriptions confirmed the transition to the symmetrical supine treatment position.

As part of the balancing and tonification prescriptions, **SP3** was checked and compared to SP5 metal + SP9 water; the metal + water combination tested favorably, as evidenced in the pulse. LU5 water (to combine with LU8 metal) was checked and tested unfavorably, as evidenced in the pulse. KD7 metal (to combine with KD10 water) was checked and tested favorably, as evidenced in the pulse. The transition to symmetry and reduction in heat-clearing acupoints signified substantial progress in CS2's healing journey.

PLANNING STEP FIVE: ASSESS THE CORRESPONDING TESTING LOCATIONS

CS2's symptoms and meridian balance had improved. Therefore, the gallbladder and liver testing locations were checked again, and the levels of pain, discomfort, and muscle tightness were significantly diminished compared to the first appointment. The testing locations with corresponding signs of organ/meridian dysfunction included:

- right rib cage liver-referred discomfort
- bilateral LV2 and LV8 alarm points painful
- right UB43-UB44 upper body muscle memory region less tight and painful

PLANNING STEP SIX: TEST ESSENTIAL OILS

The same two manufactured products containing essential oils were tested and used again to provide pain relief and a bioidentical hormone precursor for repair of the nerves.

Appointment #5 Treatment Stage

TREATMENT STEP ONE: APPLY ESSENTIAL OILS

The essential oil lotions were applied the same as at the first and subsequent appointments. A thin layer of hormonal lotion was applied first to CS2's spine in the upper back and neck area, the occipital area below the hairline, outside the right ear, and over the scar on the right calf. Then a thin layer of the pain-relief lotion was applied atop the hormonal lotion.

TREATMENT STEP TWO: REGULATE THE AUTONOMIC NERVOUS SYSTEM

New acupoints to regulate the ANS further supported her transition to symmetry: 3 acupoints between CV10 and CV13 regulated the ANS and relaxed the master alarm points on the right side.

TREATMENT STEP THREE: TREAT THE TWO ROOTS

Needled the liver balancing and tonification prescriptions bilaterally LV4, LV3, SP5 + SP9, LU8, KD10, and LV8.

TREATMENT STEP FOUR: SUPPORT THE ROOT

The supporting acupoints needled included KD7 (additional individual metal point), TB5 (yang linking extra-vessel controlling and luo-connecting acupoint), and a line of 4 scalp ashi acupoints between the motor and sensory regions of the brain on the right side only. The corresponding left side acupoints caused increased tension and pain in the master alarm points, indicating the right side was weaker and the left side did not need to be strengthened.

Appointment #5 Post-Treatment Stage

TEST SUPPLEMENTS AND HERBS

No supplements or herbs were tested.

TEST ESSENTIAL OILS TO USE BETWEEN APPOINTMENTS

CS2 continued to apply the essential oil lotions twice daily, as recommended in the first session.

Appointment #6 Follow-up

SUBJECTIVE INFORMATION

CS2 returned for a follow-up appointment three weeks later. She said the nerve pain had resolved, and she has had no pain since the last appointment. She had a mild cold with clear post-nasal drip and fatigue that began a few days prior.

OBJECTIVE INFORMATION

Pulse - slightly choppy overall, wiry and forceful in the LU/LI and HT/SI positions, and deep in the KD/UB position
Tongue - thin white coat with pink full body and reduced vertical center crack

ASSESSMENT

The assessment changed to represent current cold virus and constitutional weakness.
TCM: exterior-wind cold, qi stagnation, depressive heat, blood stasis, and blood deficiency
Body-Feedback: first trisection discord

PLAN

The plan changed to represent current cold virus and constitutional weakness.
Treatment principle: release exterior-wind cold, rectify qi to resolve depressive heat, transform blood stasis, nourish blood, and harmonize the first trisection.

Appointment #6 Pre-Treatment Planning Stage

PLANNING STEP ONE: ASSESS FOR ASYMMETRY

Visual assessment of the hips, feet, and shoulders indicated symmetry at this appointment. The right knee and ankle aligned with the left foot's resting position. There was mild pain when pressing the master alarm points, but slightly more intense on the right side. The tension in her neck muscles was the same side to side; however, the right-side neck muscles felt broader and thicker.

PLANNING STEP TWO: REGULATE THE AUTONOMIC NERVOUS SYSTEM

Checking the abdomen decreased the tightness at TB15, SI13, and GB21 on the right and indicated supine as the optimal treatment position. The wood and metal regions on the abdomen regulated the ANS at this appointment.

PLANNING STEPS THREE AND FOUR: DETERMINE THE BALANCING AND SEDATION OR TONIFICATION PRESCRIPTIONS

Based on the new symptoms related to a common cold, along with the most excessive pulse positions, the following exclusive shu-points were tested to the pulse bilaterally to determine this treatment's root prescription: GB34, LV3, LU10, LI5, HT3, and SI2. The right wrist's pulse positions became slightly slippery to balanced when pressing LI5, the large intestine balancing, and the tonification acupoints on the right and left sides. The same root prescriptions confirmed a symmetrical supine treatment position.

As part of the balancing and tonification prescriptions, **ST36** was checked and compared to ST45 metal and ST44 water; the metal + water combination tested favorably, as evidenced in the pulse. **GB41** was checked and compared to GB44 metal + GB43 water; the metal + water combination tested favorably, as evidenced in the pulse. The increase in heat-clearing acupoints reflected her propensity to be affected by pathogenic heat.

PLANNING STEP FIVE: ASSESS THE CORRESPONDING TESTING LOCATIONS

CS2's nerve pain symptoms and asymmetry had resolved. Her acute immune symptoms were new at this appointment and her root prescription was symmetrical. Therefore, the large intestine testing locations were checked for pain, discomfort, and muscle tightness. The testing locations with corresponding signs of organ/meridian dysfunction included:

- bilateral LI10 immune system alarm point tender
- bilateral LI5 meridian alarm point tender
- bilateral Iliotibial-band-referred tightness and pain

PLANNING STEP SIX: TEST ESSENTIAL OILS

The Large Intestine Meridian Balancing and Organ Supporting blends were tested individually to the master alarm points on the right side, and both blends released tension and discomfort. The blends were then checked together by placing both bottles on the upper abdomen, and together, they further reduced tightness and pain in the master alarm points.

First Trisection Discord Root Large Intestine Deficiency

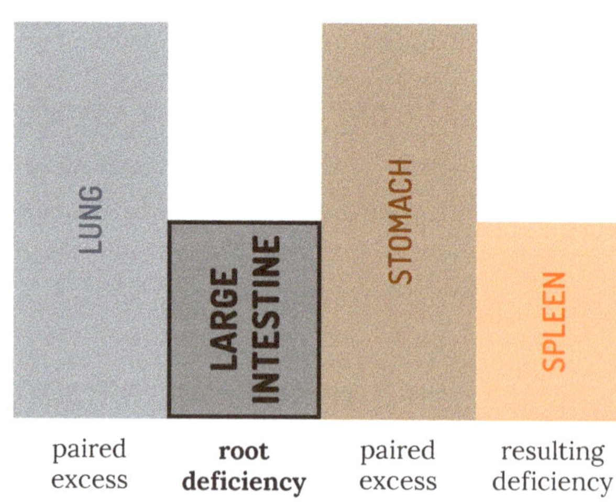

Appointment #6 Treatment Stage

TREATMENT STEP ONE: APPLY ESSENTIAL OILS

Applied 6 drops each of the Large Intestine Meridian Balancing and Organ Supporting blends to the soles of the feet.

TREATMENT STEP TWO: REGULATE THE AUTONOMIC NERVOUS SYSTEM

The acupoints that regulated the ANS at the first appointment released the tightness in the master alarm points at this appointment again. The ANS was regulated by needling 3 acupoints along a diagonal line in both the upper right (wood) and lower left (metal) quadrants of the abdomen for a total of 6 acupoints.

TREATMENT STEP THREE: TREAT THE TWO ROOTS

On both sides, needled the large intestine balancing and tonification prescriptions LI5, LI3, GB44 + GB43, SI5, ST45 + ST44, and LI11.

TREATMENT STEP FOUR: SUPPORT THE ROOT

The supporting acupoints needled included KD9 (xi-cleft point for yin linking extra-vessel), PC6 (controlling point for yin linking extra-vessel and luo-connecting point), LV5 (luo-connecting point), and 4 acupoints in a line in the scalp motor ashi region bilaterally (indicating improved brain health).

Root Large Intestine Tonification Prescription

STEP 1: LI5 is the restraining fire shu-point on the large intestine meridian.

STEP 2: LI3 is the restraining wood shu-point on the large intestine meridian.

STEP 3: **GB41** is the yang wood horary shu-point that engenders fire (compare **GB41** to GB44 metal + GB43 water combination for pathogenic heat).

STEP 4: SI5 is the yang imperial-fire horary shu-point that restrains metal.

STEP 5: **ST36** is the yang earth horary shu-point that tonifies metal (compare **ST36** to ST45 metal + ST44 water combination for pathogenic heat).

STEP 6: LI11 is the earth shu-point on the large intestine meridian that tonifies metal.

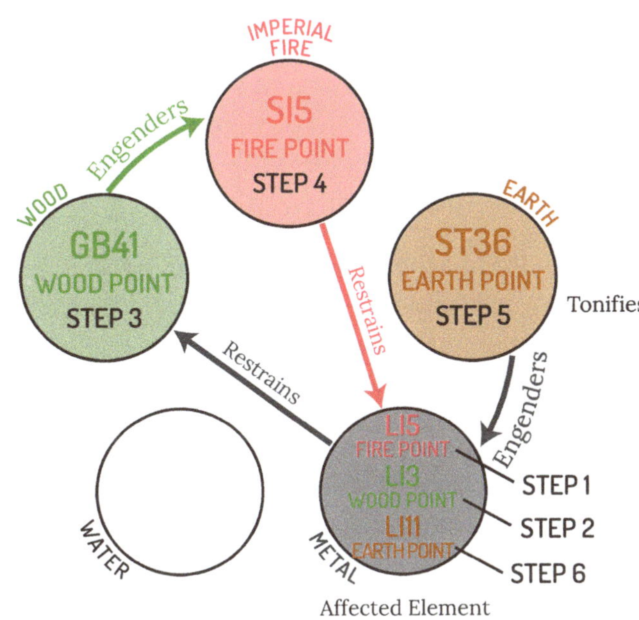

Appointment #6 Post-Treatment Stage

TEST SUPPLEMENTS AND HERBS

No supplements or herbs were tested.

TEST ESSENTIAL OILS TO USE BETWEEN APPOINTMENTS

CS2 can use the essential oil lotions, as needed, for topical relief and regeneration.

CS2 Conclusion Summary

At the initial appointment, CS2 presented with significant pathogenic heat and inflammation affecting the head, which indicated her body was unable to complete the healing process. Body-Feedback testing demonstrated local needling of the scalp points was beneficial and tolerated at later appointments when her body could complete the inflammatory cycle. The wiry and forceful KD/UB and LU/LI pulse positions indicated pathogenic heat and dysfunction in the endocrine and immune systems, which likely resulted from age-related hormone deficiency that failed to provide the needed hormones to complete a healthy inflammatory cycle.

After the first session, CS2 experienced temporary improvement and improved blood flow in the head, which indicated the treatment approach was successful. She needed more time for the hormone lotion to provide the raw materials to complete a healthy inflammatory cycle. The accelerated healing after the second treatment held longer, as the hormone reserves started to build up from the topical lotion.

At multiple appointments, several of the liver and gallbladder testing locations were painful and tense bilaterally, which indicated the wood element dysfunction was likely present before the shingles outbreak. Pathogenic heat in the liver and gallbladder meridians may have caused a weakness for the shingles virus to attack the nerves affecting the right temporal area around the ear.

The pain and muscle tightness in the liver and gallbladder testing locations slowly diminished throughout CS2's first three appointments. Beginning with the fourth treatment, CS2 experienced dull pain following her acupuncture session for one week while the nerves repaired. The transition from sharp to dull nerve pain indicated accelerate healing. Once a healthy inflammatory cycle resulted in repaired nerves, her pain resolved.

Her age-related, naturally lower hormone levels, along with several meridians affected by pathogenic heat, required additional time for healing to occur. At the fifth appointment, CS2 had a significant improvement in pain and discomfort in the individual testing locations and a corresponding reduction in heat-clearing acupoints. This indicated her body was able to complete a healthy inflammatory cycle with regeneration that resulted from increased hormone reserves, the cooling and nourishing properties of the metal + water acupoints, and the essential oil products.

At the last appointment, CS2's abdominal acupoints to regulate the ANS reverted to the original diagonal line to harmonize wood and metal. The acute cold virus caused the abdominal acupoints to regress from the symmetrical combination along the conception vessel to an asymmetrical diagonal line. This change indicated her constitutional weakness occurs in two elements: wood and metal. The wood element may reflect the liver's diminished ability to generate hormones due to age or genetics. CS2's immune system response to the acute infection depleted her hormone reserves. The metal element may reflect the immune system's challenge in completing a healthy inflammatory cycle due to a lack of hormones or genetics. The increase in metal + water combinations at this session may also indicate a genetic weakness causing dysfunction in the inflammatory response.

At her last treatment, I recommended acupuncture as needed in the future. CS1 indicated that she would return if she had a health concern. Family members have reported CS2 has been doing well, and she has continued downhill skiing.

CHAPTER 24

Case Study Three: Symmetrical Prone

Appointment #1 New Client Assessment

Case Study Three (CS3) was a male, age 41 at the first appointment, with a very active lifestyle that included playing sports, bicycling, and active duty in the military. He has had major surgeries on both knees due to sports injuries, a deviated septum, varicose veins removed twice, mononucleosis at age fifteen, and tonsils removed as a child. He has been receiving chiropractic treatments, dry needling, acupuncture with a different provider, and massage therapy for many years. CS3 lived a healthy lifestyle, used non-toxic personal care products, and ate only organic foods prepared at home.

CS3's health history form had four symptoms indicated in the wood element section. This did not match his presenting complaint of lower back pain and immune deficiency according to five-element theory. His healthy, but over-active, lifestyle may have both benefited certain aspects of the wood element and challenged others. Determining his root balancing prescription was key to properly assessing the cause of CS3's back pain and immune weakness, along with monitoring his progress. His treatments focused on testing acupoint prescriptions, essential oils, and supplements to alleviate back pain and strengthen the immune system.

SUBJECTIVE INFORMATION

CS3 scheduled acupuncture to address long-term lower back pain and a Methicillin-resistant Staphylococcus Aureus (MRSA) infection on the skin and in the lymph nodes. The MRSA infection began after a standard physical with a medical doctor two years prior. The lower back pain, which had become worse over the years, was a result of intense athletics, an automobile accident at age nineteen, and a bicycle crash at age thirty-three, which included a broken clavicle and concussion. A chiropractor indicated CS3 had a condition called "flat spine," where the standard s-curve in the lumbar area of the spine was underdeveloped and caused additional pressure on the discs in the lower back.

BODY-FEEDBACK for Health, LLC

Confidential Health History

Name Case Study #3

Please Check All That Apply

METAL ELEMENT

○ Frequent colds, rhinitis, or sinusitis
○ Allergies, asthma, or autoimmune conditions
○ Frequent cough, post-nasal drip, or congestion
○ Dry skin or sensitive skin
○ Hives, eczema, or rashes
○ Constipation, loose stools, irregular bowels
○ Colon polyps or history of any type of cancer
● Low back or hip pain worse in the morning
○ Shortness of breath or exercise induced asthma
● Cold sores or herpes or other viral infections
○ Easily disappointed or offended
○ Sadness, low self-esteem, or excessive grief

WATER ELEMENT

○ Frequent, urgent, or difficult urination
○ Swollen or puffy ankles or feet
○ Low energy or needs more than 8 hours sleep
○ Low libido, sex drive, or reduced sexual function
○ Kidney stones, disease, or dysfunction
○ Forgetful or poor short term memory
○ Low back pain worse at end of day
○ Headaches or migraines triggered by fatigue or hormone changes
○ Adrenal or thyroid dysfunction (hyper or hypo)
○ Scoliosis, osteoarthritis, osteoporosis, osteopenia
○ Hormonal imbalances or endocrine dysfunction
○ Fearful, depression, or lack of motivation

WOOD ELEMENT

● Muscle tension, cramps, tightness
● Sensitive to noise, strong odors, and tastes
○ Dry, red, or weak eyes
○ Coarse or brittle hair or nails or premature gray hair
● Tendon, ligament, or meniscus weakness or pain
○ Fibromyalgia or all over joint pain
○ Numbness and tingling with sleep or inactivity
○ Seizures, tremors, or Parkinson's
○ Pain or tightness in right shoulder or side of neck
○ Bloating, diarrhea, or stomach pains after eating
○ Headaches or migraines triggered by stress
● Anger, irritability, or easily frustrated

EARTH ELEMENT

○ Muscle weakness or lack of strength
○ All over puffiness or water retention
● Bruises easily, varicose, or spider veins
○ Low energy or fatigue after eating
○ Hypo or hyper thyroid function
○ Indigestion, bloating, or gas
● Craves sugar, sweets, or carbohydrates
○ Neck pain or left sided pain in body
○ Diabetes, pre-diabetes, or hypoglycemia
○ Pain that worsens with cold or damp weather
○ Headaches or migraines triggered by weather
○ Easily worried or upset with changes or obsessive

FIRE ELEMENT

○ Insomnia, difficulty sleeping, or waking early
○ Excessive dreaming or nightmares
○ Dry skin and increased desire for fluids
○ Heart palpitations or irregular heartbeat
○ Easy flushing, red type acne, dislike heat
○ Hot flashes or night sweats
○ Heart disease or family history of
○ Anxiety, restlessness, panic attack, or mind racing with physical exhaustion
○ High blood pressure or Low blood pressure
○ Pain in sacrum, SI joint, or tailbone
○ Mouth sores, bleeding gums, or burning tongue
○ Headaches triggered by heat or excessive sun

MINISTERIAL FIRE ELEMENT

○ High-pitched ringing or congestion in the ears
○ Headaches or migraines that move around in head
○ Swollen lymph nodes or chronic infections
○ Chronic sinus or ear congestion
○ Stiff movements or general tightness
○ Belching, burping, or heartburn
○ Difficulty losing weight or obesity in family
○ Polycystic ovarian syndrome or ovarian cysts
○ Cystic acne, boils, or cysts
○ Sciatic pain or tailbone pain
○ Overly optimistic or unrealistic
○ Feeling oppressed or unable to make changes

www.Body-Feedback.com 608·535·9144 2014 Yahara Place, Madison WI 53704

Flat back spinal misalignment

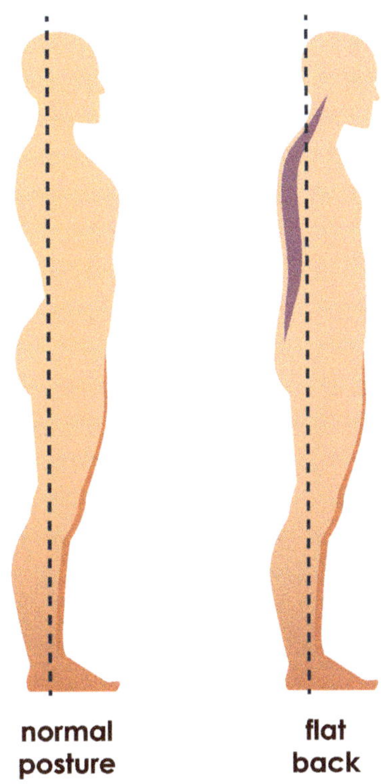

ID 170807204 © Greenni | Dreamstime.com

CS3 often woke up in the morning with severe lower back pain that improved after getting up and walking around. The lower back pain was worse when he stood for long periods. The MRSA had infected several lymph nodes and caused small spots on the skin that rotated around the body. The infection improved after using high doses of a liquid allicin supplement purchased online, and when he tried to reduce the dose, the MRSA worsened. CS3 was on a high dose of the liquid allicin, which cost $130 per month, and when he tried to reduce the dose, the MRSA worsened. He said his treatment goals were to come off this medication and be free of the chronic MRSA and to manage the back pain.

OBJECTIVE INFORMATION

Examination of CS3's lumbar spinal alignment in a standing position indicated misalignment of the sacroiliac joint and a forward-tilted sacrum. The muscles over the lumbar vertebrae area were warm to touch, soggy, and had broken blood vessels.

Pulse - overall slightly wiry to wiry and forceful in the KD/UB and PC/TB positions

Tongue - thin white coating with a slightly thin, red body

ASSESSMENT

TCM: blood heat, blood stasis, phlegm, wei qi deficiency, and qi stagnation with depressive heat

Body-Feedback: second trisection discord with tai-yang dysfunction (due to lower back pain originating from structural development rather than aging, along with chronic immune weakness)

PLAN

Treatment principle: cool blood, transform blood stasis and phlegm, tonify wei qi, rectify qi to resolve depressive heat, harmonize the second trisection, and tonify tai-yang.

Appointment #1 Pre-Treatment Planning Stage

PLANNING STEP ONE: ASSESS FOR ASYMMETRY

CS3 immediately questioned why he was not lying facedown to work on his back when asked to lie on the treatment table faceup. I explained to CS3 that an evaluation of the meridian system would occur in the faceup position first to gather information. Visual assessment of the hips, feet, and shoulders indicated symmetry. TB15 and GB21 were painful upon palpation and tight bilaterally. His posterior neck muscles felt overdeveloped, and his anterior neck muscles felt underdeveloped. His neck muscles were tight, painful, and bilaterally symmetrical.

PLANNING STEP TWO: REGULATE THE AUTONOMIC NERVOUS SYSTEM

Checking the abdomen increased the tightness at TB15 and GB21, indicating prone as the optimal treatment position at this appointment.

PLANNING STEPS THREE AND FOUR: DETERMINE THE BALANCING AND SEDATION OR TONIFICATION PRESCRIPTIONS

Based on the location of CS3's back pain, an imbalance in the kidney, urinary bladder, large intestine, or governing extra-vessel meridians could have been the root prescription. His most excessive pulse positions at this appointment were KD/UB and PC/TB, which correspond with adrenal dysfunction (likely caused by a chronic infection and over-active lifestyle). His health history form indicated a wood element imbalance, which would mostly likely be the gallbladder meridian based on his symptoms. The first appointment tested the following exclusive shu-points to the pulse bilaterally to determine this treatment's root prescriptions: KD3, UB60, GB34, LI5, and SI2 (for small intestine deficiency prescription that includes SI3 controlling acupoint for the governing extra-vessel). The pulse improved the most and became slightly slippery to balanced when pressing UB60, the urinary bladder balancing prescription, and the sedation prescription bilaterally. Testing the same acupoints for both sides of the body confirmed a symmetrical prone treatment position. As part of the balancing prescription, **ST36** was checked and compared to ST45 metal + ST44 water; **ST36** tested favorably, as evidenced in the pulse. As part of the sedation prescription, **GB41** was checked and compared to GB44 metal + GB43 water; **GB41** tested favorably, as evidenced in the pulse.

PLANNING STEP FIVE: ASSESS THE CORRESPONDING TESTING LOCATIONS

CS3's symptoms indicated he had a structural misalignment since childhood. Therefore, both the urinary bladder and governing testing locations were checked for pain, discomfort, and muscle tightness. The assessment of the testing locations occurred with CS3 in the supine position by sliding my hand underneath his back.

The testing locations with corresponding signs of organ/meridian dysfunction included:

- bilateral urinary bladder-referred tightness in erector spinae muscles
- bilateral bladder organ-referred pain and heat and over the sacrum
- bilateral UB57-UB58 lower body muscle memory region tight and painful
- bilateral urinary bladder-referred tightness in peroneal tendon
- bilateral urinary bladder-referred tightness in peroneus longus muscle
- bilateral UB40 organ alarm point tender
- bilateral hypothalamus-referred pain and tightness along the occiput tight
- bilateral urinary bladder-referred tightness in teres major muscle

PLANNING STEP SIX: TEST ESSENTIAL OILS

The Urinary Bladder, Kidney, Small Intestine, and Governing Vessel Meridian Balancing blends were tested individually to the neck muscles. The Governing Vessel Meridian Balancing Blend released the most tension and pain in the neck and erector spinae muscles, TB15, and GB21.

Because the treatment position was going to be prone, CS3 turned over before looking for phlegm nodules. He requested a pillow to place under his hips to reduce pain while in this position. Two thick pillows under the hips allowed CS3 to lay comfortably prone. The pillows under the hips elongated the disc space in the lumbar spine that allowed for deeper needling under the spinous process of each lumbar vertebrae.

PLANNING STEP SEVEN: CHECK FOR PHLEGM NODULES

Three palpable phlegm nodules were found in the lower back along PSIS on the left and right sides.

Second Trisection Discord Root Urinary Bladder Excess

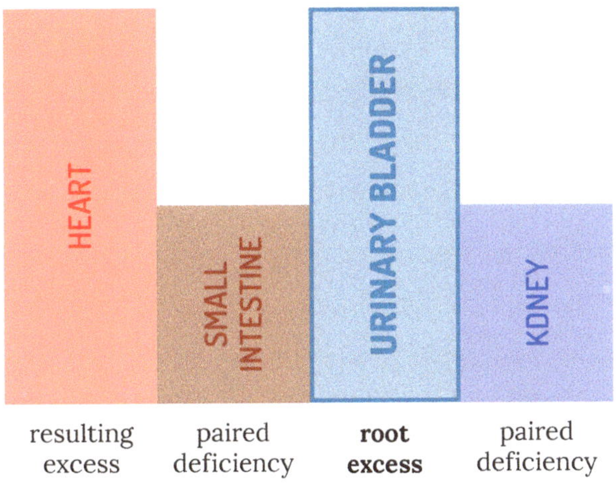

Appointment #1 Treatment Stage

TREATMENT STEP ONE: APPLY ESSENTIAL OILS

Applied 12 drops of the Governing Vessel Meridian Balancing Blend along the upper border of the PSIS and the inner UB meridian (planning to needle directly over the spine).

TREATMENT STEP TWO: REGULATE THE AUTONOMIC NERVOUS SYSTEM

Because CS3's lower back pain was the presenting complaint, each spinous process level was pressed, starting with L5 and then up the spine. The ANS was regulated by needling directly below the spinous processes of L1-L5, T3, and T5 vertebrae. Four needles surrounded each of the phlegm nodules.

TREATMENT STEP THREE: TREAT THE ROOT

Needled the urinary bladder balancing and sedation prescriptions UB40, UB60, SI5, **ST36**, UB65, and **GB41**.

TREATMENT STEP FOUR: SUPPORT THE ROOT

Needled supporting acupoints, including LI4 (yuan-source for metal element), ST37 (large intestine lower he-sea), ST39 (small intestine lower he-sea), KD9 (xi-cleft for yin linking extra-vessel), and SP6 (group luo-connecting).

Root Urinary Bladder Sedation Prescription

STEP 1: UB40 is the restraining earth shu-point on the urinary bladder meridian.

STEP 2: UB60 is the restraining fire shu-point on the urinary bladder meridian.

STEP 3: SI5 is the yang fire horary shu-point that engenders earth.

STEP 4: **ST36** is the yang earth horary shu-point that restrains water (compare **ST36** to ST45 metal + ST44 water combination for pathogenic heat).

STEP 5: UB65 is the wood shu-point on the urinary bladder meridian that sedates water.

STEP 6: **GB41** is the yang wood horary shu-point that sedates water (compare **GB41** to GB44 metal + GB43 water combination for pathogenic heat).

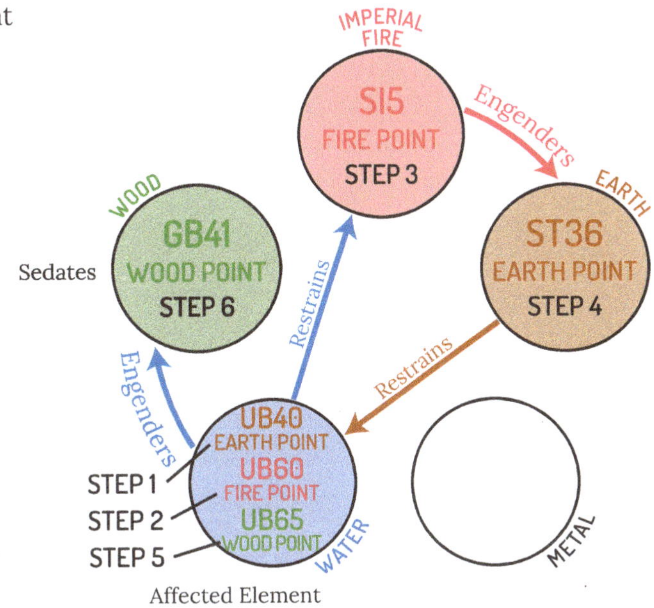

Appointment #1 Post-Treatment Stage

TEST SUPPLEMENTS AND HERBS

After the needles were removed, CS3 turned over into the supine position for testing of supplements. CS3 brought to this appointment the liquid allicin and a dairy-cultured probiotic, and both released tension in the neck muscles, GB21, and TB15. A Chinese herbal formula to cool blood and target bacteria released the most tension from the neck muscles, GB21, and TB15 when comparing three appropriate formulas. An anti-pathogenic, spore-cultured probiotic and a multimineral complex including iodine (compared to one without iodine) to support detoxification and immune functions further released the tension from the neck muscles, GB21, and TB15.

TEST ESSENTIAL OILS TO USE BETWEEN APPOINTMENTS

Peppermint, spearmint, and wintergreen oils were checked to the neck muscles to determine which oil to use to increase cellular cleansing of the phlegm nodules. A custom roll-on blend was recommended that included 3 ml of vegetable carrier oil with 5 drops of spearmint and 20 drops of the Governing Vessel Meridian Balancing Blend to apply to the nodules once daily. An essential oil deodorant released tightness at TB15 and GB21 and included anti-pathogenic properties.

Recommended 3 capsules of the Chinese herbal formula and ½ dose of the liquid allicin together on an empty stomach first thing in the morning and mid-afternoon.

Recommended 3 capsules of the multimineral complex with breakfast.

Recommended 2 capsules of spore-cultured probiotic before bed on an empty stomach.

Recommended switching to an essential oil deodorant due to swollen lymph nodes in the armpits and applying the custom roll-on blend directly over the nodules in the lower back.

Recommended follow-up appointments every two weeks for the next two months and then monthly follow-up appointments for maintenance.

Appointment #2 Follow-up

SUBJECTIVE INFORMATION

CS3 returned for a follow-up appointment two weeks later. He said his lower back pain had reduced since the initial treatment and his back muscles and knees felt stronger. The MRSA infection had fewer red spots on the skin that had appeared and resolved quickly, and the swollen lymph nodes were reduced in size. He had decided to reduce the liquid allicin to a ½ dose every other day. He had felt queasy after taking the mineral supplement with breakfast for the first week and thereafter felt fine. CS3 followed all other recommendations from the first appointment.

OBJECTIVE INFORMATION

Pulse - overall slightly wiry to wiry and forceful in the LV/GB, KD/UB, and PC/TB positions
Tongue - thin white coating with a slightly thin, red body

ASSESSMENT

The assessment remained the same as at the first appointment.
TCM: blood heat, blood stasis, phlegm, wei qi deficiency, and qi stagnation with depressive heat
Body-Feedback: second trisection discord with tai-yang dysfunction (due to lower back pain originating from structural development rather than aging, along with chronic immune weakness)

PLAN

The plan remained the same as at the first appointment.
Treatment principle: cool blood, transform blood stasis and phlegm, tonify wei qi, rectify qi to resolve depressive heat, harmonize the second trisection, and tonify tai-yang.

Appointment #2 Pre-Treatment Planning Stage

PLANNING STEP ONE: ASSESS FOR ASYMMETRY

The pain at TB15 and GB21 upon palpation had reduced since the last appointment. CS3's neck muscles were less tight and painful, and the difference in the development between anterior and posterior was less noticeable. His neck muscles were bilaterally symmetrical.

PLANNING STEP TWO: REGULATE THE AUTONOMIC NERVOUS SYSTEM

Checking the abdomen increased the tightness at TB15 and GB21, indicating prone as the optimal treatment position at this appointment.

PLANNING STEPS THREE AND FOUR: DETERMINE THE BALANCING AND SEDATION OR TONIFICATION PRESCRIPTIONS

Based on the last appointment and this appointment's most excessive pulse positions, the following exclusive shu-points were tested to the pulse bilaterally to determine this treatment's root prescription: KD3, UB60, and GB34. The pulse improved the most and became slightly slippery to balanced when pressing UB60, the urinary bladder balancing prescription, and the sedation prescription bilaterally. Testing the same acupoints for both sides of the body confirmed a symmetrical prone treatment position. As part of the balancing prescription, **ST36** was checked and compared to ST45 metal + ST44 water; **ST36** tested favorably, as evidenced in the pulse. As part of the sedation prescription, **GB41** was checked and compared to GB44 metal + GB43 water; the metal + water combination tested favorably, as evidenced in the pulse, and indicated pathogenic heat in the meridian.

PLANNING STEP FIVE: ASSESS THE CORRESPONDING TESTING LOCATIONS

The same urinary bladder and governing extra-vessel testing locations were checked as at the first appointment. The assessment of the testing locations occurred with CS3 in the supine position by sliding my hand underneath his back. There was a mild reduction in pain, discomfort, and muscle tightness in a few locations compared to the last appointment. The testing locations with corresponding signs of organ/meridian dysfunction included:

- bilateral urinary bladder-referred tightness in erector spinae muscles
- bilateral bladder organ-referred tenderness over the sacrum
- bilateral UB57-UB58 lower body muscle memory region tight and painful
- bilateral urinary bladder-referred tightness in peroneal tendon
- bilateral urinary bladder-referred tightness in peroneus longus muscle
- bilateral UB40 organ alarm point tender
- bilateral hypothalamus referral area along the occiput tight and painful
- bilateral urinary bladder-referred tightness in teres major muscle

PLANNING STEP SIX: TEST ESSENTIAL OILS

The Governing Vessel Meridian Balancing blend was tested to the neck muscles, and the tension or discomfort did not change. Because CS3 was using this blend daily and it did not further improve the pulse, other oils were tested. The pathogenic heat in the gallbladder requiring the metal + water substitution suggested checking the Gallbladder Organ Supporting Blend, and it reduced the muscle tension in the neck and erector spinae muscles. A bottle of copaiba essential oil was tested with the Gallbladder Organ Supporting Blend together for additional heat-clearing and nourishing properties. This combination released the most tension and pain in the neck and erector spinae muscles, TB15, and GB21.

Because the treatment position was going to be prone again, CS3 turned over before rechecking the phlegm nodules. CS3 asked for a third pillow under the hips to lay comfortably prone.

PLANNING STEP SEVEN: CHECK FOR PHLEGM NODULES

There was noticeably improved integrity of the muscle surrounding the three palpable phlegm nodules in the lower back along PSIS on the left and right sides.

Appointment #2 Treatment Stage

TREATMENT STEP ONE: APPLY ESSENTIAL OILS

Applied 8 drops of the Gallbladder Organ Supporting Blend and 4 drops of copaiba along the upper border of the PSIS and the inner UB meridian (planning to needle directly over the spine).

TREATMENT STEP TWO: REGULATE THE AUTONOMIC NERVOUS SYSTEM

Again, each spinous process level was pressed, starting with L5 and then up the spine. The ANS was regulated by needling directly below the spinous processes of L1-5, T2, T3, T7, T9, and T10 vertebrae. Three needles surrounded each of the phlegm nodules.

TREATMENT STEP THREE: TREAT THE ROOT

Needled the urinary bladder balancing and sedation prescriptions UB40, UB60, SI5, **ST36**, UB65, and GB44 + GB43.

TREATMENT STEP FOUR: SUPPORT THE ROOT

Needled supporting acupoints, including LI4 (yuan-source for metal element), ST37 (large intestine lower he-sea), ST39 (small intestine lower he-sea), LV6 (xi-cleft for liver), and SP6 (group luo-connecting).

Appointment #2 Post-Treatment Stage

TEST SUPPLEMENTS AND HERBS

After the needles were removed, CS3 turned over into the supine position to retest the new supplements. All herbs and supplements were tested together and further released the tension from the neck muscles, GB21, and TB15. This confirmed all of the supplements were compatible.

TEST ESSENTIAL OILS TO USE BETWEEN APPOINTMENTS

Phlegm nodules take months to reduce in size. Therefore, continuing the same custom essential oil roll-on blend from the first appointment was recommended and no other oils were tested.

Recommended 3 capsules of the Chinese herbal formula on an empty stomach first thing in the morning and mid-afternoon. CS3 added a ½ dose of the liquid allicin every other day taken at the same time as the herbs.

Recommended 3 capsules of the multimineral complex with breakfast.

Recommended 2 capsules of spore-cultured probiotic before bed on an empty stomach.

Recommended continuing the essential oil deodorant due to swollen lymph nodes in the armpits and applying the custom roll-on blend directly over the nodules in the lower back.

Appointment #3 Follow-up

SUBJECTIVE INFORMATION

CS3 returned for another follow-up appointment three weeks later. He noticed increased back tightness that began over the last few days and could tell the previous treatment benefits began declining after two weeks. He stated some stiffness in the knees and neck first thing in the morning upon waking, even though the lower back felt better. He had experienced increased stress at work over the previous two weeks. The MRSA continued to improve since the last appointment with reduced swelling of the lymph nodes and only small whiteheads on the skin with little to no pain. CS3 followed all other recommendations from the first appointment.

OBJECTIVE INFORMATION

Pulse - overall slightly wiry to wiry and forceful in the KD/UB position
Tongue - thin white coating with a slightly thin, red body with small cracks in the center

ASSESSMENT

The assessment remained the same as at the first appointment.
TCM: blood heat, blood stasis, phlegm, wei qi deficiency, and qi stagnation with depressive heat
Body-Feedback: second trisection discord with tai-yang dysfunction (due to lower back pain originating from structural development rather than aging, along with chronic immune weakness)

PLAN

The plan remained the same as at the first appointment.
Treatment principle: cool blood, transform blood stasis and phlegm, tonify wei qi, rectify qi to resolve depressive heat, harmonize the second trisection, and tonify tai-yang.

Appointment #3 Pre-Treatment Planning Stage

PLANNING STEP ONE: ASSESS FOR ASYMMETRY

The pain at TB15 and GB21 upon palpation had reduced since the last appointment. CS3's neck muscles were less tight and painful, and the difference in the development between anterior and posterior was less noticeable. His neck muscles were bilaterally symmetrical.

PLANNING STEP TWO: REGULATE THE AUTONOMIC NERVOUS SYSTEM

Checking the abdomen increased the tightness at TB15 and GB21, indicating prone as the optimal treatment position at this appointment.

PLANNING STEPS THREE AND FOUR: DETERMINE THE BALANCING AND SEDATION OR TONIFICATION PRESCRIPTIONS

Based on the last appointment and this appointment's only excessive pulse position, UB60 was tested. The pulse improved and became slightly slippery to balanced when pressing UB60, the urinary bladder balancing prescription, and the tonification prescription bilaterally. At this appointment, the prescription changed from sedation to tonification. As part of the balancing prescription, **ST36** was checked and compared to ST45 metal + ST44 water; **ST36** tested favorably, as evidenced in the pulse. As part of the tonification prescription, LI2 water (to combine with LI1 metal) was checked and tested unfavorably, as evidenced in the pulse.

PLANNING STEP FIVE: ASSESS THE CORRESPONDING TESTING LOCATIONS

The same urinary bladder and governing extra-vessel testing locations were checked as at the first two appointments. The assessment of the testing locations occurred with CS3 in the supine position by sliding my hand underneath his back. There was reduction in pain, discomfort, and muscle tightness in a few locations compared to the last appointment. The testing locations with corresponding signs of organ/meridian dysfunction included:

- bilateral urinary bladder-referred tightness in erector spinae muscles
- bilateral bladder organ-referred tenderness over the sacrum
- bilateral UB57-UB58 lower body muscle memory region tight
- bilateral urinary bladder-referred tightness in peroneal tendon
- bilateral urinary bladder-referred tightness in peroneus longus muscle
- bilateral UB40 organ alarm point tender
- bilateral hypothalamus-referred pain and tightness along the occiput tight
- bilateral urinary bladder-referred tightness in teres major muscle

PLANNING STEP SIX: TEST ESSENTIAL OILS

The Governing Vessel Meridian Balancing blend was tested to the neck muscles, as there was no lingering pathogenic heat in the gallbladder, and it reduced tension and discomfort in the neck muscles, TB15, and GB21.

Because the treatment position was going to be prone again, CS3 turned over before rechecking the phlegm nodules. CS3 used pillows again under the hips to lay comfortably prone.

PLANNING STEP SEVEN: CHECK FOR PHLEGM NODULES

The muscle surrounding the three palpable phlegm nodules on each side continued to feel stronger and the nodules felt softer.

Second Trisection Discord Root Urinary Bladder Deficiency

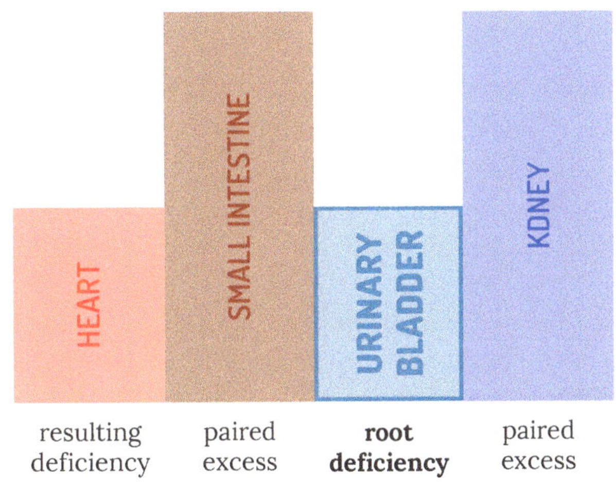

Appointment #3 Treatment Stage

TREATMENT STEP ONE: APPLY ESSENTIAL OILS

Applied 12 drops of the Governing Vessel Meridian Balancing Blend along the upper border of the PSIS and the inner UB meridian (planning to needle directly over the spine).

TREATMENT STEP TWO: REGULATE THE AUTONOMIC NERVOUS SYSTEM

Again, each spinous process level was pressed, starting with L5 and then up the spine. The ANS was regulated by needling directly below the spinous processes of L1-5, T2, T3, T7, T9, and T10 vertebrae. Three needles surrounded each of the phlegm nodules.

TREATMENT STEP THREE: TREAT THE ROOT

Needled the urinary bladder balancing and tonification prescriptions UB40, UB60, SI5, **ST36**, LI1, and UB67.

TREATMENT STEP FOUR: SUPPORT THE ROOT

Because the GB44 metal + GB43 water metal combination was included in the last treatment, these acupoints were checked to the pulse at this appointment; they caused the pulse to become wiry and forceful, indicating no pathogenic heat in the gallbladder meridian at this appointment. The supporting acupoints needled included GB40 (yuan-source for wood element), ST37 (large intestine lower he-sea), ST39 (small intestine lower he-sea), and SP6 (group luo-connecting).

Second Trisection Discord Root Urinary Bladder Tonification Prescription

STEP 1: UB40 is the restraining earth shu-point on the urinary bladder meridian.

STEP 2: UB60 is the restraining fire shu-point on the urinary bladder meridian.

STEP 3: SI5 is the yang fire horary shu-point that engenders earth.

STEP 4: **ST36** is the yang earth horary shu-point that restrains water (compare **ST36** to ST45 metal + ST44 water combination for pathogenic heat).

STEP 5: LI1 is the yang metal horary shu-point that tonifies water.

STEP 6: UB67 is the metal shu-point on the urinary bladder meridian that tonifies water.

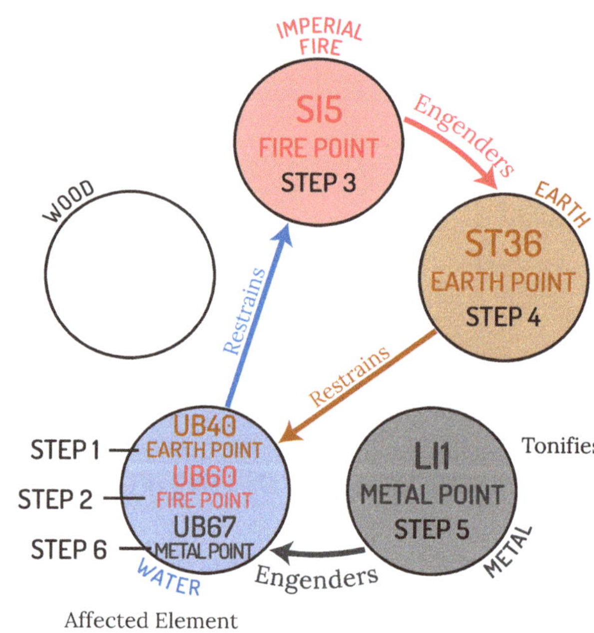

Appointment #3 Post-Treatment Stage

TEST SUPPLEMENTS AND HERBS

After the needles were removed, CS3 turned over into the supine position to retest the supplements. All herbs and supplements were tested together and further released the tension from the neck muscles, GB21, and TB15. This confirmed all of the supplements were compatible.

TEST ESSENTIAL OILS TO USE BETWEEN APPOINTMENTS

Phlegm nodules take months to reduce in size. Therefore, continuing the same custom essential oil roll-on blend from the first appointment was recommended and no other oils were tested.

Recommended 4 capsules of the Chinese herbal formula on an empty stomach first thing in the morning and mid-afternoon. CS3 combined a ¼ dose of the liquid allicin every other day with the herbs until he finished his bottle.

Recommended 3 capsules of the multimineral complex with breakfast.

Recommended 2 capsules of spore-cultured probiotic before bed on an empty stomach.

Recommended continuing the essential oil deodorant and applying the custom roll-on blend directly over the nodules in the lower back.

Appointment #4 Follow-up

SUBJECTIVE INFORMATION

CS3 returned for another follow-up appointment three weeks later. He had noticed increased back tightness and muscle spasms that began after a long and strenuous bicycle ride about ten days prior. The lymph system and MRSA spots on the skin were almost resolved with the reduced liquid allicin. Prior to the Body-Feedback treatments, reducing the allicin resulted in an increase in MRSA symptoms. The current liquid allicin supplement would run out before the next appointment, and he requested changing over to a less expensive allicin product.

OBJECTIVE INFORMATION

Pulse - overall slightly wiry to wiry and forceful in the KD/UB position
Tongue - thin white coating with a slightly thin, red body with small cracks in the center

ASSESSMENT

The assessment remained the same as at the first appointment.
TCM: blood heat, blood stasis, phlegm, wei qi deficiency, and qi stagnation with depressive heat
Body-Feedback: second trisection discord with tai-yang dysfunction (due to lower back pain originating from structural development rather than aging, along with chronic immune weakness)

PLAN

The plan remained the same as at the first appointment.
Treatment principle: cool blood, transform blood stasis and phlegm, tonify wei qi, rectify qi to resolve depressive heat, harmonize the second trisection, and tonify tai-yang.

Appointment #4 Pre-Treatment Planning Stage

PLANNING STEP ONE: ASSESS FOR ASYMMETRY

The pain at TB15 and GB21 upon palpation reduced since the last appointment. The development of CS3's neck muscles was normal between the anterior and posterior sides.

PLANNING STEP TWO: REGULATE THE AUTONOMIC NERVOUS SYSTEM

Checking the abdomen increased the tightness at TB15 and GB21, indicating prone as the optimal treatment position.

PLANNING STEPS THREE AND FOUR: DETERMINE THE BALANCING AND SEDATION OR TONIFICATION PRESCRIPTIONS

Based on the last appointment and this appointment's only excessive pulse position, UB60 was tested. The pulse improved and became slightly slippery to balanced when pressing UB60, the urinary bladder balancing prescription, and the sedation prescription bilaterally. At this appointment, the prescription reverted back to sedation. As part of the balancing prescription, **ST36** was checked and compared to ST45 metal + ST44 water; **ST36** tested favorably, as evidenced in the pulse. As part of the sedation prescription, **GB41** was checked and compared to GB44 metal + GB43 water; the metal + water combination tested favorably, as evidenced in the pulse, and indicated pathogenic heat in the meridian.

PLANNING STEP FIVE: ASSESS THE CORRESPONDING TESTING LOCATIONS

The same urinary bladder and governing extra-vessel testing locations were checked as at the first two appointments. The assessment of the testing locations occurred with CS3 in the supine position by sliding my hand underneath his back. There was a significant reduction in pain, discomfort, and muscle tightness in a few locations compared to the last appointment. The testing locations with corresponding signs of organ/meridian dysfunction included:

- bilateral urinary bladder-referred tightness in mid to lower erector spinae muscles
- bilateral UB57-UB58 lower body muscle memory region tight
- bilateral hypothalamus-referred tightness along the occiput

PLANNING STEP SIX: TEST ESSENTIAL OILS

The Governing Vessel and Urinary Bladder Meridian Balancing blends and the Gallbladder Organ Supporting Blend were tested to the neck muscles individually. The Governing Vessel and Urinary Bladder Meridian Balancing blends reduced tension and discomfort in the neck muscles, TB15, and GB21 when checked individually and together.

Because the treatment position was going to be prone again, CS3 turned over before rechecking the phlegm nodules. CS3 used pillows again under the hips to lay comfortably prone.

PLANNING STEP SEVEN: CHECK FOR PHLEGM NODULES

The muscle surrounding the three palpable phlegm nodules on each side continued to feel stronger and the nodules felt softer.

Appointment #4 Treatment Stage

TREATMENT STEP ONE: APPLY ESSENTIAL OILS

Applied 8 drops of the Governing Vessel Meridian Balancing Blend and 8 drops of the Urinary Bladder Meridian Balancing Blend along the upper border of the PSIS and the inner UB meridian (planning to needle directly over the spine).

TREATMENT STEP TWO: REGULATE THE AUTONOMIC NERVOUS SYSTEM

Again, each spinous process level was pressed, starting with L5 and then up the spine. The ANS was regulated by needling directly below the spinous processes of L1-5, T2, T3, and T7 vertebrae. Three needles surrounded each of the phlegm nodules.

TREATMENT STEP THREE: TREAT THE ROOT

Needled the urinary bladder balancing and tonification prescriptions UB40, UB60, SI5, **ST36**, UB65, and GB44 + GB43.

TREATMENT STEP FOUR: SUPPORT THE ROOT

Needled supporting acupoints, including LI4 (yuan-source for metal element), ST37 (large intestine lower he-sea), ST39 (small intestine lower he-sea), and LV5 (luo-connecting for the liver).

Appointment #4 Post-Treatment Stage

TEST SUPPLEMENTS AND HERBS

After the needles were removed, CS3 turned over into the supine position to retest the supplements. Rechecking the herbs, minerals, and spore-cultured probiotics indicated released tension from the neck muscles, GB21, and TB15. A new high-quality and less expensive allicin capsule tested beneficial individually and together with the herbs.

TEST ESSENTIAL OILS TO USE BETWEEN APPOINTMENTS

Phlegm nodules take months to reduce in size. Therefore, continuing the same custom essential oil roll-on blend from the first appointment was recommended and no other oils were tested.

Recommended rotating every other day: 4 capsules of the Chinese herbal formula with 2 of the new allicin capsules on an empty stomach first thing in the morning.

Recommended 3 capsules of the multimineral complex with breakfast.

Recommended 2 capsules of spore-cultured probiotic before bed on an empty stomach.

Recommended continuing the essential oil deodorant due to swollen lymph nodes in the armpits and applying the custom essential oil roll-on blend directly over the nodules in the lower back.

Appointment #5 Follow-up

SUBJECTIVE INFORMATION

CS3 returned for a follow-up appointment four weeks later. CS3 reported no muscle spasms in the lower back and only some aches and tightness after bicycling and when waking in the morning. He was going to start a new job the following week and expected some increased stress with the transition. There were no new MRSA spots on the skin and the lymph nodes were undetectable.

OBJECTIVE INFORMATION

Pulse - overall slightly wiry to wiry and forceful in the SP/ST and PC/TB positions
Tongue - thin white coating with a slightly thin, red body, and the cracks in the center resolved

ASSESSMENT

The assessment was changed from the last appointment. The blood heat, blood stasis, and wei qi deficiency were removed because of resolving the MRSA.
TCM: Qi stagnation with depressive heat and phlegm
Body-Feedback: second trisection discord with tai-yang dysfunction (due to lower back pain originating from structural development rather than aging, along with a history of immune weakness)

PLAN

The plan was adjusted to remove cool blood, transform blood stasis, and tonify wei qi from the last appointment.

Treatment principle: Rectify qi to resolve depressive heat, transform phlegm, harmonize the second trisection, and tonify tai-yang.

Appointment #5 Pre-Treatment Planning Stage

PLANNING STEP ONE: ASSESS FOR ASYMMETRY

This step was skipped and CS3 used pillows again under the hips to lay comfortably prone for the planning stage.

PLANNING STEP TWO: REGULATE THE AUTONOMIC NERVOUS SYSTEM

TB15 and GB21 released tightness when pressing directly under the L1 to L5 spinous processes and indicated prone as the optimal treatment position at this appointment.

PLANNING STEPS THREE AND FOUR: DETERMINE THE BALANCING AND SEDATION OR TONIFICATION PRESCRIPTIONS

UB60 was the only exclusive shu-point tested. The pulse improved and became slightly slippery to balanced when pressing UB60, the urinary bladder balancing prescription, and the tonification prescription bilaterally. At this appointment, the prescription changed again to tonification. As part of the balancing prescription, **ST36** was checked and compared to ST45 metal + ST44 water; **ST36** tested favorably, as evidenced in the pulse. As part of the tonification prescription, LI2 water (to combine with LI1 metal) was checked and tested unfavorably, as evidenced in the pulse.

PLANNING STEP FIVE: ASSESS THE CORRESPONDING TESTING LOCATIONS

The same urinary bladder and governing extra-vessel testing locations were checked as at the first appointment. The only remaining testing location with slight muscle tightness was the erector spinae muscle group in the lower back.

PLANNING STEP SIX: TEST ESSENTIAL OILS

The Governing Vessel and Urinary Bladder Meridian Balancing blends and the Gallbladder Organ Supporting Blend were tested to the neck muscles individually. Only the Governing Vessel Meridian Balancing blend reduced tension and discomfort in the neck muscles, TB15, and GB21.

PLANNING STEP SEVEN: CHECK FOR PHLEGM NODULES

The muscle surrounding the three palpable phlegm nodules on each side continued to feel stronger and the nodules were smaller and soft.

Appointment #5 Treatment Stage

TREATMENT STEP ONE: APPLY ESSENTIAL OILS

Applied 12 drops of the Governing Vessel Meridian Balancing Blend along the upper border of the PSIS and the inner UB meridian (planning to needle directly over the spine).

TREATMENT STEP TWO: REGULATE THE AUTONOMIC NERVOUS SYSTEM

Again, each spinous process level was pressed, starting with L5 and then up the spine. The ANS was regulated by needling directly below the spinous processes of L1-5, T3, T5, and T7 vertebrae. Three needles surrounded each of the phlegm nodules.

TREATMENT STEP THREE: TREAT THE ROOT

Needled the urinary bladder balancing and tonification prescriptions UB40, UB60, SI5, **ST36**, LI1, and UB67.

TREATMENT STEP FOUR: SUPPORT THE ROOT

Needled supporting acupoints, including GB44 metal + GB 43 water combination, ST37 (large intestine lower he-sea), ST39 (small intestine lower he-sea), and LV5 (luo-connecting for liver).

Appointment #5 Post-Treatment Stage

TEST SUPPLEMENTS AND HERBS

After the needles were removed, CS3 turned over into the supine position to retest the supplements. All herbs and supplements were tested together and further released the tension from the neck muscles, GB21, and TB15. This confirmed all of the supplements were compatible and beneficial.

TEST ESSENTIAL OILS TO USE BETWEEN APPOINTMENTS

The phlegm nodules were reduced in size. Recommended continuing the same custom essential oil roll-on blend from the first appointment, and no other oils were tested.

Recommended rotating every other day: 2 capsules of the Chinese herbal formula with 2 of the new allicin capsules on an empty stomach first thing in the morning. The herbs were being reduced in preparation for discontinuing after appointment #6.

Recommended 3 capsules of the multimineral complex with breakfast.

Recommended 2 capsules of spore-cultured probiotic before bed on an empty stomach.

Recommended continuing the essential oil deodorant to maintain resolution of swollen lymph nodes in the armpits and applying the custom roll-on blend directly over the nodules in the lower back.

CS3 Conclusion Summary

CS3 continued to improve and strengthened his immune system. After appointment #6, he discontinued the Chinese herbal formula, and a few MRSA spots on the skin started to reappear. He continued 2 capsules of herbs every other day for another six weeks, and then he was able to stop with no resurgence of symptoms. He felt most comfortable continuing to take 1 allicin capsule, 2 spore-cultured probiotics, and 3 capsules of minerals daily, along with vitamin D in the winter as long-term nutritional support.

As a result of CS3's healthy lifestyle and previous holistic care, the Body-Feedback treatments immediately focused on his constitutionally weak tai-yang six-level pair and second trisection discord. The structural abnormality in the lower back, causing the lack of curve, likely developed either in utero or during early childhood. CS3's neck alignment and cervical spinal curvature was normal, which indicated the root of the structural imbalance was the sacrum and lower back. Either the excessive forward-tilting pelvis caused the lumbar spine to accommodate by lacking the standard curve, or the lack of normal curve in the lumbar spine caused the sacrum to tilt forward. His long-distance bicycle rides may have exacerbated CS3's misalignment of the sacrum and lower back.

CS3 indicated that the lower back symptom relief lasted longer with the Body-Feedback style of acupuncture than the other therapies he has tried. He noticed the lower back pain starting to return after four to five weeks if he missed his monthly treatment. Over time and with long-term maintenance treatments, signs of a standard curve in the lower back started to form.

The governing vessel (*du mai*) and yang heel vessel (*yang qiao mai*) control the spinal column through the tai-yang six-level pair. There was likely a genetic component to the tai-yang six-level pair root dysfunction, as the Governing Vessel Meridian Balancing Blend provided more relief than the Urinary Bladder Meridian Balancing Blend. A strong extra-vessel component in Body-Feedback treatments indicates genetic involvement in the root dysfunction. Varicose veins can result from either misalignment of the sacrum or genetics. CS3's tai-yang six-level dysfunction with extra-vessel involvement demonstrates genetic and structural components to his varicose vein pathology.

The natural progression of healing for CS3 depended on supporting the second trisection discord through the root urinary bladder treatments. Long-term maintenance treatments for CS3 support his healthy cellular aging and neuro-regeneration. He has indicated that he feels better emotionally, has more endurance, and has experienced fewer seasonal cold and flu pathogens while maintaining regular treatments.

CHAPTER 25

Case Study Four: Asymmetrical Prone

Appointment #1 New Client Assessment

Case Study Four (CS4) was a female, age 58 at the first appointment, with pain in multiple areas due to scoliosis from childhood and arthritis that had developed recently. Her pain typically reduced with stretching, yoga, and salt baths, and it increased with heavy lifting, driving, extended sitting, and sometimes forward bending. She could have problems sleeping while traveling or experiencing heightened pain.

At age forty-five, CS4 had a mild stroke due to a heart defect. She experienced migraines that became severe just before the stroke occurred. The residual issues from the stroke included pain in the left forearm (along the pericardium meridian), left-handed numbness (which could become disabling with excessive stress), and difficulty recalling words. Excessive vibration from her lawnmower had triggered the left-hand symptoms. In addition, she had food allergies to gluten, dairy, and egg, along with a chronic fungal infection in her thumbnails.

CS4's major surgeries included abdominal surgery for infertility, fibroid removal, post-ectopic pregnancy surgery, heart repair, and corrective foot surgery in her early twenties due to bunions. She had nerve damage on the right foot caused by the corrective bunion surgery. Before the foot surgery, CS4 had knee pain and excessive wear in knee joints due to foot misalignment, which improved after the foot surgery. Significant traumas included abdominal trauma as a teenager and three automobile accidents (one causing a broken collar bone and one a head injury).

CS4's scoliosis and the severity of symptoms affecting different areas of her body implied asymmetry. The health history form had two symptoms indicated in each of the metal, water, and wood elements. This same number of symptoms checked in three different elements suggested several different possibilities for the left and right sides' root asymmetrical treatment. CS4's constitutional weakness was likely one of these three elements, which required time to confirm due to her age and length of time affected by scoliosis.

BODY-FEEDBACK for Health, LLC

Confidential Health History

Name Case Study 4

Please Check All That Apply

METAL ELEMENT

- ○ Frequent colds, rhinitis, or sinusitis
- ● Allergies, asthma, or autoimmune conditions - food
- ○ Frequent cough, post-nasal drip, or congestion
- ○ Dry skin or sensitive skin
- ○ Hives, eczema, or rashes
- ○ Constipation, loose stools, irregular bowels
- ○ Colon polyps or history of any type of cancer
- ● Low back or hip pain worse in the morning
- ○ Shortness of breath or exercise induced asthma
- ○ Cold sores or herpes or other viral infections
- ○ Easily disappointed or offended
- ○ Sadness, low self-esteem, or excessive grief

WATER ELEMENT

- ○ Frequent, urgent, or difficult urination
- ○ Swollen or puffy ankles or feet
- ○ Low energy or needs more than 8 hours sleep
- ○ Low libido, sex drive, or reduced sexual function
- ○ Kidney stones, disease, or dysfunction
- ○ Forgetful or poor short term memory
- ● Low back pain worse at end of day depends on activity
- ○ Headaches or migraines triggered by fatigue or hormone changes
- ○ Adrenal or thyroid dysfunction (hyper or hypo)
- ● Scoliosis, osteoarthritis, osteoporosis, osteopenia
- ○ Hormonal imbalances or endocrine dysfunction
- ○ Fearful, depression, or lack of motivation

WOOD ELEMENT

- ● Muscle tension, cramps, tightness
- ○ Sensitive to noise, strong odors, and tastes
- ○ Dry, red, or weak eyes
- ○ Coarse or brittle hair or nails or premature gray hair
- ○ Tendon, ligament, or meniscus weakness or pain
- ○ Fibromyalgia or all over joint pain
- ○ Numbness and tingling with sleep or inactivity
- ○ Seizures, tremors, or Parkinson's
- ● Pain or tightness in right shoulder or side of neck
- ○ Bloating, diarrhea, or stomach pains after eating
- ○ Headaches or migraines triggered by stress
- ○ Anger, irritability, or easily frustrated

EARTH ELEMENT

- ○ Muscle weakness or lack of strength
- ○ All over puffiness or water retention
- ○ Bruises easily, varicose, or spider veins
- ○ Low energy or fatigue after eating
- ○ Hypo or hyper thyroid function
- ○ Indigestion, bloating, or gas
- ● Craves sugar, sweets, or carbohydrates
- ○ Neck pain or left sided pain in body
- ○ Diabetes, pre-diabetes, or hypoglycemia
- ○ Pain that worsens with cold or damp weather
- ○ Headaches or migraines triggered by weather
- ○ Easily worried or upset with changes or obsessive

FIRE ELEMENT

- ○ Insomnia, difficulty sleeping, or waking early
- ○ Excessive dreaming or nightmares
- ○ Dry skin and increased desire for fluids
- ○ Heart palpitations or irregular heartbeat
- ○ Easy flushing, red type acne, dislike heat
- ○ Hot flashes or night sweats
- ○ Heart disease or family history of
- ○ Anxiety, restlessness, panic attack, or mind racing with physical exhaustion
- ○ High blood pressure or Low blood pressure
- ○ Pain in sacrum, SI joint, or tailbone
- ○ Mouth sores, bleeding gums, or burning tongue
- ○ Headaches triggered by heat or excessive sun

MINISTERIAL-FIRE ELEMENT

- ○ High-pitched ringing or congestion in the ears
- ○ Headaches or migraines that move around in head
- ○ Swollen lymph nodes or chronic infections
- ○ Chronic sinus or ear congestion
- ○ Stiff movements or general tightness
- ○ Belching, burping, or heartburn
- ○ Difficulty losing weight or obesity in family
- ○ Polycystic ovarian syndrome or ovarian cysts
- ○ Cystic acne, boils, or cysts
- ○ Sciatic pain or tailbone pain
- ○ Overly optimistic or unrealistic
- ○ Feeling oppressed or unable to make changes

www.Body-Feedback.com 608-535-9144 2014 Yahara Place, Madison WI 53704

CS4 was informed that the most effective treatment approach to resolve her pain required two sets of needles: one facedown, then another faceup. Needling the spine for 10-15 minutes first while in the facedown position would address the curvature. After those needles were removed, another set of acupoints would be treated in a faceup treatment position to address her other concerns. She was instructed to schedule an extra 15 minutes with her follow-up appointments to accommodate two sets of needles.

SUBJECTIVE INFORMATION

CS4 scheduled acupuncture to address pain in multiple areas, including her shoulders, back, and right hip from scoliosis, along with her hands and feet from arthritis. The hip pain had recently increased, which made entering and exiting her vehicle more difficult. Scoliosis from early childhood caused her chronic shoulder and back pain. The arthritis pain in her hands flared up with excessive use and when her dog pulled on the leash during walks.

CS4 experienced increased insomnia due to recent pain and travel. Her digestion was sensitive to processed, high-fat, and non-organic foods (in addition to her food allergies), which resulted in abdominal cramping and urgent, loose, bowel movements. She was concerned about her heart condition and noticed a dull recurring pain on the left side of her chest. She has been taking supplements, including fiber, dairy-cultured probiotic, and fish oil, along with over-the-counter medications of aspirin and Tylenol as needed.

OBJECTIVE INFORMATION

Pulse - slightly thin and wiry overall, wiry and forceful in the SP/ST and PC/TB positions, and thin and deep in the HT/SI position
Tongue - thin glossy coat, pink full body, deep vertical center crack, and red speckles (inflamed taste buds)

ASSESSMENT

TCM: blood, essence, and qi deficiency, blood stasis, qi stagnation with depressive heat
Body-Feedback: second and third trisection discord

PLAN

Treatment principle: nourish blood and essence, tonify qi, transform blood stasis, move qi to resolve depressive heat, and harmonize the second and third trisections.

Appointment #1 Side #1 Pre-Treatment Planning Stage

SIDE #1 PLANNING STEP ONE: ASSESS FOR ASYMMETRY

As CS4 walked to the treatment room, spinal asymmetry was apparent from her uneven gait, which revealed a significant difference in her shoulder and hip alignment. Because scoliosis likely caused her pain, careful assessment and priority was given to the immediate treatment of her spinal alignment with the first set of needles. With moderate to severe scoliosis, optimizing the spinal alignment with acupuncture and essential oils first regulates the ANS and allows for masterful treatment results.

Examination of the spine identified an S-curve pattern with the most significant right-side curve between thoracic vertebrae three to seven (apex at thoracic five) and a mild right-side curve from lumbar vertebrae three to five. The spine had smaller left-side curves between cervical vertebrae six and thoracic vertebrae one, and again between thoracic vertebrae ten to lumbar vertebrae one. GB21, TB15, and SI13 were significantly more tight and painful on the right side.

SIDE #1 PLANNING STEP TWO: REGULATE THE AUTONOMIC NERVOUS SYSTEM

Pressing the outer edge of each curve's peak along the lateral border of the erector spinae muscles inward towards the spine decreased the tightness at GB21, TB15, and SI13 testing locations on the right, and confirmed prone as the optimal treatment position at this appointment.

SIDE #1 PLANNING STEPS THREE, FOUR, AND FIVE: DETERMINE THE BALANCING AND SEDATION OR TONIFICATION PRESCRIPTIONS AND ASSESS THE CORRESPONDING TESTING LOCATIONS

These were skipped during this prone first-side pre-treatment stage and addressed during the supine second-side pre-treatment stage.

SIDE #1 PLANNING STEP SIX: TEST ESSENTIAL OILS

Essential oils were tested in the prone position to apply over the spine before inserting the first set of needles. Based on CS4's concerns about her heart and scoliosis, the Heart, Urinary Bladder, and Governing Vessel Meridian Balancing and Heart Organ Supporting blends were tested individually by resting the bottles on her lumbar vertebrae and checking the right side's master alarm points. Because she was in the prone position, it was acceptable to set the oils on the draping sheet used to cover her lower body. The Urinary Bladder and Governing Vessel Meridian Balancing blends were tested, as they correspond with spinal issues; however, they caused increased tightness in the testing locations. The Heart Meridian Balancing and Organ Supporting blends released the most tension in the master alarm points on the right side when tested together.

SIDE #1 PLANNING STEP SEVEN: CHECK FOR PHLEGM NODULES

There were small, palpable phlegm nodules in the lower back along the right side PSIS. The area felt warm to touch, which indicated pathogenic heat or inflammation on the right side of the lower back.

Appointment #1 Side #1 Treatment Stage

SIDE #1 TREATMENT STEP ONE: APPLY ESSENTIAL OILS

Applied 6 drops each of the Heart Meridian Balancing and Organ Supporting blends directly over the spine since the needling was along the outer border of the erector spinae muscles.

SIDE #1 TREATMENT STEP TWO: REGULATE THE AUTONOMIC NERVOUS SYSTEM

The ANS was regulated by needling along the outermost scoliosis curves on the right and left sides of the spine, and along the right upper border of the PSIS.

On the right side, transverse needles were inserted at the edge of the erector spinae muscles towards the spine at T4, T5, T6, L4, L5, and along the upper border of the PSIS above the nodules.

On the left side, transverse needles were inserted at the edge of the erector spinae muscles towards the spine at C7, T1, T11, and T12. The first set of needles were retained for 10 minutes.

SIDE #1 TREATMENT STEPS THREE AND FOUR: TREAT THE ROOT AND SUPPORT THE ROOT

These were skipped during this prone first-side treatment and addressed during the supine second-side treatment.

SIDE #1 POST-TREATMENT STAGE

This occurred after the supine second-side treatment was completed.

Appointment #1 Side #2 Pre-Treatment Planning Stage

SIDE #2 PLANNING STEP ONE: ASSESS FOR ASYMMETRY

After removing the first set of needles, CS4 turned over into the supine position. The right hip, knee, and ankle were rotated externally with the right foot lying closer to the table. Her neck muscles felt broader, thicker, and tighter on the right lateral side while smaller and weaker on the left lateral side. She had tenderness at CV15 and around the xiphoid process.

SIDE #2 PLANNING STEP TWO: REGULATE THE AUTONOMIC NERVOUS SYSTEM

This was completed during the prone first-side planning steps.

SIDE #2 PLANNING STEPS THREE AND FOUR: DETERMINE THE BALANCING AND SEDATION OR TONIFICATION PRESCRIPTIONS

After the first set of needles, CS4's pulses were reassessed; the PC/TB and LV/GB positions were wiry and excess and indicated a possible root third trisection discord. Based on the health history form, the heart essential oils blends tested, and the excessive pulse positions, the following bilateral exclusive shu-points were tested to the pulse of the right and left wrists to determine each side's root prescription: HT3, LV3, GB34, LU10, LI5, KD3, UB60, PC3, and TB2. The right wrist's pulse positions became slightly slippery to balanced when pressing LV3, the liver balancing prescription, and the tonification prescription on the right side, along with HT3, the heart balancing prescription, and the tonification prescription on the left side. The tension and pain in her master alarm points on the right side also diminished when pressing on these acupoints. The root prescriptions from two different trisections frequently occur with intricate health conditions.

As part of the balancing prescription on the right side, **SP3** was checked and compared to SP5 metal + SP9 water; the metal + water combination tested favorably, as evidenced in the pulse, and indicated pathogenic heat. The left side's root heart deficiency prescription contained no metal + water substitution points to test.

SIDE #2 PLANNING STEP FIVE: ASSESS THE CORRESPONDING TESTING LOCATIONS

The root prescriptions to correct CS4's asymmetry corresponded with the imperial-fire and wood elements. Therefore, the liver, gallbladder, heart, and small intestine testing locations were checked for pain, discomfort, and muscle tightness.

The testing locations with corresponding signs of organ/meridian dysfunction included:

- right rib cage and scapula shared regions with liver- and gallbladder-referred pain
- left scapula heart-referred pain
- bilateral liver-referred discomfort at sternal attachment of pectoralis major muscle
- bilateral gallbladder-referred discomfort in the anterior head of the deltoid muscle
- left small intestine-referred discomfort in quadriceps muscles
- bilateral LV8 organ and LV2 fire alarm points painful
- bilateral GB34 organ alarm points
- bilateral HT3 organ and HT8 fire alarm points painful

SIDE #2 PLANNING STEPS SIX AND SEVEN: TEST ESSENTIAL OILS AND CHECK FOR PHLEGM NODULES

These occurred during the prone first-side planning steps.

Second and Third Trisection Discord

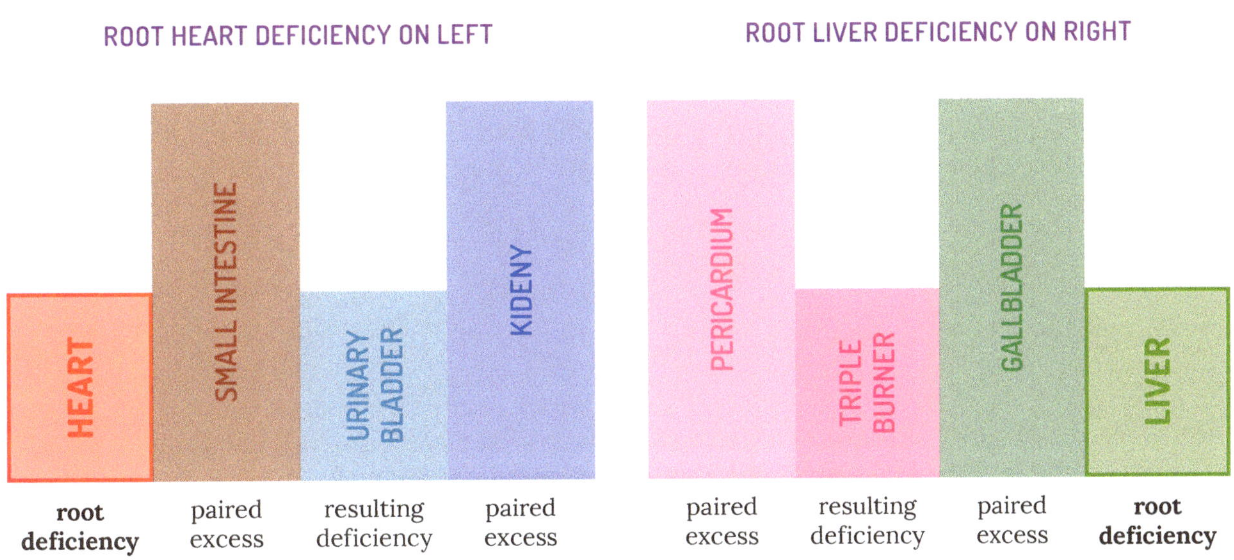

Appointment #1 Side #2 Treatment Stage

SIDE #2 TREATMENT STEP ONE: APPLY ESSENTIAL OILS

CS4 had foot pain and prior foot surgeries. Therefore, 3 drops each of the Heart Meridian Balancing and Organ Supporting blends were also applied to the soles of the feet during the supine second-side treatment.

SIDE #2 TREATMENT STEP TWO: REGULATE THE AUTONOMIC NERVOUS SYSTEM

This occurred during the prone first-side treatment.

SIDE #2 TREATMENT STEP THREE: TREAT THE TWO ROOTS

On the right side, needled the liver balancing and tonification prescriptions LV4, LV3, SP5 + SP9, LU8, KD10, and LV8.

On the left side, needled the heart balancing and tonification prescriptions HT3, HT4, LU8, KD10, LV1, and HT9.

SIDE #2 TREATMENT STEP FOUR: SUPPORT THE ROOT

Both sides' root prescriptions included LU8 metal and KD10 water shu-points. The additional individual metal and water points were checked bilaterally by pressing LU5 water and KD7 metal, which caused the pulse to become more wiry and forceful, indicating these meridians were not affected by pathogenic heat. Testing additional individual water and metal acupoints can occur during the planning stage when checking the acupoint prescriptions or during the support-the-root treatment stage. CS4 required complex root treatments that included a variety of acupoints on both sides; therefore, a minimal number of supporting points were needled during this treatment step.

On the right side, PC6 (controlling point for the yin linking extra-vessel) released additional tension in the corresponding master alarm points.

On the left side, SP4 (controlling point for the penetrating extra-vessel) released additional tension in the corresponding master alarm points.

By needling the controlling and linking points for the paired extra-vessels, these points reconnect the pair and powerfully address the genetic components associated with the heart condition and scoliosis.

Root Heart Tonification Prescription on left

STEP 1: HT3 is the restraining water shu-point on the heart meridian.

STEP 2: HT4 is the restraining metal shu-point on the heart meridian.

STEP 3: LU8 is the yin metal horary shu-point that engenders water.

STEP 4: KD10 is the yin water horary shu-point that restrains imperial-fire.

STEP 5: LV1 is the yin wood horary shu-point that tonifies imperial-fire.

STEP 6: HT9 is the wood shu-point on the heart meridian tonifies imperial-fire.

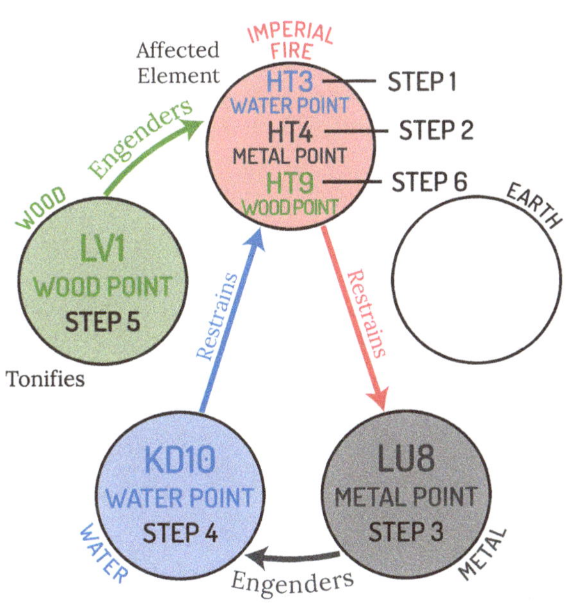

Root Liver Tonification Prescription on right

STEP 1: LV4 is the restraining metal shu-point on the liver meridian.

STEP 2: LV3 is the restraining earth shu-point on the liver meridian.

STEP 3: **SP3** is the yin earth horary shu-point that engenders metal (compare **SP3** to SP5 metal + SP9 water combination for pathogenic heat).

STEP 4: LU8 is the yin metal horary shu-point that restrains wood.

STEP 5: KD10 is the yin water horary shu-point that tonifies wood.

STEP 6: LV8 is the water shu-point on the liver meridian that tonifies wood.

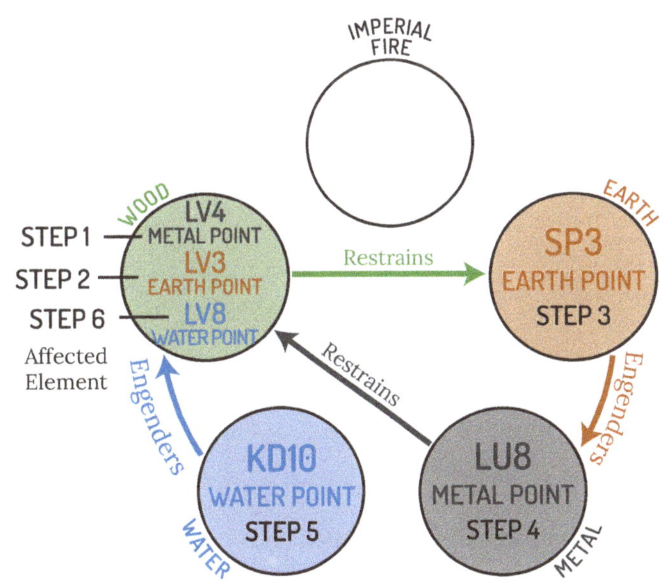

Appointment #1 Post-Treatment Stage

TEST SUPPLEMENTS AND HERBS

CS4 did not bring her supplements with her. The brand of probiotics she was taking is dairy-cultured. Because she has a dairy intolerance, all three types (dairy, yeast, and soil) of cultured probiotics were tested. The dairy- and soil-cultured probiotics caused the neck muscles and master alarm points to become very painful and tight. The yeast-cultured probiotic released tension in the master alarm points on the right side. The supplement inositol supports healthy liver function and the cardiovascular system, and reduces anxiety. An inositol supplement also tested beneficial for the heart-testing locations by releasing pain under the left scapula and reducing pain on the right side of the rib cage in the liver referral area.

TEST ESSENTIAL OILS TO USE BETWEEN APPOINTMENTS

Individual essential oils for pain relief were tested to use between appointments, which included the following: frankincense, copaiba, clove, wintergreen, peppermint, and spearmint. Frankincense and copaiba tested favorably, as evidenced by released tension and tightness in the master alarm points on the right. Frankincense supports the cardiovascular system and relieves discomfort from arthritis. Copaiba has restorative properties that encourage a healthy inflammatory cycle. Both of these oils have harmonizing properties, which will allow their healing benefits to adjust.

CS4 expressed an interest in using rosemary essential oil to address her long-term fungal infection in the thumbnails. The rosemary released tension in the master alarm points on the right by itself and also when tested together with frankincense and copaiba for compatibility.

Recommended taking 1 tablet of inositol with breakfast and dinner.

Recommended taking 2 capsules of yeast-cultured probiotics with dinner or before bed.

Recommended applying a custom roll-on blend of 50% carrier oil, 25% frankincense, and 25% copaiba to any area of pain, including the neck, lower back, and right hip as needed.

Recommended applying 1 drop of rosemary oil directly to the thumbnail and using an organic, fragrance-free lotion as needed.

Recommended follow up appointments weekly for six weeks and then every two weeks until the pain is significantly reduced.

Appointment #2 Follow-up

SUBJECTIVE INFORMATION

CS4 returned for a follow-up appointment after four weeks because of limited scheduling availability. Her right hip had reduced discomfort after applying the essential oils and continued increased pain when sitting in the car. Her right shoulder felt better, and her range of motion during yoga improved. The arthritis pain in hands was lessened with the essential oils. She reduced the amount of Tylenol she had been taking for pain by 50%. She experienced cramping and diarrhea after she ate dried fruit. She had increased diarrhea after starting the probiotic and inositol, and she reduced the probiotic dose in half and felt fine.

OBJECTIVE INFORMATION

Pulse - slightly thin and wiry overall to wiry and forceful in the LV/GB, SP/ST, and PC/TB positions
Tongue - thin glossy coat, pink full body, deep vertical center crack (red speckles no longer apparent)

ASSESSMENT

The multiple trisection discord changed from the first appointment to a single trisection with root prescriptions in the same element. The assessment was updated after the treatment to reflect the changes.
TCM: blood, essence, and qi deficiency, blood stasis, qi stagnation with depressive heat
Body-Feedback: first trisection discord with earth element dysfunction

PLAN

The plan was updated after the treatment to reflect the changes.
Treatment principle: nourish blood and essence, tonify qi, transform blood stasis, move qi to resolve depressive heat, harmonize the first trisection, and optimize the earth element.

Appointment #2 Side #1 Pre-Treatment Planning Stage

SIDE #1 PLANNING STEP ONE: ASSESS FOR ASYMMETRY

CS4 had moderate scoliosis that required months of treatment to result in noticeable structural improvements. Assessing her spine while regulating the ANS with essential oils and needles in the prone treatment position monitored the changes in her spine at most appointments.

Examination of the spine identified a reduction in muscle tightness around the S-curve pattern. The most significant right-side curve was between thoracic vertebrae three and seven (apex at five), and a mild right-side curve at lumbar vertebrae three to five. The spine had smaller left-side curves between cervical vertebrae six and thoracic vertebrae one, and again between thoracic vertebrae ten and lumbar vertebrae one. GB21, TB15, and SI13 on the right were significantly tighter and more painful on the right side.

SIDE #1 PLANNING STEP TWO: REGULATE THE AUTONOMIC NERVOUS SYSTEM

The same treatment approach as at appointment #1 regulated the ANS. Pressing the outer edge of each curve's peak along the lateral border of the erector spinae muscles inward towards the spine decreased the tightness at GB21, TB15, and SI13 testing locations on the right, and confirmed prone as the optimal treatment position at this appointment.

SIDE #1 PLANNING STEPS THREE, FOUR, AND FIVE: DETERMINE THE BALANCING AND SEDATION OR TONIFICATION PRESCRIPTIONS AND ASSESS THE CORRESPONDING TESTING LOCATIONS

These were skipped during this prone first-side and addressed during the supine second-side.

SIDE #1 PLANNING STEP SIX: TEST ESSENTIAL OILS

The Heart Meridian Balancing and Organ Supporting blends were tested again in the same manner as at the first appointment. In the prone position, the bottles of oils were placed in the lower back on the draping sheet used to cover CS4's lower body. The blends were tested individually, and only the Heart Meridian Balancing Blend released the tension in the master alarm points bilaterally.

SIDE #1 PLANNING STEP SEVEN: CHECK FOR PHLEGM NODULES

There were no changes in the small, palpable phlegm nodules in the lower back along the right side PSIS. However, the area felt normal in temperature, which indicated little to no pathogenic heat or inflammation on the right side of the lower back.

Appointment #2 Side #1 Treatment Stage

SIDE #1 TREATMENT STEP ONE: APPLY ESSENTIAL OILS

Applied 12 drops of the Heart Meridian Balancing Blend directly over the spine, as the needling was along the outer border of the erector spinae muscles.

SIDE #1 TREATMENT STEP TWO: REGULATE THE AUTONOMIC NERVOUS SYSTEM

The ANS was regulated by needling along the outermost scoliosis curves on the right and left sides of the spine, and along the right upper border of the PSIS.

On the right side, transverse needles were inserted at the edge of the erector spinae muscles towards the spine at T4, T5, T6, L4, and L5, and along the upper border of the PSIS above the nodules.

On the left side, transverse needles were inserted at the edge of the erector spinae muscles towards the spine at C7, T1, T11, and T12. These needles were retained for 10 minutes.

SIDE #1 TREATMENT STEPS THREE AND FOUR: TREAT THE ROOT AND SUPPORT THE ROOT

These were skipped during this prone first-side treatment and addressed during the supine second-side treatment.

SIDE #1 POST-TREATMENT STAGE

This occurred after the supine second-side treatment was completed.

Appointment #2 Side #2 Pre-Treatment Planning Stage

SIDE #2 PLANNING STEP ONE: ASSESS FOR ASYMMETRY

After removing the first set of needles, CS4 turned over into the supine position. The right hip, knee, and ankle were rotated externally with the right foot lying closer to the table. Her neck muscles (broader, thicker, and tighter on the right lateral side while smaller and weaker on the left lateral side) and tenderness at CV15 were the same as at the first appointment.

SIDE #2 PLANNING STEP TWO: REGULATE THE AUTONOMIC NERVOUS SYSTEM

This was completed during the prone first-side planning steps.

SIDE #2 PLANNING STEPS THREE AND FOUR: DETERMINE THE BALANCING AND SEDATION OR TONIFICATION PRESCRIPTIONS

Based on the last appointment and the most excessive pulse positions at this appointment, the following bilateral exclusive shu-points were tested to the pulse of the right and left wrists to determine each side's root prescription: HT3, LV3, GB34, SP1, ST43, PC3, and TB2. The right wrist's pulse positions became slightly slippery to balanced when pressing ST43, the stomach balancing prescription, and the tonification prescription on the right side. The left wrist's pulse positions became slightly slippery to balanced when pressing SP1, the spleen balancing prescription, and the sedation prescription on the left side. The tension and pain in CS4's master alarm points on the right side also diminished when pressing on these acupoints. The transition from the last appointment's two root prescriptions in different trisections to two root prescriptions within the earth element indicated progress.

The left side's root spleen excess prescription contained no metal + water substitution points to test. On the right side, as part of the balancing prescription, **GB41** was checked and compared to GB44 metal + GB43 water; **GB41** tested favorably, as evidenced in the pulse.

PLANNING STEP FIVE: ASSESS THE CORRESPONDING TESTING LOCATIONS

The spleen and stomach testing locations were checked to correspond with the new root prescriptions. The neck muscles and master alarm points are closely related to the earth element testing locations, and there was a slight reduction in pain, discomfort, and muscle tightness from the last appointment.

The testing locations with corresponding signs of organ/meridian dysfunction included:

- left anterior rib cage spleen-referred pain
- stomach-referred pain along the lineal alba above the umbilicus
- right spleen-referred tightness in the upper trapezius muscle
- left stomach-referred pain and tightness in anterior neck flexor muscles
- right ST36 organ alarm point painful
- bilateral SP9 organ alarm point painful

SIDE #2 PLANNING STEPS SIX AND SEVEN: TEST ESSENTIAL OILS AND CHECK FOR PHLEGM NODULES

These occurred during the prone first-side planning steps.

First Trisection Discord

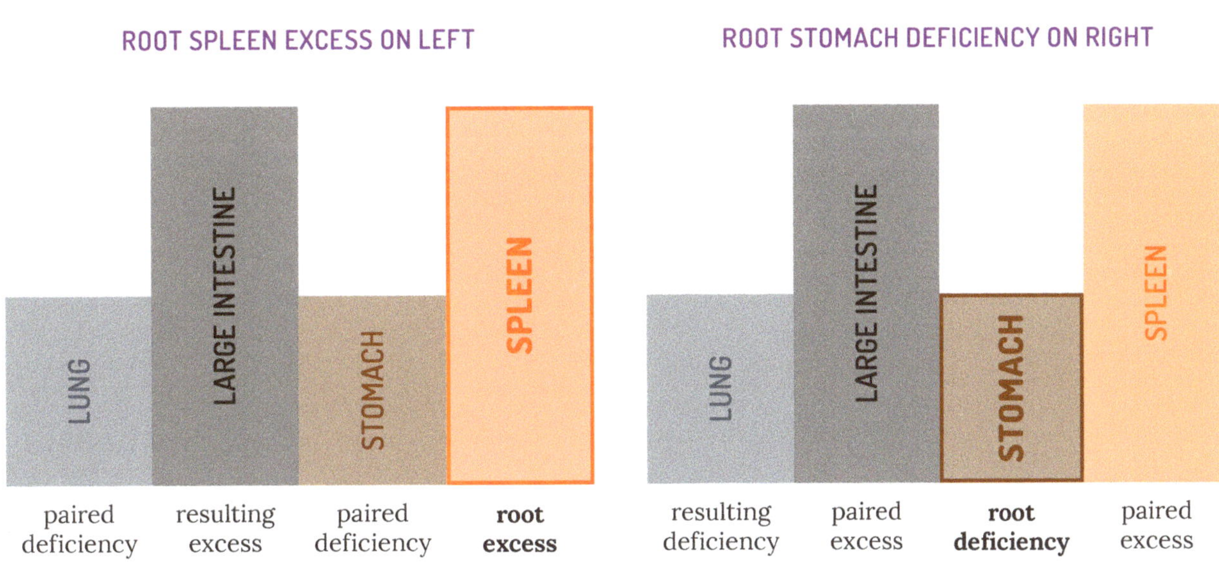

Appointment #2 Side #2 Treatment Stage

SIDE #2 TREATMENT STEP ONE: APPLY ESSENTIAL OILS

Applied 6 drops of the Heart Meridian Balancing Blend to the soles of the feet during the side #2 supine treatment.

SIDE #2 TREATMENT STEP TWO: REGULATE THE AUTONOMIC NERVOUS SYSTEM

This occurred during the prone first-side treatment.

SIDE #2 TREATMENT STEP THREE: TREAT THE TWO ROOTS

On the left side, first needled the spleen balancing and sedation prescriptions SP1, SP9, LV1, KD10, SP5, and LU8.

On the right side, needled the stomach balancing and tonification prescriptions ST43, ST44, UB66, **GB41**, SI5, and ST41.

TREATMENT STEP FOUR: SUPPORT THE ROOT

On the left side, testing the additional individual metal and water points by pressing LU5 water and KD7 metal caused the pulse to become more wiry and forceful, indicating these meridians were not affected by pathogenic heat or inflammation. TB5 (controlling point for the yang linking extra-vessel) and GB40 (yuan-source point) released additional tension in the master alarm points on the left.

On the right side, testing the additional individual UB67 metal point caused the pulse to become more wiry and forceful, indicating this meridian was not affected by pathogenic heat or inflammation. PC6 (controlling point for the yin linking extra-vessel), KD6 (controlling point for the yin heel extra-vessel), LV5 (luo-connecting point), and LI10 (immune system point) released additional tension in the master alarm points on the right.

Root Spleen Sedation Prescription on left

STEP 1: SP1 is the restraining wood shu-point on the spleen meridian.

STEP 2: SP9 is the restraining water shu-point on the spleen meridian.

STEP 3: KD10 is the yin water horary shu-point that engenders wood.

STEP 4: LV1 is the yin wood horary shu-point that restrains earth.

STEP 5: SP5 is the metal shu-point on the spleen meridian that sedates earth.

STEP 6: LU8 is the yin metal horary shu-point that sedates earth.

Root Stomach Tonification Prescription on right

STEP 1: ST43 is the restraining wood shu-point on the stomach meridian.

STEP 2: ST44 is the restraining water shu-point on the stomach meridian.

STEP 3: UB66 is the yang water horary shu-point that engenders wood.

STEP 4: **GB41** is the yang wood horary shu-point that restrains earth (compare **GB41** to GB44 metal + GB43 water combination for pathogenic heat).

STEP 5: SI5 is the yang imperial-fire horary shu-point that tonifies earth.

STEP 6: ST41 is the fire shu-point on the stomach meridian that tonifies earth.

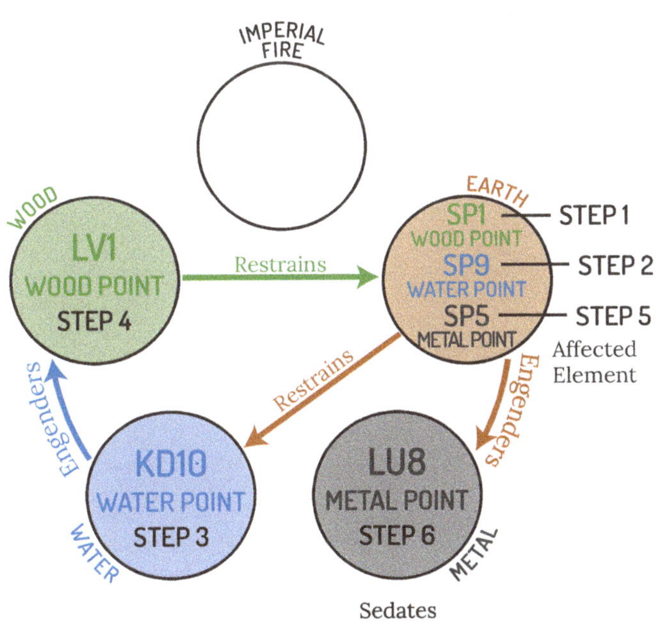

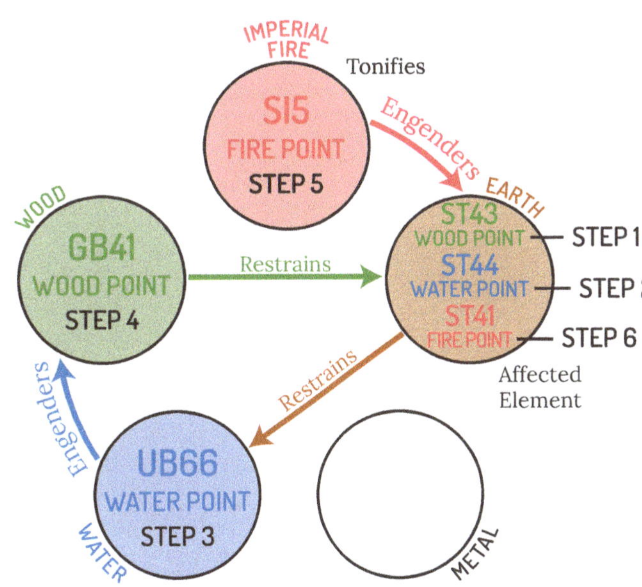

Appointment #2 Post-Treatment Stage

TEST SUPPLEMENTS AND HERBS

Testing the inositol and probiotics released tightness in the neck muscles and master alarm points on the right.

TEST ESSENTIAL OILS TO USE BETWEEN APPOINTMENTS

Testing the roll-on blend containing frankincense and copaiba, along with the rosemary oil, released tension in the neck muscles and tightness in the master alarm points on the right.

Recommended taking 1 capsule of yeast-cultured probiotics with dinner or before bed.

Recommended taking 1 tablet of inositol with breakfast and dinner.

Recommended applying the custom roll-on blend of 50% carrier oil, 25% frankincense, and 25% copaiba to any area of pain, including the neck, lower back, and right hip as needed.

Recommended applying 1 drop of rosemary oil directly to the thumbnail and using an organic, fragrance-free lotion as needed.

Recommended follow-up appointments weekly for six weeks and then every two weeks until the pain is significantly reduced.

Appointments #3 through #6

Weekly treatments for appointments #3, #4, and #5 focused on harmonizing the digestive system and treating the right hip with local ashi acupoints and electrostimulation. The pain in the hands, upper back, neck, and shoulders was significantly reduced. The only lingering pain was in the right lower back and hip after driving. Treatments for appointments #3, #4, and #5 occurred as two-sided. The ANS was regulated by needling the lateral curves of the spine during the first side. The supine side-two set of needles treated the small and large intestine prescriptions. Appointments #3 and #4 treated the small intestine balancing and sedation acupoints on the right, and large intestine balancing and tonification acupoints on the left.

At appointment #5, the small intestine prescription transitioned from sedation to tonification acupoints on the right, and the large intestine balancing and tonification acupoints on the left remained the same. The post-treatment stage of appointment #5 included recommending one-sided posture exercises to address the curvature in the back and seat adjustments to her vehicle. Between appointments #5 and #6, there were significant structural changes in CS4's spinal alignment and reduced pain in the right lower back and hip.

At appointment #6, CS4 had additional muscle soreness resulting from the posture exercises. Therefore, stationary cupping along the tight muscle regions lateral to the scoliosis curves regulated the ANS instead of needles. The root prescriptions and supporting acupoints were determined first using the pulse. On the right, the pericardium balancing and sedation prescriptions tested favorably and influenced her rib cage, shoulder, and hip alignment. On the left, the heart balancing and tonification prescriptions influenced her sacroiliac joint and alignment of pelvis and jaw.

A combination of stationary and sliding cupping regulated the ANS first. Gentle sliding cupping released general muscle soreness and tightness. Stationary cups released the tightest muscles along the apex of spinal curves for the duration of the appointment. Needling the pericardium sedation prescription on the right (PC3, PC5, LU8, KD10, PC7, and **SP3**) occurred first. Next, the heart deficiency prescription on the left (HT3, HT4, LU8, KD10, LV1, and HT9) was needled. The supporting acupoints included GB25 and L5 ashi on the right side, and SP4, T11, T12, and sacrum ashi on the left side.

Appointment #7 Follow-up

CS4 transitioned to one-sided treatments for most sessions going forward. She also began testing favorably for the supine treatment position, as evidenced by the master alarm points relaxing when pressing down on the abdomen for treatments #7 and #8. The shift from prone and two-sided treatments to supine one-sided indicated substantial progress in resolving the asymmetry in her meridian system and reducing the scoliosis pain.

SUBJECTIVE INFORMATION

CS4 returned for another follow-up appointment three weeks later. Her hip pain was much better except when sitting in the car for extended periods. She felt an overall positive change, was sleeping more comfortably, and was able to walk longer distances. Her digestion was healthier; she tolerated more foods without discomfort, and her food allergy symptoms were less intense and resolved faster. CS4 asked for a referral to a gentle chiropractor to further help with the spinal alignment.

OBJECTIVE INFORMATION

Pulse - overall slightly wiry, forceful, and balanced in all positions
Tongue - thin glossy coat, pink full body, deep vertical center crack (red speckles no longer apparent)

ASSESSMENT

The trisection discord and root element dysfunction changed from the last appointment. CS4's symptoms of blood stasis and qi stagnation (pain in multiple sites) was almost completely resolved and there were no metal + water combinations needed at this appointment. The assessment was updated after the treatment to reflect these changes.
TCM: blood, essence, and qi deficiency
Body-Feedback: third trisection discord with wood element dysfunction

PLAN

The plan was updated after the treatment to reflect the changes.
Treatment principle: nourish blood and essence, tonify qi, harmonize the third trisection, and optimize the wood element.

Appointment #7 Pre-Treatment Planning Stage

PLANNING STEP ONE: ASSESS FOR ASYMMETRY

CS4's right hip, knee, and ankle had a slight external rotation with the right foot lying closer to the table. Her neck muscles felt broader, thicker, and tighter on the right lateral side while slightly smaller on the left lateral side. The discomfort upon palpation at CV15 was reduced.

PLANNING STEP TWO: REGULATE THE AUTONOMIC NERVOUS SYSTEM

For the first time, checking the abdomen showed a decreased in the tightness at TB15, SI13, and GB21 on the right and indicated supine as the optimal treatment position at this appointment.

PLANNING STEPS THREE AND FOUR: DETERMINE THE BALANCING AND SEDATION OR TONIFICATION PRESCRIPTIONS

Since the root point prescriptions changed at most appointments, and her pulse was balanced, the common meridians treated in the past were checked. The following bilateral exclusive shu-points were tested to the right and left wrist's pulse to determine each side's root prescription: LV3, GB34, SP1, ST43, HT3, and PC3. The right wrist's pulse positions became slightly slippery to balanced when pressing GB34, the gallbladder balancing prescription, and the tonification prescription on the right side, along with LV3, the liver balancing prescription, and the tonification prescription on the left side. The tension and pain in her master alarm points on the right side also diminished when pressing on these acupoints.

As part of the balancing prescription on the right side, **ST36** was checked and compared to ST45 metal + ST44 water; **ST36** tested favorably, as evidenced in the pulse. As part of the balancing prescription on the left, **SP3** was checked and compared to SP5 metal + SP9 water; **SP3** tested favorably, as evidenced in the pulse. There were no signs of pathogenic heat at this appointment.

PLANNING STEP FIVE: ASSESS THE CORRESPONDING TESTING LOCATIONS

The root prescriptions to correct CS4's asymmetry corresponded with the wood element. Therefore, the liver and gallbladder testing locations were checked for pain, discomfort, and muscle tightness.

The testing locations with corresponding signs of organ/meridian dysfunction included:

- right rib cage and scapula shared regions with combined liver- and gallbladder-referred pain
- bilateral liver-referred discomfort at the sternal attachment of pectoralis major muscle
- bilateral gallbladder-referred discomfort in the anterior head of the deltoid muscle
- bilateral LV8 organ and LV2 fire alarm points tender
- left GB34 organ alarm points tender

PLANNING STEP SIX: TEST ESSENTIAL OILS

The Liver and Gallbladder Organ Supporting and Meridian Balancing blends were tested individually by resting the bottle on the draping cloth on her upper abdomen. Only the Gallbladder Organ Supporting blend released tightness in the master alarm points on the right. Copaiba tested favorably, both individually and when added to the Gallbladder Organ Supporting blend.

PLANNING STEP SEVEN: CHECK FOR PHLEGM NODULES

Because there was a steady improvement in the phlegm nodules, they were not checked at this appointment with CS4 in the supine position.

Third Trisection Discord

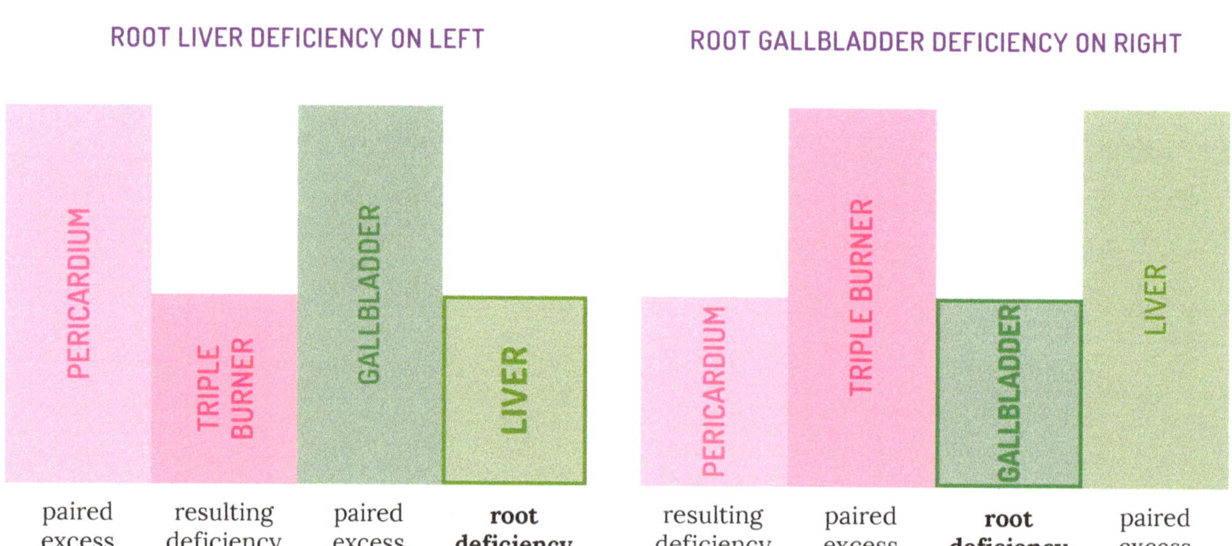

Appointment #7 Treatment Stage

TREATMENT STEP ONE: APPLY ESSENTIAL OILS

Applied 4 drops of the Gallbladder Organ Supporting blend plus 2 drops of copaiba to the sole of each foot.

TREATMENT STEP TWO: REGULATE THE AUTONOMIC NERVOUS SYSTEM

Pressing on the scalp motor-sensory area released tension in the neck muscles and at the master alarm points better than at the abdominal points. Needling 4 acupoints anterior to the scalp-motor-line on the right and 4 acupoints posterior to the scalp-sensory-line on the left regulated the ANS, as evidenced by the release in muscle tightness in the master alarm points bilaterally.

TREATMENT STEP THREE: TREAT THE ROOT

On the right side, needled the gallbladder balancing and tonification prescriptions GB44, GB34, **ST36**, LI1, UB66, and GB43.

On the left side, needled the liver balancing and tonification prescriptions LV4, LV3, **SP3**, LU8, KD10, and LV8.

TREATMENT STEP FOUR: SUPPORT THE ROOT

On the right, the additional individual water shu-point was checked by pressing on LI2, which caused the pulse to become more wiry and forceful. The supporting acupoints needled included TB5 (controlling point for the yang linking extra-vessel), KD9 (xi-cleft point for the yin linking vessel), ST37 (large intestine lower he-sea), and ST39 (small intestine lower he-sea).

On the left, the additional individual metal and water points were checked by pressing LU5 water and KD7 metal, which caused the pulse to become more wiry and forceful. The supporting acupoints needled included PC6 (controlling point for the yin linking extra-vessel) and SP10 (blood nourishing).

Root Liver Tonification Prescription on left

STEP 1: LV4 is the restraining metal shu-point on the liver meridian.

STEP 2: LV3 is the restraining earth shu-point on the liver meridian.

STEP 3: **SP3** is the yin earth horary shu-point that engenders metal (compare **SP3** to SP5 metal + SP9 water combination for pathogenic heat).

STEP 4: LU8 is the yin metal horary shu-point that restrains wood.

STEP 5: KD10 is the yin water horary shu-point that tonifies wood.

STEP 6: LV8 is the water shu-point on the liver meridian that tonifies wood.

Root Gallbladder Tonification Prescription on right

STEP 1: GB44 is the restraining metal shu-point on the gallbladder meridian.

STEP 2: GB34 is the restraining earth shu-point on the gallbladder meridian.

STEP 3: **ST36** is the yang earth horary shu-point that engenders metal (compare **ST36** to ST45 metal + ST44 water combination for pathogenic heat).

STEP 4: LI1 is the yang metal horary shu-point that restrains the wood element.

STEP 5: UB66 is the yang water horary shu-point that tonifies wood.

STEP 6: GB43 is the water shu-point on the gallbladder meridian that tonifies wood.

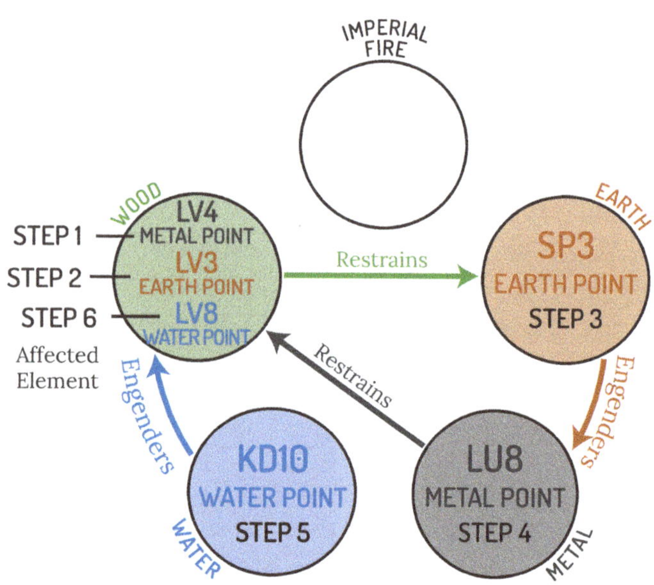

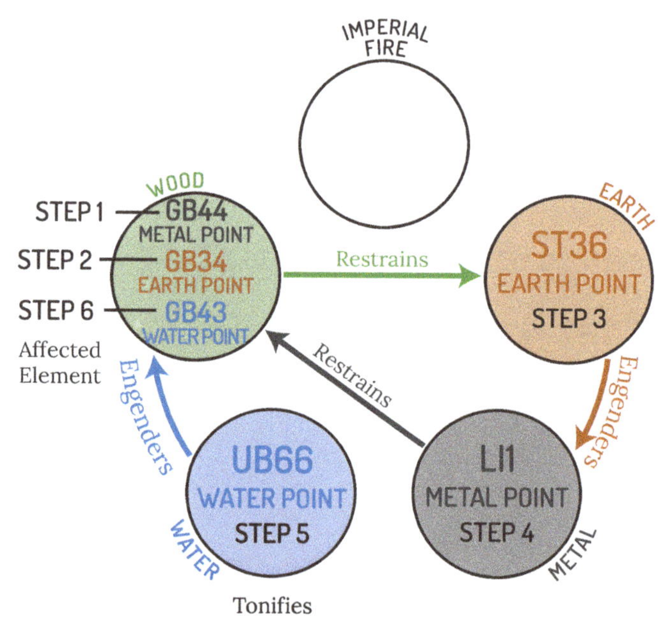

Appointment #7 Post-Treatment Stage

TEST SUPPLEMENTS AND HERBS

CS4 requested that I check calcium, magnesium, and vitamin D supplements for her. GB21, TB15, and SI13 on the right relaxed by placing the multi-mineral complex with iodine (compared to one without iodine) and the vitamin D with K (compared to one without K) on the upper abdomen. The beneficial supplements were combined with the inositol and probiotics to check for compatibility; together, they released tightness in the neck muscles and master alarm points on the right.

TEST ESSENTIAL OILS TO USE BETWEEN APPOINTMENTS

Balsam fir essential oil was checked and released tightness in the neck muscles, GB21, TB15, and SI13 on the right. Balsam fir supplies additional raw materials to encourage tissue regeneration, and it was added to the existing roll-on blend containing frankincense and copaiba. The combination of oils, along with the rosemary oil, released tension in the neck muscles and tightness in the master alarm points on the right.

Recommended taking 3 capsules of the multi-mineral complex with breakfast.

Recommended taking 1 capsule of vitamin D with K with breakfast.

Recommended taking 1 tablet of inositol with breakfast and dinner.

Recommended taking 1 capsule of yeast-cultured probiotics with dinner or before bed.

Recommended applying a custom roll-on blend of 40% carrier oil, 20% balsam fir, 20% frankincense, and 20% copaiba to any area of pain, including the neck, lower back, and right hip as needed.

Recommended applying 1 drop of rosemary oil directly to the thumbnail and using an organic, fragrance-free lotion as needed.

Appointment #8 Follow-up

CS4 returned for appointment #8 three weeks later with mild sinus congestion after an upper respiratory infection. The supine treatment position regulated the ANS and included LI20, ST7, and GV23. The root treatments were large intestine deficiency on the left and stomach deficiency on the right (yang-ming pair). The essential oils used in the treatment were the Stomach and Large Intestine Meridian Balancing Blends.

Appointment #9 Follow-up

SUBJECTIVE INFORMATION

CS4 returned for another follow-up appointment three weeks later. She began chiropractic treatments and noticed her body symmetry was better. Her pain and digestive symptoms continued to improve steadily. At this appointment, her hip and back were very sore from an adjustment a few days prior.

OBJECTIVE INFORMATION

Pulse - overall slightly wiry and forceful in the LU/LI, SP/ST, and LV/GB positions
Tongue - thin glossy coat, pink full body, deep vertical center crack (red speckles no longer apparent)

ASSESSMENT

The assessment remained the same as at the seventh and for all subsequent appointments.
TCM: blood, essence, and qi deficiency
Body-Feedback: third trisection discord with wood element dysfunction

PLAN

The plan remained the same as at the seventh and for all subsequent appointments.
Treatment principle: nourish blood and essence, tonify qi, harmonize the third trisection, and optimize the wood element.

Appointment #9 Pre-Treatment Planning Stage

PLANNING STEP ONE: ASSESS FOR ASYMMETRY

CS4's right hip, knee, and ankle had a slight external rotation with the right foot lying closer to the table. Her neck muscles felt broader, thicker, and tighter on the right lateral side while slightly smaller on the left lateral side. The discomfort upon palpation at CV15 was reduced.

PLANNING STEP TWO: REGULATE THE AUTONOMIC NERVOUS SYSTEM

Checking the outer edge of each curve's peak along the lateral border of the erector spinae muscles inward towards the spine decreased the tightness at GB21, TB15, and SI13 on the right, and confirmed prone as the optimal treatment position at this appointment.

PLANNING STEPS THREE AND FOUR: DETERMINE THE BALANCING AND SEDATION OR TONIFICATION PRESCRIPTIONS

Based on the excess pulse positions, the following bilateral exclusive shu-points were tested to the pulse of the right and left wrists to determine each side's root prescription: LU10, LI5, SP1, ST43, LV3, and GB34. The right wrist's pulse positions became slightly slippery to balanced when pressing LI5, the large intestine balancing prescription, and the tonification prescription on the right side, along with LV3, the liver balancing prescription, and the tonification prescription on the left side. The tension and pain in her master alarm points on the right side also diminished when pressing on these acupoints.

As part of the balancing prescription on the right, **ST36** was checked and compared to ST45 metal + ST44 water; **ST36** tested favorably, as evidenced in the pulse. **GB41** was checked and compared to GB44 metal + GB43 water; the metal + water combination tested favorably, as evidenced in the pulse. As part of the balancing prescription on the left side, **SP3** was checked and compared to SP5 metal + SP9 water; the metal + water combination tested favorably, as evidenced in the pulse. There were increased signs of pathogenic heat and inflammation at this appointment.

PLANNING STEP FIVE: ASSESS THE CORRESPONDING TESTING LOCATIONS

The root prescriptions to correct CS4's asymmetry corresponded with the metal and wood elements. Therefore, the liver, gallbladder, lung, and large intestine testing locations were checked for pain, discomfort, and muscle tightness.

The testing locations with corresponding signs of organ/meridian dysfunction included:

- right rib cage and scapula shared regions with combined liver- and gallbladder-referred pain
- bilateral liver-referred discomfort in the at sternal attachment of pectoralis major muscle
- bilateral gallbladder-referred discomfort in the anterior head of the deltoid muscle
- right large intestine-referred discomfort in quadratus lumborum muscle
- bilateral LV8 organ and LV2 fire alarm points tender
- left GB34 organ alarm points tender
- right LI11 organ and LI5 meridian alarm points tender

PLANNING STEP SIX: TEST ESSENTIAL OILS

Because CS4 had increased pain in the right hip and lower back, the custom-blended oils were checked by resting the combination of bottles on the draping cloth on her lower back. The combination of the balsam fir, frankincense, and copaiba released the tension in the quadratus lumborum muscle and iliotibial band on the right side.

PLANNING STEP SEVEN: CHECK FOR PHLEGM NODULES

The palpable phlegm nodules on the right side of the PSIS were slightly enlarged and felt warm to the touch, which indicated recent inflammation.

First and Third Trisection Discords

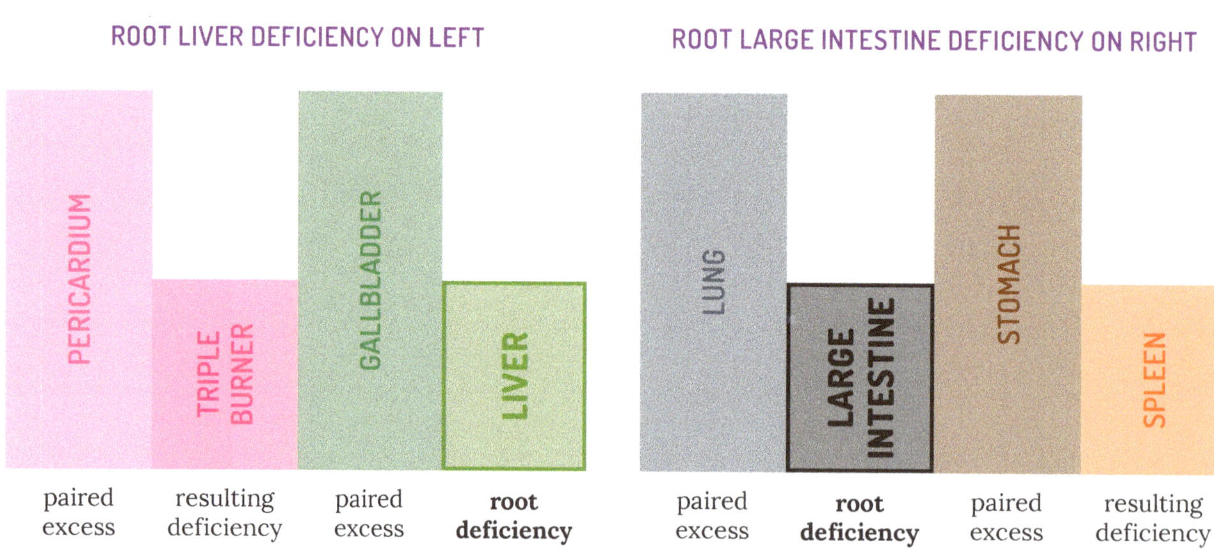

Appointment #9 Treatment Stage

The back acupoints were needled first in the prone position since CS4 was experiencing increased back and hip pain, and the root prescription's acupoints were easier to needle in the supine position. After removing the first set of needles, the root prescriptions and supporting acupoints were inserted in the supine position.

TREATMENT STEP ONE: APPLY ESSENTIAL OILS

Applied 6 drops each of balsam fir, frankincense, and copaiba directly over the spine and along the upper border of the PSIS on the right side.

TREATMENT STEP TWO: REGULATE THE AUTONOMIC NERVOUS SYSTEM

Each spinous process level was pressed, starting with L5 and then up the spine. The ANS was regulated by needling L5 ashi, around the posterior border of the greater trochanter (where multiple muscle groups attach at the hip socket), and directly below and lateral to the spinous processes of L5, L4, T9, T8, and T7 on the right, along with sacrum ashi and directly below and lateral to the spinous processes of C7, C6, C5, and C4 on the left. These back acupoints were significantly different from the previous treatments, which indicated a positive structural change had occurred. The back acupoints were retained for 15 minutes.

TREATMENT STEP THREE: TREAT THE ROOT

CS4 turned over into the supine position for the root treatments.

On the right side, needled the large intestine balancing and tonification prescriptions LI5, LI3, GB44 + GB34, SI5, **ST36**, and LI11.

On the left side, needled the liver balancing and tonification prescriptions LV4, LV3, SP5 + SP9, LU8, KD10, and LV8.

TREATMENT STEP FOUR: SUPPORT THE ROOT

No additional acupoints were added to support the root. The additional individual LU5 water and KD7 metal shu-points were pressed and caused the pulse to become more wiry and forceful. The extensive back treatment addressed the local areas of pain as supporting points.

Root Liver Tonification Prescription on left

STEP 1: LV4 is the restraining metal shu-point on the liver meridian.

STEP 2: LV3 is the restraining earth shu-point on the liver meridian.

STEP 3: **SP3** is the yin earth horary shu-point that engenders metal (compare **SP3** to SP5 metal + SP9 water combination for pathogenic heat).

STEP 4: LU8 is the yin metal horary shu-point that restrains wood.

STEP 5: KD10 is the yin water horary shu-point that tonifies wood.

STEP 6: LV8 is the water shu-point on the liver meridian that tonifies wood.

Root Large Intestine Tonification Prescription on right

STEP 1: LI5 is the restraining fire shu-point on the large intestine meridian.

STEP 2: LI3 is the restraining wood shu-point on the large intestine meridian.

STEP 3: **GB41** is the yang wood horary shu-point that engenders fire (compare **GB41** to GB44 metal + GB43 water combination for pathogenic heat).

STEP 4: SI5 is the yang imperial-fire horary shu-point that restrains metal.

STEP 5: **ST36** is the yang earth horary shu-point that tonifies metal (compare **ST36** to ST45 metal + ST44 water combination for pathogenic heat).

STEP 6: LI11 is the earth shu-point on the large intestine meridian that tonifies metal.

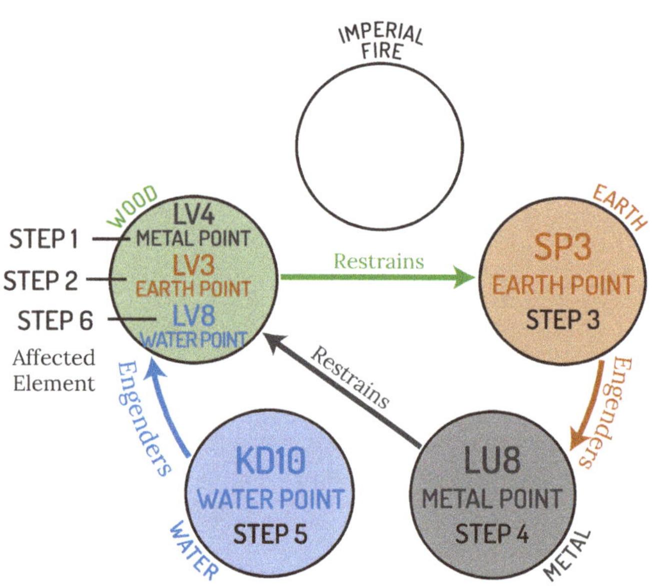

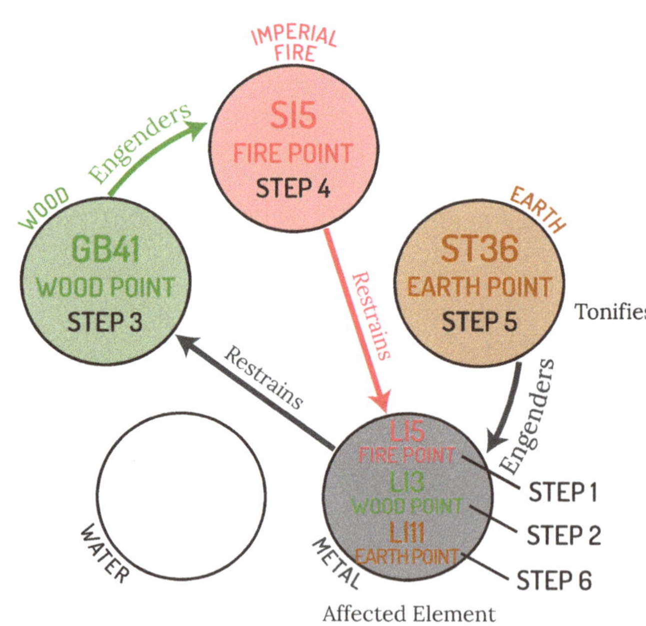

Appointment #9 Post-Treatment Stage

TEST SUPPLEMENTS AND HERBS

No supplements were tested at this appointment.

TEST ESSENTIAL OILS TO USE BETWEEN APPOINTMENTS

No additional essential oils were tested at this appointment.

Recommended taking 3 capsules of the multi-mineral complex with breakfast.

Recommended taking 1 capsule of vitamin D with K with breakfast.

Recommended taking 1 tablet of inositol with breakfast and dinner.

Recommended taking 1 capsule of yeast-cultured probiotics with dinner or before bed.

Recommended applying a custom roll-on blend of 40% carrier oil, 20% balsam fir, 20% frankincense, and 20% copaiba to any area of pain, including the neck, lower back, and right hip as needed.

Recommended applying 1 drop of rosemary oil directly to the thumbnail and using an organic, fragrance-free lotion as needed.

Appointment #10 and #11 Follow-ups

At appointment #10, CS4 had increased digestive and food allergy symptoms, and she received an asymmetrical supine wood element treatment. At appointment #11, CS4 received her first of many symmetrical and supine treatments with the gallbladder or liver as the root treatment the majority of the time. When CS4 traveled, and during the holidays, she often required a root large intestine tonification treatment.

CS4 Conclusion Summary

At appointment #1, there was a relationship between the root liver and heart deficiencies, causing the multiple trisection discord. The third trisection's root liver deficiency caused the gallbladder and pericardium to become excess. According to the twenty-four-hour organ clock, gallbladder excess can negatively affect the organ opposite it, which can induce heart organ/meridian deficiency. The heart corresponds with thoracic vertebrae five, which was the apex of CS4's most pronounced scoliosis curve, and likely related to her heart defect (either resulting from it or caused by it). The combination of the paired gallbladder excess and root heart deficiency pattern may have been a predominant factor that predisposed CS4 to a stroke (internal liver-wind) as a result of her heart defect.

The extra-vessels have a strong influence on scoliosis and asymmetry. CS4's first appointment included the controlling points for the yin linking extra-vessel on the right (PC6) and the penetrating vessel on the left (SP4), which strengthened their paired relationship to reunite the left and right sides of the body. The second appointment incorporated several controlling points for the extra-vessels: yang linking (TB5) on the left side, and yin linking (PC6) and yin heel (KD6) on the right side. Treating these acupoints during the early appointments assisted her body to resolve the meridian asymmetry.

CS4 has had a healthy diet and lifestyle that contributed to her rapid progress and ability to reduce the scoliosis curvature. Her healing journey (represented by the natural progression of healing) started with the wood and imperial-fire elements at the first appointment. At appointment #2, she progressed to the next weakest element, earth. The root spleen excess on the left and stomach deficiency on the right (extreme dysfunction within the same element) could have resulted from complex or long-standing symptoms.

Appointments #3 through #6 focused on harmonizing the immune and digestive systems to address the food allergies and intolerances, which affected the first and second trisections. The large intestine deficiency (first trisection) may have resulted in small intestine excess (second trisection), or vice versa. The underlying heart deficiency predisposed the small intestine to excess pathology.

Appointment #7 was the first time CS4's constitutional or genetic wood element dysfunction was the focus of the treatment. However, at that time, this inherent wood element weakness was unknown due to the recent positive structural changes, immune dysfunction, and digestive symptoms, which caused her root prescriptions to change frequently. Her wood element dysfunction likely caused the first trisection organ dysfunction affecting the immune and digestive systems, according to the twelve earthly branches.

Beginning with appointment #9, one of the root prescriptions treated at each session usually included the liver or gallbladder (wood element). Beginning with appointment #11, CS4 transitioned to symmetrical supine treatments that rotated between the liver and gallbladder, along with sedation and tonification the majority of the time. Choline was incorporated to support the liver and gallbladder organs directly. CS4 understood that this transition to symmetry in the meridian system represented significant improvements in health, and her spinal alignment improved dramatically. The positive benefits of these structural changes will be substantial as CS4 continues to age and will change the course of her life for the better.

APPENDIX 1

Master Summary Worksheet

FIRST TRISECTION	LUNG	LARGE INTESTINE	STOMACH	SPLEEN
Muscle Associations	Serratus anterior Deltoids Coracobrachialis	Iliotibial band Hamstrings Quadratus lumborum	Pectoralis-clavicle Neck flexors Brachioradialis	Latisimus dorsi Upper trapezius Triceps
Organ Referral	Below lateral end of clavicle bone	Lower right abdomen	Lineal alba above umbilicus	Left lower rib cage
Meridian balancing Points	LU10 FIRE LU11 WOOD LV1 WOOD **HT8 FIRE (HT4+HT3)**	LI5 FIRE LI3 WOOD **GB41 WOOD (GB44+GB43)** SI5 FIRE	ST43 WOOD ST44 WATER UB66 WATER **GB41 WOOD (GB44+GB43)**	SP1 WOOD SP9 WATER LV1 WOOD KD10 WATER
Sedation points	LU5 WATER KD10 WATER	LI2 WATER UB66 WATER	ST45 METAL LI1 METAL	SP5 METAL LU8 METAL
Tonification points	**SP3 EARTH (SP5+SP9)** LU9 EARTH	**ST36 EARTH (ST45+ST44)** LI11 EARTH	SI5 FIRE ST41 FIRE	**HT8 FIRE (HT4+HT3)** SP2 FIRE

SECOND TRISECTION	HEART	SMALL INTESTINE	URINARY BLADDER	KIDNEY
Muscle Associations	Subscapularis	Quadriceps Abdominals	Peroneus Erector spinae	Psoas
Organ Referral	Left shoulder blade	Ribcage-abdominal attachment	Above pubic bone	Mid to low back/ inner thigh
Meridian balancing Points	HT3 WATER HT4 METAL LU8 METAL KD10 WATER	SI2 WATER SI1 METAL LI1 METAL UB66 WATER	UB40 EARTH UB60 FIRE SI5 FIRE **ST36 EARTH (ST45+ST44)**	KD3 EARTH KD2 FIRE **HT8 FIRE (HT4+HT3)** **SP3 EARTH (SP5+SP9)**
Sedation points	HT7 EARTH **SP3 EARTH (SP5+SP9)**	SI8 EARTH **ST36 EARTH (ST45+ST44)**	UB65 WOOD **GB41 WOOD (GB44+GB43)**	KD1 WOOD LV1 WOOD
Tonification points	LV1 WOOD HT9 WOOD	**GB41 WOOD (GB44+GB43)** SI3 WOOD	LI1 METAL UB67 METAL	LU8 METAL KD7 METAL

THIRD TRISECTION	PERICARDIUM	TRIPLE BURNER	GALLBLADDER	LIVER
Muscle Associations	Gluteus medius Piriformis	Teres minor	Anterior deltoid Fascial adhesions	Pectoralis-Sternal attachment
Organ Referral	Diaphragm and entire rib cage	Side line of torso	Right side of lower edge of rib cage	Right side of front of rib cage
Meridian balancing Points	PC3 WATER PC5 METAL LU8 METAL KD10 WATER	TB2 WATER TB1 METAL ST45 METAL UB66 WATER	GB44 METAL GB34 EARTH **ST36 EARTH (ST45+ST44)** LI1 METAL	LV4 METAL LV3 EARTH **SP3 EARTH (SP5+SP9)** LU8 METAL
Sedation points	PC7 EARTH **SP3 EARTH (SP5+SP9)**	TB10 EARTH **ST36 EARTH (ST45+ST44)**	GB38 FIRE SI5 FIRE	LV2 FIRE **HT8 FIRE (HT4+HT3)**
Tonification points	LV1 WOOD PC9 WOOD	**GB41 WOOD (GB44+GB43)** TB3 WOOD	UB66 WATER GB43 WATER	KD10 WATER LV8 WATER

APPENDIX 2

Body-Feedback Point Prescriptions with Supporting Options

LUNG

LUNG BALANCING: LU10, LU11, LV1, **HT8** (compare HT4 metal + HT3 water)

LUNG SEDATION: LU5, KD10

OPTIONAL SEDATION SUPPORT: KD7, SP4, TB5, UB62, ST34, GB40

LUNG TONIFICATION: **SP3** (compare SP5 metal + SP9 water), LU9

OPTIONAL TONIFICATION SUPPORT: KD6, UB62, TB5, KD8, KD9, TB8, GB40

LARGE INTESTINE

LARGE INTESTINE BALANCING: LI5, LI3, **GB41** (compare GB44 metal + GB43 water), SI5 Large intestine sedation: LI2, UB66

OPTIONAL SEDATION SUPPORT: UB67, PC6, SP4, TB5, KD9, LV5, ST40

LARGE INTESTINE TONIFICATION: **ST36** (compare ST45 metal + ST44 water), LI11

OPTIONAL TONIFICATION SUPPORT: KD6, SP4, UB62, KD9, LV5, PC6, SP6

STOMACH

STOMACH BALANCING: ST43, ST44, UB66, **GB41** (compare GB44 metal + GB43 water)

STOMACH SEDATION: ST45, LI1

OPTIONAL SEDATION SUPPORT: UB67, LI2, KD6, LU7, PC6, TB5, LV5

STOMACH TONIFICATION: SI5, ST41

OPTIONAL TONIFICATION SUPPORT: UB67, KD6, PC6, TB5, LV5, LI4

SPLEEN

SPLEEN BALANCING: SP1, SP9, LV1, KD10

SPLEEN SEDATION: SP5, LU8

OPTIONAL SEDATION SUPPORT: LU5, KD7, PC6, TB5, UB62, GB40

SPLEEN TONIFICATION: **HT8** (compare HT4 metal + HT3 water), SP2

OPTIONAL TONIFICATION SUPPORT: KD7, LU7, TB5, UB62, LI4, GB40

HEART

HEART BALANCING: HT3, HT4, LU8, KD10

HEART SEDATION: HT7, **SP3** (compare SP5 metal + SP9 water)

OPTIONAL SEDATION SUPPORT: KD7, LU5, TB5, UB62, GB40

HEART TONIFICATION: LV1, HT9

OPTIONAL TONIFICATION SUPPORT: KD7, LU5, SP4, TB5, UB62, GB39

SMALL INTESTINE

SMALL INTESTINE BALANCING: SI2, SI1, LI1, UB66

SMALL INTESTINE SEDATION: SI8, **ST36** (compare ST45 metal + ST44 water)

OPTIONAL SEDATION SUPPORT: UB67, LI2, KD6, LU7, SP4, KD9

SMALL INTESTINE TONIFICATION: **GB41** (compare GB44 metal + GB43 water), SI3

OPTIONAL TONIFICATION SUPPORT: UB67, LI2, KD6, LU7, SP4, KD8

URINARY BLADDER

URINARY BLADDER BALANCING: UB40, UB60, SI5, **ST36** (compare ST45 metal + ST44 water)

URINARY BLADDER SEDATION: UB65, **GB41** (compare GB44 metal + GB43 water)

OPTIONAL SEDATION SUPPORT: LU7, PC6, TB5, LI4, LV5, SP4, SP6

URINARY BLADDER TONIFICATION: LI1, UB67

OPTIONAL TONIFICATION SUPPORT: LI2, LU7, PC6, SP4, TB5, SP6, SP8

KIDNEY

KIDNEY BALANCING: KD3, KD2, **HT8** (compare HT4 metal + HT3 water), **SP3** (compare SP5 metal + SP9 water)

KIDNEY SEDATION: KD1, LV1

OPTIONAL SEDATION SUPPORT: LU7, TB5, UB62, SI6, ST40, GB35

KIDNEY TONIFICATION: LU8, KD7

OPTIONAL TONIFICATION SUPPORT: LU5, TB5, SI7, GB37

PERICARDIUM

PERICARDIUM BALANCING: PC3, PC5, LU8, KD10

PERICARDIUM SEDATION: PC7, **SP3** (compare SP5 metal + SP9 water)

OPTIONAL SEDATION SUPPORT: KD7, LU5, UB62, GB40

PERICARDIUM TONIFICATION: LV1, PC9

OPTIONAL TONIFICATION SUPPORT: KD7, LU5, SP4, UB62, GB39

TRIPLE BURNER

TRIPLE BURNER BALANCING: TB2, TB1, ST45, UB66

TRIPLE BURNER SEDATION: TB10, **ST36** (compare ST45 metal + ST44 water)

OPTIONAL SEDATION SUPPORT: ST44, UB67, KD6, LU7, SP4, KD4

TRIPLE BURNER TONIFICATION: **GB41** (compare GB44 metal + GB43 water), TB3

OPTIONAL TONIFICATION SUPPORT: ST44, UB67, KD6, LU7, SP4, SP8

GALLBLADDER

GALLBLADDER BALANCING: GB44, GB34, **ST36** (compare ST45 metal + ST44 water), LI1

GALLBLADDER SEDATION: GB38, SI5

OPTIONAL SEDATION SUPPORT: LI2, KD6, LU7, PC6, SP4, TB5, UB62, KD9, SP6

GALLBLADDER TONIFICATION: UB66, GB43

OPTIONAL TONIFICATION SUPPORT: UB67, LI2, KD6, LU7, PC6, SP4, TB5, SP6

LIVER

LIVER BALANCING: LV4, LV3, **SP3** (compare SP5 metal + SP9 water), LU8

LIVER SEDATION: LV2, **HT8** (compare HT4 metal + HT3 water)

OPTIONAL SEDATION SUPPORT: LU5, KD6, TB5, UB62, KD9, LI4

LIVER TONIFICATION: KD10, LV8

OPTIONAL TONIFICATION SUPPORT: LU5, KD7, PC6, TB5, UB62, PC4

APPENDIX 3

Master Point Locations Charts

LATERAL SIDE OF FOREARM

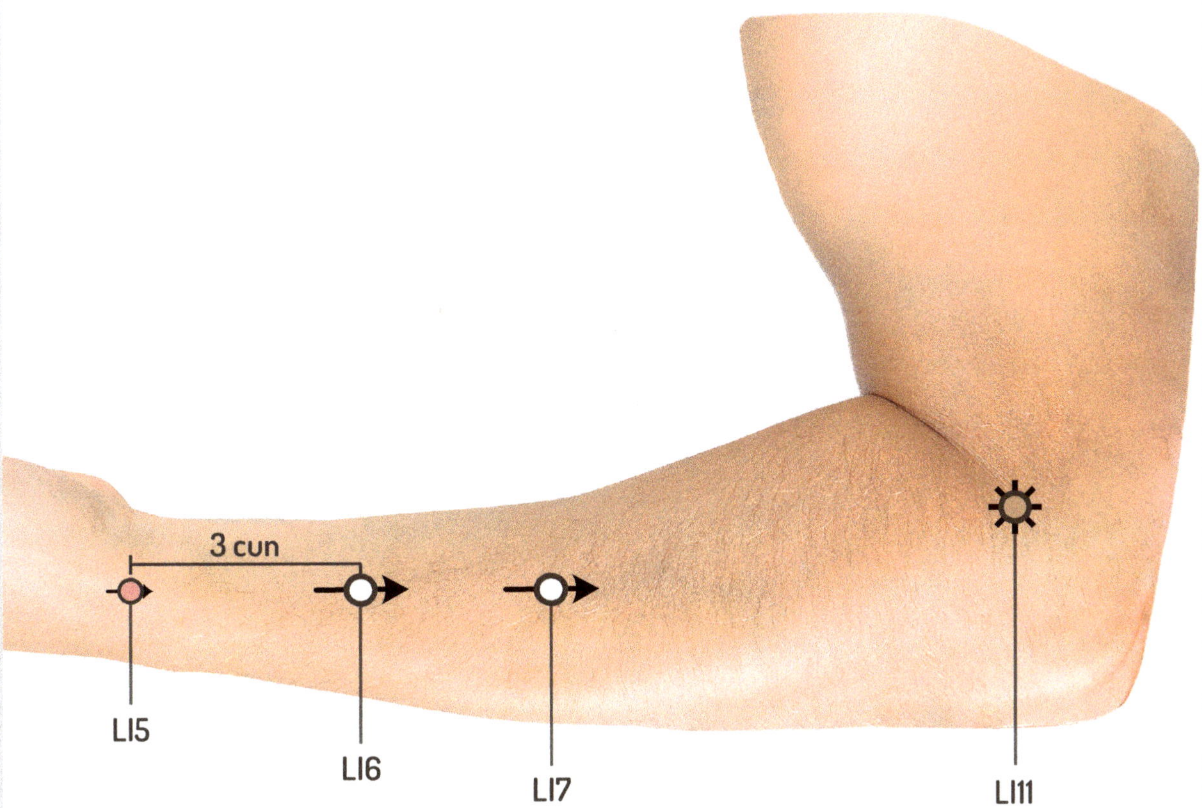

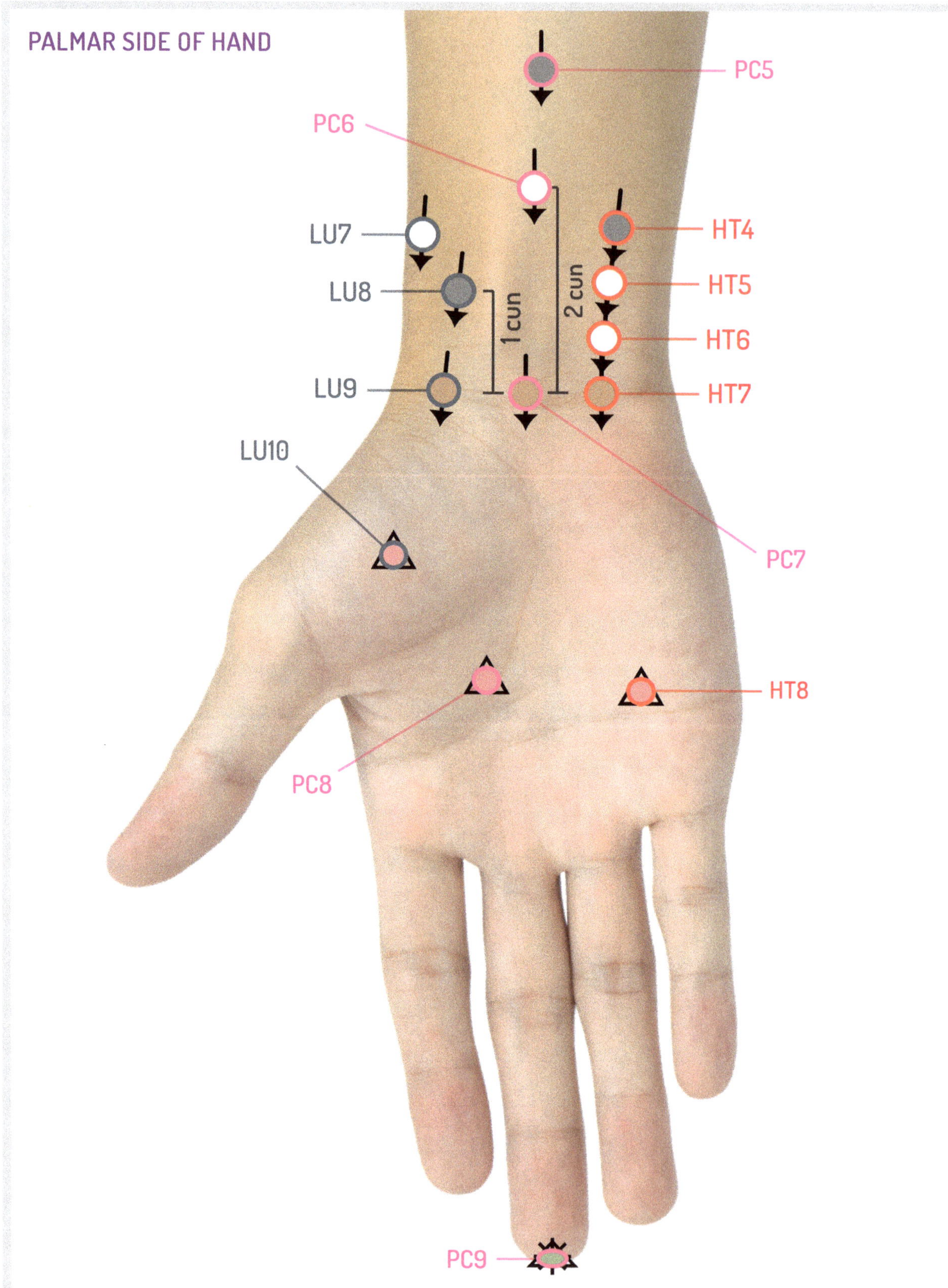
PALMAR SIDE OF HAND
PC5
PC6
LU7
HT4
LU8
2 cun
HT5
1 cun
HT6
LU9
HT7
LU10
PC7
HT8
PC8
PC9

RADIAL SIDE OF HAND

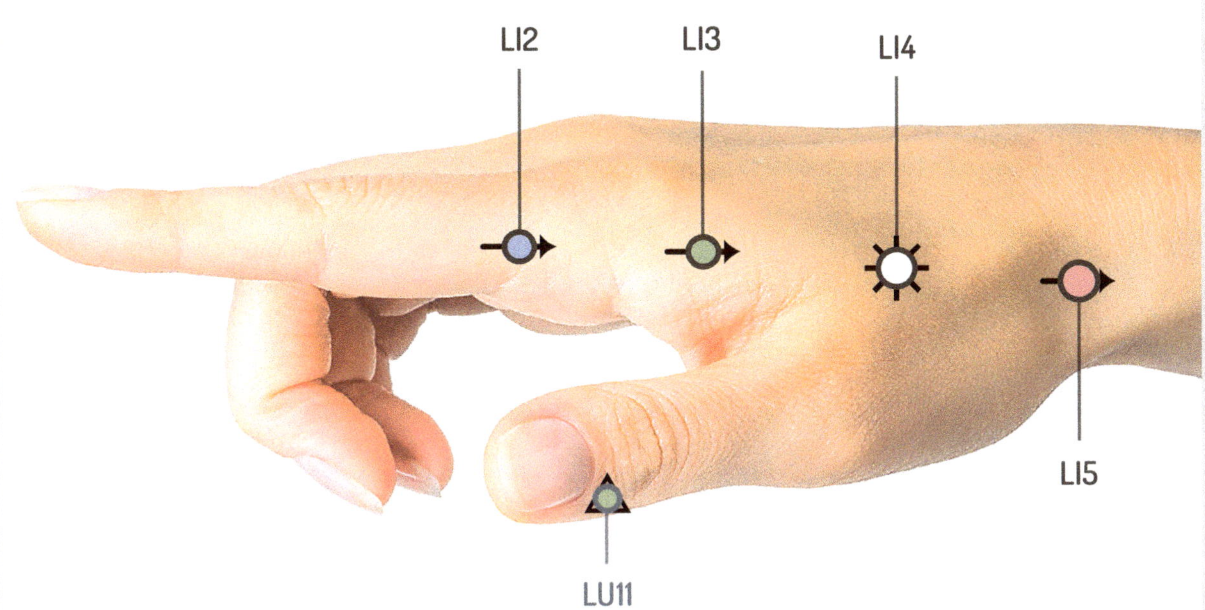

ULNAR SIDE OF HAND

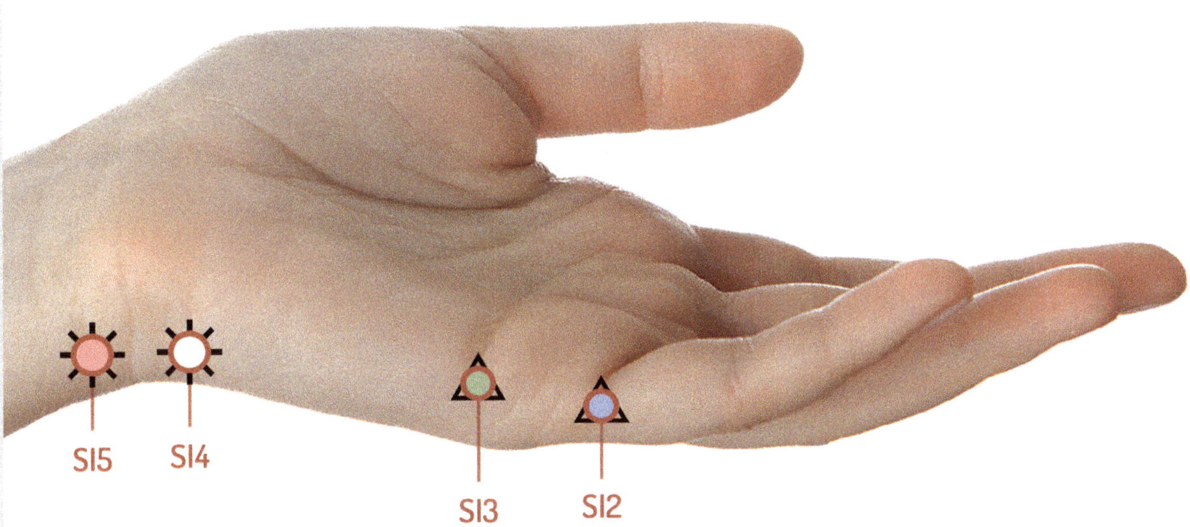

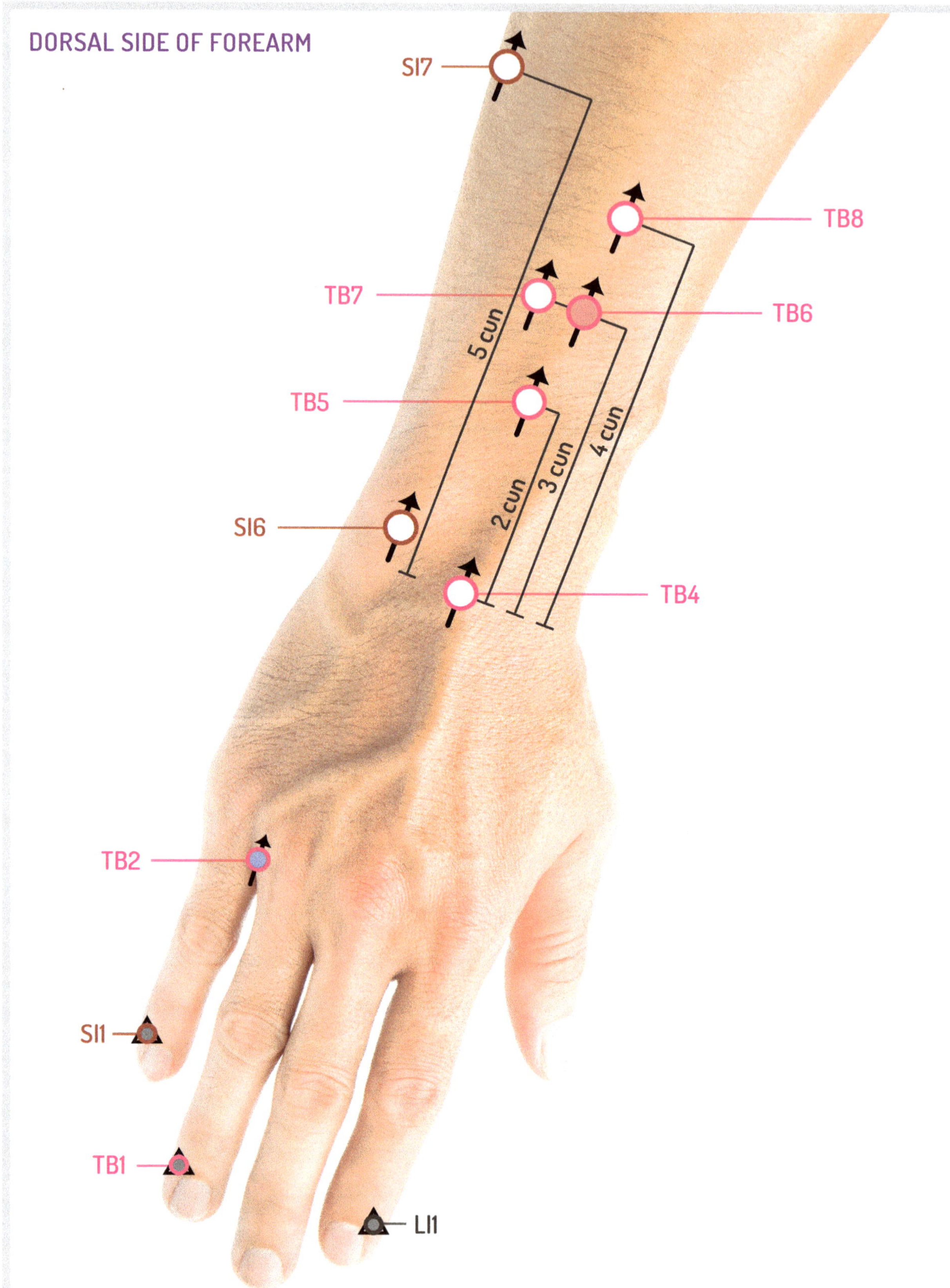
DORSAL SIDE OF FOREARM
SI7
TB8
TB7
TB6
5 cun
TB5
4 cun
3 cun
2 cun
SI6
TB4
TB2
SI1
TB1
LI1

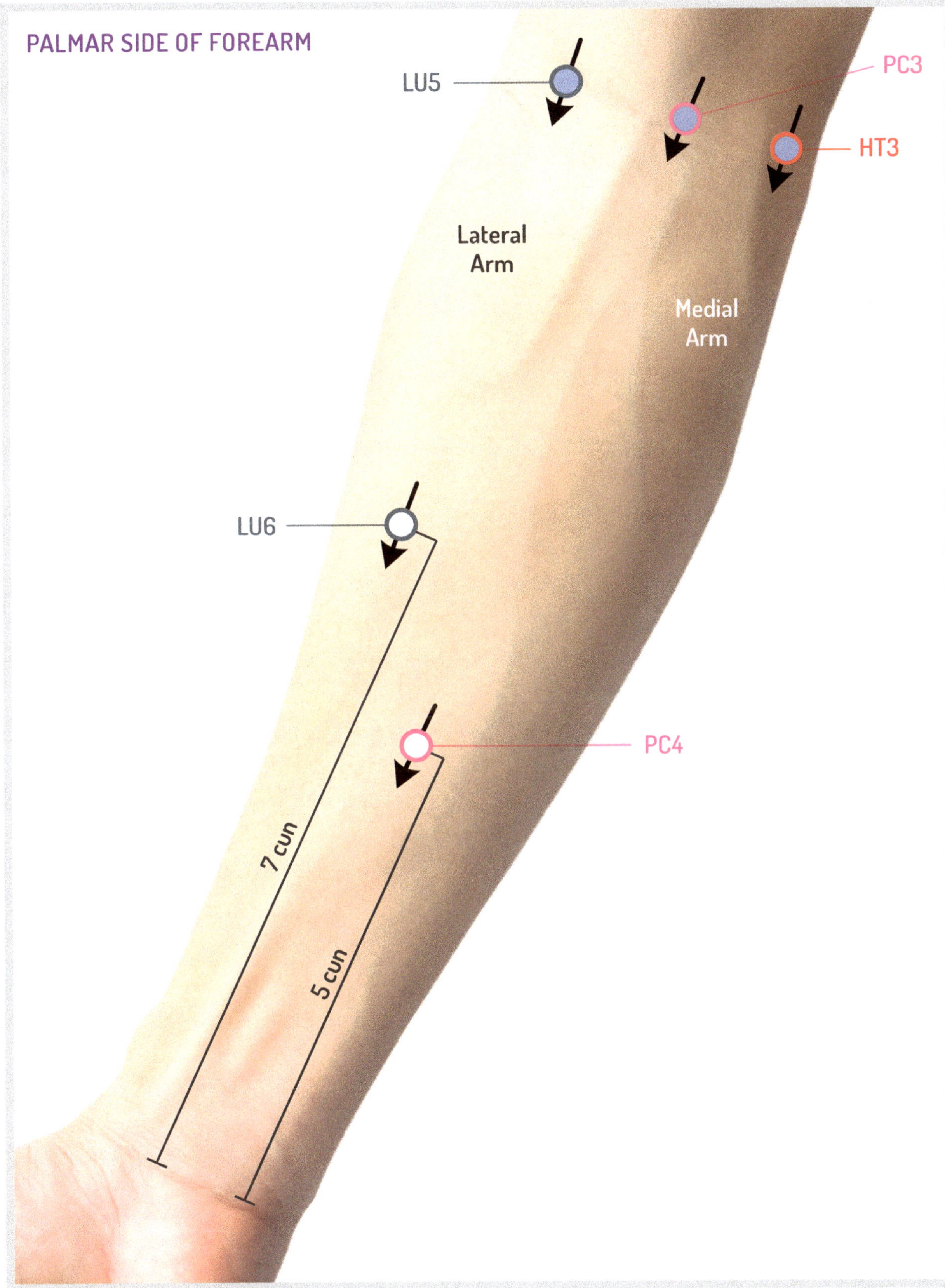
PALMAR SIDE OF FOREARM
LU5
PC3
HT3
Lateral Arm
Medial Arm
LU6
PC4
7 cun
5 cun

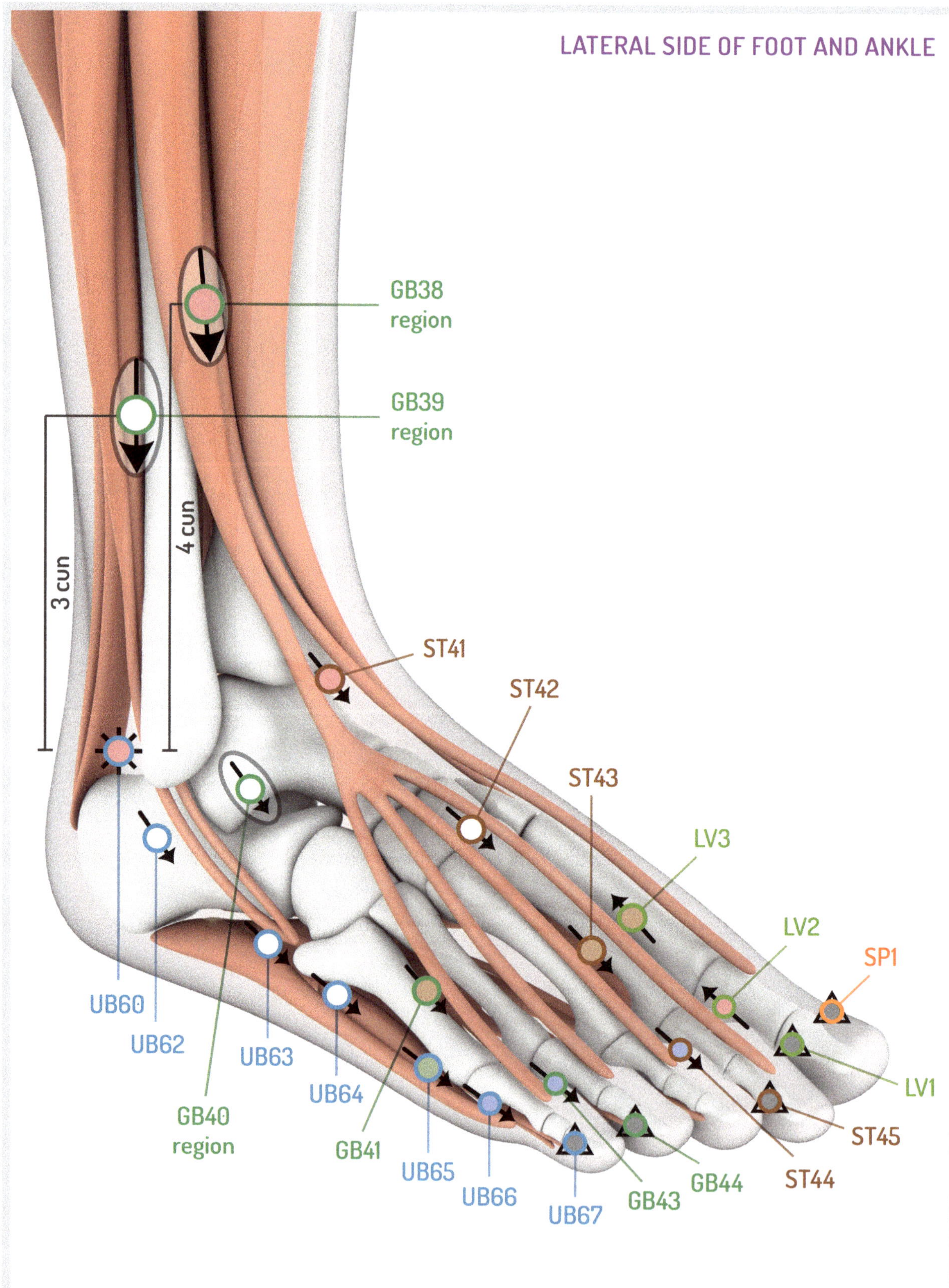
LATERAL SIDE OF FOOT AND ANKLE
GB38
region
GB39
region
3 cun
4 cun
ST41
ST42
ST43
LV3
LV2
SP1
LV1
ST45
ST44
GB44
GB43
UB67
UB66
UB65
GB41
UB64
UB63
UB62
UB60
GB40
region

MEDIAL SIDE OF ANKLE

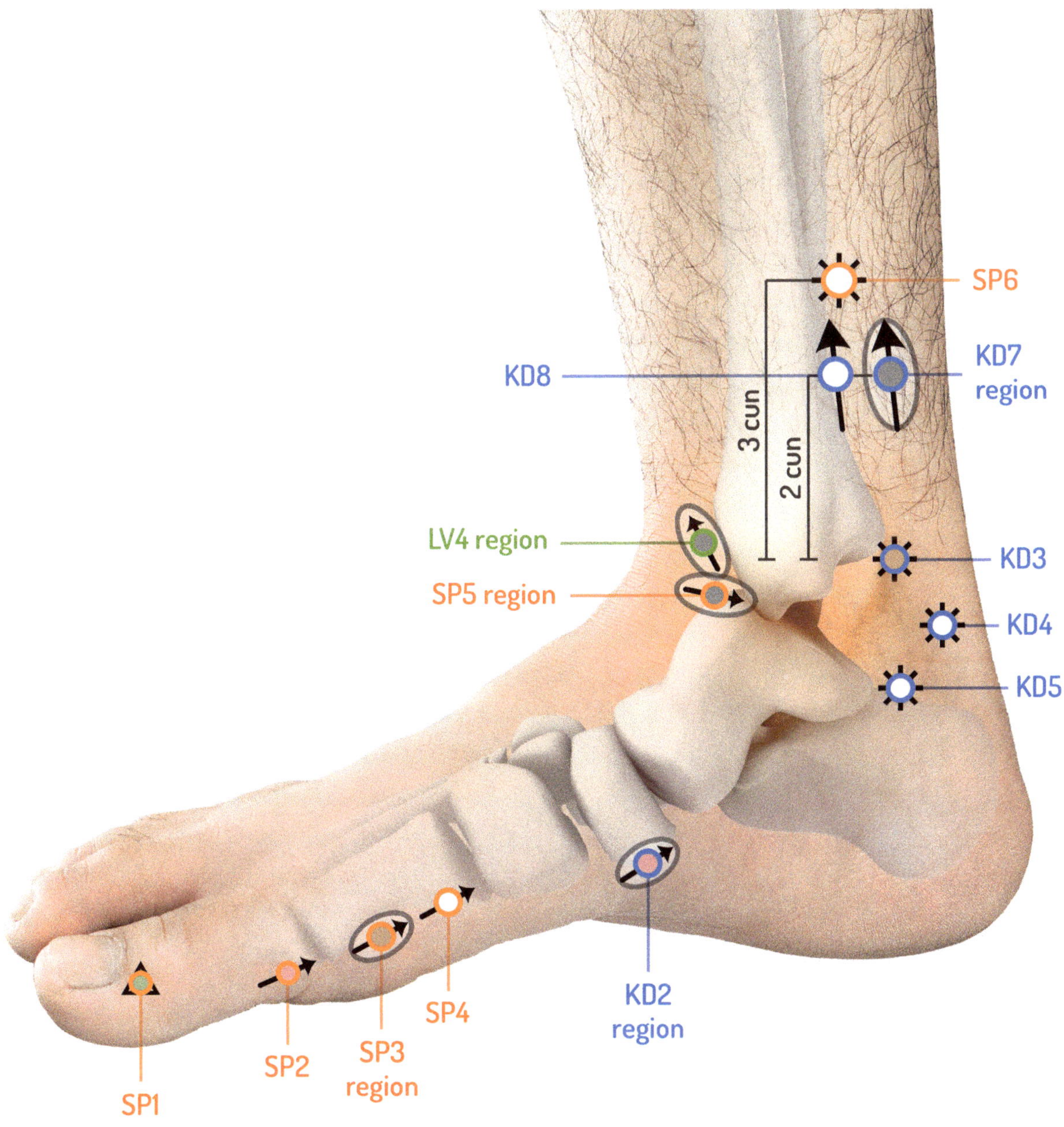

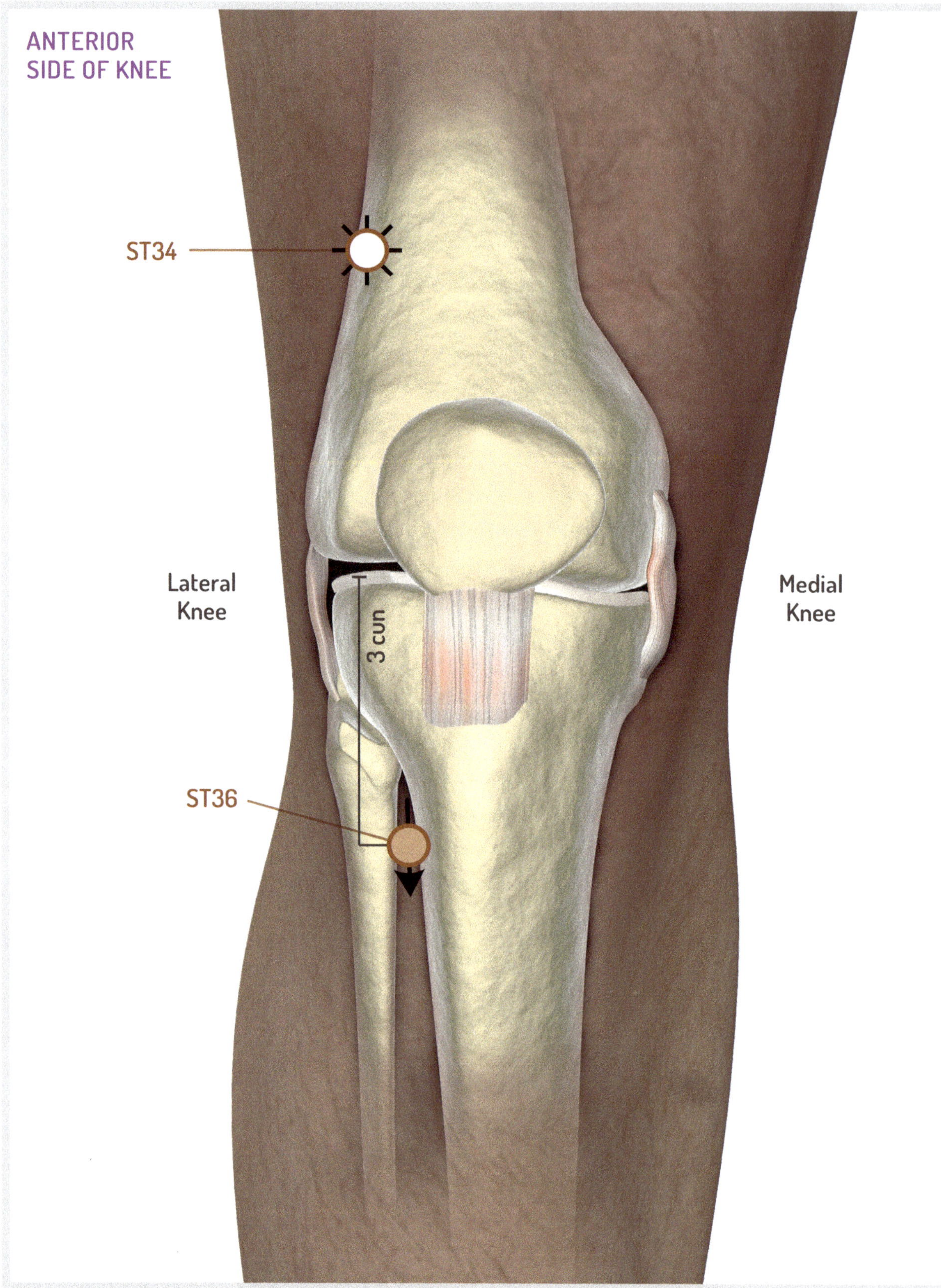
ANTERIOR
SIDE OF KNEE
ST34
Lateral
Knee
Medial
Knee
3 cun
ST36

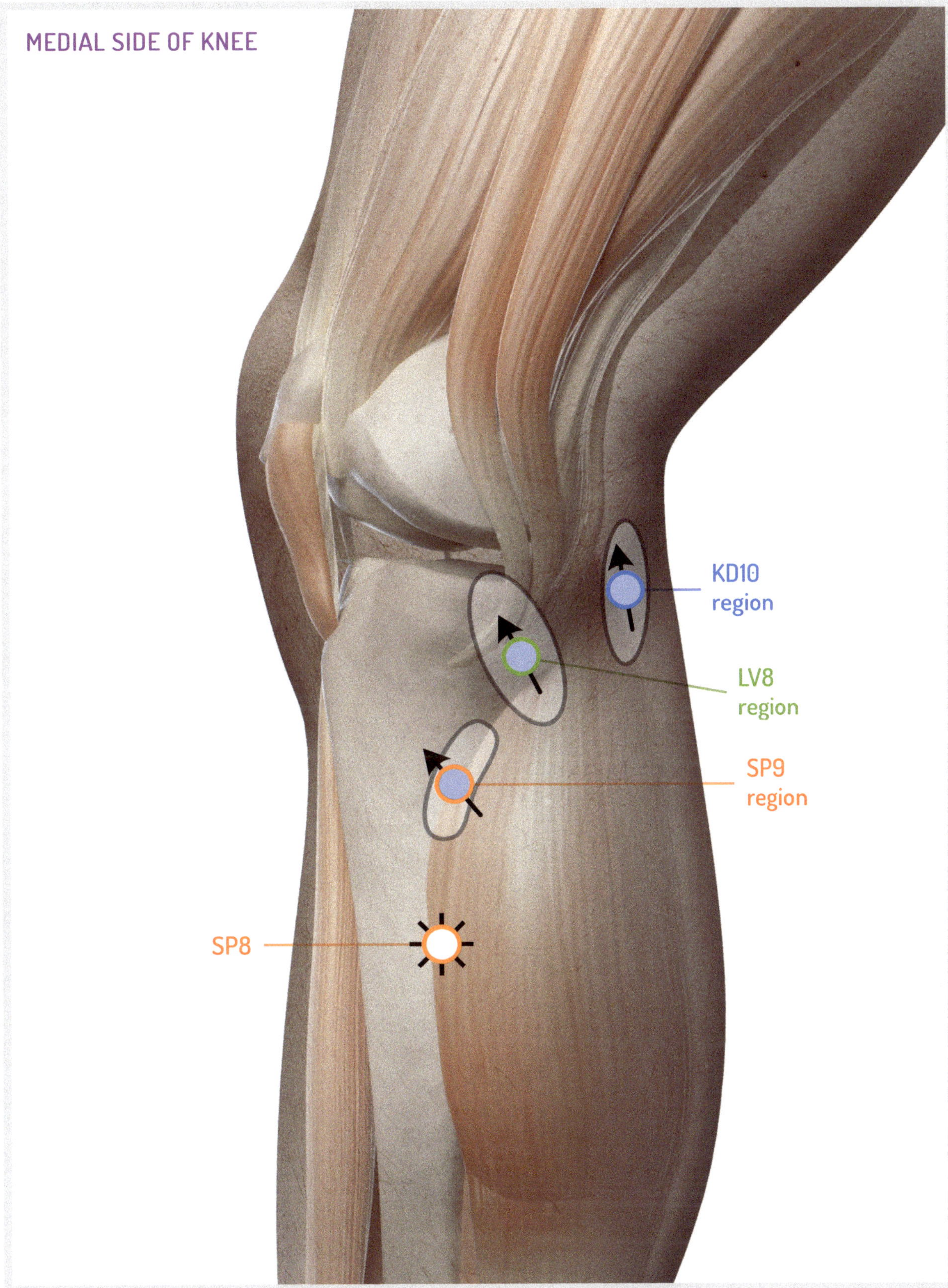
MEDIAL SIDE OF KNEE
KD10
region
LV8
region
SP9
region
SP8

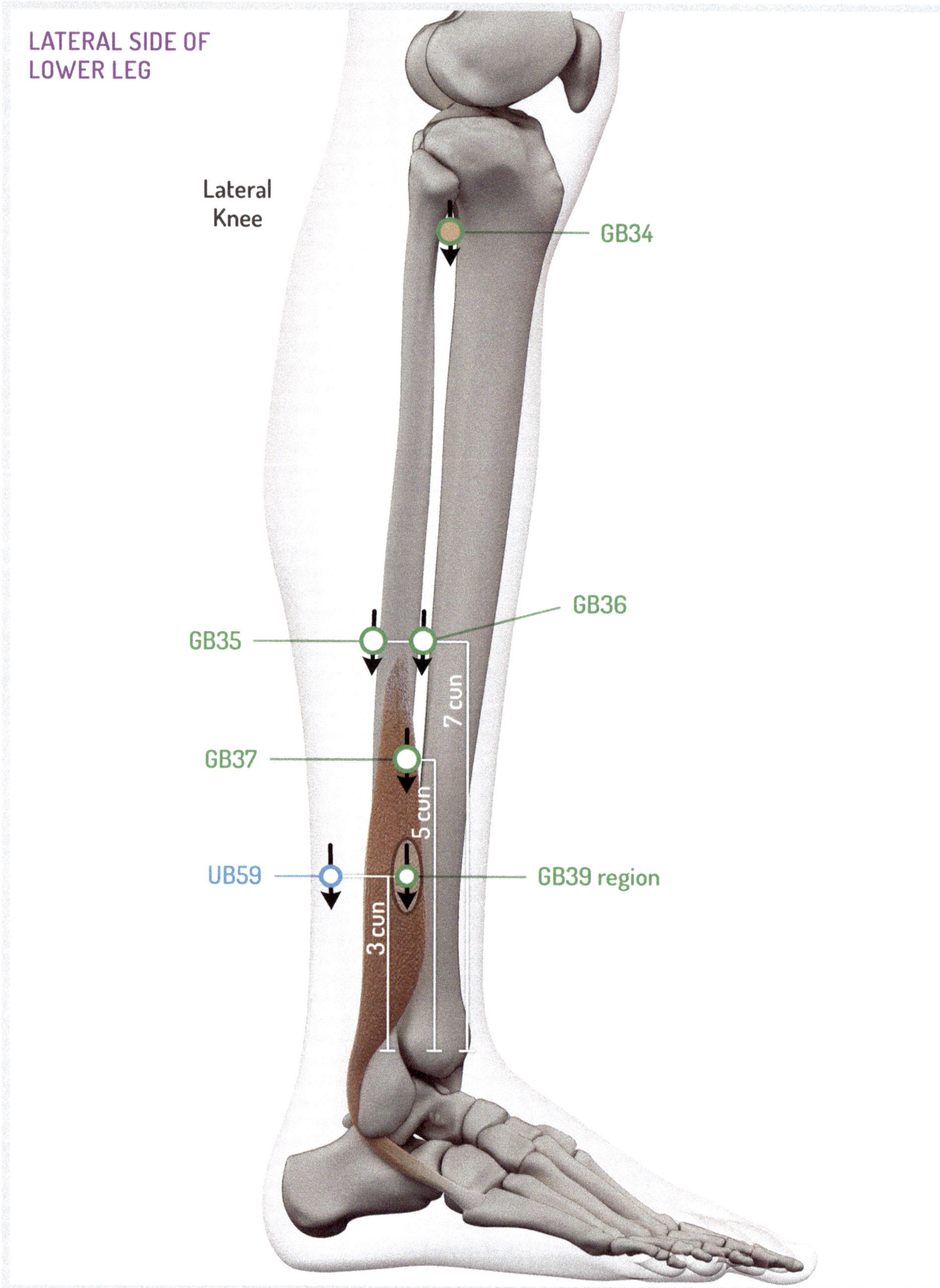
LATERAL SIDE OF LOWER LEG
Lateral Knee
GB34
GB36
GB35
7 cun
GB37
5 cun
UB59
GB39 region
3 cun

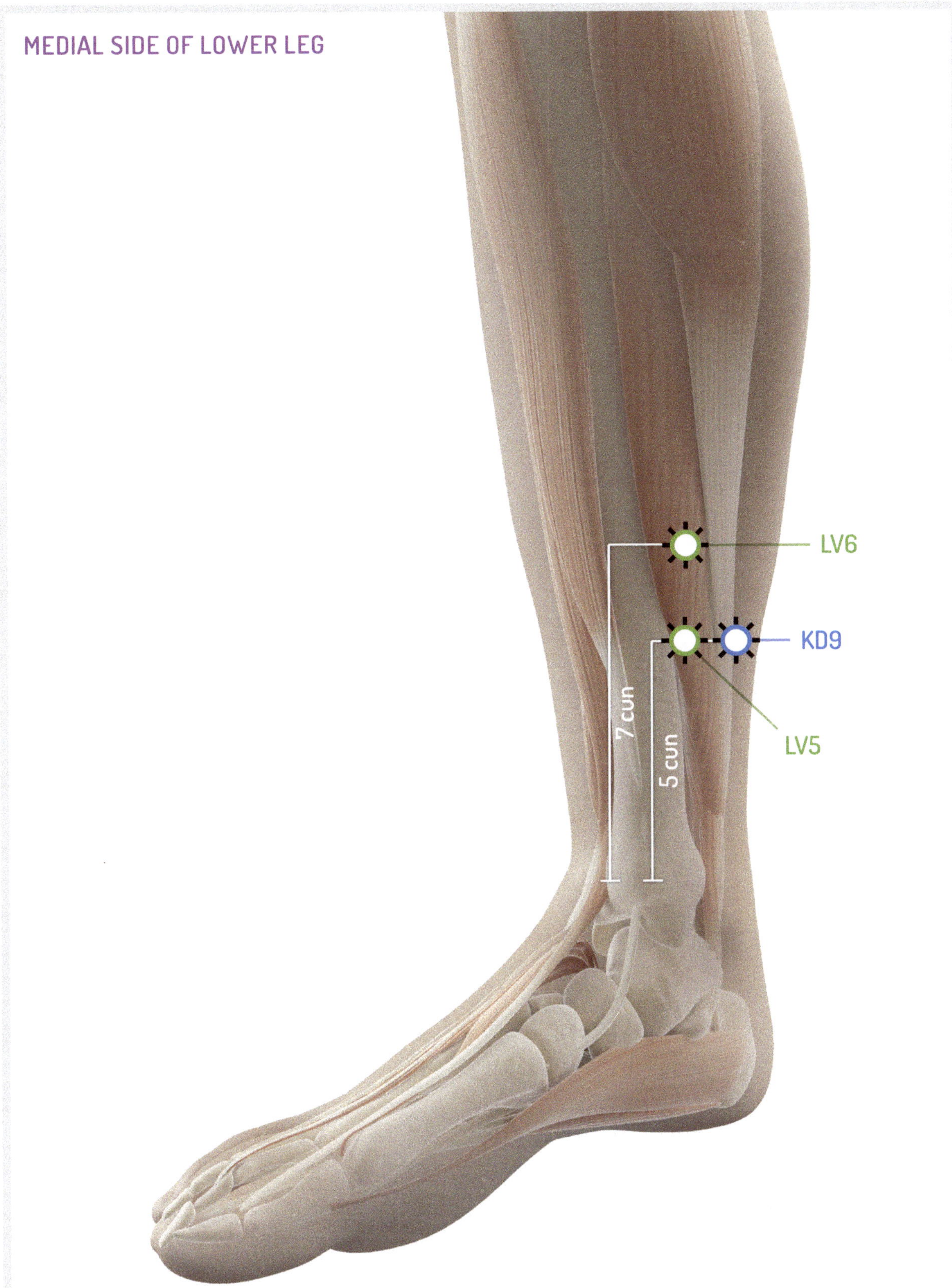
MEDIAL SIDE OF LOWER LEG
LV6
KD9
LV5
7 cun
5 cun

ANTERIOR SIDE OF LOWER LEG

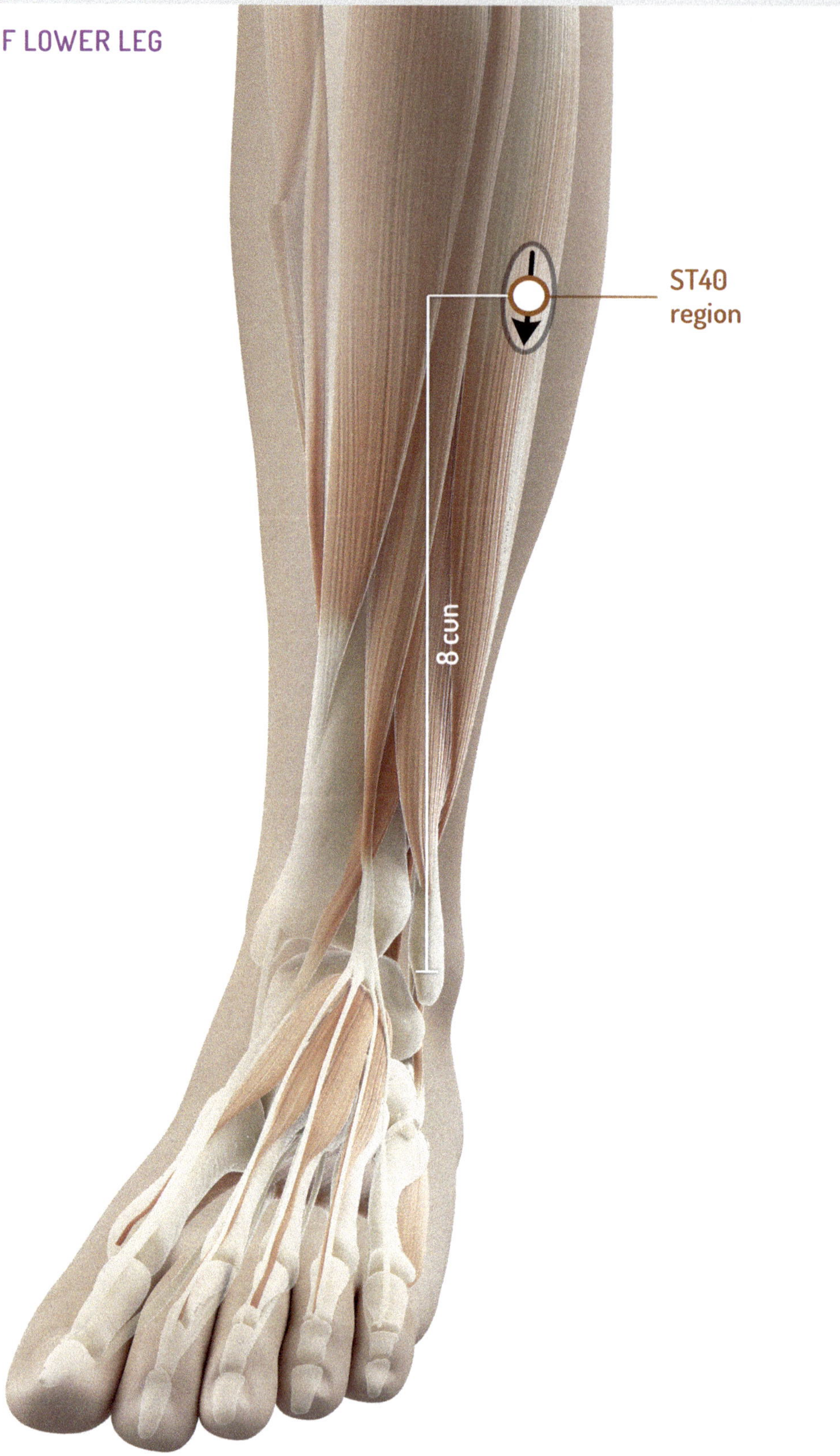

Notes

1 Maoshing Ni. *The Yellow Emperor's Classic of Medicine: A New Translation of the Neijing Suwen with Commentary* (Boston: Shambhala Publications, 1995), 300.

2 Ibid., 240.

3 Ibid., 27.

4 Ibid., 28.

5 Ibid.,17.

6 Nigel Wiseman and Fend Ye, A *Practical Dictionary of Chinese Medicine* (Brookline: Paradigm Publications, 1998), 705-706.

7 Nigel Wiseman and Andrew Ellis, *Fundamentals of Chinese Medicine* (Brookline: Paradigm Publications, 1995), 2-4.

8 Ni, *The Yellow Emperor's Classic of Medicine*, 295.

9 Ibid., 16.

10 Ibid., 19.

11 Ibid., 293.

12 Wiseman and Ellis, *Fundamentals*, 228-235.

13 Rachel Morello-Frosch et al., "Environmental Chemicals in an Urban Population of Pregnant Women and Their Newborns from San Francisco," *Environmental Science & Technology*, 50, no. 22 (2016): 12464-12472.

14 U.S. Food & Drug Administration, "FDA Extends Compliance Date for Certain Uses of Partially Hydrogenated Oils in Food; Denies Petition for Certain Uses of PHOs," May 18, 2018, https://www.fda.gov/food/cfsan-constituent-updates/fda-extends-compliance-date-certain-uses-partially-hydrogenated-oils-food-denies-petition-certain.

15 Richard Feit and Paul Zmiewski, *Acumoxa Therapy Reference & Study Guide* (Brookline: Paradigm Publications, 1989), 27.

16 Wang Ju-Yi and Jason Robertson, "Channel Palpation," *Journal of Chinese Medicine*, no. 83 (2007):18-24.

17 C.M.S. Plowright, et al., "Floral Guidance of Learning a Preference for Symmetry by Bumblebees," *Animal Cognition* 20, no. 6 (2017): 1115-1127, https://link.springer.com/article/10.1007%2Fs10071-017-1128-0 (accessed February 19, 2018).

18 Brent A. Berger et al., "Geometric Morphometrics Reveals Shifts in Flower Shape Symmetry and Size Following Gene Knockdown of CYCLOIDEA and ANTHOCYANIDIN SYNTHASE," BMC *Plant Biology* 17, no. 205 (2017), https://bmcplantbiol.biomedcentral.com/articles/10.1186/s12870-017-1152-x (accessed February 19, 2018).

19 Anthony C. Little, Benedict C. Jones, and Lisa M. DeBruine, "Facial Attractiveness: Evolutionary Based Research," *Philosophical Transactions of the Royal Society B: Biological Sciences*, 366,1571 (2011): 1638–1659, PMC, Web, 19 Feb. 2018.

20 Ibid.

[21] L. K. McCorry, "Physiology of the autonomic nervous system," *American Journal of Pharmaceutical Education* 71(4) (2007): 78. doi:10.5688/aj710478, https://www.ncbi.nlm.nih.gov/pmc/articles/PMC1959222/ (accessed June 30, 2019).

[22] Ibid.

[23] J.B. Furness, et al., "The Enteric Nervous System and Gastrointestinal Innervation: Integrated Local and Central Control," *Microbial Endocrinology: The Microbiota-Gut-Brain Axis in Health and Disease, Advances in Experimental Medicine and Biology* 817, (Springer, New York, NY 2014): 39-71, https://link.springer.com/chapter/10.1007%2F978-1-4939-0897-4_3.

[24] Philip Strandwitz, "Neurotransmitter Modulation by the Gut Microbiota," *Brain Research* 1693, Part B, (2018): 128-133, ISSN 0006-8993, https://doi.org/10.1016/j.brainres.2018.03.015 (accessed June 30, 2019).

[25] V. RajMohan and E. Mohandas, "The Limbic System," *Indian Journal of Psychiatry* 49 (2007):132-9, http://www.indianjpsychiatry.org/text.asp?2007/49/2/132/33264 (accessed 2019 Jun 30).

[26] Vijaita Syngle et al., "Predictors of Autonomic Neuropathy in Rheumatoid Arthritis," *Autonomic Neuroscience: Basic and Clinical* 201: 54-59, https://www.autonomicneuroscience.com/article/S1566-0702(16)30116-3/fulltext.

[27] Angela Spontelli Gisselman et al., "Musculoskeletal Overuse Injuries and Heart Rate Variability: Is There a Link? *Medical Hypotheses* 87:1-7, https://www.medical-hypotheses.com/article/S0306-9877(15)00457-0/fulltext.

[28] Ihori Kobayashi et al., "The Impact of Posttraumatic Stress Disorder Versus Resilience on Nocturnal Autonomic Nervous System Activity as Functions of Sleep Stage and Time of Sleep," *Physiology & Behavior* 164, Part A, 2016, 11-18, ISSN 0031-9384, https://doi.org/10.1016/j.physbeh.2016.05.005.

[29] Muhammad Abid Azam et al., "Individuals with Tension and Migraine Headaches Exhibit Increased Heart Rate Variability During Post-stress Mindfulness Meditation Practice but a Decrease During a Post-stress Control Condition – A Randomized, Controlled Experiment," *International Journal of Psychophysiology* 110 (2016): 66-74, ISSN 0167-8760, https://doi.org/10.1016/j.ijpsycho.2016.10.011.

[30] Peng An et al., "'Qufeng Tongluo' Acupuncture Prevents the Progression of Glomerulonephritis by Decreasing Renal Sympathetic Nerve Activity," *Journal of Ethnopharmacology* 155, Issue 1 (2014): 277-284, ISSN 0378-8741, https://doi.org/10.1016/j.jep.2014.05.019.

[31] Soo-Byeong Kim et al., "Use of Pupil Size to Determine the Effect of Electromagnetic Acupuncture on Activation Level of the Autonomic Nervous System," *Journal of Acupuncture and Meridian Studies* 7, Issue 3:122-132.

[32] In-Seon Lee , et al., "Fear of Acupuncture Enhances Sympathetic Activation to Acupuncture Stimulation," *Acupuncture in Medicine* 31 (2013):276-281.

[33] Mitsuhiro Denda, "Newly Discovered Olfactory Receptors in Epidermal Keratinocytes Are Associated with Proliferation, Migration, and Re-Epithelialization of Keratinocytes," *Journal of Investigative Dermatology* 134, Issue 11: 2677-2679.

[34] RajMohan and Mohandas, "The Limbic System," 132-9.

[35] Nasra Naeim Ayuobet al., "*Ocimum Basilicum* Improve Chronic Stress-induced Neurodegenerative Changes in Mice Hippocampus," *Metabolic Brain Disease* 33 (2018): 795, https://doi.org/10.1007/s11011-017-0173-3 (accessed June 22, 2019).

[36] Pao-Ju Chen et al., "Effects of Aromatherapy Massage on Pregnant Women's Stress and Immune Function: A Longitudinal, Prospective, Randomized Controlled Trial," *The Journal of Alternative and Complementary Medicine* 23, no.10, Oct 2017, http://doi.org/10.1089/acm.2016.0426.

[37] A. Salamati, S. Mashouf, and F. Mojab, "Effect of Inhalation of Lavender Essential Oil on Vital Signs in Open Heart Surgery ICU," *Iranian Journal of Pharmaceutical Research: IJPR* 16(1) (2017): 404–409.

[38] C. Collet et al., "Autonomic Nervous System Correlates in Movement Observation and Motor Imagery," *Frontiers in Human Neuroscience* 7 (2013) :415. doi: 10.3389/fnhum.2013.00415, PubMed PMID: 23908623; PubMed Central PMCID: PMC3726866, https://www.frontiersin.org/articles/10.3389/fnhum.2013.00415/full (accessed June 30, 2019).

[39] N. Watanabe, J. Reece, and B. I. Polus, (2007), "Effects of Body Position on Autonomic Regulation of Cardiovascular Function in Young, Healthy Adults," *Chiropractic & Manual Therapies* 15 (2007): 19. doi: 10.1186/1746-1340-15-19, https://chiromt.biomedcentral.com/articles/10.1186/1746-1340-15-19 (accessed June 30, 2019).

[40] Müzeyyen Arslan et al., "Wet Cupping Therapy Restores Sympathovagal Imbalances in Cardiac Rhythm," *The Journal of Alternative and Complementary Medicine* 20, no. 4, https://doi.org/10.1089/acm.2013.0291 (published online: 16 Apr 2014).

[41] Duane T. Lowe, "Cupping Therapy: An Analysis of the Effects of Suction on Skin and the Possible Influence on Human Health," *Complementary Therapies in Clinical Practice* 29 (2017): 162-168, https://doi.org/10.1016/j.ctcp.2017.09.008.

[42] Ni, *The Yellow Emperor's Classic of Medicine*, 101.

[43] Manyong Park and Sungchul Kim, "A Modern Clinical Approach of the Traditional Korean Saam Acupuncture," *Evidence-Based Complementary and Alternative Medicine* 2015: Article ID 703439 (8 pages), http://dx.doi.org/10.1155/2015/703439.

[44] Ibid.

[45] Ni, *The Yellow Emperor's Classic of Medicine*, 35.

[46] Park and Kim, "A Modern Clinical Approach of the Traditional Korean Saam Acupuncture," 2.

[47] Feit and Zmiewski, *Acumoxa Therapy*, 138.

[48] Ni, *The Yellow Emperor's Classic of Medicine*, 102.

[49] Denda, "Olfactory Receptors," 2677-2679.

[50] Giovanni Maciocia, *Obstetrics & Gynecology in Chinese Medicine* (New York, NY: Churchill Livingstone Medical Division of Pearson Professional Limited, 1998), 24.

[51] Ibid.

[52] Ni, *The Yellow Emperor's Classic of Medicine*, 237-238.

[53] M. Schumacher, P. Robel, E. Baulieu, "Development and Regeneration of the Nervous System: A Role for Neurosteroids" (Part 1 of 2), Dev Neurosci 1996;18:6-13. doi: 10.1159/000111391.

[54] M.E. Chávez-Delgado, et al., "Ultrastructural analysis of guided nerve regeneration using progesterone- and pregnenolone-loaded chitosan prostheses." J. Biomedical Materials Research, 74B (2005): 589-600. doi:10.1002/jbm.b.30243.

[55] X. Yang, et al., "Dihydrotestosterone Treatment Accelerates Autograft Reversal Sciatic Nerve Regeneration in Rats," Neurochemical Research 43, 659–668 (2018), https://doi.org/10.1007/s11064-018-2466-2.

[56] B. Bielecki, et al., "Unexpected central role of the androgen receptor in the spontaneous regeneration of myelin," Proc Natl Acad Sci U S A. 2016, 113(51):14829–14834. doi:10.1073/pnas.1614826113.

Bibliography

An, Peng, et al. "'Qufeng Tongluo' Acupuncture Prevents the Progression of Glomerulonephritis by Decreasing Renal Sympathetic Nerve Activity." *Journal of Ethnopharmacology*, vol. 155, no. 1, 2014, pp. 277-284. ISSN 0378-8741. doi.org/10.1016/j.jep.2014.05.019.

Arslan, Müzeyyen, et al. "Wet Cupping Therapy Restores Sympathovagal Imbalances in Cardiac Rhythm." *The Journal of Alternative and Complementary Medicine* vol. 20, no. 4, 2014. doi.org/10.1089/acm.2013.0291.

Ayuob, Nasra Naeim, et al. "*Ocimum Basilicum* Improve Chronic Stress-Induced Neurodegenerative Changes in Mice Hippocampus." *Metabolic Brain Disease*, vol. 33, 2018, p. 795. doi.org/10.1007/s11011-017-0173-3. Accessed 22 June 2019.

Azam, Muhammad Abid, et al. "Individuals With Tension and Migraine Headaches Exhibit Increased Heart Rate Variability During Post-Stress Mindfulness Meditation Practice but a Decrease During a Post-Stress Control Condition – a Randomized, Controlled Experiment." *International Journal of Psychophysiology*, vol. 110, 2016, pp. 66-74. doi.org/10.1016/j.ijpsycho.2016.10.011. (www.sciencedirect.com/science/article/pii/S0167876016307346).

Berger, Brent A. et al. "Geometric Morphometrics Reveals Shifts in Flower Shape Symmetry and Size Following Gene Knockdown of CYCLOIDEA and ANTHOCYANIDIN SYNTHASE." *BMC Plant Biology*, vol. 17, no 205, 2017. bmcplantbiol.biomedcentral.com/articles/10.1186/s12870-017-1152-x. Accessed 19 Feb 2018.

Chen, Pao-Ju, et al. "Effects of Aromatherapy Massage on Pregnant Women's Stress and Immune Function: A Longitudinal, Prospective, Randomized Controlled Trial." *The Journal of Alternative and Complementary Medicine*, vol. 23, no. 10, 2017. doi.org/10.1089/acm.2016.0426. Accessed ahead of print.

Collet C, et al. "Autonomic Nervous System Correlates in Movement Observation and Motor Imagery." *Frontiers in Human Neuroscience*, vol.7, p. 415, 2013. doi: 10.3389/fnhum.2013.00415. Accessed 30 June 2019. (www.frontiersin.org/articles/10.3389/fnhum.2013.00415/full).

Denda, Mitsuhiro. "Newly Discovered Olfactory Receptors in Epidermal Keratinocytes Are Associated with Proliferation, Migration, and Re-Epithelialization of Keratinocytes."

Feit, Richard and Paul Zmiewski. *Acumoxa Therapy Reference & Study Guide*. Paradigm Publications, 1989.

Furness John B., et al. "The Enteric Nervous System and Gastrointestinal Innervation: Integrated Local and Central Control." *Microbial Endocrinology: The Microbiota-Gut-Brain Axis in Health and Disease, Advances in Experimental Medicine and Biology. Advances in Experimental Medicine and Biology*, vol. 817, Springer, 2014, pp. 39-71. doi.org/10.1007/978-1-4939-0897-4_3. (link.springer.com/chapter/10.1007%2F978-1-4939-0897-4_3).

Gisselman, Angela Spontelli, et al. "Musculoskeletal Overuse Injuries and Heart Rate Variability: Is There a Link?" *Medical Hypotheses*, vol. 87, 2016, pp.1-7. www.medical-hypotheses.com/article/S0306-9877(15)00457-0/fulltext.

Journal of Investigative Dermatology, vol. 134, no. 11, 2014, pp. 2677-2679.

Kim, Soo-Byeong et al. "Use of Pupil Size to Determine the Effect of Electromagnetic Acupuncture on Activation Level of the Autonomic Nervous System." *Journal of Acupuncture and Meridian Studies*, vol. 7, no. 3, pp. 122-132.

Kobayashi, Ihori, et al. "The Impact of Posttraumatic Stress Disorder Versus Resilience on Nocturnal Autonomic Nervous System Activity as Functions of Sleep Stage and Time of Sleep." *Physiology & Behavior*, vol. 164, part A, 2016, pp. 11-18. doi.org/10.1016/j.physbeh.2016.05.005. (www.sciencedirect.com/science/article/pii/S0031938416302165).

Lee In-Seon, et al. "Fear of Acupuncture Enhances Sympathetic Activation to Acupuncture Stimulation." *Acupuncture Medicine*, vol. 31, 2013, pp. 276-281.

Little, Anthony C., Benedict C. Jones, and Lisa M. DeBruine. "Facial Attractiveness: Evolutionary Based Research." *Philosophical Transactions of the Royal Society B: Biological Sciences*, vol. 366, no. 1571, 2011, pp. 1638-1659.

Lowe, Duane T. "Cupping Therapy: An Analysis of the Effects of Suction on Skin and the Possible Influence on Human Health." *Complementary Therapies in Clinical Practice*, vol. 29, 2017, pp. 162-168. doi.org/10.1016/j.ctcp.2017.09.008.

Maciocia, Giovanni. *Obstetrics & Gynecology in Chinese Medicine*. Churchill Livingstone Medical Division of Pearson Professional Limited, 1998.

Matsumoto, Kiiko and David Euler. *Kiiko Matsumoto's Clinical Strategies: In the Spirit of Master Nagano, Volume 1*. Kiiko Matsumoto International, 2002.

McCorry L. K. "Physiology of the Autonomic Nervous System." *American Journal of Pharmaceutical Education*, vol. 71, no. 4, 2007, p. 78. doi:10.5688/aj710478. Accessed 30 June 2019. (www.ncbi.nlm.nih.gov/pmc/articles/PMC1959222/).

Meramour, Michelle. *Supporting Your Acupuncture Meridian System: How to Recover Your Health by Choosing the Best Food, Supplements, and Essential Oils*. Body-Feedback for Health, 2017.

Meramour, Michelle and Heather Ensworth. *Higher Vibrational Living: Through Astrology, Essential Oils and Chinese Medicine*. Body-Feedback for Health, 2018.

Morello-Frosch, Rachel, et al. "Environmental Chemicals in an Urban Population of Pregnant Women and Their Newborns from San Francisco." *Environmental Science & Technology*, vol. 50, no. 22, 2016, pp. 12464-12472.

Ni, Maoshing. *The Yellow Emperor's Classic of Medicine: A New Translation of the Neijing Suwen with Commentary*. Shambhala Publications, 1995.

Park, Manyong and Sungchul Kim. "A Modern Clinical Approach of the Traditional Korean Saam Acupuncture." *Evidence-Based Complementary and Alternative Medicine*, vol. 2015, 2015. Article ID 703439. dx.doi.org/10.1155/2015/703439.

Plowright, Catherine M.S., et al. "Floral Guidance of Learning a Preference for Symmetry by Bumblebees." *Animal Cognition*, vol. 20, no. 6, 2017, pp. 1115-1127. link.springer.com/article/10.1007%2Fs10071-017-1128-0. Accessed 19 Feb 2018.

RajMohan V. and E. Mohandas. "The Limbic System." *Indian Journal of Psychiatry*, vol. 49, no. 2, 2007, pp. 132-139. www.indianjpsychiatry.org/text.asp?2007/49/2/132/33264. Accessed 30 Jun 2019.

Salamati, Armaiti, Soheyla Mashouf and Faraz Mojab. "Effect of Inhalation of Lavender Essential Oil on Vital Signs in Open Heart Surgery ICU." *Iranian Journal of Pharmaceutical Research*, vol. 16, no. 1, 2017, pp. 404–409.

Strandwitz, Philip. "Neurotransmitter Modulation by the Gut Microbiota." *Brain Research*, vol. 1693, part B, 2018, pp. 128-133. doi.org/10.1016/j.brainres.2018.03.015. Accessed 30 June 2019. (www.sciencedirect.com/science/article/pii/S0006899318301501).

Syngle, Vijaita, et al. "Predictors of Autonomic Neuropathy in Rheumatoid Arthritis." *Autonomic Neuroscience: Basic and Clinical*, vol. 201, pp. 54-59. www.autonomicneuroscience.com/article/S1566-0702(16)30116-3/fulltext.

U.S. Food & Drug Administration. "FDA Extends Compliance Date for Certain Uses of Partially Hydrogenated Oils in Food; Denies Petition for Certain Uses of PHOs." May 18, 2018. www.fda.gov/food/cfsan-constituent-updates/fda-extends-compliance-date-certain-uses-partially-hydrogenated-oils-food-denies-petition-certain.

Wang, Ju-Yi and Jason Robertson. "Channel Palpation." *Journal of Chinese Medicine* no. 83, 2007, pp. 18-24.

Watanabe, Nobuhiro, John Reece and Barbara Polus. "Effects of Body Position on Autonomic Regulation of Cardiovascular Function in Young, Healthy Adults." *Chiropractic & Osteopathy*, vol. 15, no.19, 2007. doi:10.1186/1746-1340-15-19. Accessed 30 June 2019. (chiromt.biomedcentral.com/articles/10.1186/1746-1340-15-19).

Wiseman, Nigel and Andrew Ellis, *Fundamentals of Chinese Medicine*. Paradigm Publications, 1995.

Wiseman, Nigel. and Fend Ye. A *Practical Dictionary of Chinese Medicine*. Paradigm Publications, 1998.

Index

B

C

U

X

Y

About the Author

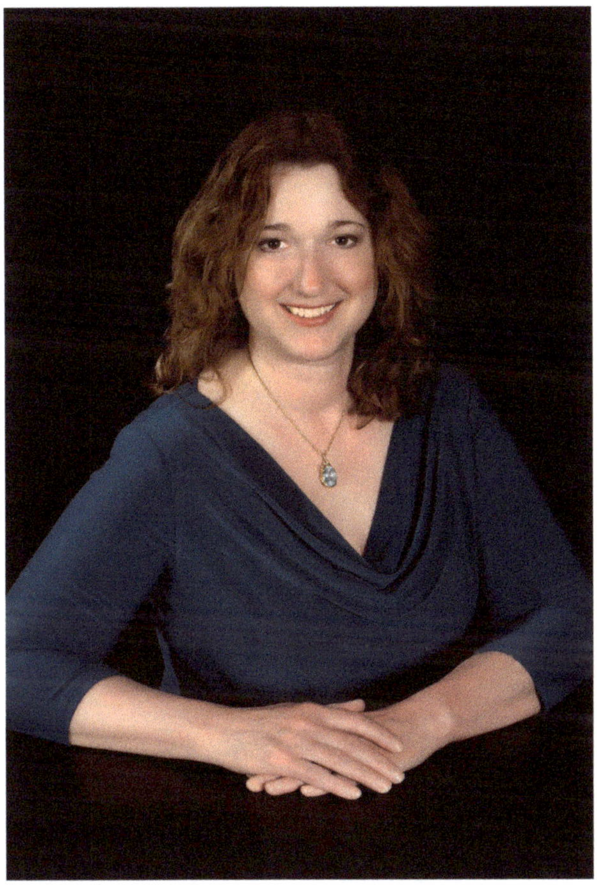

Michelle Meramour, MSOM, CA

Michelle Meramour is a practicing acupuncturist in Madison, Wisconsin with a focus in fertility enhancement and pregnancy care. She created the Body-Feedback treatment style to systematically integrate classical acupuncture and palpation techniques with modern-day advancements in medicine.

Ms. Meramour graduated Magna Cum Laude from the Midwest College of Oriental Medicine in September 2002 with a Master of Science in Oriental Medicine (MSOM). She continued her post-graduate training directly under Bob Flaws at the Blue Poppy Institute in Boulder, Colorado and completed the two-year Chinese medical gynecology certification program in September 2004.

In 2017, Ms. Meramour published *Supporting Your Acupuncture Meridian System*. In 2018, she co-authored *Higher Vibrational Living through Astrology, Essential Oils, and Chinese Medicine* with Heather Ensworth, PhD., which received the Best Aromatherapy Book award in 2020 from the Spiritual Book Awards in London, England.

Teaching is a passion of Ms. Meramour's. She has taught numerous classes through the Lotus Institute of Integrative Medicine (eLotus.org) and the body-feedback.com website. Her hands-on workshops provide direct supervision to practitioners learning the Body-Feedback system. Ms. Meramour has published articles on fertility enhancement with *Conceiving Concepts* and *Achieving Families* and has served as a guest speaker for RESOLVE: The National Infertility Association.

Ms. Meramour, née Michelle Steffens, grew up in a northern suburb of Chicago. At age fourteen, she moved to Clearwater, Florida and developed a love of the ocean, spending many weekends swimming at beaches along the Gulf of Mexico. She returned to the Chicago area to attend acupuncture college. Prior to publishing her first book, she adopted her professional name, Michelle Meramour, which is a perfect fit because it means sea of love in French–*mer amour*. In her free time, Ms. Meramour enjoys spending time with her husband and two sons. She enjoys an active lifestyle of downhill skiing, golfing, traveling, snorkeling, and, of course, swimming in the ocean.

For more information about Michelle Meramour and the Body-Feedback system visit **body-feedback.com**. Ms. Meramour loves to hear from her students and can be contacted at **michelle@body-feedback.com**.

www.ingramcontent.com/pod-product-compliance
Lightning Source LLC
LaVergne TN
LVHW071413210926
848486LV00004B/264